Introductory Nutrition and Diet Therapy

J.B. Lippincott Company / Philadelphia

London   Mexico City   New York   St. Louis
São Paulo   Sydney

Introductory Nutrition and Diet Therapy

Marian Maltese Eschleman, M.S., R.D.

Coordinator, Nutrition Program
The Mercer Regional Medical Group
(A Health Maintenance Organization)
Trenton, New Jersey;
Formerly Nutrition Consultant,
New Jersey State Department of Health;
Instructor of Nutrition, School of Nursing and
Chief Therapeutic Dietitian, Saint Joseph's Hospital,
Paterson, New Jersey

Sponsoring Editor: Bernice Heller
Manuscript Editor: Martha Hicks-Courant
Indexer: Kathleen Garcia
Art Director: Tracy Baldwin
Designer: Dariel Mayer
Production Supervisor: N. Carol Kerr
Production Assistant: Martha Hicks-Courant
Compositor: Progressive Typographers
Printer/Binder: R.R. Donnelley & Sons Company

Eschleman, Marian Maltese.
  Introductory nutrition and diet therapy.

  Bibliography: p.
  Includes index.
  1. Nutrition. 2. Diet therapy. I. Title.
[DNLM: 1. Diet therapy. 2. Nutrition. QU 145 E738i]
QP141.E77 1984   613.2   83-12035
ISBN 0-397-54241-0

The author and publisher have exerted every effort to ensure that drug selection and
dosage set forth in this text are in accord with current recommendations and practice at
the time of publication. However, in view of ongoing research, changes in government
regulations, and the constant flow of information relating to drug therapy and drug
reactions, the reader is urged to check the package insert for each drug for any change in
indications and dosage and for added warnings and precautions. This is particularly
important when the recommended agent is a new or infrequently employed drug.

To my husband, Ned, whose trust, encouragement, and willing sacrifices are largely responsible for this book.

I am also deeply grateful to my sister, Rosemary Maltese, whose boundless help has lightened, immeasurably, the task of writing.

Preface

Introductory Nutrition and Diet Therapy aims to fill the need for a nutrition text that emphasizes practical applications — those aspects of nutrition and diet therapy that are of direct concern to the health worker and the client. The book was written for nursing students, dietetic technicians, and students in the many health technology courses that include a nutrition component, such as dental hygiene, dental assisting, physical therapy, and respiratory therapy, to name a few. It can also be used in refresher courses.

Attention is focused on major health concerns, so that the topics, whether related to normal or to therapeutic nutrition, are relevant to student goals. Discussions of nutrients have been kept straightforward, to be understood by students who have not taken a course in biochemistry. Much effort and interest have gone into making the book as up-to-date as possible. The reader will find discussions of such recent topics as the new classification of diabetics; bulimia (recognized as a syndrome in 1980); aspartame (the protein-based sweetener); generic labeling of supermarket items; the sodium–hypertension controversy; and the newest (1983) Metropolitan Life Insurance Company height–weight tables.

The unifying thread of this book is the use of "keys" in every chapter to help the student identify significant concepts, skills, and behaviors. "Key Ideas" summarize the essential points of the chapter. "Keys to Practical Application" translate theory into practice, identifying desirable attitudes, insights, approaches, and action. "Key Terms" are a glossary of new terms the student needs to know. And "Keys to Learning" present thought-provoking questions.

Introductory Nutrition and Diet Therapy is divided into four parts. Part One, "Nutrition in the Community," is devoted to explaining the relationship of nutrition and the community environment, including social and economic aspects. The student becomes aware of the meanings of food — social and cultural as well as chemical or sensual — to be better prepared to work with clients toward the enhancement of their nutritional status.

The reader will note a departure from the traditional sequence in that hospital food service and client feeding are covered in the first part of the book. This was done to afford background information for the student's early clinical experience, in which client feeding is frequently a first assignment. Nevertheless, this topic can easily be read at a later point in the course.

The essential nutrients are presented in Part Two, "The Role of Nutrients in the Maintenance of Normal Health," which opens with an overview of nutrient functions to unify the concepts of cellular nutrition. Considerable emphasis is placed on food sources of nutrients, knowledge of which is basic to practical application. An abstract understanding of the properties and functions of nutrients is of little value unless the student can readily identify food sources and incorporate them into the client's diet.

Relevant concerns of the public also come into the discussion. For example, the material on carbohydrates is followed by such topics as overconsumption of sugars, dental caries, dietary fiber and its lack, low-carbohydrate reducing diets, and diseases requiring carbohydrate modification. The purpose of these brief discussions is to help the student connect the study of nutrients to dietary goals.

Part Three, "Nutrition in the Life Cycle," translates the information of the preceding two parts into practical terms. This section discusses

topics such as choosing foods that meet nutritional requirements in various stages of life; fast foods; U.S. Dietary Goals; the prudent diet; culture, lifestyle, and nutrition; vegetarianism; teenage pregnancies; diet in infancy and old age; food additives; and food management and food safety.

Diet therapy is addressed in Part Four, "Diet Modifications During Illness." The opening chapter relates the scientific method of problem solving to client-centered nutritional care. Nutrition education, as an essential part of that care, is stressed. Techniques that promote learning, and the student's role in nutrition education, are covered. The practical aspects of diet therapy, such as the purchase and the preparation of food, are discussed. Included also is the most recently available information on en-

teral and parenteral feeding, diet in cancer, fiber-modified diets, and drug–nutrient interactions.

In this text, persons receiving nutritional care services are referred to as *clients*. This is because they are viewed as consumers of health services with the rights and responsibilities this term implies. Moreover, since these consumers may be well persons or sick persons, the use of the term is appropriate. For the sake of clarity, the client is referred to as "he" (except in the obvious case of pregnancy or maternity), and the caregiver as "she." The use of these words is nonevaluative.

I welcome suggestions and critical comments from readers.

Marian Maltese Eschleman, M.S., R.D.

Acknowledgments

I wish to express my sincere appreciation to those who provided assistance and encouragement during the writing of this text. I am grateful to Margaret Zealand, B.S., M.P.H., formerly State Nutrition Consultant, New Jersey State Department of Health; and Joan Birchenall, R.N., M.Ed., Director, Bureau of Occupational Programs, New Jersey Department of Education, for encouraging me to accept the challenge of writing this text and for their assistance and suggestions at the onset. I am also indebted to the educators who have reviewed the manuscript: Carolyn Waltzer, R.N., M.A., Parkersburg Community College, West Virginia; Genevieve Smith, R.N., M.S.N., formerly of Sussex County Vocational–Technical School, New Jersey; and Ray Gick, R.N., M.S.N., Gloucester County Community College, New Jersey. The many valuable suggestions of these reviewers have been incorporated into the text.

I have been especially privileged to have the support and expert guidance of Bernice Heller, Editor, whose innovative ideas have added immeasurably to the book. I am also grateful to other members of the Lippincott staff: to David Miller, Vice President and Editor, for his support and assistance in the initial stages of manuscript preparation, and to Mary Murphy, Secretary, for her efficient and generous assistance.

Lastly, I wish to express my gratitude to my children, Thomas and Annemarie, for their patience and to acknowledge the example of diligence and perseverance provided by my dear and loving parents, Mary and the late Thomas Maltese.

Contents

Nutrition in the Community

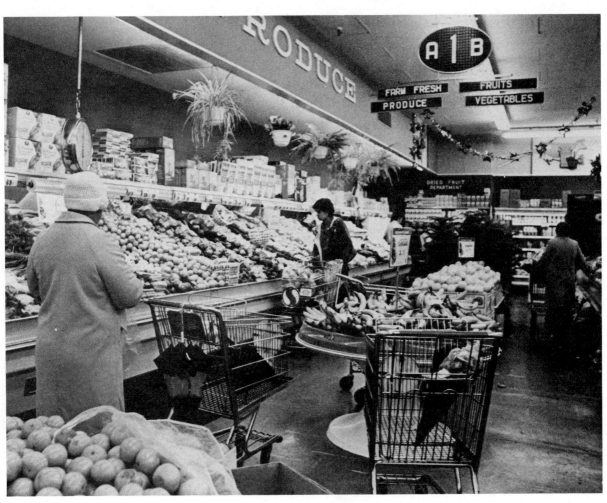

1

Current Nutritional Concerns

KEY TERMS

chronic   Long-term; when applied to diseases, means those that have symptoms of long duration and are frequently incurable.

client   The receiver of health care; replaces the word *patient,* which usually implies illness.

health care   Includes care aimed at prevention and the achievement of good health as well as care provided during illness.

health care delivery system   An organization of functions and services by which health care is made available to persons; includes such aspects as manner of financing, place of care, and types of services provided.

nutrition   The science of food and its relationship to health and disease, and the processes by which the body ingests, absorbs, transports, uses, and excretes food substances.

nutritional care   The application of the science of nutrition to the care of people.

obesity   Excessive deposit and storage of fat in the body.

sedentary   Involving mostly sitting; little physical activity.

The subject of nutrition in today's world is both exciting and bewildering. It is exciting because the consumer is awakened, more than ever before, to the importance of adequate nutrition. He has a new appreciation of its relationship to the quality of life. He is convinced that the person who is well nourished is better able to concentrate, to learn, to do physical activity, to produce work, and to resist disease. Perhaps you, like so many Americans, want to know more about nutrition. You may be asking: "What is a healthful diet?" "Do I need to take vitamin pills?" "Is our food supply safe?" "Can diet prevent heart disease?"

Exciting new trends in health care are highlighting the importance of nutrition education. We are living in a period of time when much attention is focused on the prevention of disease. The focus has changed because our health problems have changed. In the past, infectious diseases such as smallpox, diphtheria, bacterial pneumonia, and tuberculosis were the killer diseases. Today, Americans are faced with early death and disability from accidents and chronic

3

Table 1-1. How Healthy is Your Life-Style?

Risk Category	No Risk	Slight Risk
Smoking	Do not smoke or have stopped for at least 10 years	Fewer than 10 cigarettes or 5 pipes or cigars a day
Alcohol	Nondrinker	Stopped drinker
Trimness	Lean	Slightly plump
Physical Activity	Walk more than 2 miles a day or climb 20 or more flights of stairs a day	Walk 1.5–2 miles a day or climb 15–20 flights of stairs a day
Prescription Drugs	Take medication with doctor's consent following orders carefully	Take medication daily without side-effects
Nonprescription Drugs	Use occasionally only for short periods. Heed label warnings	
Alcohol and Driving—Boats, Cars, Motorcycles, Snowmobiles	Never drink. Drive only with safety aids—seat belt, helmet, life jacket	Never drive after drinking without safety aids
Motor Vehicle Safety	Always wear seat belt	Wear seat belt more than half of the time
Water Safety—Swimming and Boating	Qualified expert	Know how to swim and the safety rules
Blood Cholesterol	Less than 180	180–220
Blood Pressure	120/80 or less	120/80–140/90
Blood sugar	Less than 120 2 hours after a meal of syrup and pancakes	Between 110 and 130 2 hours after meals; checked every 3 months
For Women Only		
Breast Check for Lumps	Monthly self-exam and yearly check by physician	Monthly self-exam but no doctor's exam
Pap Smear	Every year	Every 3 years

(After Blueprint for Health, Volume XXVII, Number 1: "Help Yourself!" Chicago, Blue Cross Association, 1978)
Note: Some risk factors are more important than others, so it is not possible to score the results of this self-analysis accurately. But for a longer and healthier than average life, try to change your health habits so you will be in the categories on this page rather than the opposite one.

(long-term) diseases. The individual can do more to prevent these causes of death and disability than modern medicine can do to fight them once they occur.

Improved nutrition is one of the most important tools in disease prevention. Improved diet was a very important factor in conquering the infectious diseases of the past. Today it is just as important in preventing or delaying the onset of chronic disease. Diet is associated with

a number of chronic diseases that are leading causes of death: heart and blood vessel diseases, diabetes, and cirrhosis of the liver. Obesity (excessive fatness) is a diet-related health problem that contributes to the occurrence or severity of a number of chronic diseases. Our present nutrition problems are related mostly to excess—excess calories, sugar, fat, and salt.

Of course, nutrition is not the only factor over which we have some control. Lack of exer-

Substantial Risk	Heavy Risk	Dangerous Risk
Half pack a day	1 pack a day	2 or more packs a day
Fewer than 6 drinks a week	More than 6 drinks a week	More than 2 drinks a day
Moderately obese	Considerably obese	Grossly obese
Walk only 0.5–1.5 miles a day or climb only 5–15 flights of stairs a day	Walk only 2–5 blocks a day or climb 2–4 flights of stairs a day	Walk less than 2 blocks a day or climb less than 2 flights of stairs a day
Take medication when needed with few side-effects	Use sleeping and nerve pills regularly without doctor's supervision	Without doctor's consent, mix medication with other drugs or alcohol
		Continuing use, alcohol used or auto driven despite label warnings
Drive after 2 drinks with safety aids	Drive after 2 drinks without safety aids	Drive after more than 2 drinks without safety aids
Wear seat belt as a driver half of the time	Wear seat belt as a passenger half of the time	Wear seat belt less than half of the time
Know how to swim and may swim after 1 drink or nerve drug	Do not know how to swim but use life jacket half of the time	Do not know how to swim; never use life jacket
220–280	280–320	320 and up
140/90–160/100	160/100–180/105	Above 180/105
Blood sugar more than 150 without diet control	Blood sugar more than 150 without diet control or doctor's care	Diabetes without doctor's care at less than 45 years of age
Self-exam 2–3 times a year but no doctor's exam	Doctor's exam once a year	Never
Every 4 years	Never	Never; nonmenstrual bleeding

This chart was prepared by Pamela Hall under the supervision of Drs. Lewis C. Robbins and Jack H. Hall of Methodist Hospital, Indianapolis, developers of the Health Hazard Appraisal system.

cise, smoking, too much mental and emotional stress, and alcoholism are other life-style conditions that contribute to the occurrence of these chronic diseases. (How would you rate your life-style? See Table 1-1.)

Closely related to the preventive care movement is the new emphasis on self-care. In this approach, the client himself assumes greater responsibility than in the past for managing the treatment of his chronic health problems. The diabetic, for example, may check his blood sugar in his own home and make changes in diet and insulin dose, if necessary. To accomplish this, the client (receiver of services) must be well informed, skillful, and highly motivated.

The subject of nutrition is bewildering to many people. Americans are concerned about the quality and the safety of their food supply and about their nutritional state. Because authorities do not always agree on what makes up a "healthful" diet, consumers are often confused. Uncertainty is also created when we are slow to apply what we know about nutrition to rapidly changing social conditions. Fears about

chronic diseases such as heart disease and cancer, often reported to be linked in some ways with diet, may lead people to be exploited by persons who promise simple nutritional "cures" for complex diseases.

The Challenge to the Health Worker

You, the health worker, face a clear challenge in this new environment. In today's health care setting, a deep knowledge of nutrition and great skill in helping clients apply this knowledge is required. You must be well informed so that you can offer sound nutrition information, promote good nutrition, and help the public distinguish between false and reliable information. The informed health worker also recognizes when it is necessary to refer clients to physicians, dietitians, or other resource persons for assistance with problems related to nutrition and diet. Being well informed about nutrition is also important for your own well-being and that of your family and community. Persons who understand the principles of nutrition and who are convinced of their worth will put them into practice and will encourage their families to follow them.

Nutrition is the science that deals with food eaten and how the body uses it. The study of nutrition will answer many of your questions and concerns. However, you will find that some questions cannot yet be answered and that the answers to other questions are steeped in controversy. Some of what you learn will change because of new findings by nutrition and food scientists.

What you learn in your study of nutrition is not the kind of information you will place on the "back burner." It is knowledge you can begin to use today and continue to use to advantage in both your health career and your personal life.

Current Influences on Food Habits

For a person to be an effective promoter of nutritional health, several basic elements are required: a knowledge of body requirements of food; an understanding of the cultural, social, psychological, and economic factors that help to shape a person's food habits; and a commitment to this knowledge in terms of one's own behavior (example is the best teacher). Knowing the principles of good nutrition is of little value unless this knowledge can be applied to the everyday needs and circumstances of people. Before beginning your study of nutrition, it is important to consider some of the current factors that have strong influences on how and what people eat. These challenge you to apply what you learn to an ever-changing environment.

The Changing Society

American food habits have undergone many changes as a result of the changing life-style of the American family. For example, family members may arise at different times and prepare their individual breakfasts. Some may skip breakfast. Lunch may be purchased at the factory or office cafeteria, the school cafeteria, a restaurant, or a fast-food establishment. Dinner may be hurriedly prepared, served, and eaten to accommodate family members' many other activities. Snacking may begin with the midmorning and midafternoon coffee break, to end only at bedtime. Children may get into the habit of snacking from the time they return from school until dinnertime. Are all the essential foods being provided by this fragmented style of eating? Or are foods with little nutritional value making up too large a part of the American diet?

A second change is to be seen in the increasing number of single-person households. It

has been estimated that by 1990, at least one third of all households will consist of one person. Meal patterns frequently change with this shift from family to nonfamily households. Are persons who live alone preparing well-balanced meals for themselves? Are they as motivated as those who must provide food for a family?

Of persons living alone, 45% are over 65 years of age. The over-65 population increased by 5 million in the 1970s. A further increase of 20% is anticipated in the 1980s. Persons in this age group are prone to nutritional problems caused by poor eating habits, social and economic factors, and chronic diseases.

An increase in the number of meals eaten away from home is another outgrowth of the changing American scene, especially the increased employment of women outside the home. In the 1960s, 17% of the food budget was spent on "eating out"; by the late 1970s, this had increased to 24% of the food budget.

Easy access to inexpensive fast-food establishments is one reason for the increase in "eating out." Some universities allow on-campus fast-food establishments in which students are permitted to use their meal tickets. Many school food service programs now follow this fast-food meal pattern. Fast-food meals lack variety, may be high in calories relative to the amount of nutrients they provide, and tend to be excessively high in fat. Since this trend is not likely to decline, how can we encourage better consumer choices and more variety in the foods offered?

The fast pace of life has made the use of convenience foods increasingly attractive. Some 10,000 food products confront the consumer at the supermarket. Attractive packaging and displays and ease of preparation may entice many persons to buy foods that may be nutritionally inadequate—overrefined and excessive in fats, salt, and calories.

The role of stress in food habits is under intensive study. It is widely believed that we live in a more stressful time than did our grandparents. The stress factors may be related to employment, frequency of moving from one place to another, the general pace of life, or other factors. Whatever the cause, many people find that what they eat, when they eat, and how they eat are all influenced by stress factors.

A substance dependency, whether on alcohol, drugs, tobacco, or other form may strongly influence a person's food habits. Not only the cost of these items, but also their relationship to the foods that are eaten, may be significant factors.

Although studies show that Americans are consuming fewer calories than they did before, obesity is increasing. This implies that Americans are becoming increasingly sedentary (inactive). In many cases, lack of physical activity is so extreme that weight reduction can occur only at very low calorie levels. When calories are severely restricted, it is difficult to obtain an adequate diet. Reducing food intake alone is not the answer.

The Changing Consumer

In recent years, the consumer movement has gained ground. Consumer groups have heightened public concern about the nutritional quality of food, the safety of food additives, the freshness of shelf foods, methods of pricing foods, and the role of government at all levels in protecting the safety of food. The consumer movement has increased concern for the rights of the individual and the desire of the consumer to have greater control than in the past over his fate. In the health field, the client has become a prominent member of the health team, making choices and decisions and assuming a greater role than before in managing his health problems.

Along with the growing interest in food and nutrition have arisen various types of food faddism. The consumer, frequently motivated by fear, falls prey to those who claim that so-called health foods and large doses of vitamin and mineral supplements prevent or cure dreaded chronic diseases.

The food habits of today's consumer are greatly influenced by the mass media, especially television. Children and adults alike are the targets of commercial messages aimed at persuading them to purchase various food items.

The Changing Economy

Changes in economic conditions have a strong influence on eating habits. In times of inflation and unemployment, many people may have to cut their food budget in order to meet the rising costs of such necessities as heating fuel, housing, and transportation. The amount spent for food becomes the only flexible item in their budget. When the food budget is low, nutritional needs can be met only if purchases are carefully planned and limited to those foods that provide the most food value at the lowest cost. At the same time, developing industries may help to create a group of newly rich persons who may have money available to spend on food and yet may not know how to spend it wisely. These people may increase their intake of rich foods that are low in nutritional value. Good and poor diets are found at all income levels.

Current Influences on Health Care

Combined with these many changes in life-style is a remarkable change in the health care delivery system (ways of providing health care). This system has changed from an exclusive relationship between the physician and the client to a system that includes an increasing number of allied health personnel. These personnel function as a team in providing health care to clients.

Including the client as a member of this health team is another development in the changing health care system. The on-going care required by chronic diseases, increased concern for individual rights, advances in the development of drugs and devices for use in controlling chronic diseases, and the increasing cost of health care have given impetus to this movement.

Hospitals, while still providing traditional care for the ill person, are reaching into the community with "wellness programs" geared toward preventive health care. Prevention is also the emphasis in health maintenance organizations (HMOs). An HMO is a group medical practice financed by prepaid health insurance. Unlike usual health insurance, the HMO plan covers the cost of preventive care as well as care during illness. It is modeled after group practice plans that have been in existence for many years.

Responsibilities of the Health Team

Working successfully to maintain or improve the nutritional well-being of individuals or to treat disease by means of diet requires teamwork. The physician usually prescribes the nutritional care (application of the science of nutrition) to be given and provides guidance to other members of the health team. Health personnel involved include the nurse and dietitian and the primary care assistants, such as dietary technicians, licensed vocational or practical nurses, and home health aides.

The dietitian, public health nutritionist, and community diet counselor are specialists in human nutrition. They can assist the nurse and other health workers in providing nutritional care both in the hospital and in the community. In some cases, they work directly with the client and his family. The dietary technician assists the dietitian both in the management of hospital food service and in contact with clients. The community or home health aid works under the supervision of a nurse or nutritionist. She works in the client's home, where she frequently plans and prepares meals, buys food, and, if necessary, feeds the client.

The need for nutritional services permeates many areas of health care. Included here is a brief discussion of the roles of health workers in various health care settings.

In the hospital or nursing home, the nurse sees that the client receives and eats his meals. She does all in her power to make the mealtime atmosphere as encouraging to his appetite as possible. The nurse may assist in providing nutrition education for the client. The dietitian plans the menus for both normal and therapeutic diets and supervises both the preparation and service of food. She also provides diet counseling for clients. The dietary technician may assist her by taking diet histories and participating in diet instruction.

In the ambulatory care setting, such as the clinic, health center, or physician's office, the nurse has an excellent opportunity to provide nutrition education. She sees the client periodically over an extended period of time. Because a change in food habits is usually a slow process, the nurse is able to help the client make a gradual adjustment to his diet. A dietitian is frequently available to assist. Sometimes, the dietitian is a member of the staff and provides diet counseling for clients with complex nutritional problems.

In the home, the community or public health nurse has a unique opportunity to observe food habits and the circumstances that influence them. She provides health education and/or bedside nursing care in the home and may supervise a home health aide. The public health nurse is aware, more than other members of the health team, of the effects of circumstances such as income, cultural factors, family organization, and housing on the food habits of a particular family. With a knowledge of these factors, she can provide practical and meaningful assistance. She also has the advantage of having repeated contact with families over an extended period of time. A public health nutritionist or a community diet counselor is frequently available to assist the nurse with nutritional care in the home.

In the school or day care center, the nurse has close contact with children. She may be more successful than the child's mother in influencing food habits. She may be able to help parents with their children's eating problems and may be involved in nutrition education programs for both children and parents.

In business and industry, the nurse provides nutrition education as part of preventive health programs offered to employees. She may also provide guidance to personnel who are on therapeutic diets.

KEYS TO PRACTICAL APPLICATION

Change those life-style habits that are damaging your health.

Keep in mind the everyday circumstances of your clients as you study nutrition and apply what you learn.

Look to the dietitian or diet counselor to help you with nutrition problems.

KEY IDEAS

Adequate food and sound nutrition practices are essential to good health and are key factors in the prevention of disease and recovery from illness.

Today's nutritional problems are related mostly to excess — excess calories, fat, sugar, salt, and alcohol.

Emphasis on prevention and self-care places more responsibility than in the past on the client.

The new emphasis requires that health care personnel be more involved and more knowledgeable than before in providing nutrition education.

Social changes affect the way people eat and bring about changes in patterns of eating.

To be effective, knowledge of nutrition must be applied to the everyday needs and circumstances of people.

Successfully providing nutritional care requires teamwork and involves including the client as a prominent member of the team.

The need for nutritional care permeates many areas of health care; the services of dietitians, public health nutritionists, and diet counselors are available to assist health workers with nutrition-related problems.

KEYS TO LEARNING: STUDY–DISCUSSION QUESTIONS

1. Increasing responsibility for health care is being placed on the shoulders of the consumer himself. Why?

2. From your present knowledge of the subject, discuss the ways in which nutrition is involved in achieving and maintaining good health, preventing disease, and treating illness.

3. Explain why the preventive self-care movement requires that health care personnel become more involved in nutrition education.

4. What facilities for preventive health care are available in your community? What kinds of nutrition services, if any, are provided?

5. Bring to class an example from a newspaper or magazine of one of the current influences on food habits. Explain to the class the way in which food habits may be affected by the examples you have chosen.

6. What do you hope to achieve from this study of nutrition?

Bibliography is found at the end of Part One.

2

Assessing Nutritional Needs

KEY TERMS

anthropometry   Measurement of body size (height, weight) and body composition (fat, muscle, water).

assessment   Evaluation of a person's nutritional well-being by the collection of data such as a nutrition history, physical examination, laboratory values, and x-ray studies.

culture   Beliefs, arts, and customs that make up a way of life for a group of people.

energy   Capacity to do work; body fuel provided by certain nutrients (carbohydrate, fat, and protein).

hunger   An unpleasant sensation due to inadequate intake of food.

malnutrition   A state of impaired health due to undernutrition, overnutrition, an

imbalance of nutrients, or the body's inability to utilize the nutrients ingested.

monitor   To watch over or observe for an extended period of time.

nutrients   Chemical substances supplied by food that the body needs for growth, repair, and general functioning.

nutrition   The scientific and systematic study of nutrients, the processes they undergo in the body, and the effects of food selection on nutritional well-being.

overnutrition   Excessive intake of one or more nutrients; frequently refers to excessive intake of nutrients providing energy.

undernutrition   Deficiency of one or more nutrients; may also refer to a deficiency of nutrients providing energy.

Food: Its Physiological Importance

As long as we are not hungry, does it really matter what we eat? Most of us have been warned of the dire consequences of missing breakfast or eating lunches consisting of soda and potato chips. Nevertheless, we may have skipped breakfast and satisfied our hunger with snack foods or sweets at mealtime and felt no ill effects. A person who eats poorly today will most likely live to tell the tale tomorrow. What, however, will be the long-range effects of the many todays of poor eating? Will it be anemia, with its symptoms of weakness and fatigue that sap the body of strength to enjoy life to the fullest? Will it be overweight, which is frequently damaging to emotional health and

11

which makes the individual more susceptible than normal to serious chronic diseases? Will it be premature hardening of the arteries, a condition responsible for heart attacks and strokes? Or will it be decreased resistance to disease resulting in frequent colds and infections, which take their toll on an individual's productive days?

Nutrition is the science that deals with the chemical substances in food — called *nutrients* — that the body needs for life and growth. Nutrition provides information about how much of each nutrient is needed and under what circumstances and on the types and quantities of food that will satisfy bodily needs. Foods that should not be eaten and the reasons therefor are also identified. The functions of nutrients, how they interact, what happens when there is a lack, an excess, or an imbalance in nutrients, and the processes by which the body digests, absorbs, utilizes, and excretes the end-products of food eaten are included in nutrition. Because food must be consumed to be used by the body, the psychological, social, and cultural factors that influence food selection are also to be considered. As you can see, nutrition draws upon many other sciences, including biology, chemistry, physiology, medicine, psychology, anthropology, and sociology.

The terms *nutritional status* and *malnutrition* are used frequently in this book. *Nutritional status* refers to the body's food intake and food use. *Malnutrition* is a state of impaired health resulting from undernutrition — a lack of nutrients — or from overnutrition — excessive intake of nutrients. The person who is obese, for example, is malnourished. Malnutrition may also result if the body cannot properly use the food it receives. For example, a child who has frequent bouts of diarrhea may be poorly nourished because the nutrients in the food he eats cannot be adequately absorbed from the intestinal tract.

Role of Nutrition in Growth and Development

Food maintains life. Certain chemical substances (nutrients) in food are required by the cells for growth, repair, rebuilding, and regula-

tion of function. Retarded growth and delayed sexual development result from deficiencies of certain nutrients. Severe malnutrition and infection together may result in permanent growth retardation and increased susceptibility to disease.

Though the relationship between nutrition and mental development is under intensive study, it is difficult to separate the effects of nutrition on health from those of other factors such as heredity, presence of disease, physical and emotional state, and the home environment.

Skeletal Growth and Sexual Development

Although heredity limits a person's ultimate build, his state of nutrition determines whether he will achieve his hereditary limits. The growth pattern of a child is a useful means for judging his nutritional well-being. When a child is poorly nourished, his growth rate diminishes, owing in part to a delay in bone development. Both the quality of the bone (i.e., the amount of calcium and phosphorus it contains) and its capability for growth are influenced by nutrition.

Sexual maturity appears to occur later in populations that are malnourished than in developed countries. Furthermore, in developed countries, sexual maturity occurs at an earlier age in each succeeding generation.

Mental Development

The most rapid growth of the brain occurs from 5 months before birth to 10 months after birth. At the end of the first year of life, the brain, the first organ to attain full development, has achieved 70% of its adult weight. Poorly nourished babies have fewer and smaller brain cells than babies who are adequately nourished. Whether inadequate nutrition will damage later intellectual development is not known with certainty. However, the majority of studies to date indicate that early and severe malnutrition is an important factor in deficiencies in later mental development apart from social and hereditary influences. The effects of mild or moderate un-

dernutrition on intellectual development are less clear.

Severe deficiencies of specific nutrients can cause adverse structural changes and impaired functioning of the central nervous system. Symptoms such as anxiety, irritability, depression, mental confusion, and physical and mental apathy are associated with certain deficiency diseases. Such symptoms most certainly influence learning ability. Iron deficiency anemia among school children may interfere with motivation and the ability to concentrate for extended periods of time. A study conducted by the National Heart, Lung, and Blood Institute suggests that iron deficiency states may cause a reduction in iron-containing enzymes in brain tissue, which in turn causes alterations in brain function.

Hunger, the unpleasant sensation of stomach pangs caused by insufficient food intake, can affect learning. It is possible to be poorly nourished without being hungry, because eating just about any food will relieve hunger. It is also possible to be hungry without being poorly nourished. However, persons who experience a constant sense of hunger are undoubtedly poorly nourished. Hungry children are distracted by their hunger pangs. They are frequently unable to pay attention and are thus unable to respond to educational stimulation. Very often, children who are poorly nourished come from home environments that are also poor in educational level, economic status, and motivation. These factors also influence behavior. Nevertheless, it is safe to assume that the poorly nourished person who tires easily, has little energy, and is unable to concentrate will have difficulty achieving his intellectual potential.

Malnutrition, Illness, and Chronic Disease

Undernourished persons do not tolerate illness well. They show delayed wound healing and are more susceptible than normal to infection and complications of illness.

A number of chronic diseases have been linked to diet. Populations with diets high in fat and cholesterol tend to have high blood cholesterol levels. Many scientists believe that a high blood cholesterol level promotes atherosclerosis (a form of "hardening of the arteries"), which is the underlying cause of most heart attacks and strokes. Hypertension (high blood pressure) has been associated with high intake of salt, obesity, and the use of alcohol. Hypertension increases the risk of stroke and heart disease. Obesity makes some persons more susceptible to a type of diabetes mellitus that does not require insulin. A high percentage (10–20%) of persons consuming large quantities of alcohol for extended periods of time develop cirrhosis of the liver. This serious disease, frequently fatal, is characterized by fatty deposits in the liver and damaged liver cells. Lack of fiber in the diet has been blamed for the high occurrence of diverticulosis in the United States. Diverticulosis is the condition in which abnormal sacs form at points of weakness in the intestinal wall. Lastly, diet is a basic factor in tooth decay, one of the most widespread of all chronic diseases.

Malnutrition Worldwide

Undernutrition is widespread in the developing countries of the world. It is estimated that 400 million persons suffer from serious nutritional deficiencies. In Asia, Africa, and Latin America, 25% to 30% of the population suffer from semistarvation. Millions more suffer from a serious deficiency of a specific nutrient such as iron, iodine, or vitamin A (Fig. 2-1).

Children are hardest hit. Nutritional deficiency and infection, working together, create a vicious cycle. The poorly nourished child is highly susceptible to infection, and infections are more severe and last longer in a malnourished than in a well-nourished child. The child is then more vulnerable to the next infectious disease to which he is exposed. The annual death toll due to common childhood diseases is extremely high in developing countries—15 million children under the age of 5. This represents one fourth of all the deaths throughout the world.

It may be argued that, in some parts of the world, people who have little knowledge about

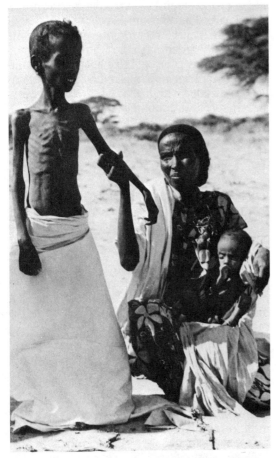

Fig. 2-1. Successive years of drought have left thousands of nomadic people suffering from severe malnutrition, like the children of this Somalian woman. (Courtesy WHO)

nutrition have survived well for generations on very limited diets. Although their food supply is limited, all of the nutrients required for good nutrition are provided in the few foods available to them. Nevertheless, the worldwide prevalence of malnutrition demonstrates that millions of people are not so fortunate.

Malnutrition in the United States

In this country, cases of severe undernutrition are the result of ignorance, extreme poverty, neglect, mental illness, or unusual environmental conditions. Although severe malnutrition is not widespread in the United States, it does exist. Malnutrition is considered a contributing factor in the high death toll among children of migrant farmers and native Americans and among the elderly.

The severe undernutrition you, the health worker, are most likely to see is the result of illness. Many illnesses interfere with appetite or with the body's ability to utilize food. In recent years, surveys have indicated that malnutrition is widespread among clients hospitalized more than 2 weeks. Much more attention is now being focused on maintaining or improving the nutritional status of clients in hospitals and other health agencies.

The United States ranks 12th among the industrialized nations of the world in number of infant deaths. Babies born to poorly nourished women and teenagers are likely to have a low birth weight. About 45% of all infant deaths occur among low-birth-weight babies. Those that survive are about twice as likely to have physical, mental, and developomental handicaps.

Most problems of nutritional deficiency in the United States are moderate in severity. Although his undernutrition is not severe enough to threaten his life, the malnourished child grows at a slower rate and is more susceptible to infection than the well-nourished child.

Overnutrition, not deficiency, is responsible for the major nutritional problems in the United States today. Heart disease, diabetes, and cirrhosis are among the diseases linked to diet. Over 1 million deaths each year are attributed to heart attack, stroke, and other diseases of the heart and blood vessels. An estimated 60 million Americans have hypertension, a condition that increases the risk of heart disease and stroke. Ten million are presumed to have diabetes. Four percent or more of American adults are alcoholics. More than 20% of the adult population is seriously overweight, a condition that also increases the risk of chronic illness.

Measuring Nutritional Status

A well-nourished person has a general appearance of vitality and well-being. He is alert, has sufficient energy to perform physical activities, and recovers rapidly from periods of stress. However, a lack of these attributes is not necessarily due to inadequate nutrition, it could be caused by nonnutritional factors such as lack of rest or emotional stress.

Generally speaking, the symptoms of the less severe type of malnutrition, the type most commonly found in the United States, are vague and difficult to detect. Nevertheless, health workers should learn to recognize the major signs of nutritional deficiency so that they can alert the physician, who can then make a detailed examination (Table 2-1).

Evaluation (assessment) of an individual's nutritional status should be done as part of a routine health check-up and to monitor the nutritional needs of high-risk clients such as

Table 2-1. Physical Signs Indicative or Suggestive of Malnutrition

Body Area	Normal Appearance	Signs Associated with Malnutrition
Hair	Shiny; firm; not easily plucked	Lack of natural shine; hair dull and dry; thin and sparse; fine, silky, and straight; color changes; can be easily plucked
Face	Skin color uniform; smooth, pink, healthy appearance; not swollen	Skin color loss; skin dark over cheeks and under eyes; lumpiness or flakiness of skin of nose and mouth; swollen face; enlarged parotid glands; scaling of skin around nostrils
Eyes	Bright, clear, shiny; no sores at corners of eyelids; membranes a healthy pink and moist; no prominent blood vessels or mounds of tissue or sclera	Eye membranes are pale or red; redness and fissuring of eyelid corners; dryness of eye membranes; dull appearance of cornea; softness of cornea; scar on cornea; ring of fine blood vessels around cornea
Lips	Smooth; not chapped or swollen	Redness and swelling of mouth or lips, especially at corners of mouth
Tongue	Deep red; not swollen or smooth	Swelling; scarlet and raw tongue; purplish color of tongue; smooth tongue; swollen sores; hyperemic and hypertrophic papillae; atrophic papillae
Teeth	No cavities; no pain; bright	May be missing or erupting abnormally; gray or black spots; cavities
Gums	Healthy; red; do not bleed; not swollen	"Spongy" and bleed easily; recede
Glands	Face not swollen	Thyroid enlargement (front of neck); parotid enlargement (cheeks become swollen)

(*continued*)

Table 2-1. (continued)

Body Area	Normal Appearance	Signs Associated with Malnutrition
Skin	No signs of rashes, swellings, dark or light spots	Dryness of skin; sandpaper feel of skin; flakiness of skin; skin swollen and dark; red swollen pigmentation of exposed areas; excessive lightness or darkness of skin; black and blue marks due to skin bleeding; lack of fat under skin
Nails	Firm; pink	Nails are spoon-shaped; brittle, ridged nails
Muscular and skeletal systems	Good muscle tone; some fat under skin; can walk or run without pain	Muscles have "wasted" appearance; baby's skull bones are thin and soft; round swelling of front and side of head; swelling of ends of bones; small bumps on both sides of chest wall (on ribs)—beading of ribs; baby's soft spot on head does not harden at proper time; knock-knees or bow-legs; bleeding into muscle; person cannot get up or walk properly
Internal Systems:		
Cardiovascular	Normal heart rate and rhythm; no murmurs or abnormal rhythms; normal blood pressure for age	Rapid heart rate; enlarged heart; abnormal rhythm; elevated blood pressure
Gastrointestinal	No palpable organs or masses (in children, however, liver edge may be palpable)	Liver enlargement; enlargement of spleen (usually indicates other associated diseases)
Nervous	Psychological stability; normal reflexes	Mental irritability and confusion; burning and tingling of hands and feet; loss of position and vibratory sense; weakness and tenderness of muscles (may result in inability to walk); decrease and loss of ankle and knee reflexes

(After Christakis G: Nutritional Assessment in Health Programs. Washington, DC, American Public Health Association, 1975)

persons with chronic disease or those living in deprived environments. Nutritional assessment is also conducted on groups of people to determine which problems are likely to exist in a given population or age group.

How do we determine whether an individual is well nourished? The physician or other health professional trained in the diagnosis of nutritional problems uses a number of tools to accurately measure an individual's nutritional status. These include clinical examination, x-ray studies, laboratory data, and food intake record and diet history.

Clinical Examination

Physical Signs

The examiner looks for physical signs and symptoms associated with malnutrition. Examination of the skin, mouth, and eyes is particularly important. Easily plucked hair, scaling skin, and sores at the corners of the mouth or eyelids are examples of signs that may be associated with nutritional deficiencies. The examiner also asks the client questions about how he functions and feels.

Anthropometric Measurements (Body Size and Composition)

Height, weight, and skinfold (fatfold) thickness are examples of measurements frequently taken to evaluate nutritional status.

Because nutritional deficiency can result in retarded growth, a child's height and weight can be compared with those of other children of the same sex, age, and body build. Growth charts have been devised by the National Center for Health Statistics (NCHS) for this purpose. If a child's measurements differ substantially from standard measurements, nutritional problems should be suspected.

Measurements of head, midarm, and abdominal circumference are also useful. Measurement of head circumference provides information about brain growth, midarm circumference about muscle mass, and abdominal circumference about water retention.

Skinfold thickness measurements provide information about fatness and leanness. The width of the fat layer that lies directly beneath the skin is measured in various places on the body with a device called a *caliper* (Fig. 2-2). Skinfold thickness measurements obtained from the client are then compared with averages for persons of the same age and sex. This method is considered to be a more accurate means of determining fatness than comparing an individual's weight-for-height with tables of average weights. The person's age at the appearance of secondary sex characteristics may also be an indication of nutritional status.

X-Ray Studies

X-ray studies are a useful tool in determining whether bones have developed as would be expected for age. As has been stated, nutrition influences the size and quality of bone as well as its rate of development. X-ray films of the wrist bones of children are particularly useful. These bones appear earlier and develop earlier in well-nourished children than in poorly nourished children. Films are also useful in detecting bone deformities caused by nutritional deficiency diseases such as rickets and scurvy. These abnormalities are the result of deficient or exces-sive intake that has existed for a long period of time.

Laboratory Data

Blood, urine, and stool tests reveal much about what foods have been eaten, the quantity of certain nutrients in body stores, and how the nutrients are being utilized. A low blood level of a particular nutrient may suggest that the body is poorly nourished in regard to that nutrient. Certain blood tests, for example, indicate the adequacy of iron intake. Laboratory tests fre-

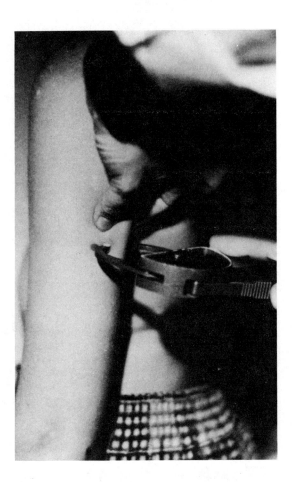

Fig. 2-2. Measuring the triceps skinfold. (Courtesy Samuel J. Fomon, M.D., Iowa City, Iowa)

quently signal a nutritional problem before outward symptoms appear.

Diet History and Food Intake Records

Information about the client's food habits can also signal the possibility of malnutrition, can serve as a check on the findings of the physical examination and laboratory tests, and provides a basis for making changes in food habits should this be necessary. Information about a client's food intake can be obtained in several ways, such as through diet recall, the food diary, and the food frequency record.

A diet recall is a record based on the client's remembrance of food items eaten during the previous 24 hours (Fig. 2-3). A food diary is a record of specific foods and the quantities con-

---

Diet Recall

What foods do you choose for your usual meals and snacks?	What specific foods have you eaten in the past 24 hours?
Morning _____	Morning _____
Noon _____	Noon _____
Night _____	Night _____
Snacks _____	Snacks _____

FOOD DIARY

Time	Place and associated activity (watching TV, talking, reading)	Who is with you?	Physical position S—Sitting St—Standing R—Reclining

Mood A—Angry B—Bored D—Depressed H—Happy N—Neutral Ner—Nervous T—Tired	Degree of Hunger 0–5 0—Not hungry 5—Very hungry	Food	Amount	Calories

Food Frequency Record

Please indicate which of the following foods you eat and how often.

	Never or hardly ever (less than once a week)	Sometimes (not daily but at least once a week)	Every day or nearly every day
Cheese, yogurt, ice cream	☐	☐	☐
Eggs	☐	☐	☐
Dried beans, peas, peanut butter	☐	☐	☐
Meat, fish, poultry	☐	☐	☐
Bread, rice, pasta, grits, cereal, tortillas, potatoes	☐	☐	☐
Fruits or fruit juices	☐	☐	☐
Vegetables	☐	☐	☐

Fig. 2-3. Forms used to assess food intake.

sumed over a certain period of time, usually 3 to 7 days. The information is recorded in the diary as soon as possible after the food has been eaten. A food frequency record is a list of food items on which the client indicates his frequency of consumption of each item. After an estimate of food intake is obtained, it is compared to a recognized standard to determine the likelihood of deficiency or excess.

In a health care facility, a dietitian or physician may request that a detailed 24-hour food intake record be kept for a client for a period of days. This record should indicate all foods and liquids consumed at meals and between meals and any foods obtained from other sources, such as those brought in by family and friends. The amount of food and fluid left on the tray is subtracted from the amount initially served. Nutrients obtained in intravenous feedings and nutrient supplements are also included.

While obtaining a diet history, a skillful interviewer will try to elicit information about environmental, cultural, economic, and behavioral factors that may affect nutritional status. Poverty, food faddism, and mental disturbance are examples of factors that can have a significant influence on nutritional status.

Food: Its Psychological Importance

Assessing an individual's need for food does not stop with an understanding of the person's physical needs. It also includes an understanding of the role of food and eating in fulfilling the person's psychological and emotional needs.

Sociologists have expressed concern about the lack in many homes of family-centered meals. At all socioeconomic levels, increasingly fewer meals are being eaten at home. It is believed that this practice could seriously weaken the stability of the family, the most basic and

important institution in our society. As one sociologist put it, "The family that eats together stays together." Although this concern focuses on children, the social aspects of eating are equally important for the elderly person. In fact, the people with whom the elderly person eats may be as important as what he eats.

You may wonder how this concern relates to your study of nutrition and ultimately to your health career. Perhaps you already know, for it does not take a very long association with hospitalized persons to appreciate the significance of meals to them. Hospitalized clients spend considerable time choosing menus, anticipating meals, and evaluating the food served them. In the anxiety that accompanies illness and hospitalization, food and food service assume great importance. To the client and his family, who may not understand the intricate tests and treatments that have been prescribed, the client's appetite and food acceptance may be one of the best indicators of his progress.

People attach meanings or labels to food. These meanings reflect a person's values and beliefs and are very stongly influenced by social factors. In nonindustrialized societies, custom is an important influence. In Western countries, fashion and accepted modes of behavior strengthened by advertising and other commercial techniques are powerful forces in food selection.

The health worker soon learns that teaching the concepts of nutrition is not a guarantee that the client will put them into practice. An acute awareness of the meanings of food is needed by health workers if they are to be successful in helping others meet their nutritional needs. If changes in food habits are necessary, they must be in harmony with the meanings that food holds for the individual.

Psychosocial Factors

From the beginning of life, food and the act of eating play a vital role in growth and development. The newborn infant's entire world centers around the eating–feeding situation. It is the basic experience through which he perceives the world around him and through which he establishes his most important relationship

—that with his mother or other caretaker. Ideally, this early eating–feeding experience conveys feelings of warmth, tenderness, and love.

As the child grows, attitudes and feelings continue to be communicated to him through food. The family mealtime is an important means of affording all members a sense of togetherness and unity. Mealtime establishes family relationships, and through it some cultural patterns are passed from one generation to the next. It also provides an occasion for parents and children to interact and to share and develop understanding.

In adulthood, warm human relationships are also fostered when food is offered. Food—even only a cup of tea or coffee—is a symbol of hospitality. We honor our friends by inviting them to eat with us. In most cultures, for a family to share a meal with someone is a strong expression of social acceptance and commitment. In ancient China, when someone fell from favor, his rice bowl was broken and he was no longer permitted to eat with the family or group.

Problems arise when mealtime is no longer shared. Aloneness is said to be the great tragedy of aging. Eating alone, as many elderly persons must, dampens the appetite and the motivation to prepare meals. To meet the problem of aloneness faced by the hospitalized person, many hospitals and other health care facilities encourage clients to eat in the company of others by making available dining rooms on various floors. Many communities offer group mealtimes for the elderly, providing social contacts for persons who would otherwise be isolated.

Reward and punishment, anxiety and depression also find expression in ways that center around food. A child's behavior may be rewarded or punished by the giving or withholding of a prized dessert or sweet. Adults may reward themselves after a particularly trying day by eating a special food or "going out" to eat. Some persons react to anxiety by overeating, and others lose their appetite. During intensive study for examinations, for example, a student may take frequent snack breaks—not because he is hungry, but because he seeks relief from tension.

Cultural Factors

Acquiring food is a basic need. However, how people meet this need varies greatly from one cultural group to another. Culture ". . . is a system of customs transmitted from one generation to the other, mainly by means of language. And among these customs none is more significant than the ways of procuring and consuming food."* Culture is learned, beginning with the earliest childhood experiences.

It is as important to consider cultural differences in this country as when dealing with a person from a foreign country. In days past, persons in the United States tended to resist the idea that there are important differences separating people. The revival of interest in native Americans, black Americans, Italian–Americans, and other cultural groups has helped to overcome this tendency and to make us more aware of cultural differences.

What is considered acceptable food by one society may be deemed inedible by another. Undoubtedly, the kinds and quantities of food available in a particular locality and the economic capacity to obtain foods are important influences. Certain plants, animals, and insects may be commonly eaten in some cultures and be taboo in others. Most Americans react negatively to the idea of eating insects, which are widely consumed by some other peoples. Many Indians starving because of a lack of rice found the wheat offered by the United States an unacceptable substitute. In World War II, Japanese prisoners were made ill when they first tried to eat the food prepared by their American captors. Only in extreme circumstances will people eat anything that is edible.

Every food in a given culture is endowed with meaning. Sometimes the meanings associated with a particular food are dramatic—for example, Americans attach vivid symbolism to such words and phrases as "Thanksgiving turkey," "champagne," "birthday cake," and

---

* Niehoff A: Food, Science, and Society, p 54. The Nutrition Foundation, 1969.

"Fourth of July picnic." Differences in sex, age, and level of sophistication may also be expressed through food likes and dislikes. A jellied fruit salad is considered feminine fare, whereas a steak-and-potatoes meal provokes thoughts of strength and manliness. Peanut butter sandwiches and hot dogs are thought to be the delight of children, whereas artichokes and lobster may be the choice of the sophisticated adult. Even the relationship between food intake and body weight is interpreted culturally. In some societies, overweight is considered natural and a sign of well-being, whereas in others, the slim, almost skeletonlike figure is held as desirable.

Religious beliefs frequently find expression in food customs. Fasting is common to many religions. Certain foods may be forbidden, such as pork to the Orthodox Jew and Moslem and beef to the Hindu. Closely akin to food habits related to religious beliefs are those associated with a life philosophy, such as the yoga diet or macrobiotics. Some people do not eat meat for philosophical reasons. Strong emotional factors are involved in the choice of these patterns.

The Hot – Cold Theory of Disease: An Example of Cultural Influence on Food Habits

An example of the effect of cultural beliefs on food habits is a type of folk medicine practiced among Latin American people known as the *hot – cold theory of disease.* Many Puerto Ricans living in the United States, especially elderly persons and recent immigrants, believe in this system of disease. Diseases are grouped into so-called hot and cold classes, and medications and foods are classified as hot, cold, or cool. Illnesses classified as cold (*frío*), such as arthritis and colds, are treated with hot medications and foods, whereas so-called hot (*caliente*) illnesses, such as rashes and ulcers, are treated with cool substances. The temperature of the food or medication is not necessarily related to its classification. For example, hot linden tea is considered a cool food, whereas cold beer, because of its alcohol content, is considered hot.

It is not difficult to imagine how these beliefs can conflict with medical advice. Puerto Rican mothers have been known to discontinue feeding formula, a hot food, in favor of cool foods such as whole milk or barley water when their infants develop rashes.

Your Personal Food Preferences

Everyone accepts certain foods and rejects others for different reasons. What are your feelings about food? Do peanut butter and jelly sandwiches give you a comfortable feeling when you are worried and anxious? Maybe they remind you of an earlier time when you felt more secure and life was less complicated. Is chocolate cake a favorite dessert, perhaps because you associate it with special family celebrations? Are peas on your "hate list" because you were forced to eat them when you were a child? Or perhaps you dislike lamb because your father wouldn't eat it and so your mother never served it.

If you have insight into your own food likes and dislikes, you will be less likely to impose your feelings on others. Moreover, you will have greater understanding and respect for preferences that differ from your own. If you are aware that you dislike lamb because it is unfamiliar to you, you are unlikely to make an unpleasant remark about the lamb being served on a client's tray. Similarly, you will be understanding of the client who uses olive oil to flavor his vegetables and the one who refuses his tray because it includes bacon. Every individual has had particular life experiences that have contributed to the formation of his food habits. This is as true for health workers as it is for the people they serve.

What the Client's Eating Behavior Tells You

By his responses to food, the client may be telling you that he is worried and afraid. He may feel insecure as his role changes from that of an independent adult to that of a person who is dependent on others in illness. He may express his feelings by being fussy about his food, by a lack of appetite, or by demands for extra attention. The hospitalized client may feel a greater need to hold onto favored foods that give him a feeling of comfort or security. He may make requests for custards and puddings or extra servings of milk, foods associated with infancy or childhood, periods of dependency and security. Some adults may refuse these same foods despite their nutritional value because they resent being dependent on others during illness and fear the loss of their independence. When under stress and in need of psychological reward, some persons eat too many sweets and desserts, foods that are frequently associated with rewards for "good behavior" in childhood. Others may express their discouragement through anorexia (lack of appetite). Providing for groups of clients to eat together in a dining room or in a solarium can help to stimulate the appetite. When anxieties are shared, problems may seem less threatening.

By his eating behavior, the client may indicate that he is dissatisfied because the hospital foods and meal patterns are so different from those to which he is accustomed. This is especially true for the client with strong cultural preferences. He may be telling us that his therapeutic diet depresses him because it is a reminder of the incurable nature of his disease. To be denied the pleasures of eating food with seasonings he likes and to keep reminding himself that he cannot have them is not easy to accept.

Health workers need to be aware of what food means to clients under different circumstances. The nurse who is aware of how her client communicates through food will be better able to help him. If changes in food habits are necessary for the client's health, these changes must respect his psychological as well as his physical needs. Food is more than nourishment for the body; it feeds the spirit as well.

KEYS TO PRACTICAL APPLICATION

What we eat does matter. Let your client know that you think good food habits are very important.

Develop an understanding of your own food habits. Why do you like some foods and dislike others?

Respect the food habits of your clients. Never display an aversion to their food preferences. Remember that these food habits hold meanings that are very important to them.

When your client is fussy, complains about food, rejects food, or overeats, try to understand what he is communicating by this behavior.

KEY IDEAS

The adverse effects of poor food habits are not immediate, but develop gradually.

Although malnutrition in the form of the classic vitamin deficiency diseases such as scurvy or beriberi is rarely seen in the United States, other less dramatic effects are widespread: growth retardation, weight loss, decreased resistance to infection, increased risk of chronic illness, depression, weakness, delayed recovery from disease, complications in newborn infants, impaired learning, and, possibly, impaired mental development.

Accurate diagnosis of nutritional problems requires that the professional use a variety of measurement techniques, including clinical examination, x-ray studies, laboratory data, and a diet history.

The meanings a person attaches to food reflect his values, beliefs, culture, and emotional state.

The health worker who understands the cultural influences that have helped to shape her own food habits will be more respectful of the food habits of her clients and more sensitive to the ways in which she and the client communicate to each other through food behaviors.

KEYS TO LEARNING: STUDY – DISCUSSION QUESTIONS

1. Discuss in class some of the nutrition problems you have observed within the community. What causes do you attribute to each of these problems?
2. Why are the effects of malnutrition, especially mild and moderate degrees of malnutrition, difficult to determine? Why is obesity considered a form of malnutrition?
3. What factors are involved in making an accurate evaluation of an individual's nutritional status?
4. Consider in class discussion the effects of the following factors on eating habits: ethnic background, religious background, anxiety, size of family, family income, hospitalization, living alone.
5. Record all the food you eat or drink for 3 days. Classify the major items (meat and meat substitutes, breadstuffs, vegetables, fruit, desserts, snack foods, beverages) into the following categories: favorite foods, foods you like, foods you tolerate, foods you do not eat (do not appear on your record).

   Try to determine why you feel as you do about each item listed. Take one item in each category and explain your feelings about that food.

Bibliography is found at the end of Part One.

3

Nutrition in the Health Care Setting

KEY TERMS

adaptive equipment Eating utensils and other commonly used items of daily living changed or adjusted in such a way as to accommodate a physical handicap.

emaciation Abnormal thinness, wasting of the flesh.

empathy The act of mentally putting oneself in the place of another person; sensitivity to the plight of another.

modified Changed from the normal to suit special needs; for example, a modified diet.

stomatitis Inflammation of the mouth.

Early in your educational program, you will have personal experience with hospital food service and the feeding of clients. This chapter has been purposely placed in the first section of the book to help prepare you for these experiences.

Your Role in the Client's Nutritional Care

Without an adequate supply of food, tissues break down. No body cell is immune to the effects of poor nutrition. Add to this the damaging effects of illness: the increased losses of energy and nutrients in the client with fever, the poor absorption of nutrients in the client with severe diarrhea, and the massive losses of fluids and nutrients in the client with extensive burns. Malnutrition prolongs illness and may even cause death. Unfortunately, more attention is frequently given to medication than to food.

The poor nutritional status of the severely underweight individual is apparent. However, it is often the apparently well-nourished client who is at high risk of developing malnutrition because his nutritional needs are overlooked. You hold a key position in maintaining and improving nutrition because you have frequent interaction with clients. Although you do not plan the diet and may not serve the tray, you may be responsible for knowing what the client eats and how he reacts to the food served him.

You may be the first person to become aware of circumstances that discourage the client from eating or of problems related to the client's understanding of his diet.

Poorly fitted dentures or a sore tongue or mouth may hinder the client's efforts to eat adequately. You may observe that food portions are too small for an adolescent boy or that a Mexican–American adult is eating little of the food served him. Conversely, you may note that a particular food is well taken by someone who generally eats poorly.

Creating a Pleasant Environment

In response to a client's questions, or as a means of encouraging him to eat, you might explain the reasons for his diet order and that the specific diet has been ordered by the physician.

You can do much to stimulate and maintain a client's appetite. Showing enthusiasm is an important factor. The person who understands his own feelings about food will make only positive remarks about the client's meal. Conversation will be cheerful and encouraging. The person who "wouldn't eat" or "wasn't hungry" may have needed the encouragement of a concerned, unhurried person. Some elderly clients may have to be made aware that it is mealtime. They may fall asleep while eating and have to be awakened and reminded to eat.

Mouth care before meals can improve the appetite of the anorexic patient. Good mouth care can help prevent stomatitis (ulcerative lesions in the mouth), which can seriously affect one's ability to eat. This condition may develop in persons receiving chemotherapy. Clients receiving tranquilizers may complain of a dry mouth. When feeding such a patient, offer sips of water before offering the food.

When the tray arrives, the client should be ready to receive it: his hands and face should have been washed, and he should be positioned at a comfortable angle. The extension table should be positioned over the bed and cleared. The meal can then be served and eaten as soon as it arrives. A tidy, well-ventilated room promotes a good appetite. The client should be screened from offensive sights.

Food Service

When a person is being cared for in the home or in a small residential or health care facility, the health worker may have some responsibilities for supervising the food service. Making the food attractive and appetizing is of the utmost importance. To the extent that the individual's diet permits, variety in the color, texture, flavor, and temperature of food adds interest and attractiveness to a meal. The use of colorful garnishes, favors for special occasions and holidays, and an occasional flower or item of interest to the client add that special touch that says someone cares.

Whether the client is served at a table or by tray, all items should be spotlessly clean: the table or tray cover, silverware, dishware, glassware, and tray card and holder. All dishware and glassware should be free of chips and cracks. Hot foods should be served hot and cold foods cold. Portions of food should be appropriate to the client's appetite. Nothing is more discouraging to a person with little appetite than to be confronted with a plate piled high with food.

If tray service is used, the tray should be large enough so that the items on it are not crowded together. The items should be placed conveniently so that they can be easily reached. Serving trays as promptly as possible will assure that the food is at its best.

Communication

Words are only one means of communication. We also communicate in nonverbal ways — by listening, by facial expressions, by our hurriedness or unhurriedness. A client frequently communicates through his reaction to the food served him. You can learn a good deal about your client's attitudes by observing his response to the food served him and by listening to what he says about it.

Any change in food service that may make the patient feel better or improve his food intake is worth trying. Sometimes you can accomplish these changes yourself. More frequently, you

must report your observations to the nursing supervisor, dietitian, or physician, depending on the circumstances.

Interpreting the Diet

You may often be the first person to become aware that the client is confused or worried about the diet prescribed for him. This situation may provide the opportunity for some informal teaching. Similarly, if the client has been given a selective menu, helping him choose items that are balanced in nutritional content and appropriate for his particular diet provides opportunity for education. You are not expected to know "all the answers" about nutrition; when asked a question you cannot answer, you should consult with the nurse in charge or the dietitian.

Assisting the Client

How much help a client will need depends on his ability to feed himself. Clients should be encouraged to feed themselves as much as possible, and most prefer to do so. Some may need assistance with cutting meat or buttering bread; others may need to be fed.

Feeding the Client

Some clients require total assistance. To feed someone successfully requires sensitivity to the feelings of the individual and an awareness of the importance of providing nourishment for someone who cannot do this for himself. Imagine that you are very weak, are depressed about your condition, and have little appetite and that you are being fed by someone who is hurried, distracted, and clearly bothered by the task.

How much food do you think you would consume? If you have empathy (*i.e.,* identify with the experiences of your client), you will be better able to provide understanding and support.

Before beginning to feed the client, position and support him so that he is comfortable and at an angle to promote easy swallowing. If it is permitted, have him in as nearly upright a position as possible. If he must stay in a prone or near-prone position, take care to prevent liquid or food from entering the trachea. A client who cannot be raised may be more comfortable lying on his side while he eats. Special positioning and feeding techniques are necessary for persons who cannot control movements of the jaw, lips, tongue, and swallowing owing to brain dysfunction.

A pleasant, unhurried manner will do much to stimulate the client's appetite. Assume a relaxed, comfortable position; sit, if possible, so that the client does not feel rushed. Ask him about his eating preferences: whether he likes to have his tea with the meal, the meat and potatoes together, and so on. Offer him small amounts of food at a time. A drinking tube, preferably a disposable one for sanitary reasons, is useful for persons who have difficulty drinking from a cup. Caution the client to take only small sips of warm liquids. If the client is permitted and able, suggest that he hold a slice of toast or roll or that he hold the drinking tube in the beverage while he sips it.

If the client cannot see, describe the food on the tray and indicate the position of each item. If the sightless client can feed himself, describe the face of a clock to indicate the position of food on the plate: for example, potatoes are at 12 o'clock, peas at 3 o'clock, and meat between 6 and 9 o'clock. If he needs to be fed, establish a method of signaling, such as moving his hand to indicate when he is ready for more food.

Some clients, such as those in traction or those who have a loss of hand or arm strength, may not need to be fed but do need some assistance. Buttering bread, cutting meat, opening milk and juice cartons and salad dressing containers, opening the shell of an egg, and placing food within reach are some things that may need to be done for these clients.

Handicapped Clients

You will encounter clients among all age groups who have physical handicaps that hamper their ability to obtain an adequate diet. Clients with such conditions as severe arthritis, Parkinson's disease, a stroke, or neuromuscular diseases such as cerebral palsy may have difficulty feeding themselves and/or may be unable to suck, chew, bite, or swallow normally.

The client should be evaluated on a regular basis to determine his nutritional needs and his physical abilities. As soon as possible, a self-feeding training program is begun to help the client do all he can for himself. Consultation with a physical therapist can provide useful information about techniques and equipment that are appropriate for the individual needs. Helping a handicapped person feed himself promotes self-esteem and helps prevent mental and physical deterioration.

A person who is being trained to feed himself needs much support and encouragement from the health team. In order to provide the necessary support and understanding, health care personnel must be sensitive to the client's feelings. He may feel frustrated by the difficulty he experiences in cutting food and opening car-

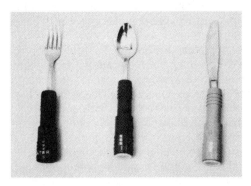

Built-up handled utensils

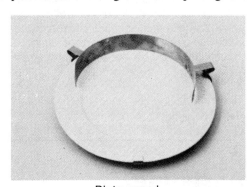

Plate guard

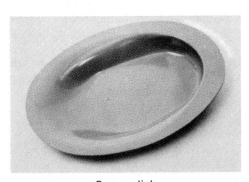

Scoop dish

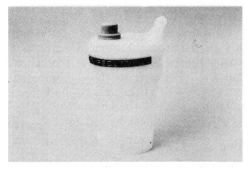

Covered plastic cup

Fig. 3-1.   Adaptive equipment used in self-feeding of the handicapped. (Hargrave M: Nutritional Care of the Physically Disabled. Minneapolis, Sister Kenny Institute, 1979) (*Continued on facing page*)

tons; embarrassed because his table manners may be unacceptable to others; too proud to ask for help; angry because of his handicaps; and isolated, especially if he is blind or deaf.

Techniques and Aids Useful in Self-Feeding. Certain techniques and equipment are beneficial in self-feeding programs. A handicapped client who cannot maintain head balance could inhale fluid or food into the lungs. To prevent this, he is positioned so that he is comfortable and stable. The use of a binder or strap at the pelvis may be helpful. Pillows and a headrest, as well as a footstool, may afford addi-

tional support. A high chair for a small child or a cutout table for an older child may provide the needed stability.

The parent of an infant having difficulty sucking is taught how to stimulate the mouth so as to encourage the sucking reflex. The infant may need to be tube-fed until he can obtain sufficient amounts of food on his own.

Neither food nor fluids can be given by mouth to the client who cannot swallow. He is fed by tube. This client should be continually evaluated to assess his ability to swallow before feeding by mouth can be started. The ability to swallow saliva is one indication of this. An ice

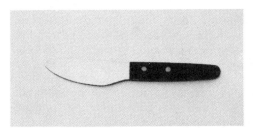

Rocker knife

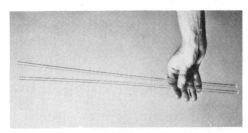

Long straw

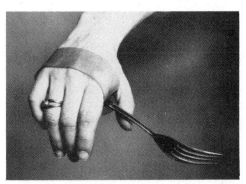

Universal cuff with utensil

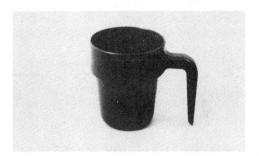

Quad-quip cup

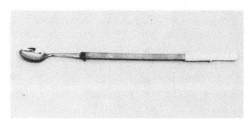

Long-handled utensils

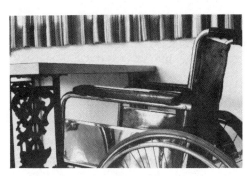

Elevated table

cube is sometimes rubbed on the skin over the throat to induce swallowing.

Physical Characteristics of Food. If the client has eating problems that involve the mouth or throat, the physical characteristics of the food —its consistency and texture—may assume great importance. Liquids are frequently very difficult to handle; soft or semisolid foods may be more easily managed. Liquids may be provided in the form of fruit ices or slush prepared by blenderizing concentrated fruit juice with ice. Some handicapped children can handle only a single texture or consistency at a time. The consistency, texture, shape, and size of the food should be suited to the needs of the individual.

Offering semisolid food in the form of finger food is useful in self-feeding programs for the elderly. Semisolids appear to be more acceptable than pureed food. It has been suggested, too, that children receiving pureed or ground food also be given the opportunity to see the foods in their customary form.

Very hard or brittle foods that do not soften quickly in the mouth should be avoided. Nuts, dry raisins, whole kernel corn and coconut are examples of such foods, which could be inhaled and cause choking.

Care must be taken to see that the client is receiving an adequate diet regardless of the consistency of the food. In an effort to provide foods of a suitable consistency, it is easy to overlook the nutritional balance of the diet.

Equipment. Adaptations in utensils can help the handicapped person eat independently. This special equipment, called *adaptive equipment,* can be purchased or can be made in the health facility or home. A long straw, a universal cuff holder, and a rocker knife are examples of equipment that require less strength than normal for self-feeding. Built-up handles make grasping easier. A plate guard, scoop dish, and covered plastic cup help the client whose coordination is poor (Fig. 3-1). A placemat, frame, or wet face cloth on which the plate can rest can turn a slick tabletop into a nonskid surface.

Bibs, which are sometimes used to protect the clothing, can cause embarrassment and

damage to the self-image of the client, as well as damage to the image the client presents to the staff and other clients. It is suggested that the vest-type of bib be used.

Hospital Food Service

The hospital food service department is responsible for providing the required diet for all clients. Meals for staff may also be a responsibility of the food service department. The chief administrative dietitian or food service manager directs the overall operation of the food service department. This includes supervision of menu planning and food purchase, preparation, and service.

Clinical dietitians are responsible for the nutritional care of clients. They work with the medical and nursing staffs to see that the nutritional needs of individual clients are met and that nutrition education is provided when necessary. Dietary technicians and diet aides or clerks assist the administrative and therapeutic dietitians. They may distribute and collect menus, serve trays, and keep records. The dietary technician may assist in taking diet histories and in teaching. The dietary staff also includes cooks, maids, porters, and receiving clerks.

The Diet Order

When the client is admitted to the hospital or other health care facility, a diet is prescribed to meet his individual needs. In most cases the physician prescribes the diet, but in some situations a nutrition specialist or a dietitian may do this. The orders may vary from "nothing by mouth" to "normal diet." The diet may be changed during the course of the client's hospital stay because of a change in his condition or because the diagnosis necessitates a modified

Breakfast SUNDAY	Luncheon SUNDAY	Dinner SUNDAY
FULL DIET	**FULL DIET**	**FULL DIET**
Mark X as large as possible in the box ☒ Portion Size: ☐ Small ☐ Regular ☐ Large	*Please No Substitutions* Portion Size: ☐ Small ☐ Regular ☐ Large	*Please Do Not Leave Menu on Tray* Portion Size: ☐ Small ☐ Regular ☐ Large
☐ ORANGE JUICE ☐ PEAR NECTAR ☐ FRESH BANANA ☐ HOMINY GRITS ☐ SPECIAL K ☐ CORN FLAKES ☐ SCRAMBLED EGG ☐ EGG OMELET w/Mushroom sauce ☐ SAUSAGE LINK	☐ CREAM OF MUSHROOM SOUP ☐ ROAST BEEF w/Gravy ☐ MANICOTTI ☐ BAKED POTATO ☐ SOUR CREAM ☐ BROCCOLI SPEARS ☐ CORN SOUFFLE ☐ TOSSED SALAD Italian or Blue Cheese Dressing ☐ GRAPEFRUIT SECTIONS ☐ CHEESE CAKE ☐ JELLO	☐ CRANBERRY JUICE ☐ SHAKE 'N BAKE CHICKEN ☐ HAMBURGER ON ROLL Mustard-Catsup-Relish ☐ RICE FIESTA ☐ PEAS & CARROTS ☐ CAULIFLOWER ☐ LETTUCE & TOMATO SALAD Italian Dressing or Mayonnaise ☐ APRICOT HALVES ☐ GERMAN CHOCOLATE CAKE ☐ VANILLA PUDDING

	Breakfast			Luncheon			Dinner	
☐ SUGAR ☐ SUGAR SUB. ☐ SALT ☐ PEPPER	☐ HARD ROLL ☐ WHITE BREAD ☐ WHOLE WHEAT ☐ RYE BREAD	☐ COFFEE BLACK ☐ DECAF COFFEE ☐ HOT CHOC. ☐ TEA	☐ SUGAR ☐ SUGAR SUB. ☐ SALT ☐ PEPPER	☐ HARD ROLL ☐ WHITE BREAD ☐ WHOLE WHEAT ☐ RYE BREAD	☐ COFFEE BLACK ☐ DECAF COFFEE ☐ HOT CHOC. ☐ TEA	☐ SUGAR ☐ SUGAR SUB. ☐ SALT ☐ PEPPER	☐ HARD ROLL ☐ WHITE BREAD ☐ WHOLE WHEAT ☐ RYE BREAD	☐ COFFEE BLACK ☐ DECAF COFFEE ☐ HOT CHOC. ☐ TEA
☐ MILK ☐ SKIM MILK ☐ CREAM	☐ MARGARINE ☐ JELLY	☐ ICE TEA ☐ LEMON	☐ MILK ☐ SKIM MILK ☐ CREAM	☐ MARGARINE ☐ JELLY	☐ ICE TEA ☐ LEMON	☐ MILK ☐ SKIM MILK ☐ CREAM	☐ MARGARINE ☐ JELLY	☐ ICE TEA ☐ LEMON
NAME_____ ROOM_____			NAME_____ ROOM_____			NAME_____ ROOM_____		
DIET_____			DIET_____			DIET_____		

Fig. 3-2. Selective hospital menu for one day. (Courtesy Mercer Medical Center, Trenton, New Jersey)

Table 3-1. Routine Hospital Diets

	Regular Diet	Light or Soft Diet	Pureed Soft Diet	Full Liquid Diet	Clear Liquid Diet
Beverages	All	All	Milk and milk drinks, carbonated beverages, coffee, tea, decaffeinated coffee, cereal beverages, fruit drinks	Same as pureed soft diet	Ginger ale, tea, coffee, cereal beverages, fruit-flavored drinks (some strained fruit juices may be permitted)
Breads	All	Enriched white and refined whole wheat or rye breads, saltine and graham crackers	Enriched white bread or toast, saltine and graham crackers	None	None
Cereals	All	Refined cooked and prepared cereals	Refined cooked cereals (cornmeal, farina, rice) and oatmeal, refined prepared, cereals such as corn or rice flakes and puffed rice	Cooked refined cereals or cereal gruel	None
Desserts	All	Plain cakes (iced sparingly if desired), plain cookies, plain puddings, custard, smooth ice cream and sherbet, gelatin desserts, fruit whips	Same as light diet	Custard, gelatin desserts, rennet desserts, smooth ice cream, sherbet, pudding, popsicles	Clear flavored gelatin, popsicles
Eggs	All	All except fried	Same as light diet	Custard, egg-nog*	None
Fats	All	Butter, margarine, cream, vegetable shortening and oils, bland salad dressings, white sauce	Same as light diet	Butter, margarine, cream, vegetable oils	None
Fruit, Fruit juices	All	All fruit juices, cooked or canned fruits (without seeds, skins, coarse fiber), ripe banana, orange and grapefruit sections, peeled ripe peach or pear	All fruit juices, ripe banana, puree of cooked or canned fruits	All fruit juices, puree of cooked or canned fruit	Strained fruit juices (apple, grape, orange, cranberry, cranapple). Fruit juices sometimes omitted

* A pasteurized commercial egg-nog preparation or pasteurized dried egg powder should be used rather than fresh raw eggs. The danger of *Salmonella* infection, a type of food poisoning, exists when raw egg is used.

Table 3-1. *(continued)*

Regular Diet	Light or Soft Diet	Pureed Soft Diet	Full Liquid Diet	Clear Liquid Diet
Meat, Fish, Poultry, Cheese				
All	Tender beef, lamb, veal, liver, lean pork, chicken, turkey, fish, seafood (prepared any way except highly seasoned, fried, or pickled), cottage cheese, cream cheese, mild cheddar or processed cheese	Pureed or finely ground beef, lamb, veal, lean pork, chicken, turkey, and fish served in broth or cream sauce; cottage cheese, cream cheese, mild cheddar or processed cheese	Mild cheese sauce, pureed meat added to broth or cream soup	None
Potato or Substitutes				
All	White and sweet potatoes, hominy, rice, spaghetti, macaroni, noodles	Mashed or well-cooked white potato, mashed sweet potato, hominy, rice, spaghetti, macaroni, noodles (if client able to masticate)	Mashed potato in cream soup	None
Soups				
All	Broth-based and cream soups made from foods allowed	Broth soups and cream soups made with pureed foods	Consommé, broth, bouillon, strained cream soup made from foods allowed	Clear broth, consommé
Sugar, Sweets				
All	Sugar syrup, honey, clear jelly, fruit butters, plain sugar or chocolate candy in moderation	Same as light diet (except no chocolate)	Honey, sugar, syrup, clear sugar candy	Sugar, honey, syrup, clear sugar candy
Vegetables, Vegetable Juices				
All	All vegetable juices, raw lettuce, cooked or canned tender vegetables, including asparagus tips, beets, carrots, green and wax beans, eggplant, mushrooms, peas, pumpkin, spinach, squash, tomatoes, pureed lima beans, and corn	All vegetable juices, puree of the following cooked vegetables: asparagus, beets, green and wax beans, carrots, corn, lima beans, peas, pumpkin, spinach, squash, tomatoes	All vegetable juices, pureed vegetables in cream soup	None

(After Dietary Department Staff, University of Iowa Hospitals and Clinics: Recent Advances in Therapeutic Diets. Ames, Iowa State University Press, 1979)

diet. Modified diets (also called *therapeutic diets*) are diets that have a specific purpose in the treatment of symptoms or disease conditions.

Open communication between the dietary and nursing departments is absolutely essential to successful food service. Neither can provide for the nutritional needs of the client without the help of the other. The nurse communicates to the dietitian the special needs of the patient. The dietitian plans meals around the permitted foods and sees that they are served. The two share responsibility for helping the client achieve a positive attitude toward his diet and for educating him in dietary matters.

The Diet Manual

Diet plans are compiled in the diet manual. They specify the kinds and frequently the amounts of food that will be served when a particular diet is ordered. This avoids misunderstandings by physician, nurse, or dietitian. A copy of the diet manual is usually available at the nurses' station. The diets are described in technical terms and are intended for use by the health care team. They usually are not appropriate for distribution to clients. Materials used in diet counseling are adapted from diets in the manual and are adjusted to the needs and preferences of clients. Diet manuals often differ. You should become familiar with the diets served in the hospital where you work.

Selective Menus

Most hospitals offer a daily menu from which a patient can make selections (Fig. 3-2). Two or more items are offered for each course. For example, for dinner there may be a choice of roast pork or salisbury steak, mashed or baked potatoes, and tossed green salad or Waldorf salad. Sometimes the client on a therapeutic diet is also offered a selective menu. The client indicates his selections on the printed menu the day before the meal. Some clients need assistance in making choices, and some may need help marking their menus.

Selective menus have considerably improved the acceptance of foods in hospitals and other health care institutions. The client can choose, and in most cases his food preferences are accommodated. Where selective menus are not used, allowance should be made for food preferences. Even minor choices such as whether to have tea, coffee, or cocoa with a meal or jelly and butter or margarine with toast can do much to make a meal more enjoyable.

Selective menus are effective in client teaching. For example, if the client repeatedly selects a less-than-adequate diet, he needs assistance. He needs information on how to make proper selections from the menu. If the selective menu is the basis of a modified diet, the client needs instruction to make appropriate choices for his diet. His selections can serve as a test of his understanding of the diet and as an aid in follow-up instruction.

Routine Hospital Diets

The diets served in most hospitals are usually classified into two categories: routine hospital diets and modified (or therapeutic) diets. The routine hospital diets consist of the normal, soft, full liquid, and clear liquid diets (Tables 3-1 and 3-2). Some hospitals may offer a light diet, a step between the soft and regular diets.

The diabetic diet, reducing diet, and restricted fat diet are classified as modified or therapeutic diets. This classification is somewhat misleading for two reasons. First, all diets, whether normal or modified, are important in therapy from the standpoint of healing and recovery. Second, the routine soft and liquid diets also qualify as modified diets, differing mainly in texture and consistency from the normal diet.

Because most hospitalized persons are placed on routine hospital diets, a knowledge of these diets would be useful to you at this point. However, to understand nutritional needs during illness, you need first to understand normal nutrition. After you have studied normal nutrition, reference again will be made to this chapter.

Table 3-2. Typical Menus for Routine Hospital Diets

Regular	Light or Soft Diet	Pureed Soft Diet	Full Liquid Diet
Breakfast			
Orange	Orange sections	Orange juice	Orange juice
Oatmeal with milk or cream	Oatmeal with milk or cream	Oatmeal with milk or cream	Strained oatmeal gruel with cream
Soft-cooked egg	Soft-cooked egg	Soft-cooked egg	Eggnog
Whole-wheat toast	Refined whole-wheat toast	Refined white toast	Coffee with cream and sugar
Butter	Butter	Butter	10:00 a.m.: Applesauce
Milk	Milk	Milk	
Coffee with cream and sugar	Coffee with cream and sugar	Coffee with cream and sugar	
Dinner			
Vegetable soup	Vegetable soup	Strained vegetable soup	Cream of potato soup
Roast beef sirloin	Roast beef sirloin	Ground beef sirloin	Tomato juice
Mashed potato	Mashed potato	Mashed potato	Pureed peaches
Buttered peas	Buttered peas	Pureed peas	Vanilla ice cream
Tomato salad with French dressing	Tomato juice	Tomato juice	Milk
Whole-wheat bread	Refined rye bread	White bread	3:00 P.M.: Malted milk or flavored yogurt
Butter	Butter	Butter	
Butter pecan ice cream	Vanilla ice cream	Vanilla ice cream	
Milk	Milk	Milk	
Supper			
Creamed chicken on biscuit	Creamed chicken on rice	Creamed ground chicken on rice	Grape juice
Buttered carrots	Buttered carrots	Buttered pureed carrots	Cream of chicken soup
Head of lettuce salad with French dressing	Shredded lettuce salad with French dressing	White bread	Pureed cherries
Whole wheat bread	Refined whole-wheat bread	Butter	Chocolate milk shake
Butter	Butter	Pureed cherries	9:00 P.M.: Hot cocoa
Canned cherries	Canned cherries	Angel food cake	
Angel food cake	Angel food cake	Milk	
Milk	Milk	Tea with sugar and cream	
Tea with cream and sugar	Tea with cream and sugar		

Routine hospital diets are as follows:

Regular (full or general diet)

Normal, adequate diet

All foods permitted; pastries, fried foods, and spices in moderation

Soft (light diet)

Offered during the recovery phase to clients who cannot tolerate highly seasoned, fried, or raw foods

Omits fried, highly spiced, high-fiber foods and raw fruits and vegetables

Pureed soft

Offered to clients who have undergone surgery or have swallowing difficulties, gastrointestinal conditions, or extreme weakness

Very soft diet consisting of ground or pureed meats, pureed fruits and vegetables, and soft desserts

Omits spicy, gas-forming, and fried foods

Dental soft

For dental problems that give rise to difficulty in chewing or when facial muscles should not be used, as after eye surgery

Includes all easily chewed foods: ground meats, tender fruits and vegetables, finely chopped raw fruits and vegetables; all seasonings and methods of preparation are permitted

Full liquid

For persons who are acutely ill with infection or gastrointestinal disturbances or who are weak and whose strength must be conserved

Consists of foods that are liquid at room temperature, such as milk, soup, ice cream, gelatin, refined cooked cereals, or strained cooked cereal gruels; egg in soft custard or egg-nog (made with pasteurized powdered egg, not raw egg, to avoid the possibility of *Salmonella* infection, a type of food poisoning)

Clear liquid

Offered following surgery

Includes only broth, tea, black coffee, flavored gelatin, ginger ale; some strained fruit juices may be permitted; no milk or milk products are permitted

See Table 3-1 for a summary of foods included in routine hospital diets and Table 3-2 for typical menus.

KEYS TO PRACTICAL APPLICATION

Be aware of what each one of your clients eats and how he reacts to the food served.

When a client eats poorly, try to find out why, and communicate your findings to the nurse in charge.

Be positive. Show enthusiasm for the food served; be cheerful and encouraging at mealtime.

Have the client ready for his meal when the tray arrives: hands and face washed; mouth care provided, if necessary; client positioned properly; and room environment made conducive to a good appetite.

Remember that your attentiveness, facial expressions, and hurriedness or unhurriedness convey, as much as words do, how much you care.

Circulate among your clients at mealtime; they frequently need help cutting meat and opening milk and juice cartons and condiment containers.

When you feed a client, let him know that you consider this an important assignment worthy of your time.

Be sensitive to the feelings of frustration, embarrassment, anger, dependence, and isolation that a handicapped client with feeding problems is likely to feel.

Use adaptive equipment, if available, or make your own, to help the handicapped person feed himself.

Be aware that the nutritional needs of clients can be met only when good communication exists between the nursing and dietary departments.

KEY IDEAS

Attending to the nutritional needs of the client deserves high priority.

The nurse holds a key position in meeting the nutritional needs of clients. Her responsibilities include creating an environment conducive to good appetite, promoting good communication with the client and with the health team, and assisting in nutrition education.

Providing for the nutritional care of clients requires teamwork; good communication among the various members of the health team is essential.

Feeding situations that involve helplessness or handicapping conditions require a special sensitivity and empathy for the feelings the client is likely to experience and an awareness of the importance of providing adequate nourishment for him.

Positioning techniques, changes in the texture and consistency of food, and adaptive equipment are useful in feeding the handicapped.

Hospital diets fall into two general categories: routine hospital diets and modified diets. The routine hospital diets include the regular, soft, full liquid, and clear liquid diets; the modified diets include such diets as the diabetic, fat-restricted, and reducing diets.

KEYS TO LEARNING: STUDY–DISCUSSION QUESTIONS

1. The appetite of a client is affected not only by his physical condition but also by what he hears, sees, smells, and tastes. What can the nurse do to provide an environment that promotes a good appetite?

2. Close your eyes and imagine that you are helpless and are about to be fed by a member of the nursing staff. How do you think you would feel about having to be fed? What would you expect of the person feeding you?

    Imagine that you are recovering from a stroke and being trained to feed yourself. What feelings would you be likely to experience?

3. Examine the diet manual used in your hospital. Where in the clinical areas is the manual usually kept? Compare the routine hospital diets in this manual with those listed in Table 3-1. What are the differences, if any? With the help of your instructor, discuss possible reasons for these differences.

4. Discuss in class the importance of good communication between the nursing staff and dietary staff. Who suffers as a result of poor communication?

5. What adaptive equipment useful in self-feeding of the handicapped is available in your hospital? Make a display of this equipment and explain the usefulness of each item.

Bibliography is found at the end of Part One.

Bibliography

Chapter 1. Nutrition and Health: Current Concerns

Books and Pamphlets

Aziz, S: The world food situation today and in the year 2000. Proceedings of the World Food Council of 1976, Ames, Iowa State University Press, 1977

Blue Cross Association: Help Yourself. Chicago, Blue Cross Association, 1978

Frankle RT, Owen AY: Nutrition in the Community. St. Louis, CV Mosby, 1978

Lowenberg ME, Todhunter EN, Savage JR, Lubowski IL: Food and People. New York, John Wiley & Sons, 1979

Mayer J, Dwyer JT, Dowd K, Mayer L: Food and Nutrition Policy in a Changing World. New York, Oxford University Press, 1979

New York Times Staff: Give Us This Day. New York, Arno Press, 1975

Periodicals

Connor WE: Too much or too little—The case for preventive nutrition. Am J Clin Nutr 32:1975, 1979

Cunningham RM: Keeping them well is good business, too. Hospitals 53:19:94, 1979

Etzwiler DD: Teaching allied health professionals about self-management. Diabetes Care 3:121, 1980

Green LW: How to evaluate health promotion. Hospitals 53:19:106, 1979

Harper AE: Science and the consumer. J Nutr Ed 11:171, 1979

Hegsted DM: Nationwide food consumption survey—Implications. Family Economics Review U.S. Department of Agriculture, Spring, 1980

Jonas S: Hospitals adopt new role. Hospitals 53:19:84, 1979

McGinnis JM: Prevention—Today's dietary challenges. J Am Diet Assoc 77:129, 1980

Tolpin HG: Economics of health care. J Am Diet Assoc 76:217, 1980

Vickery DM: Is it a change for the better. Hospitals 53:19:87, 1979

Zafferblatt SM, Wilbur CS, Pinsky JL: Understanding food habits. J Am Diet Assoc 76:9, 1980

Chapter 2. Assessing Nutritional Needs

Books and Pamphlets

Butterworth CE, Weinsier RL: Malnutrition in hospital patients: Assessment and treatment. In Modern Nutrition In Health and Disease. Goodhart RS, Shils MS (eds): Philadelphia, Lea & Febiger, 1980

Fomon SJ: Nutritional Disorders of Children—Prevention, Screening, and Follow-Up. DHEW Publication No. (HSA) 77-5104, 1977

Food and Nutrition Board, National Academy of Sciences: The Relationship of Nutrition to Brain Development and Behavior. Washington, DC, National Research Council, June, 1973

Hargrave M: Nutritional Care of the Physically Disabled. Minneapolis, Sister Kenny Institute, 1979

Hodges RE: Nutrition in Medical Practice. Philadelphia, WB Saunders, 1980

Mason M, Wenberg BG, Welsch PK: The Dynamics of Clinical Dietetics. New York, John Wiley & Sons, 1977

Niehoff, A: Food, Science, and Society. New York, The Nutrition Foundation, Inc., 1969.

Seventh Report of the Director, National Heart, Lung and Blood Institute, National Institute of Health. Washington, DC NIH Publication No 80-1672, November, 1979

Suitor CW, Hunter MT: Nutrition: Principles and Application in Health Promotion, 2nd ed. Philadelphia, JB Lippincott, 1984

Wilson ED, Fisher KH, Garcia PA: Principles of Nutrition. New York, John Wiley & Sons, 1979

Woodburn JM, Fitch MM: Feeding Programs and the Handicapped Child. Published by the authors, 1978

Periodicals

Baird PC, Schutz HG: Life-style correlates of dietary and biochemical measures of nutrition. J Am Diet Assoc 76:228, 1980

Bushman L, Russell R, Warfield L et al: Malnutrition among patients in an acute-care veterans facility. J Am Diet Assoc 77:462, 1980

Crane NT, Green NR: Food habits and food preferences of Vietnamese refugees living in northern Florida. J Am Diet Assoc 76:591, 1980

Day ML, Lentner MJ: Food acceptance patterns of Spanish-speaking New Mexicans. J Nutr Ed 10:3:121, 1978

Foley C, Hertzler AA, Anderson HL: Attitudes and food habits—A review. J Am Diet Assoc 75:13, 1979

Gambert SR, Guansing AR: Protein–calorie malnutrition in the elderly. J Am Geriatr Soc, 28:272, 1980

Harfouche JK: "Psycho-social aspects of breast feeding, including bonding. Food and Nutrition Bulletin 2:2, 1980

Harwood A: The hot–cold theory of disease—Implications for treatment of Puerto Rican patients. JAMA 216:1153, 1971

Raeburn JA, Kondl M, Lau D: Social determinants in food selection. J Am Diet Assoc 74:637, 1979

Salmond SW: How to assess the nutritional status of acutely ill patients. Am J Nurs 80:922, 1980

Willard MD, Gilsdorf RB, Price RA: Protein–calorie malnutrition in a community hospital. JAMA 243:1720, 1980

Chapter 3. Nutrition in the Health Care Setting

Books and Pamphlets

Anderson L, Turkki P, Mitchell H et al: Nutrition in Health and Disease, 17th ed. Phhiladelphia, JB Lippincott, 1982

Dietary Department Staff of the University of Iowa Hospitals and Clinics: Recent Advances in Therapeutic Diets. Ames, Iowa State University Press, 1979

Hargrave M: Nutritional Care of the Physically Disabled. Minneapolis, Sister Kenny Institute, 1979

Howard RB, Herbold NH: Nutrition In Clinical Care. New York, McGraw-Hill, 1978

Mason M, Wenberg BG, Welsch PK: The Dynamics of Clinical Dietetics. New York, John Wiley & Sons, 1977

Woodburn JM, Fitch MM: Feeding Programs and the Handicapped Child. Bothell, WA, Woodburn & Fitch, 1978

Periodicals

Allaire B: Staff skills in patient/family relations grow. Hospitals 53:22:92, 1979

Howard J: Dehumanization in health care. Am J Nurs 80:719, 1980

Salmond SW: How to assess nutritional status of acutely ill patients. Am J Nursing 80:922, 1980

Zimmerman BN: Human question vs. human hurry. Am J Nurs 80:719, 1980

Part Two

The Role of Nutrients in the Maintenance of Normal Health

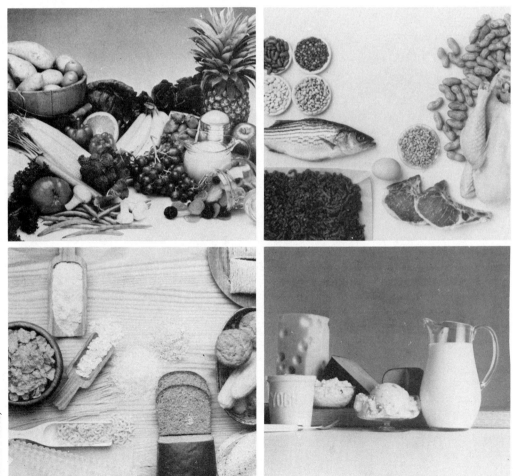

(USDA Photos)

Food and Its Functions

KEY TERMS

catalyst A substance that causes or speeds up a chemical change without being changed itself.

enzyme A substance, usually a protein, that is formed in living cells and brings about chemical changes. The enzyme itself remains unchanged.

extracellular Outside the cell.

intracelluar Inside the cell.

kilocalorie (kcal) The unit of heat that measures the energy values of food or the energy needs of the body; represents the amount of heat required to raise the temperature of 1 kilogram (kg) of water 1°C.

Although there are more than 50 known nutrients, all are easily classified into six categories as follows: carbohydrates, proteins, fats, vitamins, minerals, and water. Fiber also plays a role in the diet. However, it is not considered a nutrient because it is not absorbed by the bloodstream.

Most foods contain more than one nutrient group. Milk, for example, contains water, protein, carbohydrate, fat, the mineral calcium, and the vitamins A, riboflavin, thiamine, and niacin. However, foods are usually identified by the amount of protein, carbohydrate, or fat they contain. A food that contains more protein than fat or carbohydrate is known as a protein food. For example, fish is a protein food; in contrast, bacon is considered a fat food, although it contains some protein. This classificiation is useful, yet there are many exceptions. Peanut butter is usually classified as a protein food; however, it contains significant amounts of fat and carbohydrate as well as protein. Beef is usually considered a protein food; however, some fatty cuts of beef, such as the steak or rib portion, may contain more fat than protein.

For the cells to be nourished, food eaten must be changed to a form they can use. This is done by the digestive system. Once food has been reduced to its simplest form, it passes through the intestinal tract into the blood and lymph. By means of the circulatory system, the nutrients finally reach the extracellular fluid — the fluid outside each individual cell. From this extracellular fluid, the cell selects the nutrients it needs.

The waste products that result from cellular activity are released into the extracellular fluid and enter the bloodstream to be excreted from the body, primarily through the lungs and kidneys.

Functions of Nutrients

The nutrients perform three basic functions. Each class of nutrients is involved in one or more functions as follows: Building and maintaining body tissue (water, proteins, fats, carbohydrates, mineral elements); Furnishing energy (carbohydrates, fats, proteins); Regulating body processes (water, vitamins, mineral elements, proteins, fats, carbohydrates).

Building and Maintaining Tissue

Water makes up one half to two thirds of the weight of an adult. It is an essential part of every cell and is the basic substance of blood, lymph, and body secretions. All body cells require protein. Fat rounds the body contours and provides protective padding and support for vital organs. Calcium and phosphorus are deposited in bones and teeth. Various minerals are found in body tissues. Carbohydrate occurs in only small amounts. Even when the body has reached its final growth, there is continual exchange of material composing the cells.

Furnishing Energy

Carbohydrates, fats, and protein are used by the body as fuel. Providing energy is a main function of carbohydrates and fats. Protein provides energy when carbohydrates and fats do not meet the body's energy needs.

The energy value of food or the energy needs of the body are measured in units called *calories.* Calories are a measure of the amount of heat produced by ingested food. The large calorie, or kilocalorie (kcal), is the amount of heat required to raise 1 kg (1000 g) of water 1°C. The small calorie is the unit of energy used in chemistry and physics. It is one thousandth of a large calorie. The calorie used in nutrition always represents the large calorie.

The body requires energy for its ongoing activities. These include not only such obvious activities as breathing and walking but also the infinite number of "hidden" tasks carried on by the trillions of body cells.

Regulating Body Processes

The cell has been aptly described as a chemical factory. The chemicals the cell produces are called *enzymes.* An enzyme is a protein that directs the activities of the cell. Enzymes are catalysts, that is, they cause chemical reactions to occur but do not themselves change.

Vitamins combine with specific proteins to form enzymes. Minerals are also involved in the production of enzymes.

In addition to enzymes, the body produces other substances that act as regulators. For example, in the blood is an iron-containing substance, hemoglobin, that transports oxygen to the cells.

Water is an important regulator, for all chemical reactions in the body take place in its presence. Also, as the basic ingredient of body fluids, water permits nutrients to be digested, absorbed, and circulated to the cells, and it provides for the elimination of waste products. Water also regulates body temperature.

Cellular Nutrition

Each cell, such as a blood cell or a nerve cell, has its own work or specific activity to do. Each cell also has its specific nutritional needs; the nutrient needs of one type of cell differ from those of another. Adequate nutrition of all the cells is the final goal, for the health of the cells determines the health of the tissues, which in turn determines the health of the organs and systems of the body.

Nutrients Work Together

Like the cells, the nutrients each have their own special part to play. However, they cannot function independently. The functions of the nutrients are related one to the other in a very complex fashion. Any changes in the consumption of one nutrient may lead to changes in the activity of others. For example, the absorption of calcium depends upon the supply of vitamin D. Calcium, in turn, is needed for the absorption of vitamin B_{12}.

Nutrient Storage

Some nutrients can be stored in the body. This reserve supply is called upon when food intake is low, as in illness, or when need is increased, as in pregnancy. Excessive amounts of nutrients that cannot be stored are excreted, principally in the urine.

The ability to store certain nutrients is not always an advantage. Obesity can result from excessive caloric intake; harmful effects may also result when there is too much of certain vitamins and minerals. Toxic (poisonous) effects have resulted from excessive intake of vitamins A and D in the form of vitamin supplements. As in the case of vitamins, excessive intake of minerals is usually due not to the food itself but to minerals that contaminate the food supply. For example, in the past, copper poisoning developed from deteriorating copper tubing through which sodas and other fountain drinks were served.

How Deficiency Diseases Develop

Inadequate intake of nutrients does not produce immediate, dramatic effects. At first, the body goes through a period of exhausting its reserves. This time varies from a few hours in the case of proteins to as much as 7 years for calcium. During this period of depletion, the body attempts to cope with the deficiency. Eventually, the individual cells become depleted of the nutrient, and the symptoms of deficiency disease become evident. Such diseases as scurvy, beriberi, pellegra, and simple goiter are deficiency diseases.

Nutrient Standards

U.S. Recommended Daily Dietary Allowances

How much of each nutrient is required by the body is the subject of intensive and continual study. In the United States, standards of nutrition are set by the Committee on Dietary Allowances appointed by the Food and Nutrition Board of the National Research Council. The committee recommends for all age levels the amounts of nutrients that will keep the normal population well nourished. The committee recommendations are published in a table, Recommended Daily Dietary Allowances (RDA); (Table 4-1). This table is revised periodically to reflect new information.

The RDA is a guide, not a requirement. Individuals differ in their precise nutritional requirements. To take into account these differences among normal persons, the RDA provides a "margin of safety." That is, they set the allowances high enough to cover the needs of most healthy persons. They provide not only for individual differences but also for some storage of nutrients as a means of protection during periods of stress.

U.S. Dietary Goals

Another set of dietary recommendations, the U.S. Dietary Goals, was published in 1977 by the Select Committee on Nutrition and Human Needs of the United States Senate. The goals were issued because many nutritionists and physicians expressed concern about American eating habits. They felt that these habits were promoting the potential for various chronic diseases.

Table 4-1. Food and Nutrition Board, National Academy of Sciences – National Research Council Recommended Daily Dietary Allowances,* Revised 1980 Designed for the maintenance of good nutrition of practically all healthy people in the U.S.A.

	Age (years)	Weight (kg)	Weight (lb)	Height (cm)	Height (in)	Protein (g)	Fat-Soluble Vitamins Vitamin A (μg RE)†	Fat-Soluble Vitamins Vitamin D (μg)‡	Fat-Soluble Vitamins Vitamin E (mg α-TE)§
Infants	0.0–0.5	6	13	60	24	kg × 2.2	420	10	3
	0.5–1.0	9	20	71	28	kg × 2.0	400	10	4
Children	1–3	13	29	90	35	23	400	10	5
	4–6	20	44	112	44	30	500	10	6
	7–10	28	62	132	52	34	700	10	7
Males	11–14	45	99	157	62	45	1000	10	8
	15–18	66	145	176	69	56	1000	10	10
	19–22	70	154	177	70	56	1000	7.5	10
	23–50	70	154	178	70	56	1000	5	10
	51+	70	154	178	70	56	1000	5	10
Females	11–14	46	101	157	62	46	800	10	8
	15–18	55	120	163	64	46	800	10	8
	19–22	55	120	163	64	44	800	7.5	8
	23–50	55	120	163	64	44	800	5	8
	51+	55	120	163	64	44	800	5	8
Pregnant						+30	+200	+5	+2
Lactating						+20	+400	+5	+3

(Recommended Dietary Allowances. Washington, DC, National Academy of Sciences, 1980)

* The allowances are intended to provide for individual variations among most normal persons as they live in the United States under usual environmental stresses. Diets should be based on a variety of common foods in order to provide other nutrients for which human requirements have been less well defined.

† Retinol equivalents. 1 retinol equivalent = 1 μg retinol or 6 μg β carotene. See text for calculation of vitamin A activity of diets as retinol equivalents.

‡ As cholecalciferol. 10 μg cholecalciferol = 400 IU of vitamin D.

§ α-tocopherol equivalents. 1 mg d-α tocopherol = 1 α-TE. See text for variation in allowances and calculation of vitamin E activity of the diet as α-tocopherol equivalents.

Water-Soluble Vitamins							Minerals					
Vita-min C (mg)	Thia-min (mg)	Ribo-flavin (mg)	Niacin (mg NE)‖	Vita-min B-6 (mg)	Fola-cin* (μg)	Vitamin B-12 (μg)	Cal-cium (mg)	Phos-phorus (mg)	Mag-nesium (mg)	Iron (mg)	Zinc (mg)	Iodine (μg)
35	0.3	0.4	6	0.3	30	0.5**	360	240	50	10	3	40
35	0.5	0.6	8	0.6	45	1.5	540	360	70	15	5	50
45	0.7	0.8	9	0.9	100	2.0	800	800	150	15	10	70
45	0.9	1.0	11	1.3	200	2.5	800	800	200	10	10	90
45	1.2	1.4	16	1.6	300	3.0	800	800	250	10	10	120
50	1.4	1.6	18	1.8	400	3.0	1200	1200	350	18	15	150
60	1.4	1.7	18	2.0	400	3.0	1200	1200	400	18	15	150
60	1.5	1.7	19	2.2	400	3.0	800	800	350	10	15	150
60	1.4	1.6	18	2.2	400	3.0	800	800	350	10	15	150
60	1.2	1.4	16	2.2	400	3.0	800	800	350	10	15	150
50	1.1	1.3	15	1.8	400	3.0	1200	1200	300	18	15	150
60	1.1	1.3	14	2.0	400	3.0	1200	1200	300	18	15	150
60	1.1	1.3	14	2.0	400	3.0	800	800	300	18	15	150
60	1.0	1.2	13	2.0	400	3.0	800	800	300	18	15	150
60	1.0	1.2	13	2.0	400	3.0	800	800	300	10	15	150
+20	+0.4	+0.3	+2	+0.6	+400	+1.0	+400	+400	+150	††	+5	+25
+40	+0.5	+0.5	+5	+0.5	+100	+1.0	+400	+400	+150	††	+10	+50

‖ 1 NE (niacin equivalent) is equal to 1 mg of niacin or 60 mg of dietary tryptophan.

* The folacin allowances refer to dietary sources as determined by *Lactobacillus casei* assay after treatment with enzymes (conjugases) to make polyglutamyl forms of the vitamin available to the test oganism.

** The recommended dietary allowance for vitamin B$_{12}$ in infants is based on average concentration of the vitamin in human milk. The allowances after weaning are based on energy intake (as recommended by the American Academy of Pediatrics) and consideration of other factors, such as intestinal absorption.

†† The increased requirement during pregnancy cannot be met by the iron content of habitual American diets nor by the existing iron stores of many women; therefore the use of 30–60 mg of supplemental iron is recommended. Iron needs during lactation are not substantially different from those of nonpregnant women, but continued supplementation of the mother for 2–3 months after parturition is advisable in order to replenish stores depleted by pregnancy.

The U.S. Dietary Goals recommend that Americans avoid excessive calorie intake; reduce consumption of refined and processed sugars, fats, cholesterol, and salt; and increase consumption of starches and "naturally occurring" sugars (fruits, vegetables). Many authorities support these dietary goals, whereas others believe there is not enough evidence linking diet to chronic diseases.

The U.S. Dietary Goals are listed in Chapter 13. We will refer to them as we discuss the various nutrients and food groups mentioned in the "goals."

Tables of Food Composition

Tables of food composition list various foods and indicate the nutrient content of each. You need to understand the nutritional composition of foods so you can determine the following: the nutritional value of one food compared with another; the nutritional value of a particular diet for comparison with a standard such as the RDA; what foods must be included in, limited in, or omitted from diets to meet specific needs such as high protein, restricted sodium, or high iron.

The values given in a table of food composition are approximate, not exact. They represent the average value of a number of samples of the food analyzed in a laboratory. Many factors, such as the climate in which the foodstuff was grown, the method of processing, and the method of preparation, have a bearing on nutritional value. For this reason, the nutritive values given for a particular food may differ in various tables. However, such differences are usually slight. (See the Appendix for a table of food composition.)

In the study of nutrition, as in other sciences, the metric system of weights and measures is used instead of the customary pounds and quarts. The United States is currently the only industrialized nation in the world not using the metric system. However, American children are learning the metric system in school.

KEYS TO PRACTICAL APPLICATION

Don't expect the effects of poor eating habits to be felt immediately, but be assured that prolonged poor eating habits will take their toll.

Be suspicious when any foods are promoted as miracle foods.

Be cautious about the use of vitamin and mineral supplements; changes in the intake of one nutrient affect the functioning of other nutrients, and excess amounts of some nutrients can be toxic.

KEY IDEAS

Nutrients, chemical substances in food needed by the body, are classified into the following categories: carbohydrates, proteins, fats, vitamins, minerals, water.

Nutrients provide for growth and maintenance of the body, furnish energy, and regulate body processes.

Adequate nourishment of the body as a whole is dependent upon adequate nutrition of the cell, the basic unit of life.

The functions of the various nutrients are interrelated; changes in the consumption of one nutrient leads to changes in the activities of others.

Some nutrients can be stored, providing a reserve supply but also presenting the danger of toxic effects due to excessive intake.

Deficiency diseases develop slowly. The body first attempts to adjust to a

reduced supply of the involved nutrient(s), and eventually symptoms of disease appear.

The Recommended Dietary Allowances (RDA) represent the opinion of an expert committee as to the amounts of energy and nutrients that will keep the population of the United States well nourished.

The U.S. Dietary Goals aim to correct food habits that, in the opinion of some authorities, are exposing Americans to the risk of certain chronic diseases.

KEYS TO LEARNING: STUDY – DISCUSSION QUESTIONS

1. Discuss in class the meaning of "interrelationships of nutrients" and "storage of nutrients." In light of these explanations, what is your opinion of the practice of taking vitamin, mineral, and other nutrient supplements without a physician's advice?

2. What are the advantages of recommending the consumption of nutrients in quantities that provide a "margin of safety"?

Bibliography is found at the end of Part Two.

Digestion and Absorption

KEY TERMS

absorption The transfer of nutrients from the intestinal tract to the bloodstream.

amylase An enzyme that digests carbohydrate.

chyme The semifluid mass formed by the mixing and partial digestion of food in the stomach.

digestion The chemical breakdown of complex nutrient molecules to a form that can be utilized by the cells. This is accomplished mainly through the action of enzymes found in digestive fluids.

emulsification The production of a liquid substance in which small globules of one liquid such as a fat are dispersed evenly throughout a second liquid.

epithelium The tissue that forms the outer part of the skin and lines the blood vessels and the passages that lead to the outside of the body.

hydrolysis A chemical reaction in which a large molecule is split up into simpler compounds by the addition of water.

lamina propria The connective tissue in the villus that is supplied with blood and lymph vessels.

lipase An enzyme that digests fat.

metabolism The total of all the chemical and biological processes that take place in the body.

mucus A fluid with a slippery consistency that is secreted by mucous membranes and glands; lubricates and protects the gastrointestinal mucosa.

peristalsis Rhythmic muscular contractions of the gastrointestinal tract that break food up into smaller particles, mix these particles with digestive fluids, and move the food along the intestinal tract.

protease An enzyme that digests protein.

pylorus The opening of the stomach into the duodenum.

pyloric sphincter A ringlike muscular valve located between the stomach and the small intestine; determines the length of time food stays in the stomach.

villus A fingerlike projection of the mucosa that lines the small intestine and is supplied with blood and lymph vessels. The epithelial cells of each villus have tiny rodlike projections that form what is called the *brush border*.

To be used by the body cells, nutrients must first be digested, that is, broken down into molecules. Once food is digested, the nutrients move from the digestive tract into the bloodstream in a process called *absorption*. The absorbed nutrients are then transported by the blood, lymph, and tissue fluids to the cells. The cells use the nutrients for energy or for the production of body tissue and regulatory compounds, such as enzymes, hormones, and body fluids.

Digestion

It is obvious that the functioning of the gastrointestinal tract has an important influence on nutritional status. The following review of digestion is therefore necessary to the study of nutrition.

The Digestive Tract

The digestive tract is a long, unbroken muscular tube passing through the body beginning at the mouth and ending at the anus (Fig. 5-1). The tract consists of two holding or receiving areas connected by a tube (the small intestine) designed to provide close contact between the food in the tract and the circulatory system. The first of the holding areas (the stomach) receives the ingested food, and the other (the large intestine) collects the indigestible waste. Strong rings of muscle, called *sphincters,* separate one segment of the tube from another. These sphincters (valves) prevent food from passing too rapidly through the digestive tract. They also prevent regurgitation (back-up). The function of each part of the tract is dependent upon and interrelated with the functions of the other parts.

Peristalsis, the muscular activity of the digestive tract, moves the food along. Two sets of muscles control this activity. One set is circular and squeezes inward; the second set consists of muscle fibers that run the length of the tract. These two sets alternately contract and relax, creating a wavelike movement. In the stomach, a third set of muscles churns the food, reducing it to small particles and mixing it thoroughly with digestive secretions. These muscular actions are controlled by a network of nerves within the gastrointestinal wall extending from the esophagus to the anus.

The tract is lined with a mucous membrane that produces secretions. The characteristics of the mucous membrane as well as its secretions vary: the mucous lining of the stomach differs from that of the small intestine, which in turn differs from that of the esophagus and that of the large intestine. Other organs that are essential to digestion, called *accessory organs,* include the liver, the pancreas, and the gallbladder.

The digestive tract also protects the body from harmful substances that may be ingested along with food. These include parasites, bacteria, viruses, and chemical poisons. Many of these potentially harmful substances pass through the gastrointestinal tract without entering the bloodstream. They are then excreted in the feces.

The Digestive Process

Most of the protein, fat, and carbohydrate in food occurs in a form that cannot be absorbed in its original state. Within the digestive tract, the nutrients are broken down into their basic forms as follows:

$$\text{Carbohydrate} \xrightarrow{\text{is reduced to}} \text{simple sugars: glucose, fructose, and galactose}$$

$$\text{Protein} \xrightarrow{\text{is reduced to}} \text{amino acids}$$

$$\text{Fat} \xrightarrow{\text{is reduced to}} \text{fatty acids and glycerol}$$

Some vitamins must also be broken down before they can be absorbed.

Digestion is accomplished by simultaneous mechanical and chemical means. The muscular movement of the gastrointestinal tract prepares the food for chemical digestion by breaking it into small particles (increasing the surface area) and mixing these particles with digestive fluids. Emulsification, (the suspension of one substance in another) prepares fats and fatlike materials for chemical breakdown. This occurs in the small intestine through the action of bile salts. The bile coats the tiny fat particles and prevents them from coming together and forming larger particles. In this way, the surface area of the fat is increased so that the digestive fluids have greater access to the fat molecules. Bile salts are produced by the liver and released in the bile.

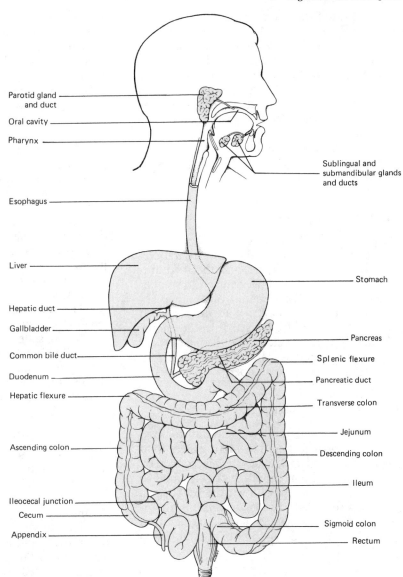

Fig. 5-1. Digestive tract. (Chaffee EE, Lytle IM: Basic Physiology and Anatomy, 4th ed. Philadelphia, JB Lippincott, 1980)

The chemical breakdown of carbohydrates, proteins, and fats to their basic forms involves the process of hydrolysis. Hydrolysis is the addition of water to each molecule resulting in the splitting of the molecule into simpler compounds. In the case of very large molecules, hundreds of much smaller molecules are formed. In contrast, simple sugars such as fructose require no digestion at all.

The hydrolysis, or chemical breakdown, of nutrients is accomplished largely by the action of enzymes in digestive fluids. The enzymes are specific in their activity; for example, pepsin acts only on protein, and ptyalin acts only on starch. The enzymes involved in the digestive process are named for the substances upon which they act. For example, lipase is an enzyme that digests lipids (fats), and protease is an enzyme that digests protein. The ending *-ase* signifies *enzyme*.

Hormones are also involved in gastrointestinal activity. The mucous membranes of the

tract produce these chemical substances, which travel through the bloodstream and stimulate target glands and organs to release their secretions. The hormones are produced in the presence of specific substances; for example, the entrance of fats into the duodenum stimulates the secretion of cholecystokinin, a hormone that causes the gallbladder to contract and release bile.

Water dilutes the nutrients, which in turn promote the activity of digestive enzymes. It also promotes peristalsis.

Stages of Digestion

Digestion normally occurs in stages. Large molecules are broken down to medium-sized molecules by a specific enzyme, and the medium-sized molecules are in turn reduced to smaller molecules through the action of another enzyme. Any food materials that are not absorbed are moved onward by peristalsis to the end of the tube and are excreted. Fiber is one of these indigestible materials. Humans lack enzymes capable of breaking down fiber.

Digestion in the Mouth

Chewing aids digestion by breaking up food into smaller particles and by mixing these food particles with saliva. Saliva, which is secreted by salivary glands in the mouth, lubricates food so that it may readily pass down the esophagus. Ptyalin, also called *salivary amylase,* is an enzyme occurring in saliva. It begins the digestion of starch, breaking down some of the starches to sugars.

Digestion in the Stomach

From the esophagus, food enters the stomach, where it is temporarily stored. The digestion of carbohydrate begun in the mouth continues until the food mass mixes with hydrochloric acid.

Gastric secretions contain primarily hydrochloric acid, pepsin, and mucus. Because of the presence of hydrochloric acid, the stomach contents are highly acidic. The hydrochloric acid has several very important functions: it activates the enzyme pepsin, it prepares the protein molecule for partial digestion by pepsin, it destroys harmful bacteria, and it makes certain minerals such as iron and calcium more soluble.

Pepsin, a gastric protease, or enzyme, partially digests protein, reducing the large protein molecules to smaller molecules. (In infants and children, the enzyme rennin coagulates milk protein, making it more readily acted upon by pepsin. This enzyme is not produced in adults.) Some digestion of fats occurs as a result of the action of lipase, a fat-digesting enzyme in the stomach.

Mucus, a thick, slippery substance, protects the lining of the stomach (gastric epithelium) from being eaten away by its own digestive juices. Mucus counteracts these strong acids and forms a protective covering on the gastric epithelium.

The churning action of the stomach mixes the food with digestive juices and reduces it to a semiliquid state known as *chyme.* Peristalsis moves the chyme toward the pylorus (the opening of the stomach into the small intestine). The chyme is then gradually released into the duodenum through the pyloric sphincter.

Digestion in the Small Intestine

The small intestine, so named because of its diameter, is the longest part of the digestive tract, about 20 feet in length. It consists of three parts: the duodenum, the jejunum, and the ileum.

The duodenum receives the chyme from the stomach and mixes it with intestinal juices. The digestive fluids in the small intestine consist of bile secreted by the liver, pancreatic juice secreted by the pancreas, and intestinal juice produced by the walls of the intestine. Large quantities of mucus are secreted in the intestine to protect the intestinal lining and to lubricate the moving food mass. These fluids, which are alkaline (basic), serve to neutralize the acidity of chyme as it comes from the stomach. Most of the digestion of food takes place in the small intestine. For this reason, a person who has had all or part of his stomach surgically removed is able to survive quite well.

Carbohydrate digestion, which begins in

the mouth, is completed in the small intestine through the action of enzymes secreted by the pancreas and the intestinal mucosa. Pancreatic amylase (amylopsin) splits the remaining starch to sugar. Three enzymes in the intestinal juice —sucrase, lactase, and maltase—act on the sugars, reducing them to simple sugars, or monosaccharides, the simplest form of carbohydrate.

Protein digestion, begun in the stomach, is completed in the small intestine through the action of the enzyme trypsin in pancreatic juice and a group of enzymes known as *peptidases* in the intestinal juice. Trypsin breaks down proteins to smaller molecules. The peptidases reduce these molecules to amino acids, the form in which proteins enter the bloodstream.

Fat digestion occurs for the most part in the small intestine. Bile and a pancreatic enzyme are responsible for the digestion of fats. Liver cells continually secrete bile, which is formed from cholesterol. The bile collects in the gall-

bladder and is stored there until fatty foods enter the small intestine. When this occurs, a hormone stimulates the gallbladder to release a quantity of bile, which then flows through the bile duct to the small intestine. Bile is an emulsifier. It breaks the fat up into smaller particles so that they can be readily acted upon by enzymes.

When the gallbladder is surgically removed, there is no longer a storage place for bile. Instead, bile is continually secreted in small amounts directly into the small intestine, regardless of whether fatty foods are present. When large amounts of fat are eaten, there may not be enough bile in the intestinal tract to emulsify the fat. The fat globules tend to cluster together, and consequently the digestive enzymes take longer than normal to do their job. For this reason, some persons who have had their gallbladder removed experience discomfort after eating a high-fat meal.

The lipase called *steapsin*, which is secreted

Table 5-1. Summary of Chemical Changes in Digestion

Place of Action	Juices and Glands	Enzymes	Results of Enzyme Activity
Mouth	Saliva from salivary glands	Ptylin (salivary amylase)	Begins starch digestion
Stomach*	Gastric juice from stomach wall	Pepsin (protease)	Begins protein digestion
		Renin (protease)	Curdles milk protein
		Lipase	Breaks down emulsified fats to fatty acid and glycerol
Small intestine†	Pancreatic juice from the pancreas	Trypsin (protease)	Reduces protein to smaller molecules
		Steapsin (lipase)	Breaks down fats to fatty acids and glycerol
		Amylopsin (amylase)	Reduces starch to sugar
	Intestinal juice from the small intestine	Peptidases (proteases)	Completely breaks down protein to amino acids
		Sucrase } Maltase } Lactase }	Reduce sugars to simplest form

* Hydrochloric acid in the gastric juice softens the connective tissue of meat and activates the enzyme pepsin.
† Bile, produced by the liver, reduces fat to tiny globules so that the pancreatic lipase can more readily act upon it.

in pancreatic juice, completes the digestion of fats. Through the action of this pancreatic enzyme, fats are reduced to fatty acids and glycerol and then absorbed.

In this way, through the process of digestion, proteins, fats, and carbohydrates are reduced to their simplest forms (Table 5-1). Once reduced to these smallest forms—amino acids, fatty acids, and monosaccharides—the nutrients can be absorbed and utilized.

The time required for food material to pass through the intestine varies with the rate of peristaltic movements. Toxic materials, irritating substances, including some laxatives, and emotional stress can cause hypermotility, or abnormally rapid peristalsis. This results in diarrhea and causes the digestion and absorption of nutrients to be greatly reduced.

Absorption

Absorption is the transfer of nutrients from the gastrointestinal tract into the blood and lymph vessels. Limited amounts of water, alcohol, mineral salts, and glucose are absorbed through the lining of the stomach. However, most absorption occurs in the small intestine, with most absorptive activity occurring in the lower part of the duodenum and the first part of the jejunum. Disease conditions may seriously hinder the absorption of some nutrients. Problems may result from the lack of certain digestive enzymes or from defects in the intestinal mucosa. Celiac disease, lactose intolerance, and cystic fibrosis are examples of such disease.

The anatomy of the small intestine is uniquely suited to promoting absorption. The inner lining or mucosa of the small intestine is gathered into folds. Millions of fingerlike projections, called *villi,* cover the mucosa. The epithelial cells of the villi have a brush border consisting of thousands of tiny rodlets, or microvilli. The surface area provided by these combined structures is tremendous, estimated at 3000 square feet.

Although the villi are extremely small (0.04 inch long), each villus has a complex structure (Fig. 5-2). Beneath the epithelium of each villus is a layer of connective tissue, the lamina propria, that is supplied with small arteries and veins connected by capillaries. The villus is also supplied with lymphatic capillaries called *lacteals.*

Nutrients are transported across the epithelium into the lamina propria, where they enter the blood and lymph vessels. Some fatty acids and other fat-soluble substances, such as cholesterol and fat-soluble vitamins, are absorbed into the lacteals. They are then transported by the lymph vessels to the thoracic duct, which empties into the subclavian vein. Monosaccharides, amino acids, glycerol, mineral salts, water-soluble vitamins, and some fatty acids enter the blood capillaries and are carried to the liver by the portal vein.

Extent of Absorption

In healthy persons, practically all digested carbohydrate, protein, and fat is absorbed. Some minerals such as sodium, potassium, and iodine are also absorbed to a high degree.

Absorption of some other minerals is less complete. A well-nourished adult absorbs only about 10% of the iron, 20% to 30% of the zinc, and about 40% of the calcium ingested. Higher amounts of iron and calcium are absorbed if body stores are low or if there is greater need than normal, as in pregnancy. The mechanisms in the small intestine that regulate absorption protect the body, since excessive amounts of these minerals can be toxic.

The amount of minerals absorbed is also influenced by the form in which the minerals occur and by the presence of other substances. Iron found in flesh foods is absorbed more readily than iron from plant food. The presence of vitamin C improves the absorption of iron, whereas the presence of vitamin D increases the absorption of calcium.

Some nutrients form insoluble compounds with other substances in food. Minerals bound in these insoluble compounds are not absorbed even when body stores are low. The calcium in

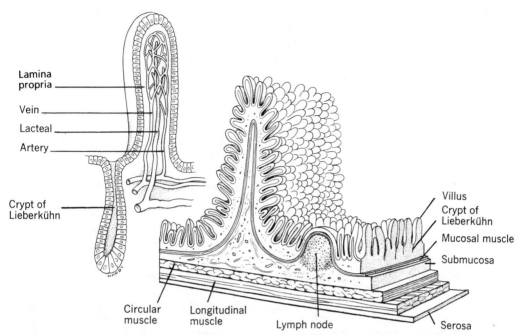

Lamina propria
Vein
Lacteal
Artery
Crypt of Lieberkühn
Villus
Crypt of Lieberkühn
Mucosal muscle
Submucosa
Circular muscle
Longitudinal muscle
Lymph node
Serosa

Fig. 5-2. Diagram of the mucous membrane of the small intestine showing numerous villi on one circular fold. At *left* is an enlarged drawing of a single villus. (Chaffee EE, Lytle IM: Basic Physiology and Anatomy, 4th ed. Philadelphia, JB Lippincott, 1980)

spinach, for example, is not absorbed, because it forms an insoluble compound with oxalate, a substance also present in spinach.

Excretion of Waste

The Large Intestine

Whatever remains of food after digestion and absorption have taken place is excreted via the large intestine. The mucous lining contains no villi, and no enzymes are secreted. The large intestine, which is 4 to 5 feet long, consists of three parts: the cecum, which receives undigested material from the small intestine; the colon, which removes most of the water content from the undigested material; and the rectum,

which temporarily stores the solid waste material, called *fecal matter,* until it is excreted.

The main function of the large intestine is to remove water from waste material and change it to a semisolid state. The feces consist of water, fiber from food, unabsorbed minerals, bacteria, mucus and other intestinal secretions, and dead cells shed by the inner lining of the gastrointestinal tract.

Digestive Disturbances

Disturbances of the gastrointestinal tract are extremely common. Hundreds of millions of dollars are spent each year on self-prescribed

medications such as antacids and laxatives. More important than this monetary loss, however, is the harm that can result from the frequent use of these self-prescribed digestive aids. Because these medications can temporarily relieve the symptoms of underlying disease, some of which may be serious, a person using them may delay seeking medical treatment. Minor disorders of the gastrointestinal tract can produce the same symptoms as serious conditions. The health worker's knowledge of the process of digestion can be a vital tool in conveying scientifically sound information.

In many cases, digestive disturbances are due to conditions that hinder the digestive process. These include poor mental and emotional states, overeating, eating of high-fat meals, insufficient chewing of food, and eating when overly tired. Respect for the factors that promote the best conditions for digestive function can do much to relieve digestive problems. Some circumstances that may help and some that may hinder digestion are described below.

Psychological Factors

Emotional stress is the primary cause of disturbances in digestive function. Fear, worry, anger, nervous fatigue, and emotional excitement can adversely affect digestive process, especially in the stomach. These stresses give rise to changes in the flow of digestive juices and in the muscular activity of the tract. Some emotions may cause hypermotility, abnormally increased movement of the tract with increased secretion of digestive juices. Others may cause hypomotility, depressed or abnormally slow movement of the digestive tract. A person's emotional state may inhibit mucus secretions in the duodenum. Such inhibition is believed to be a factor in the development of duodenal ulcers.

A lack of appetite frequently accompanies a depressed emotional state. A person may be so certain that various foods will disagree with him that his apprehension actually causes discomfort after he eats these foods.

A peaceful environment, cheerful companionship, and attractively served food all promote good digestion. The dinner table is not the place for controversy or scolding. In a hospital setting, mealtimes are not appropriate for unpleasant procedures, sights, smells, or sounds.

"Indigestion"

Pain or discomfort in the abdominal region or chest is often referred to as *indigestion* or *poor digestion*. This discomfort is usually not caused by foods that are hard to digest but by emotional factors or other conditions that adversely affect digestion.

The typical American diet is almost completely digested: 98% of the carbohydrates, 95% of the fat, and 92% of the proteins are digested. The digestion of carbohydrate is reduced to about 85% in diets that contain large amounts of the indigestible fiber found in fruits, vegetables, and whole-grain cereals, such as vegetarian diets.

However, some foods are more slowly digested than others, remaining in the stomach longer. This slowing of the digestive process may be caused by the nature of the food itself, the size of the meal, the way it is cooked, or the manner in which it is eaten. We frequently think that foods that are digested slowly are those that are hard to digest.

Foods that are gulped and not chewed properly can slow the digestive process and cause distress. Large lumps of food require more churning action by the stomach and more time for the hydrochloric acid and enzymes to do their work. Foods that by nature are more slowly digested than others are more satisfying because they delay the emptying of the stomach and have greater "staying" power. Such foods are said to have a high satiety value. Carbohydrate foods leave the stomach first, followed by protein and then fat. Fats and foods rich in fat, especially mixtures of protein and fat, such as meat, milk, and eggs, have a high satiety value. It is no wonder that a person who eats a breakfast of juice, toast, and coffee is hungry by mid-morning. The addition of an egg or a glassful of milk will improve the satiety value of this breakfast. Foods containing excessive amounts

of fat, especially fried foods, may cause digestive discomfort because of the long time required to digest them.

Under normal conditions, the body can digest almost any food or combinations of food without any trouble. True allergic reactions to foods do exist but are relatively rare. Foods that can be eaten separately should not cause discomfort when eaten together. This applies to the eating of seafood in the same meal with milk products and to other widely held taboos. However, if a person always avoids certain foods to prevent discomfort, he may be masking the symptoms of a serious disorder.

Gastric Acidity

The stomach is normally acidic. As we have seen, this strongly acidic environment has important functions in the digestive process. Psychological factors can stimulate the flow of gastric juice. However, the presence of food in the stomach stimulates acid gastric secretion more than anything else. Meat and meat extracts (found in meat soups and gravies), alcohol, caffeine, and substances other than caffeine in both regular and decaffeinated coffee have an especially stimulating effect on acid secretion.

Although the presence of acid in the stomach is normal and essential to proper digestion, some people produce more acid than others and tend to be susceptible to the development of ulcers. Sometimes digestive disturbances are caused by abnormally low amounts of stomach acid, which may indicate serious illness. A person suffering from such a digestive disturbance may mistake the condition for excess acidity and take antacid medications. The regular use of antacids sold over the counter is a dangerous practice. These self-prescribed medications can mask the symptoms of serious illness and delay treatment. Also, the excessive use of antacids can upset the acid–base balance in the body.

Constipation

Constipation may be caused by dehydration or intestinal disease. Uncomplicated constipation (not due to disease) is frequently a result of eating and health habits. One of the most common causes of constipation is failure to respond to the defecation reflex. Another major cause is a lack of muscle tone, characterized by inadequate muscular movements along the digestive tract. A lack of exercise and a low intake of fibrous foods contribute to this lack of tone. Frequently, the affected person resorts to the use of self-prescribed laxatives. The intestine then becomes dependent upon this artificial stimulation, and a vicious cycle results.

Medication

Some medications are irritating to the lining of the stomach and can cause discomfort if not taken with food. Among them are iron preparations, potassium, chloride, levadopa, and analgesics.

KEYS TO PRACTICAL APPLICATION

Prevent digestive disturbances by encouraging your client to

- Create as pleasant an atmosphere as possible at mealtime
- Chew food well; eat slowly
- Avoid excessive amounts of fat in a meal, especially in the form of fried food
- Eat small to moderate amounts of food at one time; large meals take longer to digest.

Advise persons who repeatedly experience digestive discomfort to see a physician.
Discourage the regular use of self-prescribed antacids; these medications can mask the symptoms of serious illness and thereby delay treatment.

KEY IDEAS

The functioning of the gastrointestinal tract greatly influences nutritional status.

The digestive tract reduces the size of nutrient particles to a form that can be absorbed and protects the body from harmful substances ingested with food.

The rhythmic muscular movements of the gastrointestinal tract and the emulsification of fats through the action of bile salts prepare food for chemical digestion, which occurs mainly by the action of enzymes.

The stomach is normally acidic; hydrochloric acid secreted in gastric juice activates pepsin, prepares protein for partial digestion by pepsin, increases the solubility of certain minerals, and destroys harmful bacteria.

Digestion occurs in stages; the chemical breakdown of nutrients and absorption take place mostly in the small intestine.

Hydrolysis results in the splitting of the nutrient molecule into simpler compounds.

The process of digestion reduces proteins to amino acids, carbohydrates to simple sugars, and fats to fatty acids and glycerol.

Almost all digested protein, fat, and carbohydrate is absorbed. The degree of absorption of some minerals is less complete, being dependent upon body stores, need, form in which the nutrient occurs, and the presence of other substances.

Whatever remains of food after digestion and absorption have taken place is excreted from the body via the large intestine; the main function of the large intestine is to remove water from waste material.

Fats and proteins are more slowly digested than carbohydrates and thus tend to delay hunger.

Poor mental and emotional states, overeating, high-fat meals, improperly chewed food, and eating when overly tired hinder the digestive process and may cause digestive disturbances.

KEYS TO LEARNING: STUDY–DISCUSSION QUESTIONS

1. What are the mechanical aspects of digestion? The chemical aspects?
2. Discuss the effects of psychological factors on the functioning of the digestive tract. What evidence do you see of these effects among your clients?
3. What are some of the common causes of gastric distress or so-called indigestion? Why is the repeated use of nonprescribed remedies a dangerous practice?
4. What is meant by the *satiety value* of food? What foods have a high satiety value? What are some of the other factors that influence the speed with which foods are digested?

Bibliography is found at the end of Part Two.

6

Energy Metabolism

adenosine triphosphate (ATP)   A high-energy compound involved in the transfer of energy within the cell.

aerobic   Requiring oxygen.

anabolism   That phase of metabolism in which new molecules are synthesized; more complex substances are made from simpler ones.

anemia   A decrease in the number of red blood cells, or hemoglobin.

basal metabolism   The amount of energy required to carry on the vital processes when the body is at rest.

basal metabolic rate (BMR)   Expression of the number of kilocalories used hourly in relation to the surface area of the body.

caloric density   The number of kilocalories in a unit of weight of a specific food.

catabolism   The chemical breakdown of more complex substances in living cells to simpler compounds with the release of energy.

coenzyme   A substance, such as a vitamin, required for the activation of some enzymes.

energy metabolism   All the chemical changes that result in the release of energy in the body.

hemoglobin   The oxygen-carrying red pigment in blood cells.

hyperthyroidism   Excessive secretion of the thyroid gland increasing the basal metabolic rate.

hypothyroidism   Deficiency of thyroid secretion resulting in a lowered basal metabolic rate.

metabolism   The total of all the chemical and biological processes that take place in the body.

nutrient density   The nutritional content of a food in relation to its caloric value; usually determined in terms of specific nutrients.

oxidation   The chemical process by which a substance combines with oxygen.

ratio   A numerical or quantitative comparison of two things.

synthesis   The process of building up; the formation of complex substances from simpler ones.

thermic effect of food   The increase in metabolism caused by the digestion, absorption, and transport of nutrients to the cells.

Metabolism is a general term that refers to all the processes by which the body cells use nu-trients to support life. These processes involve chemical changes that occur in nutrients after

they have been absorbed from the digestive tract. Metabolism has two parts: synthesis (building), and breakdown of nutrients. Synthesis involves the conversion of simple compounds into more complex molecules. This process, by which the body forms new tissue, is called *anabolism*. The breakdown of nutrients involves the reconversion of complex molecules into simpler ones. This process is called *catabolism*. The production of energy is a catabolic, or breakdown, process. Because the formation of new compounds requires energy, both catabolic and anabolic processes take place at the same time.

Anabolism and catabolism occur continuously and are normally in balance. During periods of rapid tissue growth, such as in childhood, pregnancy, and convalescence, anabolism exceeds catabolism. Some catabolic processes occur as a result of disease, injury, immobility, or aging and are not beneficial. Under these conditions, catabolism exceeds anabolism.

Energy metabolism refers to chemical changes that result in the release of energy. The light energy of the sun is converted to chemical energy in the form of carbohydrate, fat, and protein in food. The body has the ability to transform food energy from one form to another. The chemical energy of food can be converted to such forms as mechanical, electrical, and heat energy and to other forms of chemical energy in the body.

Converting Food to Energy

Carbohydrates, proteins, and fats are the nutrients that provide energy. Alcohol (ethanol), which is derived from glucose, also yields energy. Vitamins, minerals, and water do not supply energy.

Carbohydrates and fats are the body's preferred source of energy. When more protein is consumed than is needed by the body, the excess is also converted to energy. When protein intake is low, the use of body protein for tissue building and repair takes priority, provided that enough energy is available from other sources.

Oxidation

Oxygen is required for the release of the energy available in the fuel-producing nutrients, just as it is required for the complete burning of substances outside the body. The chemical process in which a substance combines with oxygen is called *oxidation*. Oxidation is also called an *aerobic* (oxygen-requiring) *process*.

The process by which energy is released within the cell involves many steps. The oxidation of proteins, fats, and carbohydrates is slow and controlled, each step requiring the assistance of a specific enzyme. Many enzymes require other substances called *coenzymes*. The coenzymes involved in energy metabolism are composed in part of the B vitamins. The vitamin thiamine, for example, is needed for the formation of a coenzyme involved in one of the steps in carbohydrate metabolism. Other nutrients, such as minerals, also act as coenzymes. Various hormones play important roles in energy metabolism. Insulin, a hormone secreted by the islets of Langerhans in the pancreas, must be present for glucose to enter the cell.

The energy that results from the oxidation of nutrients is converted to heat, which maintains body temperature, or it is temporarily held by a high-energy phosphorus-containing compound called *adenosine triphosphate* (ATP). This substance provides energy for all the work performed by the cell. Some is converted to mechanical energy needed by muscle tissue, some to electrical energy involved in the transmission of nerve impulses, and some to chemical energy needed for the synthesis of new compounds.

Normal hemoglobin levels are necessary for the efficient use of body fuel, because hemoglobin supplies oxygen to the cells. It is no surprise that persons suffering from low hemoglobin levels (anemia) become very tired with physical effort.

Disposal of End-Products of Energy Metabolism

Oxidation of the fuel-producing nutrients results in heat and other forms of energy, water, and carbon dioxide. The carbon dioxide is carried to the lungs, where it is exhaled. The water, called *metabolic water,* can be used by the body just like the water obtained from food and beverages. That portion of water that is not needed is excreted by the kidneys in the urine. Some water may also be lost in expired air or through the skin. Nitrogen, which results from the breakdown of amino acids, is synthesized into urea in the liver and is excreted by the kidneys in the urine.

Measuring Energy Production

Heat is a measure of energy produced. In nutrition, energy is measured in kilocalories (kcal). The kilocalorie represents the amount of heat required to raise 1 kg (1000 g) of water 1°C. The abbreviation *kcal* is used throughout this book.

Measuring Energy Values of Foods

How do we know how much energy a food contains? The energy value of individual foods is determined through the burning of a weighed portion of food in a bomb calorimeter. This thoroughly insulated apparatus contains a chamber in which the food is burned. The amount of heat (or kilocalories) produced by the burning of a specific food is determined by the change in the temperature of a measured amount of water that surrounds the chamber.

Approximate energy values have been established for the three fuel-producing nutrients as follows: carbohydrate, 4 kcal/g; protein, 4 kcal/g; and fat, 9 kcal/g. Alcohol (ethanol), produced from the fermentation of glucose, provides 7 kcal/g. In excessive amounts, alcohol is toxic to the body.

Because the energy value of a particular food depends upon the amount of protein, fat, and carbohydrate it contains, energy value can be estimated if the composition of the food is known. For example, a ½-cup portion of baked macaroni and cheese contains 8 g of protein, 11 g of fat, and 20 g of carbohydrate. From this information, with the fuel values given above, its approximate energy value is determined as follows:

Protein	$8 \text{ g} \times 4 =$	32
Fat	$11 \text{ g} \times 9 =$	99
Carbohydrate	$20 \text{ g} \times 4 =$	80
		211 kcal

Measuring Energy Used

How do we know how much energy the body uses? The amount of energy produced by the body can be measured directly or indirectly. In the direct method, a person is placed in an insulated heat-sensitive chamber and the heat given off by his body measured. This method is expensive, however, and used only in scientific research.

In the indirect method, a respiration apparatus is used. The amount either of oxygen consumed by the person or of carbon dioxide exhaled in a given number of minutes is recorded. From this information, the number of kilocalories produced by the body can be calculated.

Factors Influencing Energy Needs

Total energy needs are based on three factors: basal metabolism, voluntary physical activity, and the thermic effect of food.

Basal Metabolism

Basal metabolism is the energy required to carry on vital body processes at rest. These include all the activities of the cells and glands, skeletal muscle tone, body temperature, circulation,

and respiration. In persons who are generally inactive physically, basal metabolic needs make up the largest part, about two thirds, of the total energy requirement.

The basal metabolic rate (BMR) is the rate at which a person requires energy for these vital body processes.

Factors Influencing Basal Metabolic Rate

The BMR differs from person to person because of differences in body size and shape, physical condition, age, state of nutrition, presence of disease, and glandular activity.

Body composition affects heat lost by the body. The greater the skin area, the greater the amount of heat lost and the higher the BMR. A tall, slender person has more surface area and therefore a higher BMR than a shorter, stout person of the same weight.

Muscle and glandular tissue are relatively active and have a higher metabolic rate than fatty tissue. An athlete tends to have a higher BMR than a sedentary person of the same age and size. The BMR for women is about 5% lower than that for men.

Age and growth are also responsible for differences in metabolic rate. The BMR is high at birth and increases up to the age of 2 years. Thereafter it decreases, although it is still relatively high during puberty. The BMR decreases steadily after early adulthood. This decline is about 2% per decade in adults. There is a marked drop in old age, probably because of a decrease in muscle tissue. Fewer calories are needed to maintain body functions in elderly than in young persons. Coupled with this is usually a decrease in physical activity. If an adult continues to consume the same number of kilocalories as he did earlier in life, a gradual weight gain will result. This is frequently the case among middle-aged persons.

The state of nutrition, especially severe starvation or prolonged periods of inadequate kilocalorie intake, can affect BMR, because the body attempts to adapt to a decrease in intake by decreasing its metabolic rate. Disease conditions that produce fever raise the BMR in pro-

portion to the increase in body temperature. The BMR increases approximately 7% for each increase of 1°F in temperature.

Secretions of certain endocrine glands, especially those of the thyroid and adrenal glands, affect basal metabolism. In fact, they have more influence on basal energy needs than any other single factor. Thyroxine, produced by the thyroid, regulates the speed of energy metabolism, and epinephrine, from the adrenal glands, provides for the rapid conversion of glycogen (carbohydrate stored in the liver) to glucose when a source of quick energy is needed.

The BMR is usually measured by a blood test that determines the amount of protein-bound iodine (PBI) in a sample of blood. Given that iodine is found only in the secretions of the thyroid gland, this test measures the gland's hormone output. Excessive production of thyroxine, called *hyperthyroidism,* causes the rate of metabolism to be abnormally high. A reduced secretion of thyroxine, *hypothyroidism,* results in a lower than normal rate of metabolism. Pituitary hormones, which stimulate thyroid and adrenal secretions, may also affect the metabolic rate.

Physical Activity

The influence of physical activity on total caloric needs depends on the type of activity, the length of time the work is performed, and the size of the person. Unfortunately, most Americans are expending increasingly fewer kilocalories for physical activity. The activity pattern of Americans is generally light to sedentary (sedentary tasks are those conducted from a sitting position).

Type and Duration of Activity

It may be surprising to discover how few kilocalories are required for the performance of various activities (Table 6-1). People are busy with a myriad of tasks, yet because of the type of work done, they are mostly inactive physically. For example, a student may be wholly occupied

Table 6-1. Kilocalories Used in 10 Minutes of Physical Activity

Activity	Kilocalories Expended	
	Body Weight 150 Pounds	Body Weight 200 Pounds
Sleeping	12	16
Sitting (writing)	18	24
Walking downstairs	67	88
Walking upstairs	175	229
Walking 2 miles/hour	35	46
Walking 4 miles/hour	62	81
Running 5.5 miles/hour	108	142
Running 7 miles/hour	141	187
Domestic work	41	53
Golf, lawn mowing (power)	41	53
Swimming (crawl — 20 yards/minute)	38	52
Square dancing, volley ball	57	75
Racquetball	90	117
Tennis	67	92

(After Brownell KD: Behavior Therapy For Weight Control, a Treatment Manual. Copyright KD Brownell, University of Pennsylvania, 1979)

but very sedentary at the same time. Mental activity requires practically no increase in energy expenditure over the BMR. Brain cell activity is part of the BMR and does not vary whether one is sleeping or studying. Any increase in energy expenditure that results from mental work is usually due to muscle tension rather than to brain cell activity. However, persons who engage in very strenuous physical activity for prolonged periods of time may require as many as 4000 kcal to 5000 kcal a day.

The larger the body, the more energy is needed for activities that require body movement, such as walking. The energy expenditures needed for the various activities listed in Table 6-1 increase as the weight of the person increases. Fewer kilocalories are expended by persons weighing less than 150 pounds. Persons who are overweight frequently make up for the greater effort required of them for activity by becoming less active.

Thermic Effect of Food

The metabolic rate increases for about 12 hours following a meal. Digestion, absorption, transport of nutrients to the cells, and the changes the nutrients undergo all require energy. The production of heat following a meal is known as the *thermic effect* of food or the *specific dynamic action* of food. The effect varies according to the kinds and amounts of food eaten and the person's metabolic needs. The use of nutrients to build new tissue requires more energy than the breakdown of nutrients to provide energy. The thermic effect of food varies from about 6% to 10% of total energy needs.

Energy Balance

An infallible guide exists that will help you determine whether food intake is meeting energy needs. This guide is body weight. If the number of kilocalories you consume is equal to the number you use for energy, your body weight will be constant. But if you consistently consume more calories than you use for energy, you will gain weight. Excess calories are stored in the form of fat. If you usually eat less than

you need, you will lose weight. Energy must come from somewhere, so needed calories not provided by food are withdrawn from body stores.

A pound of body fat represents 3500 kcal. For every 3500 kcal lacking in the diet, 1 pound of body weight will be lost, and for every 3500 kcal excess, 1 pound of weight will be gained. It does not matter whether the excess or shortage occurs over a period of a week or a year.

Balancing energy needs with energy intake is difficult for many persons, as clearly demonstrated by the fact that obesity is a major nutritional problem in the United States. Although it may be seen in persons of any age, obesity is especially prevalent among adults. This is due for the most part to a gradual reduction in BMR

Table 6-2.   Recommended Energy Intakes*

Category	Age (Years)	Weight (lb)	Height (in)	Energy Needs (kcal)
Infants	0.0–0.5	13	24	kg × 115
	0.5–1.0	20	28	kg × 105
Children	1–3	29	35	1300
	4–6	44	44	1700
	7–10	62	52	2400
Males	11–14	99	62	2700
	15–18	145	69	2800
	19–22	154	70	2900
	23–50	154	70	2700
	51–75	154	70	2400
	76+	154	70	2050
Females	11–14	101	62	2200
	15–18	120	64	2100
	19–22	120	64	2100
	23–50	120	64	2000
	51–75	120	64	1800
	76+	120	64	1600
Pregnancy				+300
Lactation				+500

* The energy allowances in this table are from the Recommended Dietary Allowances, 9th ed. Washington, DC, National Academy of Sciences, 1980. They represent average energy needs for each age and sex group and are not recommended intakes for individuals.

together with a decrease in physical activity. While energy needs decrease, the intake of kilocalories often remains the same as it was earlier in life, when energy expenditure was greater.

Regardless of what weight reduction ads frequently imply, weight loss can occur only when the kilocalorie intake is lower than energy needs. The diet should include all the basic foods necessary to provide the essential nutrients. Portion sizes may have to be reduced and rich desserts replaced by fruits and vegetables.

For many of us, everyday living demands little physical activity. Advances in technology often reduce the physical activity required to do a task. Exercise is a valuable aid in achieving a balance between energy intake and energy output. Over a period of months or years, even small increases in daily exercise can make a difference in weight. For example, in a person who weighs 150 pounds, going up and down stairs for a total of 5 minutes a day will result in a weight loss of 12 pounds a year (if food consumption remains the same).

The Food and Nutrition Board suggests that it is better to achieve weight control by increasing physical activity than by reducing kilocalorie intake to below recommended levels. It is difficult to obtain essential nutrients and proper use of protein on diets that are low in kilocalories. Exercise has many other advantages, including beneficial effects on the cardiovascular system and improvement of the tone of the gastrointestinal tract.

Recommended Energy Allowances

Recommended energy allowances are given in Table 6-2. The adult allowances are based on light to sedentary activity. In each age category, a "reference" person, that is, a person of a given height and weight, has been used as a standard. For example, the reference man is 23 to 50 years old, weighs 154 pounds, and is 70 inches tall. Changes are required for differences due to body size or physical activity; for example, a man whose ideal weight and/or activity is higher than that of the reference man will require more kilocalories, and vice versa.

Energy needs increase during pregnancy and in infancy and childhood. These needs are discussed in Chapter 15.

Food Sources of Energy

Consumption Patterns

As mentioned, the energy value of food comes from carbohydrate, protein, and fat, with carbohydrate contributing about 45%, fat 43%, and protein 12%. Alcohol contributes a considerable number of kilocalories, as many as 1800 a day for some persons. Many authorities feel that dietary changes would be beneficial to the entire population. The U.S. Dietary Goals suggest an increase in carbohydrates (mostly from starches and naturally occurring sugars) to 58% of energy intake and a reduction in fat to 30% of energy intake.

Energy Content of Food

Foods vary greatly in energy value, depending on the proportions of energy-producing nutrients (protein, fat, carbohydrate) and the water and fiber they contain. Energy-producing nutrients make up less than 3% of a food such as lettuce and as much as 100% of a food such as cooking oil.

Because fats provide more than twice as many kilocalories per gram as either carbohydrates or proteins, foods that contain even a moderate amount of fat have a relatively high energy value. Cream, cream cheese, butter, margarine, oils, cheese, and fatty meats provide relatively large numbers of kilocalories. In contrast, because water and fiber do not yield calories, foods that contain high proportions of these substances have a low kilocalorie content. Fruits and vegetables, especially green leafy vegetables, fall into this category. Between these two extremes are foods that are intermediate in

Table 6-3.   Energy Values of Selected Foods

	Portion	Kilocalories
Fat Content:		
High fat content → high energy value		
Ground beef, broiled (10% fat)	3 oz	185
Ground beef, broiled (21% fat)	3 oz	243
Whole milk (3.3% fat)	1 cup	150
Skim milk (0.1% fat)	1 cup	85
Cottage cheese, creamed (4% fat)	½ cup	117
Cottage cheese, low fat (1% fat)	½ cup	83
Peanut butter (2 tbsp)	1 oz	190
Turkey, light meat	1 oz	55
Cheddar cheese	1 oz	115
Alcohol Content:		
High alcohol content → high energy value*		
Beer	12 oz	150
Beer, "light"†	12 oz	96–100
Manhattan	3½ oz	164
Tom Collins	10 oz	180
Water Content:		
High water content → low energy value		
Peaches, fresh, sliced	½ cup	33
Dates	½ cup	245
Grapes, fresh	2 oz	40
Raisins	2 oz	160
Fresh peas, cooked	½ cup	41
Split peas, dried, cooked	½ cup	115
Fiber Content:		
High fiber content → low energy value		
Lettuce, raw	½ cup	10
Celery, raw	½ cup	10
Endive, raw	½ cup	5
Method of Preparation:		
High-energy ingredients → high energy value		
Potato, medium, boiled (1)	4 oz	96
Potato with 1 tsp margarine	4 oz	141
Potato, French fried	4 oz	324
Hash brown	4 oz	264

(Nutritive Value of Foods, USDA Home and Garden Bulletin 72, 1981)
* Pennington J, Church HN: Food Values of Portions Commonly Used. 13th ed.
Philadelphia, JB Lippincott, 1980
† Label information

fuel value, such as lean meats, cereal foods, and starchy vegetables.

Some foods that do not contain fat but are low in water are relatively high in fuel value. These foods include sugar, dried legumes, and dried fruits. For example, a ⅔-cup portion of fresh grapes yields 67 kcal, whereas a ⅔-cup portion of raisins (dried grapes) yields 290 kcal. The kilocalorie content of hard cheese is relatively high, not only because the food has a high fat content, but also because it is a highly concentrated food with a relatively low moisture content. Table 6-3 demonstrates the influence of fat, alcohol, water, and fiber content on the energy value of selected foods.

Method of food preparation is another factor that greatly influences the energy value of food. For example, poultry and fish, which tend to be low in kilocalories, become rather high-energy dishes when fried or served with cream sauces.

To call foods *fattening* or *nonfattening* is scientifically incorrect. Whether a person gains weight depends on whether his total caloric intake exceeds his energy needs. Unfortunately, some very nutritious foods, such as potatoes, bread, and milk, have been labeled *fattening*. Potatoes are an excellent food, providing essential vitamins and minerals. A medium-sized baked potato, which yields about 90 kcal, is well worth its calories in nutrient content. It is the addition of gravy, butter, sour cream, or crumbled bacon that greatly increases its energy content.

Choosing Kilocalories Wisely

Persons who are concerned about energy balance aim to obtain all the essential nutrients and to stay within the kilocalorie level required to maintain their ideal weight. For this goal to be accomplished, the diet should be built around the most nutritious foods: milk, meat, fish, poultry, eggs, cheese, fruits, vegetables, and breads and cereals. As long as the essential nutrients are provided by these foods, additional kilocalories may be added or subtracted as individual needs change.

For many persons with a low level of physical activity, there is little room for foods that furnish chiefly kilocalories and few or no nutrients. Many Americans obtain 30% or more of their kilocalories from foods such as pure sugars, fats, and alcohol, which provide very limited amounts of vitamins and minerals. In the United States, sugar is consumed at an average of 138 pounds per person per year. Most of this sugar is consumed in hidden forms. The more kilocalories a person derives from such foods, the more likely he is to be poorly nourished.

Caloric Density and Nutrient Density

Two terms are used to describe the energy value and the nutritional value of individual foods; *caloric density,* and *nutrient density.*

Caloric density refers to the number of kilocalories per unit of weight of a specific food. One cup of lettuce, approximately 2 ounces,

Table 6-4. Index of Nutritional Quality for Eight Nutrients in Selected Foods*

Nutrient	Chicken	Carrots	Apple Pie
Protein	7.8	0.6	0.3
Vitamin A	0.27	130.2	0.2
Vitamin C	—	6.0	0.2
Thiamin	0.5	0.8	0.6
Riboflavin	1.7	1.9	0.4
Niacin	6.5	1.6	0.4
Calcium	0.1	2.0	0.1
Iron	1.4	2.0	0.3

A "nutritious food" is defined as having an INQ of at least 1 or more for four nutrients or 2 or more for two nutrients.
* The USRDA has been used for the nutrient requirement and 2000 calories as the energy requirement in the calculations.

yields 5 kcal and is said to have low caloric density; 2 ounces of cheddar cheese yield 230 kcal, and this food is of high caloric density.

Nutrient density refers to the nutritional quality of a specific food in relation to the kilocalories it supplies. A formula is used to calculate this relationship. The nutritional value of the food is expressed as *INQ* (index of nutrient quality). If the INQ is 1 or more for a nutrient, the food is considered to be an adequate source of that nutrient. If a food has an INQ of 1 or more for four nutrients or an INQ of 2 or more for two nutrients, it may be termed *nutritious* (Table 6-4).

Foods can be chosen wisely even if such precise information is not available. Knowledge of the general characteristics of different foods enables us to choose those that have a good ratio of nutrients to calories. Greens are foods of low caloric density but of high nutrient density with respect to a number of important nutrients. Carbonated beverages have a poor nutrient density for all nutrients. Peanut butter is high in caloric density but also high in nutrient density for a number of nutrients.

KEYS TO PRACTICAL APPLICATION

Choose foods that provide the most nutrients for the fewest calories.

Eat less fatty and sugary foods, and drink alcohol in moderation, if at all — these foods provide mostly kilocalories and few, if any, nutrients.

Avoid calling foods *fattening* or *nonfattening*. Whether a person gains weight depends on his total caloric intake, not on the consumption of any specific foods.

Maintain a high level of physical activity. It can help you control your weight and has many other benefits.

KEY IDEAS

Metabolism includes all the processes by which body cells use nutrients to support life. Anabolism is the use of food nutrients to build more complex substances, as in the formation of new tissue; catabolism is the breakdown of nutrients or body tissue, as in the production of energy.

Carbohydrates and fats are the preferred source of energy.

To release energy, the fuel-producing nutrients combine with oxygen (oxidation). Normal hemoglobin levels are required for sufficient oxygen to be supplied to the cell so that oxidation can take place.

Release of energy in the cells is a complex process requiring the activity of enzymes, coenzymes, and hormones.

The oxidation of carbohydrates, fats, and proteins results in heat and other forms of energy, carbon dioxide, and water. The carbon dioxide is excreted by the lungs; the water not used by the body is excreted via the skin and kidneys. When protein is used for energy, the nitrogen that results from a breakdown of amino acids is converted into urea in the liver and excreted by the kidneys.

The energy value of a particular food depends upon its protein, fat, and carbohydrate content: protein provides 4 kcal/g, fat 9 kcal/g, and carbohydrate 4 kcal/g.

A person's total energy needs are based on basal metabolism, voluntary physical activity, and the thermic effect of food.

The basal metabolic rate (BMR) is the speed

at which fuel is needed to maintain the vital body processes at rest. It is influenced by body composition, age and physical condition, state of nutrition, disease conditions, and secretions of endocrine glands.

The effect of physical activity on total caloric needs depends on the type of activity, the length of time over which it is performed, and the size of the person doing it.

Energy balance results when the number of kilocalories consumed equals the number used for energy; body weight indicates the relationship of energy intake to energy output in the person. Exercise is a valuable aid in achieving energy balance.

Foods vary in energy value depending on the proportion of energy-producing nutrients they contain: foods that contain fat or alcohol or have a low water content tend to have a relatively high energy value, lean meats, cereal foods, and starchy vegetables are intermediate in energy value, and fruits and vegetables are relatively low in energy value.

All the essential nutrients should be provided within the kilocalorie level required to maintain ideal weight; the more kilocalories a person obtains from pure sugars, fats, and alcohol, the more likely he is to be poorly nourished.

KEYS TO LEARNING: STUDY – DISCUSSION QUESTIONS

1. What are the three factors that determine a person's total energy needs? Describe each of these factors.
2. A ½-cup serving of New England clam chowder contains 4 g of protein, 5 g of fat, and 7 g of carbohydrate. Using this information, calculate the approximate energy value of this food serving.
3. Using your food diary, calculate your energy intake for one day. What is the infallible guide for determining whether your kilocaloric intake is in balance with your energy needs? Explain. What

happens to excess kilocalories?
4. Discuss the value of exercise in maintaining energy balance and in other aspects of health.
5. More than 30% of the total energy intake of many Americans consists of pure sugars, fats, and alcohol. Why are these persons apt to be malnourished?
6. Explain the fallacy in the statement "Potatoes are fattening."

Bibliography is found at the end of Part Two.

Carbohydrates

KEY TERMS

cellulose Plant fiber; a fibrous form of carbohydrate making up the framework of the plant.

complex carbohydrates A class of carbohydrates called *polysaccharides;* foods composed of starch and cellulose.

fiber A group of compounds that make up the framework of plants. Fiber includes the carbohydrate substances (cellulose, hemicellulose, gums, and pectin) and a noncarbohydrate substance called *lignin.* These compounds are not digested by the human digestive tract.

glycogen Animal starch; the form in which carbohydrate is stored in animals.

insulin A hormone that is secreted by the beta cells of the islets of Langerhans of the pancreas and that is necessary for the proper metabolism of blood sugar.

ketosis The accumulation in the body of ketones, substances that result from the incomplete metabolism of fatty acids.

"naturally occurring" sugars Sugars found in foods in their natural state; for example, glucose occurs naturally in grapes and other fruit.

refined food Food that undergoes many commercial processes resulting in the loss of nutrients.

What do intravenous glucose, tooth decay, fiber, and diabetes mellitus have in common? In one way or another, all are associated with a class of food called *carbohydrates.* Carbohydrates are composed of carbon, hydrogen, and oxygen.

Although most carbohydrates occur in plant life, a few are of animal origin. These include lactose, which is the sugar in milk, and glycogen, which is the form in which animals store sugar. Sugars, starches, and celluloses are the main forms in which carbohydrate occurs in food. Starches and sugars are the major source of energy and the cheapest and most easily utilized form of fuel for the body. Celluloses are fibrous materials that provide bulk, aiding digestion.

Worldwide, carbohydrates are the major sources of energy. The proportion of energy supplied by carbohydrates depends on agricultural and economic conditions. Most of the peoples of Asia, the Middle East, Africa, and Latin America obtain as much as 80% of their total energy from carbohydrates such as cereal grains and starchy vegetables.

Generally speaking, the proportion of carbohydrate in the diet is greater when income is low. Carbohydrates such as rice, pasta, bread,

legumes, potatoes, and other starchy vegetables are considerably less expensive than meat, poultry, eggs, and dairy products.

The kind of carbohydrate foods eaten determines the nutritional contribution made to the diet. Highly refined and overprocessed carbohydrate foods such as sugars and products made from unenriched white flour contribute little other than calories to the diet. Refined and processed foods undergo changes in processing that cause a loss of nutrients. In contrast, whole-grain and enriched carbohydrate products, fruits, and vegetables provide vitamins, minerals, and fiber as well as energy.

Classification of Carbohydrates

Carbohydrates are classified into three major types: monosaccharides, disaccharides, and polysaccharides. The monosaccharides are the simplest form of carbohydrate and are referred to as *simple sugars.* They are composed of one (mono-) carbohydrate unit. The disaccharides, called *double sugars,* are composed of two (di-) carbohydrate units. The polysaccharides contain many (poly-) carbohydrate units. The monosaccharides and disaccharides are called *sugars;* polysaccharides are called *complex carbohydrates* because they have a more intricate chemical structure.

Monosaccharides

Monosaccharides require no digestion and are readily absorbed from the intestinal wall directly into the bloodstream. The nutritionally important monosaccharides are glucose, fructose, and galactose.

Glucose, also called *dextrose,* is found widely in fruits, vegetables, and sap syrups. All other carbohydrates are transformed into glucose by the body. Glucose is the form in which carbohydrates occur in the bloodstream and is called *blood sugar.* Fructose, also called *fruit sugar,* is found in fruits, vegetables, and honey. It has the sweetest taste of all sugars. Galactose, in combination with glucose, forms lactose, the sugar in milk. A few fruits, vegetables, and legumes contain galactose; the galactose in some of these foods may not be available for absorption. During periods of lactation, glucose is changed in the body to galactose so that lactose can be produced by the mammary (breast) glands.

Disaccharides

In the process of digestion, disaccharides are reduced to monosaccharides. Three disaccharides important in nutrition are sucrose, or table sugar, powdered sugar, or brown sugar, one of the sweetest forms of sugar; maltose, or malt sugar, produced during the breakdown of starch and found in maple syrup and beer; and lactose, or milk sugar, found in the milk of mammals.

Sugars vary in sweetness and in solubility (ability to dissolve in water). The sweetness of a sugar is an important consideration when effort is made to reduce the use of sugar (as in diabetes and obesity) or to try to increase the use of sugar (when extra calories are needed and appetite is poor). Because fructose is very sweet, a small amount of it is of the same sweetness as larger amounts of table sugar for fewer calories. Although lactose is about one sixth as sweet as table sugar, it is seldom used to increase the caloric value of beverages. It is poorly soluble and tends to cause gastrointestinal discomfort when consumed in large quantities. It is important to remember, however, that regardless of how sweet they taste, all sugars have the same energy value. One teaspoon of fructose has the same energy value as 1 teaspoon of sucrose.

Polysaccharides

Polysaccharides (complex carbohydrates) must also be reduced to monosaccharides before they can be absorbed into the bloodstream. The polysaccharides important in nutrition are dextrins, starch, cellulose, and glycogen.

Dextrins occur mostly as products in the partial breakdown of starch due to enzymes or in cooking, such as in toasting bread. Starch is the chief form of carbohydrate in the diet. Cereal grains, vegetables, and other plants provide starch. Plant starches are the main source of food for humans. Cellulose is one of a group of polysaccharides that make up the framework of plants. It occurs in the stalks and leaves of all plants, in the skins of fruit and vegetables, and in the outer covering of seeds and cereals. Cellulose cannot be broken down in the human digestive tract and therefore is not absorbed. Cellulose together with other indigestible substances found in the skeletal walls of plants is commonly called *fiber* or *roughage.* Although fiber is not a true nutrient, it plays an important role in the functioning of the intestinal tract.

Other nondigestible polysaccharides found in the cell walls of plants, including pectin, agar, carrageenan, and vegetable gums, have the ability to absorb water and form a gel. This property is utilized in food processing. For example, commercial pectin made from apple peels and cores is used in the production of fruit jellies, cosmetics, and drugs; alginates and carrageenans are used in the production of ice cream to provide "body" and smooth consistency.

Glycogen, or animal starch is the form in which carbohydrate is stored in the body. Glycogen is found in liver and muscle tissue.

Utilization of Carbohydrates

Before carbohydrates can be absorbed into the bloodstream, they must be reduced to monosaccharides by the process of digestion. Table 7-1 summarizes carbohydrate digestion.

The monosaccharides are absorbed and carried by the portal circulation to the liver. In the liver, fructose and galactose are converted to glucose. Glucose is then released by the liver into the bloodstream and distributed to the cells. Any excess glucose is converted in the liver to glycogen, the form in which carbohydrate is stored. When energy is needed, the liver converts the glycogen back to glucose and releases it into the bloodstream in sufficient amounts to maintain a normal blood sugar level. Muscle tissue is also able to store glucose as glycogen. Glycogen is present in most body organs. However, the ability to form glycogen is limited. When more carbohydrate is eaten than is needed for energy or storage as glycogen, it is converted to fat and stored as fat tissue.

While glucose is being absorbed from the digestive tract, the blood sugar level rises. As the tissues take the needed glucose from the bloodstream and the liver converts glucose to glycogen, the blood sugar gradually returns to its normal level of less than 100 mg per 100 ml of venous whole blood (less than 115 mg/dl venous plasma).

The hormone insulin, produced by the beta cells of the pancreas, greatly influences the way the body uses carbohydrates and regulates the blood sugar level. When blood sugar rises, the pancreas is stimulated to produce insulin. Insulin has important functions: it regulates the use of glucose for energy by the cells, the storage of carbohydrate as glycogen in the liver, and the conversion of excess glucose to fat. Whereas insulin lowers blood sugar, other hormones cause a rise in blood sugar. Glucagon, a hormone secreted by certain cells of the islets of Langerhans in the pancreas (called *alpha cells*), raises the blood sugar level by promoting the conversion of glycogen in the liver to glucose. Other hormones, released in response to stress, raise the blood sugar level by blocking the effects of insulin and are therefore called *insulin antagonists.* These include epinephrine (from the adrenal medulla), glucocorticoids (from the adrenal cortex), and growth hormone (from the pituitary) as well as glucagon. Some persons taking glucocorticoid medications such as cortisone, prednisone, and dexamethasone develop abnormal blood sugar levels. In healthy persons, there is a balance between the two groups of hormones.

Somatostatin, the most recently discovered of the pancreatic hormones, is secreted by the

Table 7-1.   Summary of Carbohydrate Digestion

Site of Action	Carbohydrate	Enzyme	End-Product	
Mouth	Starch	Amylase in saliva (ptyalin) ⟶	Dextrins, maltose, glucose	
Small intestine	Starch	Amylase in pancreatic juice ⟶	Dextrins, maltose, glucose	
	Dextrins	⟶	Maltose, glucose	
		Enzymes in brush border of small intestine		
	Maltose	Maltase ⟶	Glucose	
	Sucrose	Sucrase ⟶	Glucose and fructose	Absorbed into the bloodstream
	Lactose	Lactase ⟶	Glucose and galactose	

delta cells of the islets of Langerhans. It reduces the production of both insulin and glucagon, and it interferes with the activity of pituitary growth hormone. The role of somatostatin in regulating blood sugar levels has not been clearly established.

Functions of Carbohydrates

Carbohydrates perform the following functions: they provide the most efficient form of energy, they form parts of certain body substances, they promote the growth of beneficial bacteria, and they provide fiber for the proper functioning of the gastrointestinal tract.

Provide Energy

Carbohydrates are the most economical and efficient source of energy. Each gram of carbo- hydrate supplies 4 kcal. One tablespoon of sugar contains 12 g of carbohydrate and yields 48 kcal (12×4 kcal = 48 kcal).

In addition to carbohydrate, protein and fat can also be used to produce energy. However, the body utilizes carbohydrate first. When not enough carbohydrate is provided, the body uses protein and fat for its energy needs. This occurs at the expense of the other functions of protein and fat. Under normal conditions, the tissue of the central nervous system can use only glucose as its form of energy, whereas skeletal muscles can use either glucose or fatty acids (fats) as fuel.

When the amount of carbohydrate con- sumed is greater than the amount needed im- mediately for energy, the excess is stored in two ways: in limited amounts as glycogen, and as body fat.

Spare Protein

Carbohydrates are needed to provide energy quickly so that the available protein can be used for building and repairing tissue. If a person does not eat enough food to meet his energy

needs, his body will burn its own tissues to supply energy. In starvation, death eventually results from the breakdown of vital body tissue. The discussion of diet in disease, in Part 4, indicates that the protein-sparing effect of carbohydrate is extremely important in disease of the kidneys and liver and following surgery.

Help the Body Use Fat Efficiently

Carbohydrates are necessary for the proper use of fats. If carbohydrate intake is low, larger than normal amounts of fat are called upon to supply energy. However, the body is unable to handle the excessive breakdown of fat. As a result, the fat does not burn completely, and certain breakdown products accumulate in the blood, causing a condition known as *ketosis.*

Are a Component of Body Substances

Carbohydrates are important components of certain body substances needed for the regulation of body processes. Heparin, a substance that prevents blood from clotting, contains carbohydrate. Nervous tissue, connective tissue, various hormones, and enzymes also contain carbohydrates. Ribose, another carbohydrate, is a part of deoxyribonucleic acid (DNA) and ribonucleic acid (RNA), the substances that carry the hereditary factors in the cell.

Encourage Growth of Useful Bacteria

Carbohydrates encourage the growth of beneficial intestinal bacteria that are involved in the production of certain vitamins and in the absorption of calcium and phosphorus.

Promote Normal Functioning of the Lower Intestinal Tract

Cellulose and other indigestible carbohydrates compose dietary fiber. Fiber absorbs and holds water, resulting in a softer, bulkier stool and faster movement through the lower intestinal tract.

Sources of Carbohydrate

Groups of food providing significant amounts of carbohydrate are cereal grains, vegetables, fruit, nuts, milk, and concentrated sweets. Milk is the only important animal source of carbohydrate. Table 7-2 compares the carbohydrate content of various foods.

Cereal Grains

Cereal grains have been the staple food of humans since prehistoric times. Worldwide, rice is the most widely used cereal. It is the basic food for over half of the world's population, including the peoples of Asia, the Near East, and some Latin American and African countries. Wheat, the next most common cereal, is most widely used in Europe and the Americas. Corn is widely used in Mexico, Latin America, and the southern United States. Rice and products made from cereal grains, such as breads and other baked goods, breakfast cereals, and macaroni products, contribute substantial amounts of carbohydrate to the American diet.

Milled Grains

The milling of wheat to produce a pure white flour results in the removal of bran and the germ layers of the grain, those parts that contain most of the vitamins and minerals. Similarly, much of the vitamin and mineral content of rice is lost in the milling of white rice. Oat products retain more of the original grain kernel than do other processed cereals and thus lose fewer nutrients. Cereals that have the outer layers of the kernel removed by milling are called *refined cereals.*

Table 7-2. Comparison of Carbohydrate Content of Selected Foods

Food	Serving Size	Carbohydrate Content
Milk	1 cup	12 g
Cheddar cheese	1 ounce	Trace
Creamed cottage cheese	½ cup	3 g
Grapefruit	½ cup	12 g
Banana	1	26 g
Dried prunes	5 large	29 g
Bread	1 slice	13 g
Oatmeal, cooked	½ cup	12 g
Cornflakes	¾ cup	15 g
Macaroni	½ cup	16 g
Rice	½ cup	20 g
Asparagus	½ cup	3 g
Mashed potato	½ cup	19 g
Split peas	½ cup	21 g
Peanut butter	2 tbsp	6 g
Walnuts	¼ cup	5 g
Sunflower seeds	¼ cup	7 g
Sugar	1 tbsp	12 g
Yellow cake with icing	1/16th 8″ cake	40 g
Apple pie	1/7th 9″ pie	51 g

(Nutritive Value of Foods. USDA Home and Garden Bulletin 72, 1981)

Because breads and cereals are basic foods, measures were taken some years ago to improve the nutritional quality of refined wheat products through *enrichment,* the addition of nutrients. The label *enriched* on flour or bread means that iron and the vitamins thiamine, niacin, and riboflavin within amounts specified by law have been added. Most white flour, white bread, pasta products, such as macaroni, noodles, and spaghetti, and ready-to-eat cereals are enriched.

The practice of enriching refined grain products has been expanded to include corn and rice products. In the southern United States, laws requiring enrichment of corn products have been enacted. Enriched rice, which is fortified with thiamine, niacin, and iron, is widely available in the United States. Converted rice also has a higher nutritional value than unenriched rice. It is a wise practice to read the labels on cereal cartons and purchase only enriched products.

Whole-Grain vs. Enriched White Bread

The milling of wheat eliminates at least 20 nutrients. Enrichment restores only four of these.

Some of the nutrients not replaced, including vitamin B_6, folacin, and zinc, are lacking in many American diets. In addition, enriched white bread lacks fiber, which whole-grain bread contains. Yet enriched white bread is not a totally worthless food as some have claimed. It does have nutritional value.

Fruit

Fruits are a less concentrated source of carbohydrate than cereals because of their high water content. Cantaloupe and watermelon are the lowest in carbohydrate content; banana is one of the highest. Dried fruits such as prunes, dried apricots, raisins, dates, and figs have a much higher concentration of sugar than fresh fruit because of their low moisture content. Most canned fruits and some frozen fruits are packed in a sugar syrup, which increases their carbohydrate content. The plantain, a fruit related to the banana, must be cooked before being eaten. In tropical countries in which they are an important source of carbohydrate, plantains are part of the main course of the meal. Avocados and olives are high in fat and low in carbohydrate.

Vegetables

Vegetables contain carbohydrate in the forms of starch, sugar, and cellulose. Because of their high water and fiber content, vegetables that represent the leaf, flower, or stem of the plant are low in carbohydrate. These include the green leafy vegetables, celery, asparagus, cauliflower, broccoli, and brussels sprouts. The roots, tubers, and seeds of plants have a higher starch and sugar content and less water. These include potatoes of all kinds, beets, carrots, turnips, parsnips, peas, lima beans, dried beans, and lentils.

Nuts

Although nuts are noted for their fat and protein content, they also contain 10% to 27%

carbohydrate. Peanut butter is approximately 15% digestible carbohydrate. (Peanuts are actually legumes, although we usually think of them as nuts.)

Sugar and Sweets

Sucrose, or common table sugar, is processed from either sugarcane or beet sugar. Sugar is 100% carbohydrate and yields 4 kcal/g but contains no other nutrients. For this reason, sugar and foods high in sugar content—jellies, jams, candy, cake, cookies, and sugar-sweetened soft drinks—are "empty calories."

Honey, maple syrup, and brown sugar add variety in flavor to the diet. They are slightly more nutritious than table sugar, but the quantities of vitamins and minerals they contain are too small to make an important contribution to the diet. Molasses contains a significant amount of iron, 1.2 mg per tablespoon. Blackstrap molasses supplies 3.2 mg of iron per tablespoon; however its strong flavor limits its use. Molasses also provides B vitamins and calcium.

Read lables to determine sugar content of various products. If sucrose, dextrose, lactose, fructose, honey, or syrup appears first in the list of ingredients, there is a large amount of sugar in the product.

Milk and Milk Products

Fresh cow's milk contains carbohydrate in the form of lactose. Cottage cheese contains about half the lactose of an equal quantity of milk. Hard cheeses contain only traces.

Dietary Fiber

The polysaccharides that cannot be digested by humans are sources of dietary fiber. The best sources are whole-grain breads and cereals, especially those containing bran; leafy vegetables; legumes; vegetables and fruits with skins and seeds; and nuts and seeds. Unprocessed bran is sometimes added to food in small amounts to increase the fiber content.

Recommended Carbohydrate Intake of Americans

The Food and Nutrition Board has made no specific recommendations for carbohydrate. About 100 g of digestible carbohydrate per day is needed to pervent ketosis and the excess breakdown of tissue protein, and to supply glucose to the central nervous system. The total carbohydrate in the following foods equals this amount: 2 slices of bread, ½ cup of potato, 2 glasses of milk, and 2 servings of fruit. However, desirable amounts of carbohydrate are considerably higher than these minimal levels. In fact, the U.S. Dietary Goals (see Chapter 13) recommend a sizable increase in the carbohydrate intake of Americans.

Suggestions that carbohydrate intake be increased meet with considerable resistance from the general public. Carbohydrates are frequently thought to be "fattening," but this is a misconception. Carbohydrates provide 4 kcal/g, the same as protein. Fats yield 9 kcal/g, more than twice as much as either carbohydrate or protein. Protein foods are usually higher in kilocalories than carbohydrate foods because protein is usually combined with fat in most foods (meat, cheese, eggs, peanut butter). Complex carbohydrates and naturally occurring sugars as are found in fruits, vegetables, whole grain breads and cereals, dried peas and beans, and seeds and nuts provide many essential vitamins and minerals and fiber, in addition to kilocalories.

Refined sugars and sugars in processed foods are perhaps deserving of the "fattening" label. People tend to overeat these foods, which frequently take the place of more nutritious foods in the diet.

Carbohydrates and Health

Knowledge of the sources of carbohydrate, their characteristics, and their nutritional value will help you both in the prevention of disease (as in dental caries) and in the treatment of disease involving the utilization of carbohydrate (as in diabetes mellitus). It will also help you correct widespread misunderstandings about this group of foods.

Overconsumption of Sugars

Excessive sugar intake is a contributing factor in the widespread occurrence of obesity in the United States. Consumption of table sugar, syrups, and jelly has decreased since 1974, but consumption of sugar in processed food and soft drinks has increased. In addition to its presence in obviously sugary foods such as cake, cookies, and pies, sugar is also found in an endless number of other products, such as cereals, soups, canned vegetables, tomato sauce, and luncheon meats. Table 7-3 gives the sugar content of some popular foods. If the 630 kcal of sugar ingested daily by the average American are "extra" kilocalories over and above the individual's energy needs, they will produce a weight gain of over 1 pound per week.

Dental Disease

Sugar consumption promotes tooth decay (dental caries) and gum disease. Sugar-rich foods are used by bacteria in the mouth to form acids. These acids dissolve tooth enamel and irritate the gums. The form of the sweets and the frequency with which they are eaten are more important than the total amounts eaten as far as dental disease is concerned. Sugary foods that tend to stick to the surface of the teeth, such as caramels, gum drops, glazed doughnuts and

Table 7-3. Hidden Sugar

The approximate sugar content of popular foods expressed in teaspoons:

100 grams sugar = 20 teaspoons = ½ cup = 3½ oz = 400 kcal

Food	Quantity	Sugar (tsp)
Candy*		
Chocolate bar	1, average size	7
Chocoalte cream	1, average size	2
Chocolate fudge	1½″ sq. (*15/lb*)	4
Chocolate mints	1, medium (*20/lb*)	3
Marshmallow	1, average (*60/lb*)	1½
Chewing gum	1 stick	½
Cakes and cookies		
Chocolate cake	1/12 cake (*2-layer, iced*)	15
Angel food cake	1/12 large cake	6
Sponge cake	1/10 average cake	6
Cream puff (iced)	1, average, custard-filled	5
Doughnut, plain	3″ diameter	4
Macaroons	1 large or 2 small	3
Gingersnaps	1 medium	1
Molasses cookies	3½″ diameter	2
Brownies	2″ × 2″ × ¾″	3
Ice cream		
Ice cream	⅛ quart (½ cup)	5–6
Sherbet	⅛ quart (½ cup)	6–8
Pie		
Apple	⅙ medium pie	12
Cherry	⅙ medium pie	14
Raisin	⅙ medium pie	13
Pumpkin	⅙ medium pie	10
Soft drinks		
Sweet carbonated beverage	1 bottle, 8 oz	4⅓
Ginger ale	6-oz glass	3⅓
Milk drinks		
Chocolate	1 cup, 5 oz milk	6
Cocoa	1 cup, 5 oz milk	4
Egg-nog	1 glass, 8 oz milk	4½

(continued)

Table 7-3   (*continued*)

The approximate sugar content of popular foods expressed in teaspoons:

100 grams sugar = 20 teaspoons = ½ cup = 3½ oz = 400 kcal

Food	Quantity	Sugar (tsp)
Spreads and sauces		
Jam	1 level tbsp	3
Jelly	1 level tbsp	2½
Marmalade	1 level tbsp	3
Syrup, maple	1 level tbsp	2½
Honey	1 level tbsp	3
Chocolate sauce (thick)	1 tbsp	4½
Cooked fruits		
Peaches, canned in syrup	2 halves, 1 tbsp syrup	3½
Rhubarb, stewed, sweetened	½ cup	8
Applesauce (unsweetened)	½ cup, scant	2
Prunes, stewed, sweetened	4 to 5, medium 2 tbsp juice	8
Dried fruits		
Apricots, dried	4 to 6 halves	4
Prunes, dried	3 to 4 medium	4
Dates, dried	3 to 4, stoned	4½
Figs, dried	1½ to 2, small	4
Raisins	¼ cup	4
Fruits and fruit juices		
Fruit cocktail	½ cup, scant	5
Orange juice	½ cup, scant	2
Pineapple juice, unsweetened	½ cup, scant	2⅗
Grapefruit juice, unsweetened	½ cup, scant	2⅕
Grapefruit, commercial	½ cup, scant	3⅔

(Joseph L: Foods and drinks that will cause you the fewest cavities. Today's Health, October, p 42, 1973)

* Candy is from 75% to 85% sugar. Popular candy bars are likely to weigh from 1 to 5 ounces and may contain 5 to 20 teaspoons of sugar. Adapted from current publications on food values.

jelly, are the worst offenders. Honey, crude brown sugar, and molasses, as well as glucose, fructose, and lactose, seem to promote decay as much as refined table sugar.

Frequent use of sugary foods throughout the day is more harmful than consumption of an equal amount of sugar once or twice a day. Every time bacteria on the tooth surface are exposed to sweets, they produce acid for a period of 20 to 30 minutes. Other factors, such as dental hygiene and fluoridation of water, are also important in dental health.

Lack of Fiber

The increased use of convenience foods, which are made from highly refined ingredients, has resulted in the pattern of diets that are very low in fiber. Lack of fiber in the diet has been linked to diseases of the colon and other chronic illnesses. A high-fiber diet has proved useful in reducing the symptoms of chronic constipation and diverticulosis (see Chap. 25).

Fad Diets

Low-carbohydrate reducing diets that promote the use of fats and severely restrict or eliminate carbohydrate can cause serious harm. As previously discussed, when there is too little carbohydrate, fat is not burned completely, and a condition known as *acidosis* (also called *ketosis*) results. Excessive quantities of water and sodium are excreted, body tissue breaks down, and there is a general deterioration in physicial condition.

Abnormal Utilization of Carbohydrates

In several disease conditions, the body is unable to use carbohydrates normally. The most common is diabetes mellitus, in which the cells are unable to burn glucose for energy at a normal rate. This causes the quantity of glucose entering the cell to decrease and therefore the quantity of sugar circulating in the blood to increase. Diabetes may be due to a lack of insulin or to an unknown cause that inhibits the functioning of insulin (see Chap. 21).

Lactose intolerance is due to a deficiency of the enzyme lactase which is necessary for the digestion of lactose (milk sugar). The condition is uncommon in infancy. However, many persons lose their ability to digest milk sugar in adulthood. These persons suffer from cramps, diarrhea, and flatulence after drinking milk (see Chap. 25).

In galactosemia, the liver is unable to convert the sugar galactose to glucose. This disorder, which occurs in infancy, is caused by the lack of a certain enzyme. Digestive disturbances, physical and mental retardation, and cataracts are some of the consequences of the disease (see Chap. 28).

Alcohol Abuse

Alcohol is produced by the fermentation of glucose. It is considered a foodstuff, since it yields 7 kcal/g. One fluid ounce of 100 proof alcohol (50% alcohol) contains 12 g of alcohol, or 84 kcal. Alcohol does not require digestion and is absorbed intact from the gastrointestinal tract. It is water-soluble and immediately disperses throughout the body fluids.

Chronic alcohol abuse creates serious physiological, psychological, and social problems for an estimated 9 million Americans. The chronic alcoholic may eat poorly because of a lack of money to support an adequate diet or because alcohol depresses his appetite. Excessive alcohol intake can seriously impair the functioning of the liver and cause disorders of the nervous system.

KEYS TO PRACTICAL APPLICATION

Encourage the use of whole-grain cereals and breads.

When using refined cereal products, be sure they are enriched.

Reduce the amount of all types of sugars you eat; they provide only calories and no vitamins and minerals.

Substitute starches for fats and sugars; choose foods that are good sources of fiber and starch, such as whole-grain

bread and cereals, fruits and vegetables, beans, peas, and nuts.

Remember that, from the standpoint of tooth decay, how often you eat sugar is as important as how much sugar you eat.

Check labels for clues of sugar content; foods listing sugar of any type first on the ingredient label contain a large amount of sugar.

Correct misconceptions that carbohydrates are "fattening."

Reject diets that severely restrict carbohydrates; they can cause serious harm.

KEY IDEAS

Carbohydrates are the chief form of energy for the people of the world.

Starches, sugars, and cellulose (fiber) are the main forms of carbohydrate in food.

The kind of carbohydrate selected for consumption determines the nutritional contribution to the diet: whole grains, enriched cereal products, fruits, and vegetables provide vitamins, minerals, and fiber; sugars, sweets, and unenriched refined cereals provide little other than energy.

Carboydrates are classified as monosaccharides (simple sugars), disaccharides (double sugars), and polysaccharides (mainly starches).

All carbohydrates must be reduced to single sugars (monosaccharides) before they can be absorbed into the bloodstream.

Glucose is the form in which carbohydrates circulate in the bloodstream. All carbohydrate is converted to glucose in the body. It can also be formed from protein.

The hormone insulin lowers blood sugar and greatly influences the utilization of carbohydrate and the regulation of the blood sugar level. Some other hormones, notably glucagon, raise the blood sugar level.

Carbohydrate is the body's most economical and efficient source of energy.

Carbohydrate in excess of the body's energy needs is stored in limited amounts in the liver and muscle; amounts in excess of these needs is converted to fat and stored as fat tissue.

Carbohydrate spares protein, which then can be used for tissue building and repair rather than energy.

Some carbohydrate is needed for the proper utilization of fat; in the absence of carbohydrate, fats are not completely burned, and ketosis results. Severe restriction of carbohydrate in reducing diets can cause serious damage.

Carbohydrates are important components of certain substances needed for regulating body processes; they also encourage the growth of beneficial bacteria, which are involved in the production of certain vitamins and in the absorption of calcium and phosphorus.

Fiber promotes normal functioning of the lower intestinal tract; consumption of fiber tends to be low in the American diet.

Food sources of carbohydrate include cereal grains, fruits, vegetables, nuts, milk, and concentrated sweets.

Milling of cereal grains results in the loss of vitamins and minerals; however, the nutritional quality of milled (refined) cereal products is improved by enrichment, the addition of iron and the vitamins thiamine, niacin, and riboflavin.

Overconsumption of sugar promotes obesity and dental caries and frequently leads to a diet of poor nutritional quality.

A high-fiber diet has proved useful in reducing the symptoms of some disorders of the colon.

Diabetes mellitus, lactose intolerance, and galactosemia are examples of diseases in

which carbohydrates are not utilized normally.
Other than its caloric value of 7 kcal/g,

alcohol provides no nutrients; the chronic alcoholic is frequently malnourished.

KEYS TO LEARNING: STUDY–DISCUSSION QUESTIONS

1. Keep a food diary of all you eat and drink for one day.* Include all items, even gum, candy, diet drinks, tea, and diet soda. State the amount you have eaten; for example, ½ cup of peas, 2 slices of baked ham, 1 glass (8 ounces) of whole milk, ⅛ of a 9-inch apple pie. Estimate the amount of fat and sugar used in cooking and added at the table and add these to your record. Using this record, list those foods that supply carbohydrate. Using Table A-1, in the Appendix, record the amount of carbohydrate in each food.
2. What is the function of fiber in the diet? What are good sources of fiber? What foods in your food diary contain important amounts of fiber? Do you think you are consuming an adequate amount of fiber?
3. Rank the following foods by carbohydrate content, beginning with the food that has the most carbohydrate:

    a. 1 orange
    b. 1 medium baked potato
    c. 1/12 of a devil's food cake with icing (made from a mix)
    d. 1 slice of whole-wheat bread
    e. ½ cup of summer squash, cooked (zucchini)
    f. ½ cup cooked oatmeal

    Check your answers with the carbohydrate listed for each in Table A-1 in the Appendix.

4. Rank the following vegetables by carbohydrate content, beginning with the one that has the most carbohydrate:

    a. ½ cup of green snap beans, cooked
    b. ½ cup of cooked carrots
    c. 1 baked potato
    d. 1 sweet potato
    e. 1 small stalk of broccoli, cooked

    Check your answers with Table A-1.
5. If a person's carbohydrate intake is greater than his energy needs, what happens to the excess? fattening? Explain your answer.
6. Measures have been taken to improve the nutritional quality of refined cereal products. Why has this been necessary? Explain the terms *enriched bread* and *enriched rice.* Why are whole-grain products preferable to enriched products?
7. Discuss in class the overconsumption of refined and processed sugar in the United States. What are some of the harmful effects of this trend? In dental caries, the kind of sugar and the frequency with which it is eaten appears to be more important than the total amount consumed. Explain.
8. Why are reducing diets that severely restrict carbohydrate dangerous?

Bibliography is found at the end of Part Two.

* Save this record for use in subsequent chapters.

Fats

KEY TERMS

adipose   Containing fat, like adipose tissue.

atherosclerosis   Thickening of the inside wall of arteries by soft, cellular, and fatty deposits, called *atheromas* or *atheromatous plaques,* that narrow the arteries and hinder blood flow.

cholesterol   A fatlike compound occurring in bile, blood, brain and nerve tissue, liver, and other parts of the body; occurs in animal foods; is found in fatty deposits that line the inner wall of the artery in atherosclerosis.

chylomicrons   Small particles in the blood containing fats absorbed from the intestinal tract.

fatty acids   Organic acids that combine with glycerol to form fat. Essential fatty acids are those that cannot be produced by the body and must be obtained in the diet.

hydrogenation   The addition of hydrogen to a liquid fat, changing it to a solid or semisolid state. Generally, the harder the product, the higher is the degree of saturation with hydrogen.

lecithin   A phospholipid containing choline. It is used commercially as an emulsifier. In the body, it has an important role in the absorption and transport of fat and in nerve and brain tissue. It is synthesized by the body.

lipid   Fat or a fatlike substance that is insoluble in water and contains one or more fatty acids in its chemical structure.

lipoprotein   A combination of protein with a fat.

molecule   The smallest quantity into which a specific substance may be divided.

phospholipid   A lipid that contains phosphorus, fatty acids, and a nitrogenous base; important in fat metabolism and nerve and brain tissue.

prostaglandins   A group of extremely active hormonelike compounds derived from essential fatty acids and present in many tissues; are referred to as local hormones because they are synthesized within the cell and are metabolically active locally.

satiety value   A food's ability to produce a feeling of fullness.

saturated   United with the greatest possible amount of another substance. A *saturated fatty acid* is one in which the fatty acids are filled with hydrogen atoms, containing all the hydrogen they can hold. A *monounsaturated* fatty acid is one in which two carbon atoms are joined by a double bond; hydrogen can be added to each of the carbon atoms at this double bond. *Polyunsaturated* fatty acids have two or more double bonds; here, four or more carbon atoms can take up hydrogen atoms.

steatorrhea   Excessive fat in the stool.

triglyceride   A fat formed by the combination of three fatty acids and glycerol. Most animal and vegetable fats are triglycerides.

Fats receive more public attention than any other food group. The controversy over the relationship of food fats to cardiovascular disease is now many years old, and technical terms once used only by the biochemist and members of the medical team have become a part of everyday vocabulary. Terms such as *saturated fats, polyunsaturated fats,* and *cholesterol* are now familiar to the general public. Misconceptions continue to be held, however. In this chapter, these and other terms are explained, as are the functions and sources of fats.

Fats constituted 32% of the total kilocalories consumed in the United States in the early 1900s; the current level is 42%. But it is not unusual to find persons consuming 45% to 50% of calories as fat. This change in fat consumption over the years has been attributed to increased use of butter, oil, cream, and particularly red meats such as beef, lamb, and pork.

In more recent years, the use of fat in the home has begun to decline. A nationwide study conducted by the U.S. Department of Agriculture indicates that fat in men's diets decreased from 45% in 1965 to 42% in 1977. Consumers' demands for changes in the kind and amount of fat in the diet have led to the production of such items as low-fat milk, cheese, and frozen desserts; low-cholesterol egg substitutes; and leaner meats.

Characteristics of Fats

Fats are essential nutrients composed of carbon, hydrogen, and oxygen atoms in proportions that yield high energy. *Lipid* is the scientific name for fat. It applies to a group of substances, both animal and plant, that have a greasy, oily, or waxy consistency. The main characteristics of all lipids are that they are insoluble in water and that they contain one or more fatty acids in their chemical structure.

Fatty Acids

Fat is composed mostly of fatty acids. A fatty acid is a substance made up of a chain of carbon atoms to which hydrogen atoms and some oxygen atoms are attached. The characteristics of flavor, texture, melting point, and nutritive value depend upon the kind of fatty acids a fat contains. A food fat, whether a solid or an oil, contains a mixture of fatty acids; butter, for example, contains more than 29 different fatty acids. All fats and oils, regardless of their fatty acid content, have the same energy value.

The length of the carbon chain and the number of hydrogen atoms in a fatty acid are factors that have nutritional significance.

Length of the Carbon Chain

Fatty acids are grouped according to the length of their carbon chain as follows: short-chain, 4 to 6 carbons; medium-chain, 8 to 12 carbons; and long-chain, more than 12 carbons. The length of the carbon chain affects the ease with which fats are absorbed from the intestinal tract. Long-chain fatty acids require bile salts and must combine with other substances to be absorbed. Short- and medium-chain fatty acids are more readily hydrolyzed, absorbed, and transported. Most natural fats are composed of long-chain fatty acids, which pose a problem in diseases in which fats are poorly absorbed. MCT Oil*, an oil composed of medium-chain fatty acids, is a commercial product developed for use in these malabsorption disorders.

Degree of Saturation with Hydrogen Atoms

Fatty acids are classified as saturated, monounsaturated, or polyunsaturated, depending on the degree to which hydrogen atoms are attached to the carbon atoms in the molecule. If the carbon atoms in a particular fatty acid have attached to them all the hydrogen atoms they can hold, the fatty acid is said to be *saturated.* If some hydrogen atoms are missing and the carbon atoms are joined together by double bonds,

* Mead Johnson, Evansville, Indiana 47721

the fatty acid is *unsaturated.* Fatty acids with only one double bond in their structure are called *monounsaturated.* Those with two or more double bonds are *polyunsaturated* fatty acids.

Food fats are mixtures of saturated and unsaturated fatty acids. However, if a food contains mostly saturated fatty acids, it is a saturated fat; if it contains mostly polyunsaturated fatty acids, it is a polyunsaturated fat. Saturated fats tend to be solid at room temperature and are found mostly in animal sources. Unsaturated fats occur chiefly in vegetable sources. Oils contain large amounts of unsaturated fatty acids, with the exception of coconut oil, which is highly saturated.

Important Lipids

Triglycerides

Most food fats and the fat stored in the body are chemically known as *triglycerides.* A triglyceride is a compound formed from three (tri-) molecules of fatty acids combined with one molecule of glycerol. The principal difference between fats is the combination of different fatty acids with glycerol.

Phospholipids

Phospholipids are lipids that contain fatty acids, phosphoric acid, and nitrogen. The phosphorus–nitrogen part of the molecule makes the phospholipid partially water-soluble and gives it emulsifying properties. These properties have important uses in the body, as in the transport of fats in the bloodstream. Phospholipids also play a role in the structure of cells, the formation of certain enzyme systems, and the metabolism of fats. They are also useful in the commercial processing of foods as a smoothing agent.

Lecithin is the most abundant phospholipid in the body and in foods. It is produced (synthesized) in the liver in sufficient quantities to meet bodily needs.

Lipoproteins

Lipoproteins are the form in which fats are transported in the bloodstream. Because fats are not soluble in blood, which is basically water, they combine with protein to form substances that remain suspended in blood plasma. Lipoproteins are composed of triglycerides, protein, phospholipids, and cholesterol. Lipoproteins have been classified according to the amounts of these components they contain (see Chap. 22).

Cholesterol

Cholesterol is a waxlike lipid that normally occurs in the blood and in all cell membranes. It is a major part of brain and nerve tissue. Cholesterol is necessary for normal body functioning, as a structural material in body cells, and in the production of bile salts, vitamin D, and a number of hormones, including cortisone and the sex hormones.

Some cholesterol is supplied by food, and some is synthesized by the body. The average American has a cholesterol intake of approximately 500 mg to 800 mg daily, while the body synthesizes 2 to 3 times that amount.

Heredity, diet, emotional stress, exercise, and other conditions have an effect upon blood cholesterol levels. Persons with high blood cholesterol levels appear more likely than normal to develop atherosclerosis (hardening of the arteries). Polyunsaturated fats tend to lower blood cholesterol, whereas saturated fat and cholesterol in food tend to raise blood cholesterol. Monounsaturated fats do not appear to affect blood cholesterol levels.

Utilization of Fats

Before food fats can be absorbed into the bloodstream, they must be reduced to simpler compounds. Only about one third of the fat in the intestine is completely broken down to fatty

Table 8-1.   Summary of Fat Digestion

Site of Activity	Fat	Enzyme	End Product
Mouth		None	
Stomach	Emulsified fat	Gastric lipase	Fatty acids, glycerol diglycerides, monoglycerides
Small intestine	(Bile salts emulsify fats, allowing enzymes to penetrate more easily)		
	Triglycerides, diglycerides	Pancreatic lipase	Monoglycerides, fatty acids, glycerol
			Resynthesized in intestinal mucosa to form triglycerides
			↓
			To bloodstream via lymph
			Smaller portion enters blood capillaries

acids and glycerol, the remainder being absorbed in a partially digested state. Table 8-1 summarizes fat digestion.

Bile salts attach to digested fat substances and make possible their absorption by the cells of the intestinal wall. When the fatty acids enter the cells of the intestinal mucosa, the bile salt breaks away, and the fatty acids are converted back to triglycerides. These triglycerides, formed from dietary fat, combine with protein in the intestinal wall to form lipoproteins. Lipoproteins so formed are called *chylomicrons.* The lipoproteins then pass into the lymph duct in the center of the villus and are transported by the lymph to the bloodstream. They are then carried by the portal blood system to the liver, where they are converted to other types of lipoproteins, and then to the cells, where they are burned for energy.

Normally, 95% or more of dietary fat is absorbed. When bile is absent, as in the case of gallbladder disease or cystic fibrosis, fat absorption is poor, and fat is lost in the stools (steatorrhea).

Functions of Fats

Source of Energy

Fat is the body's most concentrated source of energy. Except for the cells of the brain and central nervous system, all cells can utilize fatty acids directly as a source of energy. Fat, in all forms and from all sources, provides 9 kcal/g, more than double the amount of energy provided by an equal weight of carbohydrate or protein. However, fat is not as readily available an energy form as carbohydrate, because the production of energy from fat is a more complicated process. Fat is more of a reserve form of energy.

Reserve Fuel Supply

Fat is an essential part of every cell wall and of the membranes within the cell. In addition, a

group of specialized cells called *adipose cells* have as their main function the storage of fat. Excess kilocalories, whether from protein, carbohydrate, or fat, are stored as fat. Fat that has been deposited in fatty tissue cannot be excreted; fat stores are reduced only when the caloric value of the food eaten is less than the body's energy needs and fat is released to provide energy. Thus, some fatty tissue is desirable, since it serves as a reserve fuel supply for circumstances in which food intake is low, as in illness.

Maintenance of Temperature; Cushioning and Protection

Deposits of fat beneath the skin help to insulate the body, protecting it from excessive heat or cold. Fat rounds out the figure and pads joints and other parts of the body, such as the soles, palms, and buttocks, protecting them from outside pressure. Fat protects the vital organs, such as the heart and kidneys, by holding them in position and protecting them from physical trauma. However, when there is too much fatty tissue, the body cannot work efficiently; heat loss during hot weather is impeded, physical movements are hindered, and various serious health problems result.

Source of Essential Fatty Acids

Humans require certain polyunsaturated fatty acids for their nutritional well-being. Linoleic acid, which the body converts to other fatty acids that are required, is the most important one. The body cannot produce linoleic acid, which must therefore be supplied by food. Thus, it is called an *essential fatty acid.* Linoleic acid occurs abundantly in vegetable oils such as corn, cottonseed, sesame, safflower, soybean, and sunflower.

The essential fatty acids are required for the transportation of other fats and for the synthesis of hormonelike compounds (prostaglandins) that act as regulators. A deficiency disease results when essential fatty acids are lacking. (This will be discussed later in this chapter.) Only a small amount of linoleic acid, about 1 tablespoon of a polyunsaturated oil used in cooking, is needed to prevent deficiency. Linoleic acid in other foods provides additional amounts.

Carrier of Fat-Soluble Vitamins

Fats serve as carriers of vitamins A, D, E, and K. Conditions that interfere with the absorption or utilization of fat reduce the amount of fat-soluble vitamins available to the body.

Meal Satisfaction

Fats add flavor and taste to meals. Fats remain in the stomach longer than either protein or carbohydrate because they are digested and absorbed at a slower rate. This prolonged digestion contributes to a feeling of fullness and delays the onset of hunger pangs. Fat is said to have high satiety value ("staying" qualities).

Because of its high satiety value and concentrated energy, fat reduces the total volume of food eaten. When fat intake is limited, a large volume of nonfat food must be eaten to provide the same amount of energy and to satisfy hunger.

How Much Fat?

Only small amounts (15–25 g) of polyunsaturated fats are needed to meet the body's need for linoleic acid. Beyond this, the Food and Nutrition Board has not recommended any specific amount for the general population.

In contrast, the U.S. Dietary Goals suggest substantial changes in fat consumption for the general population. They recommend a decrease in total fat consumption to not more than 30% of total calories (about 67 g for a person consuming 2000 kcal daily). A decrease in saturated fat, a moderate increase in polyunsaturated fat, and a restriction on cholesterol to 300 mg per day is also recommended. Putting these goals into practice requires a considerable

change in the eating habits of many Americans, as discussed in Chapter 13.

Sources of Fats

Fats and oils (liquid fats) are sometimes referred to as *visible* or *invisible*. Visible fats are those that can be easily identified: butter, cream, oil, margarine, bacon, and the fat that can be seen in some cuts of meat. Invisible fat is that which is "hidden": the fat in whole milk, egg yolk, dark meat of fish and poultry, pastries, nuts, and olives, and fat intermingled with the lean of meat.

The foods that contribute fat to the diet are whole milk and whole-milk products such as cream, butter, and cheese; eggs (yolk only); meat, fish, and poultry; nuts and seeds; and vegetable oils and hydrogenated products. All vegetables and fruits (except olives and avocados), cereal grains (except wheat germ), flour, macaroni products, bread and rolls, and sugars are practically free of fat. Figure 8-1 demonstrates the fat content of various foods. Table 8-2 compares the fat content and caloric value of normal portions of various foods.

Milk and Milk Products

The minimum fat content of whole milk is set by state law. The fat content of whole milk is approximately 3.3%, or 10 g per 8-ounce cup. An 8-ounce portion of skim milk has 1 g or less of fat. Homogenized milk is whole milk processed so that the fat is dispersed in the form of tiny globules suspended throughout the milk. Yogurt is fermented milk that has the same amount of fat as the milk from which it is made. Popular fruit-favored yogurts contain fruit preserves, which add considerably to their sugar and caloric content. Even some yogurts made from low-fat milk may supply as much as 250 kcal to 270 kcal per 8 ounces because of the

addition of ingredients such as sugar and fruit preserves.

Butter and margarine have equal caloric contents. Whipped butter and whipped margarine have about one third fewer kilocalories than unwhipped products. Diet margarine contains about half the calories of regular margarine.

Cheeses made partially from skim milk are lower in fat than those made entirely from whole milk (see Table 8-2). However, even the part-skim products contain appreciable quantities of fat. Dry curd, uncreamed cottage cheese, and 1%-fat cottage cheese are low in fat.

Meat, Fish, Poultry

The total fat content of fish ranges from 1% to more than 12% by weight. Shellfish such as oysters, clams, shrimp, lobster, and scallops are practically fat-free. Mackerel, salmon, tuna, and herring are fatty fish. However, even the fish with the highest fat content is relatively low in fat when compared with some meat cuts such as market-ground hamburger, which may be 28% fat. Poultry (without the skin) is also relatively low in fat, ranging from 4% to 8%.

The quantity of fat varies with the animal and with the grade and cut of meat. The highest grades of beef, prime and choice, contain the most marbled fat (lean interlaced with fat). Because marbled fat cannot be trimmed away, it furnishes a significant source of saturated fat and calories.

The fat content of pork and lamb is approximately equal to that of beef; the range for all meats is from 6% for very lean cuts to 36% for the lean and fat of a rib roast of beef. Veal is much lower in fat. Although pork has been considered a high-fat food, pork from which visible fat has been removed is no higher in fat than other meats. Low-marbled ham is considered a lean cut of meat. Roast pork and pork chops are medium lean cuts. Pork has less saturated fat and more linoleic acid than either beef or lamb.

Luncheon meats, bacon, frankfurters, and sausage are relatively high in fat. Bologna and liverwurst are approximately 28% fat; cooked

Amounts of Fat in Average Servings

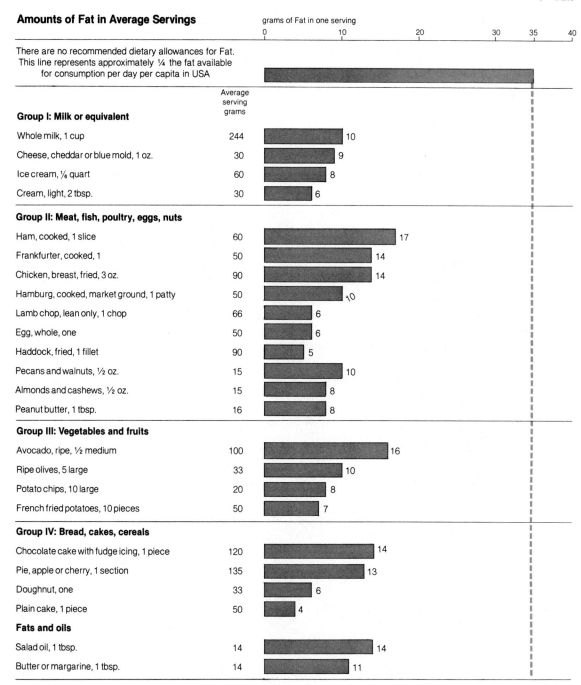

Fig. 8-1.   Fat in average servings of foods. (Anderson L, Turkki P, Mitchell H et al: Nutrition in Health and Disease, 17th ed. Philadelphia, JB Lippincott, 1982)

Table 8-2.   Fat Content of Some Common Foods

Foods	Fat Content (g)	Total kcal*
Milks and Yogurt	per cup	per cup
Skim milk (milk solids added)	1	90
Low-fat milk (1%)	3	100
Low-fat milk (2%)	5	120
Whole milk (3.3%)	8	150
Low-fat yogurt, plain	4	145
Low-fat yogurt, fruit-flavored	3	230†
Table Fats	per tablespoon	per tablespoon
Butter	12	100
Margarine	12	100
Whipped butter or margarine	8	65
Mayonnaise	11	100
Creams	per tablespoon	per tablespoon
Half & Half	2	20
Sour cream	3	30
Nondairy whipped topping (frozen)	1	15
Liquid nondairy coffee lightener	1	20
Powdered nondairy coffee lightener	1 (per tea-spoon)	10 (per teaspoon)
Desserts	per ½ cup	per ½ cup
Ice cream (11% fat)	7	135
Ice cream, soft serve	12	188
Ice milk (4.3% fat)	3	93
Sherbet	2	135‡
	per portion	per portion
Apple pie, ⅐ of 9″ pie	15	345
Danish pastry, 4¼″ diam. × 1″ deep	15	275
Doughnut, glazed 3-¾″ × 1¼″ deep	11	205
Cheese	per ounce	per ounce
Cheddar	9	115
American processed cheese	9	105
Part-skim mozzarella	5	80
Cottage cheese (4% fat)	5 (½ cup)	118
Cottage cheese (1% fat)	1 (½ cup)	82

Table 8-2.   (*continued*)

Foods	Fat Content (g)	Total kcal*
Meat, Fish, Poultry	per 3-ounce serving	per 3-ounce serving
Ham, lean and fat	19	245
Shrimp	1	100
Rib roast, lean and fat	33	375
Ground beef, 21% fat	17	235
Ground beef, 10% fat	10	185
Turkey, light meat	3	150

(Nutritive Value of Foods. USDA Home and Garden Bulletin 72, 1981)
* Total kilocalories represent the kilocalories not only from fat, but also from the protein and carbohydrate the food may contain.
† Fat content is relatively low, but sugar content raises total calories.

link or bulk pork sausage is 44% fat, and bacon is 52% fat.

Plant Sources

Vegetables and fruits, with the exception of olives and avocados, contain less than 1% fat. Avocados are about 16% fat, and ripe olives are 20% fat. Fresh coconut is 35% fat; other nuts and seeds (such as sunflower seeds) range from 60% to 70% fat. Vegetable oils are 100% fat and make a significant contribution to our fat intake.

Saturated Fats

Saturated fatty acids occur mostly in animal fats like whole milk and whole-milk products such as cream, butter, and cheese; ice cream; egg yolk; and meat fat and fatty meats such as beef, lamb, ham, pork, bacon, lard, salt pork, and beef tallow.

There are, however, three plant fats that are highly saturated: coconut oil, palm oil, and cocoa butter. Chocolate fat is equal in saturation to most saturated animal fat, about 55%, and coconut oil is more than 80% saturated.

The presence of chocolate in foods is obvious, but the presence of coconut oil or palm oil is not as easily detected and may provide a hidden source of saturated fat. Coconut oil and palm oil are low in cost and bland in flavor and therefore are used widely in commercial foods. Coconut oil is used in the manufacture of most nondairy dessert toppings and coffee lighteners. Ice milk and blended cooking oils may also contain coconut oil.

Hydrogenated Vegetable Oils

Solid vegetable shortenings and some margarines are a source of saturated fat. These are produced by a process called *hydrogenation* in which hydrogen is added to polyunsaturated vegetable oils, hardening and partially saturating the fat. Some margarines have a high percentage of polyunsaturated fat. These are described below under Polyunsaturated Fats.

Labeling

Such descriptions as "made of pure vegetable oil," "no animal fat," and "no butterfat" may lead a person to believe that a product is low in

saturated fat. However, if the product is made with coconut oil, palm oil, or hydrogenated vegetable oil, it may contain a considerable amount of saturated fat.

Federal labeling regulations help consumers make wise choices. If a claim about the fat content of a product is made, specific information must be provided about the amount of polyunsaturated and saturated fats (in grams) it contains per serving.

Polyunsaturated Fats

Polyunsaturated fatty acids occur in safflower, sunflower, corn, cottonseed, soybean, and sesame oils; salad dressings that are made from these oils (and that do not contain sour cream or cheese); special margarines that contain a high percentage of liquid oil; and fatty fish, such as mackerel, salmon, and herring.

Special margarines with a high percentage of polyunsaturated fatty acids are available. These products can be identified by a careful reading of labels. Those that list liquid oil as the first ingredient contain more polyunsaturated fat than saturated fat.

Monounsaturated Fats

Monounsaturated fats predominate in olives and peanuts and the oils made from them. Some nuts, such as pecans and Brazil nuts, contain appreciable quantities of monounsaturated fats.

Cholesterol

Cholesterol occurs only in animal foods. Organ meats, such as liver and kidneys, and egg yolk are very rich sources of cholesterol. Shrimp is moderately high. Other sources are meat, fish, poultry, whole milk, and foods made from whole milk or butter fat.

Cereals, nuts, fruits, and vegetables are free of cholesterol. However, a food may be low in cholesterol but high in saturated fat if it contains hydrogenated fats, chocolate, coconut oil, or palm oil. Saturated fat appears to be at least as important as cholesterol in controlling blood cholesterol. Don't be misled by "low cholesterol" labels on food packages, which imply that cholesterol alone plays a role.

Fat Intake and Health

Medical scientists associate the high fat content of the American diet with several major public health problems: coronary heart and blood vessel disease, obesity, and cancer of the breast and colon. However, the link between fat and cancer has not been proved, and research goes on.

Coronary heart disease is the leading cause of death in the United States. Obesity is a health hazard that increases the risk of heart disease, diabetes, and other serious illnesses.

Obesity

Excessive use of fats contributes to obesity, a major public health problem in the United States. Fats yield 2¼ times the calories of either proteins or carbohydrates. In addition, fat usually occurs in a concentrated form, whereas carbohydrate foods tend to have a high water content. For example, 1 ounce of butter (about 2 tbsp) contains approximately 200 kcal, whereas 1 ounce of snap beans contains 7 kcal. This does not mean that fats should be completely eliminated from the diet. However, fats must be chosen wisely so that those that make the greatest nutritional contribution are consumed (see Chap. 20).

Atherosclerosis

Atherosclerosis is a disease in which fatty deposits collect along the inside walls of large or medium-sized arteries. These deposits clog or narrow the passageway. If blood clots become lodged in the narrowed vessels, the blood flow to

the heart or brain may be partially or completely blocked, resulting in a "heart attack" or stroke.

The cause of atherosclerosis is unknown. However, its development appears to be influenced by many factors, including heredity, obesity, diet, high blood pressure, high plasma cholesterol level, cigarette smoking, lack of exercise, hormonal factors, stress, and certain metabolic diseases such as diabetes. High blood cholesterol, high blood pressure, and cigarette smoking appear to be the three most important risk factors in coronary heart disease.

Most authorities agree that dietary changes for persons with elevated cholesterol levels are warranted. Research continues into the effects of dietary cholesterol on persons of normal health (see Chap. 22).

Essential Fatty Acid Deficiency

A deficiency disease resulting from a lack of essential fatty acids may occur in both infants and adults. Symptoms of essential fatty acid deficiency in infants include dry and scaly skin and a slower than normal growth rate. Breast milk contains a generous amount of linoleic acid, 4 to 5 times that of evaporated milk. This may account for the low incidence of eczema and other skin conditions in breast-fed infants when compared with infants fed cow's milk. Commercial infant formulas and precooked infant cereals are good sources of essential fatty acids. Essential fatty acid deficiency in adults is characterized by dermatitis and disturbances in fat metabolism. These problems have been noted in hospitalized adults who for several months received intravenous feedings totally lacking in fat.

Gastrointestinal and Other Diseases

Fats are usually restricted in diseases that interfere with their digestion or absorption. Examples include gallbladder disease, pancreatitis, and cystic fibrosis. Fats are usually not restricted in liver disease unless the bile duct is obstructed (see Chap. 25).

Seizure Disorders

The ketogenic diet, which is high in fat and restricted in carbohydrate and protein, is prescribed for children with seizure disorders who do not respond to drug therapy. This diet produces a mild ketosis and helps reduce seizures, restlessness, and irritability (see Chap. 25).

KEYS TO PRACTICAL APPLICATION

Remember that all fat is high in calories and that excessive fat contributes to obesity.

Be aware of the sources of fat — especially hidden fat — in your diet.

Reduce your intake of total fat, saturated fat, and cholesterol. This is a sensible guide for all persons of normal health.

Read labels carefully to determine the amount and types of fat contained in the food.

Do not be misled by the "no animal fat" or "low cholesterol" label on some foods. A fat can have no cholesterol but still be highly saturated if it contains coconut oil, palm kernel oil, chocolate, or completely hydrogenated vegetable oils.

KEY IDEAS

Fatty acids are the basic units of all fats; a fat's physical characteristics and nutritional activity depend upon the kind of fatty acids it contains.

The length of the carbon chain in the fatty acid determines the ease with which fats are absorbed. Short- and medium-chain fatty acids, although in short supply in natural foods, are more readily absorbed than long-chain fatty acids.

A fat is classified as saturated, monounsaturated, or polyunsaturated according to the type of fatty acids that occur in greatest quantity in it.

Most food fats and stored body fat are triglycerides, compounds formed from three molecules of fatty acids attached to one molecule of glycerol.

Phospholipids, composed of fatty acids, phosphorus, and nitrogen, are partially soluble in water and have important emulsifying properties useful in the body and in commercial food processing.

Lipoproteins, combinations of fat and protein, are the form in which fats are carried in the bloodstream.

Cholesterol, which is involved in the production of body cells, bile salts, vitamin D, and hormones, is obtained in food and synthesized by the body. High blood cholesterol levels appear to promote atherosclerosis.

Diets rich in saturated fat and/or cholesterol lead to elevated blood cholesterol levels; polyunsaturated fats appear to lower blood cholesterol levels; monounsaturated fats have no effect.

Fat provides essential fatty acids, the most concentrated source of energy, a reserve energy supply, a carrier for fat-soluble vitamins, cushioning and insulation for the body, and meal satisfaction.

Linoleic acid must be supplied in the diet in small amounts; a lack of linoleic acid results in a deficiency disease.

Foods that contribute fat to the diet include whole milk and products containing whole milk or butterfat, such as butter, ice cream, and cheese; egg yolk; meat, fish, and poultry; nuts and seeds; vegetable oils; and hydrogenated vegetable fats (shortenings and margarine).

Saturated fats are found in whole milk and products made from whole milk; egg yolk; meat; meat fat (bacon, lard); coconut oil, palm oil, chocolate, regular margarine, and hydrogenated vegetable shortenings.

Sources of polyunsaturated fats are safflower, sunflower, corn, cottonseed, soybean, and sesame oils; salad dressings made from these oils; special margarines that contain a high percentage of liquid oil; and fatty fish such as mackeral, salmon, and herring.

Sources of monounsaturated fats are olive oil and most nuts.

Cholesterol is found only in animal foods. Organ meats and egg yolk are very rich sources; shrimp is a moderately rich source. Other sources include meat, fish, poultry, whole milk, and foods made from whole milk or butterfat.

The saturated fat content of food appears to be as important as the cholesterol content in the effect on blood cholesterol; consumers should not be misled by ''low cholesterol'' labels on food packages, which imply that cholesterol alone plays a role.

High fat intake in the United States is associated with a high incidence of obesity and coronary heart and blood vessel disease. Persons with elevated levels of blood cholesterol are more prone to atherosclerosis than normal.

Fats are usually restricted in diseases that interfere with their digestion or absorption, such as gallbladder disease and pancreatitis (inflammation of the pancreas). A high-fat diet is used in the treatment of epilepsy in children who do not respond to drug treatment.

KEYS TO LEARNING: STUDY – DISCUSSION QUESTIONS

1. In your food diary, calculate your intake of protein, fat, and carbohydrate for one day by referring to Table A-1 in the Appendix. Be sure to include the fat used in cooking and the fat and sugar used for flavoring food. These may have to be estimated. Calculate the percentage of total kilocalories that come from fat. How does this compare with the average fat consumption in the United States? With the amount of fat recommended by the U.S. Dietary Goals? (To calculate the percentage of total kilocalories derived from fat, first obtain your total daily kilocaloric intake by multiplying the grams of protein and carbohydrate by 4 and the grams of fat by 9. Then divide the fat kilocalories by the total kilocalories for the day.)

2. Classify the following as saturated, monounsaturated, or polyunsaturated: lamb chops, nondairy whipped topping, mayonnaise, olive oil, regular margarine, scrambled eggs, hamburger patty, vanilla ice cream, baked mackerel, devil's food cake with chocolate icing, corn oil, butter.

3. Rank the following foods according to fat content, listing the one with the highest fat content first:

   ½ cup of ice cream
   1 cup of whole milk
   3 ounces of sirloin steak
   20 large potato chips
   1 glazed doughnut
   2 pieces of light meat turkey
   (4 × 2 × ½'')

   Check your answer with the fat content listed for each of the above in Table A-1.

4. What are the functions of cholesterol? Is food the only source of cholesterol? Why might a label claiming that a product is ''low in cholesterol'' be misleading to the consumer who is attempting to control blood cholesterol levels?

5. Discuss in class the controversy concerning the role of fat in the development of atherosclerosis. What is the philosophy of the medical staff at your hospital — internists and pediatricians — concerning fat modification for those ''at risk'' and for the general public? A hospital staff member — physician or dietitian — might be asked to assist you in your discussion.

Bibliography is found at the end of Part Two.

Proteins

KEY TERMS

amino acids Compounds containing nitrogen that are the building blocks of the protein molecule.

antibody A protein substance produced within the body that destroys or weakens harmful bacteria.

biologic value of protein The ability of a protein to support the formation of body tissue.

complementary proteins The combination of protein foods that have opposite strengths and weaknesses in their amino acid compositions.

complete protein A protein containing all the essential amino acids.

edema Swelling; a condition in which body tissues contain an excessive amount of body fluid.

essential amino acids Amino acids that cannot be synthesized by the body and must be provided by food.

immobility The condition of being inactive owing to disability, such as that experienced by the person confined to bed or a wheelchair.

incomplete protein A protein lacking one or more of the essential amino acids or containing some of the amino acids in only very small amounts.

kwashiorkor A severe protein deficiency disease that occurs in infancy or early childhood.

lactation The secretion of milk.

marasmus A condition characterized by a loss of flesh and strength due to underfeeding; a lack of sufficient calories for a prolonged period of time.

meat analogs Food manufactured from vegetable protein that are similar to animal foods in appearance, texture, and flavor.

nonessential amino acids Amino acids that can be synthesized by the body to meet its needs.

textured vegetable protein (TVP) Protein that is drawn from plant protein, spun into fibers, and manufactured into products that imitate animal protein foods.

The word *protein* originates from a Greek word meaning "of first importance." It well deserves its name.

In areas in which protein quantity and quality are inadequate, the physical characteris- tics of whole groups of people may be affected. The increase in height among Japanese youth in recent years is an example of the effect of nutri- tion on stature. It is due to increases in both the total amount of protein and the amount of

animal protein in the Japanese diet. Similarly, Japanese–Americans who have lived in the United States for a generation or more are taller than their ancestors. Because of a limited diet, the Japanese previously did not reach their hereditary potential.

Although it is difficult to assign priorities to the various nutrients, this study of protein will show that the quality and quantity of protein in the daily diet are of extreme importance.

Composition of Protein

All protein molecules contain carbon, hydrogen, oxygen, and nitrogen. Proteins are the body's only source of nitrogen. Phosphorus and sulphur are frequently present, and some proteins may contain other elements, such as iron (in hemoglobin) and iodine (in thyroxine). The structure of protein is more varied and more complex than that of either fats or carbohydrates.

Amino Acids — The Building Blocks

Proteins are large, complex molecules made up of amino acids. During the process of digestion, proteins are broken down and released into the bloodstream as amino acids. More than 20 amino acids have been identified; they combine in many ways, so that a single protein may contain hundreds, linked together in a long chain. The genetic code within the nucleus of every cell determines the pattern in which the amino acids are arranged to form a specific protein, such as muscle protein or liver protein. These 20 or so amino acids can join together in an almost unending variety of ways to form the thousands of different proteins the body requires. Amino acids are classified into two

groups: essential, or indispensable, amino acids; and nonessential, or dispensable, amino acids.

Essential and Nonessential Amino Acids

Essential amino acids are those amino acids that cannot be synthesized by the human body and must therefore come from food. Nine amino acids are essential for the human infant: histidine, isoleucine, leucine, lysine, methionine, phenylalanine, threonine, tryptophan, and valine. Adults require all of these with the exception of histidine. Whether adults need histidine has not been definitely determined (Table 9-1).

Nonessential amino acids are those remaining amino acids that can be synthesized by the body in sufficient amounts to meet its needs.

Table 9-1. Classification of Amino Acids

Essential	Nonessential
Histidine*	Alanine
Isoleucine	Arginine
Leucine	Asparagine
Lysine	Aspartic acid
Methionine	Cysteine
Phenylalanine	Cystine
Threonine	Glutamic acid
Tryptophan	Glutamine
Valine	Glycine
	Hydroxyproline
	Proline
	Serine
	Tyrosine

* Required for infants; adult need for histidine has not been clearly established.

Protein Quality

The cells of the body are composed mainly of protein. Protein makes up the membrane surrounding the cell and also occurs within the cell. During periods of growth, such as in childhood, adolescence, and pregnancy, the number of cells increases. Protein is required for this cell growth. In addition, in all stages of life, tissue protein is constantly being broken down and must be replaced by dietary protein. Proteins are also needed for the formation of enzymes, antibodies, and hormones.

Not all dietary protein is used for tissue growth and repair. How much is used depends upon the biological value of the protein, that is, its ability to support the formation of body tissue. The biological value of a protein is determined by two factors: its amino acid make-up, and how well it is digested and absorbed.

Amino Acid Composition

Proteins that contain all the essential amino acids in the proportions needed by the body have a high biological value. They are sometimes referred to as *complete proteins.* Proteins that supply only some of the amino acids in limited amounts are of low biological value and may be referred to as *incomplete proteins.*

The production of body protein will stop once the supply of just one amino acid is exhausted. This will occur no matter how generous the amounts are of all the other amino acids left. The essential amino acids that are not used for tissue building are broken down and used for energy. The body cannot store these amino acids for use later.

Animal protein is the best-quality protein because of its similarity to human protein tissue. Egg protein is considered to have the best amino acid pattern of any food; milk protein ranks next. Gelatin is the only animal protein of poor quality. It is completely lacking in two essential amino acids and has inadequate amounts of other amino acids. Animal foods such as meat, poultry, fish, eggs, milk, and cheese provide liberal amounts of complete proteins.

Plant proteins are of a lower quality than animal proteins because they lack sufficient amounts of one or more essential amino acids. Cereal grains such as wheat and rice are low in lysine; corn is low in lysine and tryptophan; and legumes have limited amounts of methionine. Legumes (beans, peas, lentils, peanuts, and soybeans), nuts, and seeds contain the best-quality plant protein. Although of lower quality than animal proteins, plant proteins make a very important contribution to the world's protein supply, as we shall see. When mixed together appropriately, they provide high-quality protein.

Digestibility

The degree to which a protein is digested also influences its nutritional value. Animal protein is more efficiently digested than plant protein. This is because digestive enzymes have greater difficulty reaching plant cells, which are surrounded by cellulose and woody substances. Thorough chewing aids protein digestion. Method of cooking also affects digestibilty. Overheating may destroy some amino acids or may cause the formation of products resistant to digestive enzymes. Cooking with water improves the digestibility of wheat protein and rice.

Complementary Proteins

Plant proteins are not all lacking the same amino acids. When a variety of foods are eaten in a meal, one protein food may supply the

amino acid another food is lacking. A food that provides the amino acid that is absent or in short supply in another is said to *complement* the other. For example, legumes are high in lysine and low in methionine; grains are low in lysine and high in methionine. When these foods are eaten together, they complement each other and provide high-quality protein. Combinations such as beans with rice and peanut butter with bread provide high-quality protein. It is the total amino acid content of the meal that is the important factor. It is essential that the complementary proteins be eaten at the same meal (Table 9-2).

Another way to improve the quality of vegetable proteins is to serve them with small quantities of animal protein food. Bean soup with small pieces of meat and macaroni and cheese are examples of nourishing combinations (Table 9-2).

Knowledge about complementary proteins is needed by the nutrition counselor. This knowledge can be put to good use in areas in which animal protein is scarce; as the world's protein supply diminishes, an understanding of *complementarity* will become increasingly important. The proper mixing of plant protein foods can provide combinations of about the same nutritional value as high-quality animal proteins. One such product is Incaparina, developed by the Institute of Nutrition in Central America and Panama (INCAP). This all-plant product meets the growth needs of very small children, even those suffering from severe malnutrition.

Table 9-2. Improving the Nutritional Quality of Vegetable Proteins

Protein-Rich Combinations	Examples
Legumes plus grains	Macaroni and bean soup
	Beans and rice chili
	Peanut butter and bread
	Lentil soup with rice
	Baked beans with brown bread
Legumes plus seeds plus nuts	Roasted soybeans, sunflower seed, peanut snack mix
Plant protein plus small amounts of animal protein	Cereal and milk
	Lentil curry (made with yogurt)
	Bean soup with small pieces of meat
	Macaroni and cheese
	Cheese pizza

Utilization of Protein

To be absorbed, proteins must be broken down to individual amino acids or small peptides (breakdown products of protein digestion composed of only two or three amino acids). Table 9-3 summarizes protein digestion.

The products of protein digestion are released into the bloodstream as amino acids and are transported via the portal vein to the liver and then to all the body cells. Some amino acids stay in the liver to form liver tissue itself or to produce a wide variety of plasma proteins. The remaining amino acids circulate in the bloodstream, from which they are rapidly removed and utilized by the tissues.

When amino acids are broken down, the nitrogen-containing part is split off from the carbon chain. Most of the nitrogen is converted to urea in the liver and excreted via the kidneys. It is the carbon-containing portion that is utilized for energy.

Table 9-3. Summary of Protein Digestion

Place of Action	Protein	Enzyme	End-Product
Stomach	Protein	Pepsin (in acid environment) ⟶	Large peptides (polypeptides)
Small intestine	Protein, polypeptides	Trypsin (secreted by pancreas) ⟶	Polypeptides, dipeptides, amino acids
	Polypeptides, dipeptides	Peptidases (secreted by mucosal cells of small intestine) ⟶	Smaller peptides, amino acids

Enter portal blood
↓
Liver
↓
Body tissues

Functions of Protein

Tissue Maintenance and Growth

Protein is essential for the growth and maintenance of body tissue. The body is said to be in a *dynamic state,* that is, the cells are continually being broken down (catabolism) and replaced (anabolism). The rate of turnover depends on the type of tissue. Some cells, such as those in muscle tissue, turn over every few days, whereas others, such as those in bone tissue, turn over much more slowly.

Daily total protein turnover is much greater than normal protein intake. When protein tissue is broken down, amino acids are released into the plasma to be reused for building and repair. It makes no difference whether the amino acids were originally made by the body or obtained from the diet; the body uses them for the same purposes.

Normal tissue growth in infancy and childhood and during pregnancy and lactation necessitates additional amino acids over and above those needed for tissue maintenance. As has been demonstrated in many laboratory studies, in the absence of adequate protein, growth is slowed down or even stopped (Fig. 9-1). A sick person's protein needs may be simi-

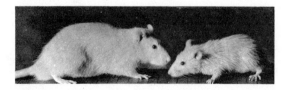

Fig. 9-1. Adequate and inadequate protein (18% vs. 4%) in rats of the same litter. This deficiency produces stunted growth but no deformities. (Anderson L, Turkki P, Mitchell H et al: Nutrition in Health and Disease, 17th ed. Philadelphia, JB Lippincott, 1982)

lar to a growing person's protein needs. Additional protein is needed to build new tissue for wound healing and for recovery from surgery, burns, fever, and other conditions that are associated with abnormally high tissue breakdown.

Formation of Regulating Compounds

Hormones, enzymes, and most other regulatory materials in the body are protein substances. Hormones such as insulin, thyroxine, and adrenalin have vital regulatory functions. Every cell contains many different enzymes, each of which is responsible for directing specific chemical reactions necessary to the cell's life processes. Another protein, hemoglobin, is responsible for carrying oxygen to the cells and carbon dioxide to the lungs.

Antibody Formation

Antibodies are proteins that assist the body in fighting infection and other toxic conditions. When the diet does not contain sufficient protein, the production of antibodies is slowed down, and susceptibility to infections is increased.

Fluid Balance

Proteins assist in regulating the fluid balance of the cells. Plasma protein molecules are so large that they cannot pass through the capillary membranes and thus remain in the blood vessels. The presence of these large molecules in the blood vessel creates the pressure needed to draw fluid back out of the cell so that it does not accumulate in the tissues. In a protein deficiency, the number of plasma proteins in the blood is reduced, and the pressure they exert is consequently also reduced. When there is insufficient pressure to remove fluid from the tissues, edema (accumulation of fluid in the tissues) results. Furthermore, hormonal changes interfere with the excretion of fluid. Edema is a symptom of severe protein deficiency.

Maintenance of Blood Neutrality

For normal function, it is essential that the blood be maintained at a nearly neutral, slightly alkaline (or basic) state. A change in pH (acidity or alkalinity), for example, can so alter enzymes that they no longer function. Certain foods can cause acids or bases (alkalies) to form. The presence of protein in the blood prevents the accumulation of too much acid or base. Proteins can serve as either acids or bases, according to body needs.

Provision of Energy

As described earlier, proteins can provide energy when kilocalories from carbohydrates and fats are too low. However, the use of protein for energy purposes is expensive in terms of both body needs and economics. If protein is used for energy, it cannot perform its many other vital functions. Most Americans consume more protein than they need. Because protein cannot be stored, the excess is converted to energy, which, if not needed, is then converted to fat. Because protein foods are the most costly foods, using protein for energy is an unnecessary expense.

Nitrogen Balance

Proteins are the body's only source of nitrogen. Each gram of nitrogen, whether in food, tissue, or urine and feces, represents 6.25 g of protein. Most of the nitrogen resulting from the breakdown of body tissue is excreted in the urine and feces. If 10 g of nitrogen are found in the urine and feces of a person within a specified period of time, it can be assumed that approximately 62.5 g of body protein were broken down during that period.

When the quantity of nitrogen from food proteins is approximately equal to the quantity lost in the feces and urine, the person is said to

be in nitrogen balance. Nitrogen balance indicates that body tissue is being adequately replaced and repaired and that there is no increase or decrease in total amount of body tissues.

In positive nitrogen balance, more nitrogen is taken in than is lost. Positive nitrogen balance is seen when new tissue is being built, as in infancy and childhood, in adolescence, in pregnancy and lactation, and during recovery from an illness or injury in which protein has been lost.

In negative nitrogen balance, more nitrogen is lost than is consumed in food protein. In other words, body tissue is breaking down faster than it is being replaced. Negative nitrogen balance is seen when protein intake is too low or of poor quality. Tissue needs for all the essential amino acids are not being met, so nitrogen is being excreted. Negative nitrogen balance also develops when a person is not consuming sufficient kilocalories to meet his energy needs. In this case, body protein is broken down to supply energy.

Body tissue breakdown due to surgery, injury, severe burns, and fever results in negative nitrogen balance, as does the inactivity imposed on bedridden patients, even when protein intake appears to be adequate. Muscles not regularly used break down rapidly and are replaced with fatty tissue. During early space explorations, astronauts experienced some breakdown of body tissue, attributed in part to weightlessness in a gravity-free environment. When exercise routines were introduced during subsequent flights, nitrogen loss diminished.

Sources of Protein

Because protein is a part of cell structure, it occurs in all foods, regardless of their source (Table 9-4). Nevertheless, the protein content of food varies widely (Fig. 9-2).

Animal sources of protein include milk and milk products (except butter), meat, fish, seafood, poultry, and eggs. Plant sources include cereals (wheat, rye, rice, corn, barley), legumes (peanuts, dry beans, dry peas, soybeans, lentils), and nuts and seeds.

Animal Sources

Meat, Poultry, Fish

Meat, poultry, and fish products are excellent sources of protein. The protein contents of beef, lamb, pork, fish, and poultry are nearly equal. Beef, the most popular meat in the United States, is wasteful when eaten excessively. Furthermore, it is high in kilocalories because of its relatively high fat content; a 3-ounce hamburger made from market-ground beef contains approximately 300 kcal.

Organs and glands (liver, kidney, brain, heart, and sweetbreads, all known as *variety meats*) are much richer in vitamins and minerals than muscle meats. Liver is very high in protein. Luncheon meats, such as spiced ham, liverwurst, bologna, and pressed meat loaves, various types of cold sausage and frankfurters, and cooked pork sausage have about half to two thirds the protein content of plain meat, fish, or poultry.

Some meats that are usually considered to be the basis of inexpensive meals may in fact be very costly sources of protein. For example, a 2-ounce portion of bologna or one frankfurter contains only 7 g of protein, whereas a 2-ounce portion of ground beef contains 14 g of protein, twice as much.

Milk and Milk Products

Milk is a less concentrated but very valuable source of protein. An 8-ounce glass of milk contains approximately 8.5 g of protein. Two 8-ounce glasses of milk provide half the daily protein recommended for a child 4 to 6 years of age. Milk should also help to satisfy adult protein needs. Fortified fresh skim milk or fortified reconstituted nonfat dry milk provide the same quantity of protein, calcium, and vitamins as fresh whole milk. Nonfat dry milk is an inexpensive source of milk protein (it costs approxi-

Table 9-4.   Comparison of Protein in Selected Foods

Food	Amount	Protein	Biologic Value of Protein
Beef round roast	3 oz	25 g	Complete
Leg of lamb	3 oz	22 g	Complete
Pork roast	3 oz	21 g	Complete
Veal cutlet	3 oz	23 g	Complete
Turkey, light meat	3 oz	28 g	Complete
Tuna in oil	3 oz	24 g	Complete
Bluefish	3 oz	22 g	Complete
Spiced ham	3 oz	13 g	Complete
Frankfurter	1 (2 oz)	7 g	Complete
Peanut butter	1 tbsp	4 g	Incomplete
Kidney beans	½ cup	7–8 g	Incomplete
Broccoli	½ cup	3 g	Incomplete
Carrots	½ cup	0.5 g	Incomplete
Applesauce	½ cup	Trace	
Orange	1	1 g	Incomplete
40% Bran Flakes	½ cup	2 g	Incomplete
Bread	1 slice	2–3 g	Incomplete
Egg	1	6 g	Complete
Nonfat dried milk	1 oz	10 g	Complete
Milk	1 cup	8 g	Complete
Cottage cheese	½ cup	14 g	Complete
Cheddar cheese	2 oz	14 g	Complete

(Nutritive Value of Foods. USDA Home and Garden Bulletin 72, 1981)

mately one third the price of fresh whole milk); in fact, it is the cheapest available source of complete protein. Its use should be encouraged when money to purchase other animal protein foods is limited.

American cheddar cheese contains 21 g of protein in a 3-ounce portion, equivalent to the amount of protein in meat. Cottage cheese contains more moisture and is therefore a less concentrated source of protein. Three ounces of cottage cheese provide about 12 g of protein. A 4-ounce portion of ice cream provides 4.5 g of protein.

Eggs

Eggs contain excellent-quality protein, one egg providing 6 g. The egg white is mostly protein and contains no fat or cholesterol.

Plant Sources

Most vegetables contain small amounts of protein. An exception is legumes, which may contain 4% to 6% protein when fresh and 7% to 9% protein in dried form. Fruits are poor sources of protein.

Amounts of Protein in Average Servings

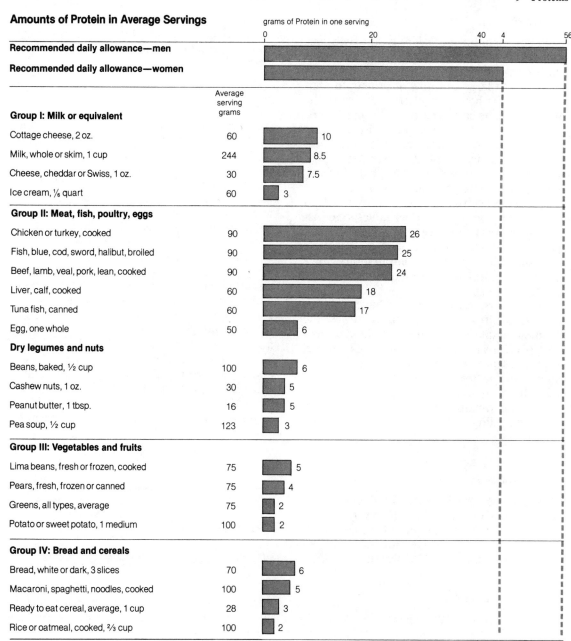

Fig. 9-2. Protein in average servings of foods. (Anderson L, Turkki P, Mitchell H et al: Nutrition in Health and Disease, 17th ed. Philadelphia, JB Lippincott, 1982)

Legumes

Legumes, including peas, lentils, kidney beans, navy beans, pinto beans, garbanzo beans (chick-peas), lima beans, soybeans, and peanuts, deposit large amounts of protein in their seeds with the help of bacteria that live in the plant roots. The bacteria are capable of converting atmospheric nitrogen to a form the plant can use. Because legumes provide much protein, they are useful meat substitutes. Lentil soup, split pea soup, chile beans, baked beans, lima bean casseroles, and peanut butter are good, low-cost substitutes for meat. Peanut butter contains 4 g of protein per tablespoon. Although the protein of legumes is not as high-quality as animal protein, it is an adequate substitute when eaten in combination with a mixed diet, particularly if it contains wheat or corn products.

In Eastern Asia, soybeans have been an important part of the diet for centuries; the Japanese obtain 12% to 13% of their protein from soybeans in the form of soy milk, cheese, flour, and sauce and from the beans themselves either dried or fresh. In the United States, soybeans have expanded from a minor crop to a major crop ranking second in value only to corn, exceeding wheat, potatoes, oats, and cotton.

Nuts and Seeds

Nuts and seeds provide substantial amounts of protein of fairly high quality. However, they are high in fat and consequently high in calories. Because they are expensive, nuts have not become an important source of protein in the diet.

Breads and Cereals

Breads and processed or cooked cereal products provide only small amounts of protein per serving. However, the wide use of these foods throughout the day makes a good contribution to the day's protein intake. A serving of cereal and one slice of toast at breakfast, two sandwiches at lunch, and two slices of bread at dinner provide 16 g of protein.

Cereal grains are the major source of protein for the world's people. Cereals eaten in a mixed diet with legumes and small amounts of animal protein provide all of the essential amino acids.

New Protein Sources

As scientists search for low-cost, protein-rich foods that will extend the world's lessening protein supply, we may note the following developments:

Textured vegetable proteins (TVP) are foods manufactured by the extraction of protein from certain oilseeds, such as soybeans, peanuts, and cottonseed, which contain no cholesterol and are low in saturated fats. The proteins are combined with colors, flavors, and other ingredients to create food products that resemble chicken, beef, tuna, sausage, bacon, and others. TVP are called *analogs* because they resemble other foods. They are useful substitutes for meat in vegetarian diets. TVP provide an inexpensive extender to ground meat.

Single-cell proteins, both microorganisms and algae, are being investigated as potential sources of protein food. Leaf protein, extracted from the leaves of many food crops such as beans and peas, is also the subject of research.

Production of Animal Protein

Most Americans associate protein with meat. In many developing countries, cereals provide 70% to 80% of the protein in the diet. Such a near-vegetarian diet is due to economic factors and a scarcity of animal foods. As income increases, the consumption of animal protein also usually increases. However, the production of animal protein is a wasteful process. Grain must be raised to feed the animals, which in turn are used as food by humans. It has been estimated

that only 15% of the protein fed to animals is converted to protein that can be eaten in the form of meat, milk, and eggs. The amount of grain required to feed the animals that supply the meat, poultry, eggs, and dairy products for one American for one year is almost a ton, enough to feed a number of humans directly. More energy is used to produce animal food than is obtained from consuming it.

Effects of Heat and Bacterial Action on Protein

Heat alters the structure but not the amino acid content of protein molecules. A protein food may be made more digestible and more palatable by cooking. Overheating may reduce digestibility.

Protein foods spoil more quickly than carbohydrate or fat foods. In the moist state in which they are generally found in foods, proteins decompose readily at room temperature. This breakdown is due to bacterial action, which may lead to the formation of poisonous substances. To prevent or delay spoilage, protein foods such as fresh meat, fish, poultry, milk, and eggs should be kept in the refrigerator.

Recommended Protein Consumption

Protein malnutrition is not a common problem in the United States. The average daily intake of protein, about 12% of total calories, is well above recommended levels. More than two thirds comes from animal sources such as meat, fish, poultry, eggs, and dairy products.

Age and body size greatly affect a person's protein needs. The larger a person is, the greater amount of living tissue there is to be maintained and repaired. Age provides an indication of whether more protein than the amount required for maintenance is needed for growth.

In 1980, the Food and Nutrition Board of the National Research Council recommended the following daily protein allowances for adults and adolescents: man (154 lb, or 70 kg), 56 g; woman (120 lb, or 55 kg), 44 g; pregnant mature woman, add 30 g; lactating woman, add 20 g; boy, 15 to 18 years (145 lb or 66 kg), 56 g; girl, 15 to 18 years (120 lb, or 55 kg), 46 g.

These recommendations are lower than the amounts of protein ordinarily consumed by Americans (Table 9-5). The recommendations of the Food and Nutrition Board represent more than minimum needs; they include a margin of safety to allow for individual differences in need and for the less than complete

Table 9-5. Protein Content of a Typical Day's Diet

Food	Amount	Protein
Milk	2 cups	16 g
Meat, fish, poultry, egg	4 oz	28 g
Vegetables		
Potato	1, medium	2 g
Other vegetables	2 servings	4 g
Fruits		
Citrus	1 serving	1 g
Other	1 serving	—
Bread	4 slices	8 g
Cereal	1 oz dry or ½ cup cooked	3 g
Butter, margarine, oil	1 tbsp or more	—
		62 g

utilization of protein in a mixed diet. The term *mixed diet* refers to a diet that provides protein from both animal and vegetable sources.

The daily recommended protein allowance is 0.8 g per kg (2.2 lb) of body weight, or approximately 0.37 g per pound. Adults over 50 years of age require at least as much protein as younger adults.

It is desirable that at least one third of the daily protein intake be derived from animal sources and that good-quality protein be included at every meal. If, for example, most of the day's protein is eaten at dinner, with very little eaten at breakfast and lunch, the body may be without an adequate source of protein for 24 hours, even though the total quantity is adequate.

Proteins and Health

The effects of protein loss during illness and injury are far-reaching. The most evident result is the wasting of muscle tissue and consequent loss of weight. Other symptoms include anemia and delayed healing of wounds and fractures. A lowering of serum protein levels and hormonal changes may result in edema, and the reduced production of antibodies makes the affected person susceptible to infection.

Protein losses occur following surgery and during serious illness and injury. The loss of protein is especially high after bone fractures, burns, and liver surgery. Persons on bed rest, especially elderly persons, lose protein even when their protein intake seems adequate. The ingestion of extra protein during convalescence promotes recovery.

Certain symptoms, such as impending hepatic coma in liver disease and chronic uremia in kidney disease, may require the restriction of protein.

Protein–Calorie Malnutrition

Protein–calorie malnutrition refers to a group of diseases caused by deficiencies of both proteins and calories and frequently accompanied by infections. A vicious cycle develops in which the malnutrition creates a susceptibility to infection and the infection further aggravates the poor nutritional condition. In children who are malnourished, common childhood diseases have very serious effects. The two major manifestations of protein–calorie malnutrition are marasmus and kwashiorkor. Protein–calorie malnutrition is the most serious and widespread deficiency disease in developing countries today.

Nutritional marasmus (wasting, emaciation) is caused by a diet severely deficient in kilocalories, as well as protein and other nutrients, for a prolonged period of time. It is seen most frequently in infants and is characterized by muscle wasting, loss of subcutaneous fat, and very low body weight.

Kwashiorkor results primarily from a deficiency of protein. A deficiency of calories is a contributing factor. Associated symptoms include retarded growth, muscle wasting, edema, depigmentation of hair and skin, enlarged liver, mental apathy, and general misery (Fig. 9-3). Children 1 to 3 years of age weaned from breast milk following the birth of a sibling or because the mother is again pregnant, are the victims. These children are abruptly weaned to a diet of grains or roots, which are difficult to digest and are poor sources of protein.

Between these two conditions are a variety of disease states that combine some of the features of each. Retarded growth is found in all forms of protein–calorie malnutrition. In general, marasmus is characteristic of urban slums and shanty towns, whereas kwashiorkor occurs most frequently in rural villages.

To prevent and treat these diseases where milk is not readily available, vegetable protein mixtures suitable for infants and young children have been developed. These mixtures are composed of locally grown foods. Incaparina, mentioned previously, is an example.

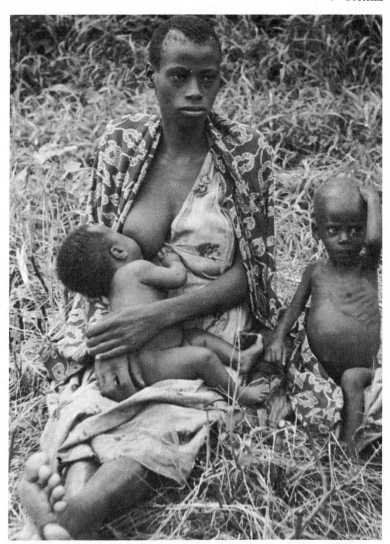

Fig. 9-3. The older child in this picture shows the protein–calorie deprivation and the malnutrition that occurred when he was "deposed" or replaced at the mother's breast by the new baby. He is subsisting on starchy foods and a few vegetables. (Courtesy John Bennett, M.D., Nutrition Unit, Ministry of Health, Kampala, Uganda)

Vegetarianism

The quantity and quality of protein in the vegetarian diets being consumed by many young adults in the United States are a cause for concern. Diets that are completely free of animal foods, including eggs and milk, are the most hazardous. With careful planning, the vegetarian diet can be made nutritionally adequate. This requires that a variety of plant foods be selected that supplement each other and thus provide all the essential amino acids. (See Chapter 14 for a more detailed discussion of vegetarianism.)

Abnormalities of Protein Metabolism

Some infants are born with the inability to produce enzymes that are necessary for the normal metabolism of certain amino acids. In one such

disease, phenylketonuria, the amino acid phenylalanine and its breakdown products build up in the blood (see Chap. 28).

A person whose digestive system is genetically unable to break down the proteins in specific foods to amino acids develops an allergy to those foods. In an allergic reaction, the body senses the offending protein as a "foreigner" and tries to reject it (see Chap. 27).

KEYS TO PRACTICAL APPLICATION

Eat moderate amounts of animal protein. Excess protein is wasteful, since the excess is converted to energy and excess energy is converted to fat. Protein food is an expensive form of energy.

Be aware of the wastefulness of using protein supplements under normal conditions. Most Americans consume more protein than they need.

Be aware that protein foods are not low in calories. They provide the same number of calories per gram as carbohydrates. Furthermore, protein foods (e.g., meats, cheese) frequently contain a good many calories from fat.

Eat some good-quality protein at each meal to provide a consistent supply of essential amino acids. Protein cannot be stored in the body.

Encourage the use of nonfat dry milk as a beverage and in cooking when funds are limited. It is the least expensive source of complete protein.

Plan some meals around complementary vegetable protein foods for variety, economy, and increased fiber.

Be aware that meals containing legumes and grains, frequently used by various nationality groups, are very nourishing.

Encourage elderly persons to eat sufficient amounts of protein. They need as much as, if not more than, younger adults.

Be aware of the importance of eating extra protein during illnesses, which cause excessive breakdown of body tissue.

KEY IDEAS

Proteins are composed of carbon, hydrogen, oxygen, and nitrogen; they provide the foundation of every body cell.

Proteins are composed of amino acids joined together in long chains.

Amino acids are classified as *essential,* those that cannot be synthesized by the body and must be obtained from food; and *nonessential,* those that can be synthesized by the body.

Whether a protein food can be used for the growth and repair of tissue depends on its biological value; proteins of high biologic value (complete proteins) contain all the essential amino acids in

adequate amounts; those of low biological value (incomplete proteins) may not supply all the essential amino acids or may supply some in limited amounts.

Animal proteins (except gelatin) are complete proteins; vegetable proteins are incomplete.

High-quality protein can result from complementary mixtures of plant proteins, in which one plant protein supplies the amino acid the other plant protein is lacking.

Protein provides for growth and maintenance of body tissues; is necessary for the

formation of substances needed to regulate body processes (e.g., hormones, enzymes); is necessary for the formation of antibodies, which help fight infection; assists in regulating fluid balance; helps maintain acid–base balance; and provides energy.

Protein in excess of body needs is converted to energy or to carbohydrate and fat; when there is a shortage of total energy, amino acids are used for energy rather than tissue building.

Body cells are in a dynamic state, continually being broken down and replaced; nitrogen balance studies compare the amount of nitrogen consumed in food with the amount lost in feces and urine to determine whether there is gain, loss, or maintenance of body tissue. In nitrogen balance, body tissues are adequately replaced and repaired; in positive nitrogen balance, new tissue is built; and in negative nitrogen balance, body tissue is broken down faster than it is replaced.

Animal sources of protein include milk and milk products, meat, fish, poultry, and eggs; plant sources include breads and cereal products, legumes, nuts and seeds, and textured vegetable protein.

Cereal grains are the primary source of protein for the majority of the world's

people; the production of animal protein is a wasteful process that will become less practical as the world's population grows.

The recommended daily protein intake for adults is 0.8 g per kg of body weight, less than the amount ordinarily consumed by Americans. At least one third of daily protein intake should be in form of animal sources, and some good-quality protein should be eaten at each meal.

Large losses of protein may occur during illness, requiring a substantial increase in protein consumption.

Protein–calorie malnutrition is the most serious and widespread deficiency disease in developing countries. The two major types are nutritional marasmus, due primarily to kilocaloric deficiency, and kwashiorkor, due primarily to deficiency of protein.

Vegetarianism requires careful planning so that a variety of complementary plant foods are eaten.

Some infants are born with an inability to metabolize phenylalanine, an essential amino acid; mental retardation results if disease is not treated.

The protein in specific foods is considered to be the cause of food allergies.

KEYS TO LEARNING: STUDY–DISCUSSION QUESTIONS

1. Using your food diary for one day, calculate your protein intake and compare your consumption of protein with the RDA for your sex and age group given in Chapter 4. Which food items on your record represent the highest-quality protein? How many grams of protein do they provide? How many grams of protein are derived from plant sources? How is the protein distributed throughout the day?
2. What are essential or indispensable amino acids? What is meant by the term

complementary proteins? Why is it such an important concept?
3. Why is it important to space the intake of good-quality protein throughout the day?
4. Protein is said to be an inefficient source of energy from both a physical standpoint and a financial one. Explain.
5. Each of the foods listed on the next page in the amounts given provides approximately 18 g of protein. Complete the chart by determining the cost of each item in your supermarket.

Food	Amount	Protein (gm)	Cost
Chicken, cooked	2 oz (figure 5 oz raw weight*)	18	
Pork and beans	1 ½ cups	18	
Flounder, cooked	2 oz (figure 4 oz raw weight*)	18	
Hamburger, market-ground, cooked	2 ½ oz (figure 3½ oz raw weight*)	18	
Bologna	5 oz	18	
Frankfurters	3, medium	18	
Sirloin steak	3 oz (figure 4 oz raw weight*, boneless)	18	
Tuna fish, canned	2 oz	18	

Which item is the least expensive source of protein? The most expensive source?

6. Exchange with your classmates recipes for meatless main dishes that are used in your family meals. Calculate the protein content of the recipes. Divide the total protein by the number of servings each recipe supplies to determine the amount of protein in one serving.

7. What are the symptoms of kwashiorkor? What age level is most likely to be affected?

8. Collect and discuss in class newspaper and magazine articles concerning international efforts to solve the problem of worldwide malnutrition.

* Raw weight allows for shrinkage and bone, if applicable. Figure the cost of sirloin steak by determining the weight of edible meat (estimate the weight of bone, or weigh the bone and subtract from the total weight of the steak).

Bibliography is found at the end of Part Two.

10

Water and Mineral Elements

KEY TERMS

electrolyte   A form of an element in body fluids that carries an electrical charge. Sodium, potassium, and chloride are common electrolytes.

homeostasis   A stable, balanced state of body fluids that maintains normal body function.

hydrolysis   A chemical reaction in which a substance is split into simpler compounds by combining with water.

hydrostatic pressure   Pressure created by fluids.

insensible   Not noticed; of which one is not aware.

interaction   Action between or among various factors.

interstitial   Pertaining to the spaces between the cells.

ions   Electrically charged molecules. Ions with a positive charge are called *cations;* those with a negative charge are called *anions.*

medium   A substance through which something acts or is done.

metabolic water   Water formed in the body as a result of metabolism.

osmosis   The passage of a solvent such as water through a semipermeable membrane from a solution of lesser concentration to one of greater concentration.

semipermeable membrane   A membrane that allows the passage of some molecules but not of others; a membrane that allows the passage of water but not some of the substances dissolved in it.

sensible   Noticed; of which one is aware.

stimulus   Something that causes another substance to react.

supplementary feedings   Food provided in addition to meals, usually for therapeutic reasons.

Water

Water, next to oxygen, is the body's most urgent need—more essential to life than food itself. Without water, nutrients would be of no value to the body. A person can survive for weeks without food but only a few days without water.

Failure to understand the role of body water contributes to health problems such as indigestion and constipation and even to needless death. For example, every year during sum-

117

mer training, several athletes die from exposure to heat. This is due to the practice of giving athletes salt while restricting their water intake, a practice condemned by the Committee on Dietary Allowances of the Food and Nutrition Board. Wearing heavy clothing that hinders the loss of body heat from the skin aggravates the problem. Another unhealthy practice among athletes is the restriction of water to control body weight. Water should be freely available to persons who have increased water loss owing to

heavy sweating. Depriving anyone of fluid intake can have very serious consequences, unless fluids are restricted for therapeutic purposes, as in some stages of kidney disease.

Water Distribution in the Body

Water makes up half to three fourths of body weight, depending on age and amount of body fat. Infants and children have a greater propor-

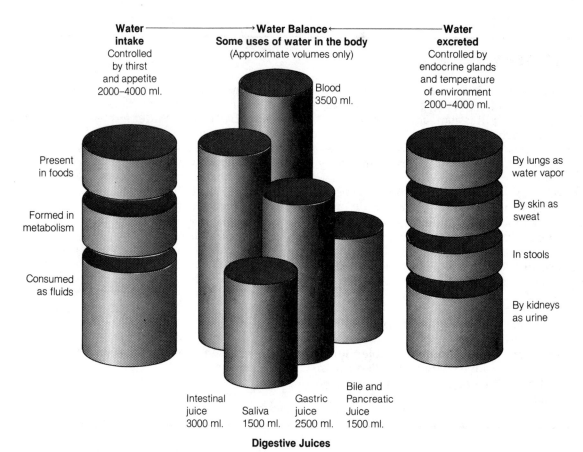

Fig. 10-1.   Use and balance of body water. Water intake and output can vary greatly between individuals and in an individual from day to day. However, healthy people can maintain water balance over a relatively large range of intakes. The daily use of water by the body greatly exceeds the daily intake. Recycling is possible because of the effective intestinal and renal reabsorption of water that flows through the intestine and the kidneys. (Anderson L, Turkki P, Mitchell H et al: Nutrition in Health and Disease, 17th ed. Philadelphia, JB Lippincott, 1982)

tion of water than older persons, and obese persons have less water than lean persons. Water is part of every body cell. This includes bone tissue, which is one third water. Water forms the basic substance of blood, lymph, and body secretions (Fig. 10-1).

Body fluids are held in compartments that are separated by semipermeable membranes. These membranes allow water to pass through yet prevent the movement of some substances from one side of the membrane to the other. Two thirds of body water is intracellular water, and one third is extracellular water.

Intracellular water, or cellular water, is located within the cell. It acts as a solvent for nutrients and for waste products produced by the cell; as an activator for biological reactions within the cell; and as a component of cell structure.

Extracellular water, water outside the cell, is divided into two body compartments: the blood vessels, and the spaces between the cells, called *interstitial spaces.* In the arteries, veins, and capillaries, as a constituent of plasma, water acts as a solvent for nutrients and for the hormones secreted by the glands. Blood vessels carry these substances to all parts of the body. Waste products such as carbon dioxide and ammonia are carried by the blood vessels to the skin, lungs, and kidneys.

The cells are surrounded by interstitial fluid. This fluid carries nutrients that have left the blood and transports them to the cell membrane, and it collects wastes and hormones secreted by the cell and delivers them to the membrane of the blood vessel.

Functions of Water

Water is essential to every organ. Its functions are as follows.

Chemical reactant

Water is the medium in which chemical reactions take place. In some cases, water acts as a catalyst; in others, water takes part in the chemical reaction. In its former role, as a solvent, water enables various substances dissolved in it to interact. For example, some substances develop an electrical charge when dissolved in water. An example of the latter role of water may be seen in the chemical reactions of digestion: the breakdown of starches to monosaccharides, the splitting of glycerol from the fatty acid molecule, and the breakdown of proteins to amino acids. A chemical reaction that requires water for the breakdown of complex compounds is called a *hydrolytic reaction,* and the process is called *hydrolysis.*

Solvent

Because very many substances dissolve in water, body fluids are capable of transporting nutrients and hormones to the cells and of carrying waste products from the cells to the lungs, skin, or kidneys.

Cell component

The intracellular water gives form and shape to the cell. When cells lose water, the cell membranes begin to collapse.

Temperature regulator

The burning of carbohydrates, fats, and protein for energy provides more heat than is needed for the maintenance of normal temperature. If temperature continued to rise without limit, cellular enzymes would eventually become inactivated, and normal function would cease. Excess heat is mainly gotten rid of through evaporation of water from the skin. Excretion of water in the form of perspiration occurs continuously; normal water loss from the skin accounts for 25% of total water loss. As a rule, a person is not aware of this insensible perspiration; he is made aware that he is perspiring only when in a hot environment or after heavy physical exercise.

Lubricant

Some body water serves as a lubricant: spinal fluid, ocular fluid, synovial fluid, and the mucous secretions of the respiratory tract, the

gastrointestinal tract, and the genitourinary tract.

Water is reused many times for different purposes. For example, the water that carries enzymes to the digestive tract also carries nutrients to the blood and the lymph. Although large quantities of water-carrying waste materials circulate through the tubules of the kidneys, most of the water and some of the useful dissolved material is reabsorbed.

Water Intake and Output

Water Output

Under normal conditions, water loss occurs in four ways: from the skin as perspiration, from the lungs as water vapor in expired air, from the kidneys as urine, and from the intestine in feces.

Table 10-1. Typical Individual Water Balance

Water Source	Volume (ml)
Intake	
Liquid foods	1300–1500
Moisture from solid foods	500–800
Water derived from oxidation of foods in the body	300–500
	2100–2800
Average	2450
Output	
Urine	1080–1650
Feces	100–150
Evaporation from the skin (sweat)	550–600
Expiration from the lungs as moist air	370–400
	2100–2800
Average	2450

(Burton BT: Human Nutrition, p 76. New York, published for HJ Heinz by McGraw-Hill, 1976)

Water loss varies from person to person. Table 10-1 indicates the average range of loss.

Water loss from the skin and lungs may be 50% to 100% higher than normal in persons living in hot, dry climates. Strenuous athletic performance or heavy work done in high environmental temperatures may increase water loss from skin and lungs 3 to 10 times. Abnormal conditions, such as diarrhea, vomiting, burns, hemorrhage, and fever, may result in large water losses.

Water Intake

Water is taken in the form of water as such; beverages, such as coffee, tea, fruit juices, and milk; and soups.

Solid foods contribute the next largest amount of water, as much as 25% to 50% of the water requirement. Some solid foods contain a high percentage of water. Fresh vegetables and fruits are 80% to 90% water; meat is 50% to 60% water; and even bread is about 35% water (Fig. 10-2).

Water formed within the body as a result of metabolism is called *metabolic water*. The burning of 100 g of fat produces 107 g of water, 100 g of carbohydrate produces 56 g of water, and 100 g of protein produces 40 g of water. Thus, the amount of water produced by the burning of fat is considerable. This metabolic water may accumulate from time to time, and its presence explains why some people experience a temporary gain in weight during weight reduction programs.

Water drunk and consumed in solid food is absorbed rapidly from the intestinal tract into the blood and lymph. Some water remains in the gastrointestinal tract and aids in waste elimination by producing a soft stool.

Recommended Water Consumption

A person's requirement for water may vary from day to day because of such factors as environmental temperature and physical activity. It is recommended that an adult in normal health take in 1 ml of water per kilocalorie

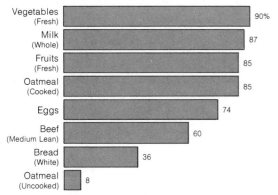

Fig. 10-2. Percentage of water in common foods. (Anderson L, Turkki P, Mitchell H et al: Nutrition in Health and Disease, 17th ed. Philadelphia, JB Lippincott, 1982)

expended; an infant, 1.5 ml/kcal. Thus, an adult burning 2000 kcal to 2500 kcal per day would require approximately 2 to 2.5 liters of fluid per day. Of this quantity, 1.25 to 1.5 liters (5 – 6 cups) should be consumed in the form of water. Persons working or living in hot environments and those engaged in heavy physical activity in high environmental temperatures or at high altitudes require more water.

Drinking water in moderate amounts before or during meals aids digestion by stimulating the flow of gastric juice.

The *sensation of thirst* is usually a reliable guide to water intake, except in infants and sick persons, especially comatose persons who cannot respond to the thirst stimulus. Some people seem to lack a thirst stimulus.

Special Situations

There are many instances in which the health worker must give special attention to the client's need for water. Since the end-products of protein metabolism are excreted by the kidneys, additional water is required for infants on high-protein formulas and for clients consuming high-protein diets or supplementary feedings. Wastes must be diluted to a certain level before the kidneys can excrete them efficiently.

Dehydration can occur rapidly in comatose clients and in disabled or elderly persons with brain impairment who are unable to respond to the sensation of thirst. Bedfast clients urinate frequently because their reclining position promotes urine production. The client may also perspire freely because he is heavily covered. Other conditions, such as fever, diabetes mellitus, vomiting, and diarrhea, and the use of various drugs, such as diuretics, also increase water need.

Minerals

Minerals are inorganic elements occurring in nature. They are inorganic because they did not originate in animal or plant life but rather from the earth's crust. Although minerals make up only a small proportion of body tissue, they are essential for growth and normal functioning (Table 10-2). Minerals are needed in such

Table 10-2.   Minerals

Macrominerals (Needed by the Body in Relatively Large Amounts)	Microminerals or Trace Minerals (Needed by the Body in Very Small Amounts)
Calcium	Chromium
Chloride	Cobalt*
Magnesium	Copper
Phosphorus	Fluoride
Potassium	Iodine
Sodium	Iron
	Manganese
	Molybdenum
	Selenium
	Zinc

* Human requirement for cobalt met by vitamin B_{12} intake. Appears to function only as an essential part of vitamin B_{12}.

small quantity that the units of milligram (mg; 0.001 g) and microgram (μg; 0.000001 g) are used.

Functions of Minerals

The functions of minerals may be broadly divided into two areas: building body tissue, and regulating body processes.

Building Body Tissue

Certain minerals, including calcium, phosphorus, magnesium, and fluorine, are components of bones and teeth. Deficiencies during the growing years cause growth to be stunted and bone tissue to be of poor quality. Adequate intake of minerals continues to be essential for the maintenance of skeletal tissue in adulthood. Potassium, sulphur, phosphorus, iron, and many other minerals are also structural components of soft tissue.

Regulating Body Processes

Components of Essential Compounds. Minerals are an integral part of many hormones, enzymes, and other compounds that regulate function. For example, iodine is required to produce the hormone thyroxine; chromium is involved in the production of insulin; and hemoglobin is an iron-containing compound. Hence, the production of these substances is dependent upon adequate intake of the involved minerals.

Some minerals serve as catalysts. For example, calcium is a catalyst in blood clotting. Some minerals act as catalysts in the absorption of nutrients from the gastrointestinal tract; the metabolism of proteins, fats, and carbohydrates; and the utilization of nutrients by the cell.

Transmitters of Nerve Impulses and Muscle Contraction. Minerals dissolved in body fluids are responsible for the transmission of nerve impulses and the contraction of muscles.

Maintainers of Water Balance. Maintenance of water balance is dependent upon the concentration of minerals in body fluids.

Maintainers of Acid–Base Balance. Minerals play an important role in the buffer systems in body fluids that help to maintain a normal acid–base balance.

Water – Mineral Balance (Homeostasis)

Despite continual change brought about by the many chemical reactions taking place within it, the healthy body maintains a balanced, stable internal environment.* A constant body temperature, water balance, and acid–base balance are maintained; heart rate, respiratory rate, and blood pressure remain within so-called normal limits. This tendency of the body to maintain a normal state despite opposing forces is known as *dynamic equilibrium* or *homeostasis*.

Practically all illnesses are a threat to this balance. Even in a healthy person, some circumstances can upset the balance, with serious consequences. Heavy physical activity on a very hot day, inadequate water intake, or a poorly balanced diet for extended periods of time can cause fluid and electrolyte disturbances.

Electrolyte Balance

Maintaining precise concentrations of electrolytes in the intracellular and extracellular fluid is a major aspect of homeostasis. Electrolytes are compounds that, when dissolved in water, dissociate (break up) into separate particles

---

* The interior of the body does not include the contents of the gastrointestinal tract.

called *ions*. The essential minerals sodium, potassium, magnesium, chloride, calcium, and phosphorus (as phosphates) are major electrolytes. Ions in solution have an electrical charge. Those particles that develop positive charges, called *cations,* include sodium, calcium, potassium, and magnesium. Negatively charged particles, called *anions,* include chloride, bicarbonate, phosphate, and sulfate. An electrolyte solution contains equal amounts of anions and cations. Milliequivalents (mEq) are the units of measure for electrolytes.

Electrolytes are required for the transmission of nerve impulses and the contraction of muscles. When a nerve is stimulated, the exchange of sodium and potassium ions across the nerve cell membrane creates a change in the electrical charge of the membrane, which passes the impulse along the nerve. Calcium ions stimulate muscular contractions; sodium, potassium, and magnesium cause muscular relaxation. The normal functioning of muscles requires an appropriate balance between these two forces. Electrolytes are also essential for maintaining water balance and acid–base balance (discussed below).

The quantity of each electrolyte in the fluid compartments must be maintained within a very narrow range, the amount differing for each electrolyte. An abnormal change in the quantity of any one electrolyte upsets the balance that exists among the other electrolytes, damaging body cells and preventing them from functioning properly.

A number of bodily mechanisms are constantly at work to maintain electrolytes at normal levels. These controls, which differ depending on the electrolyte, include the following:

Release or increased storage of minerals. For example, calcium stored in bone is released when serum calcium levels fall; deposits of calcium in the bone increase when serum calcium levels rise. These changes are regulated by hormones that are highly sensitive to changes in electrolyte concentration.

Excretion by kidneys. Hormones regulate the excretion or reabsorption of water and electrolytes by the kidneys according to need. If sodium intake exceeds body needs, water is reabsorbed and excess sodium ions are excreted.

Increased or decreased absorption from the intestinal tract. The percentage of dietary calcium absorbed from the intestinal tract is normally low. When serum calcium levels fall, a hormone stimulates increased formation of active vitamin D, which in turn increases the intestinal absorption of calcium.

Water Balance

Osmosis

Under normal conditions, fluid intake and output are in balance. Exchanges of water among various fluid compartments occur mainly as a result of osmosis. In this process, the quantity of a fluid and the direction in which it flows are determined by the quantity of electrolytes on either side of the semipermeable membrane. Water moves through the membrane to the compartment with the greater concentration of electrolytes.

Water balance between cellular fluid and interstitial fluid is regulated mainly by the potassium concentration within the cell and the sodium concentration in the interstitial spaces. If there is a loss or a gain of electrolytes in either compartment, the balance is disturbed, and more water passes into the compartment with the higher mineral concentration.

Water exchange between the blood vessels and the interstitial spaces is due to osmotic pressure and hydrostatic pressure. Osmotic pressure in the blood is determined by plasma proteins in the blood and by electrolytes in the interstitial spaces. Hydrostatic pressure is created by the pumping action of the heart on the fluid in the blood vessels. The hydrostatic pressure tends to force fluid out through the semipermeable membranes of the blood vessel walls into the interstitial spaces.

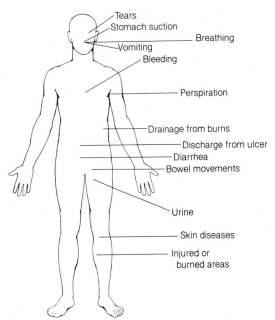

Fig. 10-3.   Ways in which water and electrolytes may be lost from the body. (Anderson L, Turkki P, Mitchell H et al: Nutrition in Health and Disease, 17th ed. Philadelphia, JB Lippincott, 1982)

Edema

The spaces surrounding the cells are more susceptible to changes in water volume than are the other fluid compartments. When too much sodium accumulates in the interstitial spaces, as occurs in congestive heart failure, more water is pulled into the interstitial compartment, and the involved area becomes swollen. This accumulation of water is called *edema*. Edema may also result from severe protein deficiency, in which the osmotic pressure exerted by proteins in the blood is lessened.

Dehydration

Excessive loss of water, dehydration, is a threat to life. Dehydration may be due to a lack of food and water or to losses of water in heavy perspiration, severe diarrhea, vomiting, hemorrhage, severe burns, or uncontrolled diabetes accompanied by frequent urination (Fig. 10-3). A 10% loss of body water is a serious threat, and a 20% to 22% loss is fatal. Dehydration is always ac-

companied by electrolyte imbalances. An infant becomes dehydrated more quickly than an older person, because there is a greater proportion of water in his body, and because much of this water is outside the cell and therefore easily lost.

Water loss due to excessive perspiration must be corrected both by an increase in the consumption of water and by sodium supplements to replace the lost sodium. If the sodium is not replaced, the sodium level will become highly dilute, with the serious consequence of heat exhaustion. (This is why persons who work in very hot environments are required to take salt tablets with fluids.) Symptoms of heat exhaustion due to dehydration are thirst, fatigue, giddiness, decreased urine output, and fever. Heat exhaustion due to sodium deficiency causes fatigue, nausea, giddiness, and exhaustion, but usually no fever.

Acid–Base Balance

Enzymes function only when the fluid within the cell is neutral (neither acid nor alkaline). Electrolytes play an important role in maintaining this specific environment. The amount of acid or alkaline (base) in a solution is expressed as *pH*. A pH of 7 is neutral; below 7 indicates acidity; above 7 indicates alkalinity. The reaction of the blood is slightly alkaline, pH 7.3 to 7.45.

This precise balance is maintained regardless of the acid-forming and alkali-forming substances resulting from metabolism. When foods are completely "burned," a residue remains. This residue is the mineral content of the food, or ash. Some ash forms acids when dissolved. Acid-forming substances predominate in meat, fish, poultry, eggs, and cereals, which for this reason are called *acid-forming* or *acid–ash foods*. Minerals that are basic in solution are found abundantly in most fruits and vegetables and are called *base-forming* or *alkaline–ash foods*. (Plums, prunes, and cranberries are the only exception. They contain an acid that is not metabolized by the body and is excreted as such.) Although milk and milk products contain both acid-forming and alkali-forming substances, alkaline substances predominate. It is

somewhat surprising that even citrus fruits, which have an acid taste because of their organic acids, are alkali-forming foods. The organic acids in citrus fruits are burned by the body, and the mineral ash that remains is alkaline in reaction. Some foods, such as pure fats, sugar, and pure starches, are neutral, since they are not sources of minerals.

Most mixed diets contain a surplus of acid-forming minerals. However, whether acid-forming or alkali-forming substances predominate, a pH of 7.3 to 7.45 must be maintained. The body has several mechanisms through which to maintain this aspect of homeostasis. In the blood are buffers—carbonates, phosphates, and proteins—that react with either excess acid or excess base to prevent changes in pH. The exhalation of carbon dioxide removes carbonic acid. The kidneys remove excessive acid and alkaline substances and produce ammonia, which neutralizes excess acid. Dietary factors alone seldom cause acid–base imbalances.

A condition known as *acidosis* results when the supply of buffers is depleted. Acidosis may be caused by starvation or by a defect in metabolism, as in advanced diabetes and in weight reduction diets that call for very low intakes of carbohydrate.

Alkalosis results from the accumulation of alkaline substances or a loss of acid. It is seen in persons who have had severe and prolonged vomiting with a heavy loss of hydrochloric acid from the stomach. The regular use of antacid medications is another cause of alkalosis.

KEYS TO PRACTICAL APPLICATION

Drink at least 5 to 6 cups of fluid daily. Drinking moderate amounts of water with meals can aid digestion.

Discourage the drinking of water with meals as a substitute for chewing. Chewing and mixing food with saliva is an important step in digestion.

Be aware of the importance of water intake for your clients, especially clients on high-protein diets; comatose clients; disabled or elderly clients with brain impairment; clients with fever, vomiting, or diarrhea; clients with increased urination due to diabetes or to the taking of drugs that increase urination; clients in hot environments; and infants.

Caution those who are in danger of upsetting the pH of the body either by low-carbohydrate fad diets or by the excessive use of antacids.

Encourage persons who are discouraged when they fail to lose weight although they are eating less. Explain that this may be caused by a temporary accumulation of metabolic water resulting from the burning of fatty tissue.

KEY IDEAS

Water is indispensable to life.

Body fluids are held in compartments in the body — two thirds within the cells, and one third outside the cells in the blood vessels and the spaces between the cells.

Water is the medium for chemical reactions; a solvent of nutrients, secretions, and waste products; a component of cell structure; a regulator of body temperature; and a lubricant.

Water is lost from skin and lungs, in urine, and in feces; it is taken in fluids and solid food; and it is a product of metabolism.

Depriving persons, including athletes, of fluid intake can have very serious consequences.

Under ordinary conditions, the total water requirement for adults is about 2 to 2½ liters daily. Of this amount, 5 to 6 cups should be consumed in the form of water.

A balanced, stable body environment called

homeostasis is required for proper body functioning; water and electrolytes play a major role in maintaining homeostasis.

A balance between fluid intake and fluid loss is reached mainly as a result of osmosis.

Water balance between fluid in the cell and fluid surrounding the cell is regulated mainly by potassium within the cell and sodium outside the cell.

Water balance between the blood vessels and the spaces around the cells is the result of osmotic pressure due to electrolytes and plasma proteins in the blood and electrolytes in the spaces around the cells. The pumping action of the blood also has an influence on water balance.

Edema occurs when sodium accumulates in the spaces between the cells or when there is severe protein deficiency, in which case the pressure exerted by proteins in the bloodstream is lower then normal.

Dehydration is a threat to life; loss of electrolytes accompanies the loss of water.

The blood maintains a slightly alkaline reaction, a pH of 7.3 to 7.45, regardless of the acid-forming and alkaline-forming substances produced by metabolism. This acid – base balance is maintained by buffers in blood, exhalation of carbon dioxide, excretion of excess acid or alkaline substances in the urine, and production of ammonia in the kidneys.

Minerals are components of body tissue and vital body compounds, transmitters of nerve impulses, stimulators of muscle contractions, and regulators of water balance and acid – base balance.

KEYS TO LEARNING: STUDY – DISCUSSION QUESTIONS

1. Estimate the amount of fluid you consumed yesterday. Include water, all beverages, milk, and soup. How does your fluid intake compare with recommended amounts? Why does the requirement for water differ from person to person?

2. How does the nurse provide for the client's need for water? What clients are most likely to require her attention in this regard?

3. Most illnesses upset the body's water and electrolyte balance. Discuss in class how this balance is threatened in those clients for whom you are providing care.

What measures have been taken to maintain or restore balance?

4. What causes edema? If dehydration is threatened as a result of profuse perspiration, why may salt tablets be advised?

5. What determines whether a food will have an acid or alkaline reaction in the body? What are some of the ways in which the body maintains a normal blood pH?

Bibliography is found at the end of Part Two.

11

Minerals, Macro and Micro

KEY TERMS

arrhythmia (*cardiac*)   Irregular heart action.

cretinism   A condition characterized by retarded mental and physical development due to a congenital lack of thyroid secretion.

endemic   Peculiar to a particular locality or population.

ferritin   An iron–phosphorus–protein complex; the form in which iron is stored in the liver, spleen, and bone marrow.

goiter   Enlargement of thyroid gland.

heme iron   Iron contained in the red pigment of blood; 40% of the total iron in animal tissue, including meat, liver, poultry, fish.

hemiplegic   Having paralysis of half of the body.

hemochromatosis   Iron storage disease.

hemosiderin   Iron-containing pigment obtained from the hemoglobin from disintegrated red blood cells; provides one means of storing iron until needed for hemoglobin formation.

hypertension   High blood pressure.

macrominerals   Minerals found in relatively large amounts in the body and needed in quantities of 100 mg or more.

microgram   0.000001 gram.

microminerals   Minerals found in small quantities in the body for which the requirement is a few milligrams or less.

nonheme iron   Sixty percent of iron in animal tissue and all the iron in plants and iron supplements.

osteoblast   A cell concerned with the formation of bone.

osteoclast   A cell concerned with the resorption (breakdown) of bone.

osteomalacia   A disease in adults in which bones become softened; caused by a deficiency of vitamin D and calcium.

osteoporosis   A disease in which calcium is lost from bones, which then fracture easily.

oxalic acid   A substance in some foods, such as spinach and Swiss chard, that combines with calcium, making the calcium insoluble and preventing its absorption.

phytates   Phosphorus compounds found in cereals that form insoluble compounds with some minerals, making them unavailable to the body.

trace elements   Minerals present in very small amounts in the body; also called *microminerals.*

Classification

Mineral elements are classified into two groups on the basis of relative amounts of each of them in the body. Minerals occurring in relatively large amounts and needed in quantities of 100 mg or more per day are called *macrominerals* (see Table 10-2). This group includes calcium, chlorine, magnesium, phosphorus, sodium, and sulfur. Minerals occurring in small amounts and needed in quantities of a few milligrams or less per day are called *microminerals* or *trace minerals* (see Table 10-2 and Table 11-1). The essential trace minerals are chromium, cobalt, copper, fluorine, iodine, iron, manganese, molybdenum, selenium, and zinc. As many as 30 other minerals occur in body tissue, among them lead, gold, and mercury. As far as is known, they are potentially harmful and are present in the body only as a result of environmental contamination. However, some trace elements formerly thought to be toxic have been found to be essential to normal body function. For example, the toxic effects of selenium were well known before its beneficial effects were discovered.

Interaction

The interactions among minerals and between minerals and other substances in the diet number in the hundreds. Absorption of iron is hindered by fiber and phosphates and promoted by ascorbic acid, copper, and meat protein. A high protein intake appears to increase the excretion of calcium, whereas vitamin D ingestion promotes the retention of calcium. These are but a few examples of mineral interactions.

Sources

In general, minerals are most abundant in unrefined foods. Processed or refined foods, such as fats, oils, sugar, and cornstarch, contain almost no minerals. Iodine, copper, and other essential trace minerals occur in some soils and drinking water and are lacking in others. Some essential minerals, including potassium, sulfur, chlorine, and sodium, are so abundant in the normal diet that deficiencies are not likely.

Nutrition authorities are concerned about the changes that have occurred in the nutritional composition of many foods in the American diet. These changes have resulted from advances in food technology and new manufacturing practices. The effects of the increased use of synthetic foods, such as textured vegetable protein, egg substitutes, and imitation fruit drinks, on the adequacy of the diet is questioned. The intake of trace minerals, some of which may not as yet have been discovered, is threatened by this trend. Excessive as well as inadequate mineral intake may result. For example, increased use of phosphate additives in food processing, although not harmful in itself, may result in changes in the calcium-to-phosphorus ratio, which in turn may adversely affect calcium metabolism.

Recommended Allowances

Because mineral interactions with other minerals and with other substances greatly affect dietary requirements, precise recommendations for mineral intake are not always possible. The 1980 RDA state recommendations for cal-

Table 11-1. Estimated Safe and Adequate Daily Dietary Intakes of Selected Minerals*

Age (Years)	Trace Elements†						Electrolytes		
	Copper (mg)	Manganese (mg)	Fluoride (mg)	Chromium (mg)	Selenium (mg)	Molybdenum (mg)	Sodium (mg)	Potassium (mg)	Chloride (mg)
Infants									
0-0.5	0.5-0.7	0.5-0.7	0.1-0.5	0.01-0.04	0.01-0.04	0.03-0.06	115-350	350-925	275-700
0.5-1	0.7-1.0	0.7-1.0	0.2-1.0	0.02-0.06	0.02-0.06	0.04-0.08	250-750	425-1275	400-1200
Children and Adolescents									
1-3	1.0-1.5	1.0-1.5	0.5-1.5	0.02-0.08	0.02-0.08	0.05-0.1	325-975	550-1650	500-1500
4-6	1.5-2.0	1.5-2.0	1.0-2.5	0.03-0.12	0.03-0.12	0.06-0.15	450-1350	775-2325	700-2100
7-10	2.0-2.5	2.0-3.0	1.5-2.5	0.05-0.2	0.05-0.2	0.10-0.3	600-1800	1000-3000	925-2775
11+	2.0-3.0	2.5-5.0	1.5-2.5	0.05-0.2	0.05-0.2	0.15-0.5	900-2700	1525-4575	1400-4200
Adults									
	2.0-3.0	2.5-5.0	1.5-4.0	0.05-0.2	0.05-0.2	0.15-0.5	1100-3300	1875-5625	1700-5100

(Recommended Dietary Allowances, 9th ed. Washington, D.C.: National Academy of Sciences, 1980)

* Because there is less information on which to base allowances, these figures are not given in the main table of RDA and are provided here in the form of ranges of recommended intakes.

† Since the toxic levels for many trace elements may be only several times usual intakes, the upper levels for the trace elements given in this table should not be habitually exceeded.

cium, phosphorus, magnesium, iron, zinc, and iodine.

General guidelines are provided for nine additional minerals. The guidelines given in Table 11-1 are called *ranges of safe and adequate intakes.* Exact recommendations are not given because of incomplete knowledge about the minerals, their interactions with other substances, and bodily regulation (absorption, excretion) of the amounts utilized. The ranges given appear to be adequate on the basis of current knowledge.

Macrominerals

Calcium

Calcium is the body's most abundant mineral. Ninety-nine percent occurs in the bones and teeth as deposits of calcium phosphates. The remaining 1%, present in the soft tissue and body fluids, has very important regulatory functions. Sixty percent of the calcium in body fluids is in ionized form, can move freely from one fluid compartment to the other, and can be filtered by the kidney.

Functions and Clinical Effects

Bone and Tooth Formation. Together with phosphorus and small amounts of other minerals, calcium provides strength and rigidity to the bones and teeth. The mineral portion of bone is largely a crystalline form of calcium phosphate. Bone salts are deposited in a strong base material consisting of protein collagen in a gelantinous substance. Small amounts of magnesium, sodium, carbonate, citrate, chloride, and fluoride are also components of bone.

Despite its hard, solid appearance, bone is active tissue, constantly being deposited and reabsorbed. In the healthy adult, the two processes are equally balanced. A turnover of about 600 mg to 700 mg of calcium occurs daily, an amount considerably greater than that absorbed

from food. The deposit of bone salts is controlled by osteoblasts, bone-forming cells, and the reabsorption (loss) of bone is controlled by osteoclasts, bone-destroying cells. In childhood, bone growth exceeds bone loss. In old age, bone loss frequently exceeds its replacement, resulting in a reduction in the amount of bone tissue (osteoporosis).

The calcium phosphate in teeth also occurs in the form of calcium phosphate crystals. However, tooth structure is much more stable than bone structure. There is little exchange of calcium in the teeth once they are formed.

Effects of Immobility. The stress of weight bearing stimulates the activity of the bone-forming cells, thus strengthening bone tissue. When an individual is bedfast or inactive for an extended period, the bones no longer receive this stimulation, so there is loss of calcium, phosphorus, and protein matrix (intercellular material). Osteoporosis may occur in a hemiplegic as early as 2 weeks following a stroke. The surplus serum calcium is excreted in the urine.

The excessive withdrawal of calcium from bone may lead to further problems. If the kidneys are unable to excrete the excess calcium, hypercalcemia, or high serum levels of calcium, results. Symptoms of this disorder include nausea, vomiting, gaseousness, headache, and reduced heart rate. In contrast, excretion of the excess calcium in the urine, or hypercalciuria, may cause the formation of bladder and kidney stones.

Blood Clotting. Calcium in the blood is needed for normal blood clotting. Vitamin K regulates the synthesis of calcium-containing proteins involved in a complex process that results in the conversion of a soluble plasma protein, fibrinogen, to a solid mass, called *fibrin,* which forms the clot.

Permeability of Cell Membranes. Calcium regulates the passage of substances across cell membranes.

Transmission of Nerve Impulses. Calcium plays a role in the transmission of nerve impulses.

Contraction and Relaxation of Muscles. Calcium is necessary for normal muscle contraction, including that of the heart.

Enzyme Activation and Absorption of Vitamin B_{12}. Calcium is an activator of certain enzymes, including pancreatic lipase, which digests fat and adenosine triphosphatase (ATPase), an enzyme involved in the release of energy for muscular activity. Calcium is also needed for the absorption of vitamin B_{12}.

Deficiency

Calcium deficiency usually goes hand in hand with inadequacies of other nutrients, such as vitamin D and phosphorus, and with other factors that affect calcium absorption and utilization. If nutrients needed for normal bone formation are insufficient, growth may be stunted; bone growth may continue, but the resulting bones and teeth will be of poor quality. The bowed legs, enlarged ankles and wrists, and narrow chest seen in rickets may result. Inadequate intake prenatally, when the teeth are being formed, may result in poor tooth structure, making teeth less resistant than normal to dental caries.

In some parts of the world, osteomalacia develops in women who have had repeated pregnancies and periods of lactation. This disease, sometimes called *adult rickets,* is characterized by poor bone calcification and resultant bone softness and flexibility. The bones are then especially susceptible to fracture (see Chap. 12).

In osteoporosis, there is gradual loss of bone resulting in a shortening of stature. Furthermore, the bones become porous and easily fractured. Symptoms arise late in life and progress more rapidly in women than in men. The disease does not appear to be due to a simple calcium deficiency; other factors, including a lack of exercise, a lack of sex hormones, and a lack or even an excess of protein, have been implicated.

Factors Affecting Calcium Balance

Bone calcium is in constant balance with plasma calcium. Maintaining a precise amount of calcium in the plasma is extremely important. A number of bodily mechanisms that maintain this crucial balance are described below.

Absorption–Excretion. Only 10% to 40% of calcium taken in is absorbed from the intestinal tract into the bloodstream. Absorption is influenced by several factors, being greatly increased during periods of rapid growth or when body stores are low. Calcium absorption is aided by adequate intake of vitamin D, an acidic environment in the upper gastrointestinal tract, and normal gastrointestinal motility. Protein, vitamin C, and lactose (milk sugar, which provides lactic acid) increase intestinal acidity, making calcium more soluble and thus more absorbable. The benefits of protein in promoting absorption may be offset by increased urinary excretion of calcium, which a high protein intake appears to cause.

Calcium absorption is hindered by excess fat in the diet or poor absorption of fat, by phytates (phosphorus compounds in cereals), and by oxalates (found in vegetables). Fatty acids, phytates, and oxalates form insoluble compounds with calcium. These compounds cannot be absorbed and are excreted in the feces. Because cocoa and chocolate also contain oxalate, their use with milk has been questioned. However, studies done on human subjects show that, in the amounts normally eaten, cocoa and chocolate do not significantly interfere with calcium absorption.

Unabsorbed calcium is excreted in the feces. Normally, small amounts of calcium are also excreted in the urine, the amount depending upon the serum level of calcium.

Storage of Calcium in Bone. As stated, calcium in the bone is in a constant state of exchange. If plasma calcium levels are high, calcium is deposited within the bone as the blood passes through it. Bone is the storehouse for calcium, to be drawn upon when serum calcium levels are low. Ideally, calcium is drawn from the trabeculae, the columns of crystalline calcium compounds at the ends of bones. When the diet is adequate in calcium, the trabeculae are well developed. However, if calcium is lacking over

an extended period of time, the trabeculae disappear, and calcium is drawn from bone itself.

Solubility Product. A specific ratio (relationship) of calcium to phosphorus is normally maintained in the blood serum owing to the relative solubility of these minerals. The solubility product of calcium and phosphorus is the result obtained when the concentration of calcium is multiplied by the concentration of phosphorus. Any increase in one of the minerals causes a decrease in the other, because this product normally remains the same. For example, excess phosphorus in the diet can create a decrease in serum calcium even though recommended amounts of calcium are being consumed. The high phosphate content of processed food may disrupt the calcium–phosphorus balance. Teenagers who drink large quantities of carbonated beverages (which are rich in phosphorus) may be prone to this problem.

Tetany, a condition characterized by uncontrolled muscular contractions (muscular spasms) and pain, results when serum calcium levels decrease below normal. It has been seen in newborns fed undiluted cow's milk, which contains a higher ratio of phosphorus to calcium than breast milk. The infant's kidneys are unable to excrete the excess phosphorus, causing the serum calcium level to drop.

Hormones. Several hormones control the plasma calcium and phosphorus levels by responding to changes in serum calcium. These include the following:

Active vitamin D exhibits hormonelike activity, increasing the absorption of calcium from the intestinal tract when the serum calcium level falls. It also controls the deposit of calcium and phosphorus in the bone. Vitamin D is converted to this active form by changes that take place in the liver and kidneys.

Parathyroid hormone (PTH), secreted by the parathyroid gland, stimulates the following changes when the serum calcium level falls: increased formation of active vitamin D, increased release of

calcium and phosphorus from the bone, increased urinary excretion of phosphorus, and decreased excretion of calcium by the kidneys. Disturbances of the parathyroid gland can cause abnormally high or abnormally low serum calcium levels.

Calcitonin is secreted by the thyroid gland in increased amounts when serum calcium levels rise. This hormone reduces serum calcium concentration by promoting the deposit of calcium in the bones.

Sources

Milk and hard cheese, such as cheddar or Swiss, are the most important food sources of calcium, accounting for about 85% percent of calcium intake in the United States. All types of milk—whole, nonfat, evaporated, and dry—are good sources of calcium. A person who cannot tolerate milk can use a soybean substitute. Including milk in puddings, custards, and creamed foods is a means of increasing intake, especially by persons who do not drink it in sufficient quantities. Butter and cream cheese, although made from milk, are not sources of calcium.

Green leafy vegetables, broccoli, dried peas and beans, and nuts are fair sources of calcium but not usually consumed frequently enough to contribute significantly to calcium intake. Among fruits, oranges are a fair source.

Canned salmon (which includes the bones), small fish such as sardines, and products made from small fish are good sources of calcium; shellfish, such as clams, oysters, and lobster, are fair sources; and meats and poultry are poor sources. Table 11-2 shows the calcium content of selected foods.

Recommended Allowances

The recommended calcium intake for children and adults throughout life is 800 mg daily; for teenagers and pregnant and lactating women, it is 1200 mg. Recommended amounts of calcium have been set rather high because of the generally high intake of protein and phosphorus in the United States.

As seen above, few foods are rich sources of

Table 11-2. Calcium and Caloric Content of Selected Foods in Portion Sizes Normally Consumed

Food	Portion Size	Calcium (mg)	Kilocalories
Milk, whole	1 cup	291	150
Milk, skim	1 cup	300	85
Cheddar cheese	1 oz	204	115
Cottage cheese, creamed	½ cup	68	118
Cottage cheese, 1% fat	½ cup	69	83
Ice cream	½ cup	88	135
Custard	½ cup	149	153
Sardines	3 oz.	372	175
Beef patty	3 oz.	10	185
Orange	1	54	65
Apple	1	10	80
Bread, white, firm-crumb	1 slice	22	65
Collards, cooked	½ cup	178	33
Kale, cooked	½ cup	103	23
Turnip greens, cooked	½ cup	126	15
Broccoli, cooked	½ cup	50	25
Potato, boiled	1	10	105
Carrots, cooked	½ cup	25	25
Dried navy beans, cooked	½ cup	48	113
Tofu (soybean curd)*	3½ oz	125	72

(Nutritive Value of Foods. USDA Home and Garden Bulletin 72, 1981)
* Tofu data from Pennington J, Church HN: Food Values of Portions Commonly Used. Philadelphia, JB Lippincott, 1980.

calcium. It is very difficult to meet recommended allowances without including adequate amounts of milk in the diet. Preschool and early school-age children should drink 1 to 1½ pints of milk a day; older children and adolescents should drink 1½ pints to 1 quart of milk daily, and adults should drink 1 pint. Some may be taken in the form of cheese or other milk prod-

ucts. Foods containing as much calcium as 8 ounces of milk are listed in Table 11-3.

Phosphorus

Phosphorus makes significant contributions, both as a component of bones and teeth and as an essential factor in regulatory processes. Phos-

Table 11-3. Foods That Contain as Much Calcium as 8 Ounces of Milk

1⅓ ounces cheddar cheese

1½ ounces processed American cheese

1⅓ cups cottage cheese

1 cup cocoa made with milk

1 cup custard

1⅓ cups ice cream

1 cup ice milk, soft serve

¾ cup homemade macaroni and cheese

1 milkshake (made with ⅔ cup milk and ½ cup ice cream)

1 cup oyster stew

1½ to 1⅔ cup canned cream soup, prepared with equal volume of milk

1 cup unflavored yogurt

phorus makes up about 1% of body weight. Eighty percent is found in the form of calcium phosphate in bones and teeth.

Functions and Clinical Effects

Bone and Tooth Formation. Phosphorus must be available for the formation of calcium phosphate, the mineral portion of bone. Poor calcification of bone can result from a lack of phosphorus as well as from a lack of calcium. However, a lack of phosphorus is most likely to result from excessive excretion of phosphorus in the urine and not from an inadequate supply in the diet. Like calcium, phosphorus is constantly being released from and built into bone tissue as a means of maintaining a normal serum level.

Energy Metabolism. Phosphorus is a component of adenosine triphosphate (ATP) and adenosine diphosphate (ADP), which control energy storage and release in the cell. ATP captures the energy released in the burning (oxidation) of protein, fat, and carbohydrate. As energy is needed, ATP is hydrolyzed (broken

down) to ADP, thus releasing energy needed to fuel reactions of metabolism.

Protein Synthesis and Genetic Coding. Phosphorus occurs in all cells as part of both ribonucleic acid (RNA) and deoxyribonucleic acid (DNA), which are essential for protein synthesis and genetic coding.

Absorption and Transport of Fats and Fatty Acids. Phosphorus combines with fats that are insoluble so that they may be absorbed from the intestinal tract and transported in the bloodstream.

Enzyme Formation. Phosphorus is a component of enzymes involved in the metabolism of proteins, fats, and carbohydrates.

Acid–Base Balance. The phosphate system is one of the principal buffers in the regulation of acid–base balance.

Deficiency

Because phosphorus is widely distributed in food, a phosphorus deficiency is rare.

Factors Affecting Phosphorus Balance

Absorption–Excretion. The amount of phosphorus in the body is controlled mostly by excretion in the urine rather than by control of absorption. By responding to changes in serum calcium levels, PTH and vitamin D hormone indirectly regulate phosphorus balance. PTH regulates the amount of phosphorus reabsorbed by the kidney. Vitamin D promotes the absorption of phosphorus from the intestinal tract.

Sources

Phosphorus is widely distributed in food and is not likely to be lacking. Meats, poultry, fish, eggs, nuts, legumes, whole-grain cereals, and milk are all good sources. Phosphate additives used in a wide variety of products, such as carbonated beverages, processed meats, cheese, dressings, and refrigerated bakery products,

contribute significant amounts of phosphorus to the diet.

Recommended Allowances

The recommended intake of phosphorus is equal to that of calcium at all ages except in infancy. During the first year of life, an intake of calcium 1½ times that of phosphorus is recommended.

In the United States, the average phosphorus intake is 1500 mg to 1600 mg daily, considerably higher than the recommendation. This high amount appears to be well tolerated as long as the vitamin D content of the diet is adequate. However, concern has been raised about the long-range effects of this unbalanced intake.

Sodium

Although attention is usually drawn to the undesirable effects of high intakes of sodium, this mineral is essential to life, playing a vital role in regulating body processes. About one third of body sodium occurs in bone tissue; most of the remaining two thirds is found in extracellular fluid.

Functions and Clinical Effects

Sodium is the principal cation (electrolyte carrying a positive charge) of the extracellular fluid. As free ionized sodium, it helps to control a number of important bodily processes.

Water Balance. Sodium acts with other electrolytes, especially potassium in the intracellular fluid, to maintain proper osmotic pressure and water balance (see Chap. 10).

When excretion of sodium is reduced, as in cardiac or kidney failure, water is retained along with the sodium. The water and sodium accumulate in the tissues, increasing the workload of the heart. Accumulation of fluid in the lungs (pulmonary edema) and in the extremities may then occur. Sodium is also retained when there is excessive secretion of adrenal hormones or when these hormones are given as medication.

Acid–Base Balance. Sodium is a base-forming element. It balances the acidic chloride and bicarbonate ions.

Transmission of Nerve Impulses and Contraction of Muscles. Together with potassium, sodium creates an electrical charge on the nerve cell membrane, which passes impulse along the nerve. It has a relaxing effect on muscle contractions, working to balance those ions that stimulate muscle contraction.

Glucose Absorption and Cell Permeability. Exchange of sodium and potassium across cell walls makes the cell membrane more permeable to other substances.

Deficiency and Excess

Sodium deficit is as serious as sodium excess. Heavy losses may occur in cystic fibrosis, in kidney disease, in diseases of the adrenal glands, in severe diarrhea and vomiting, with excessive and prolonged sweating, and with the use of diuretics. Symptoms of sodium deficiency include nausea, giddiness, apathy, exhaustion, abdominal and muscle cramps, vomiting, and finally respiratory failure if the sodium is not replaced.

Too much dietary salt over a long period of time has been associated with the development of hypertension. At present, there is considerable controversy as to how strong this relationship is. Research indicates that other nutrients, such as calcium, potassium, magnesium, and essential fatty acids, may also have a role in the development of hypertension. Some persons appear to inherit a sensitivity to sodium, making them more prone than normal to hypertension. (See Chap. 23.)

Factors Affecting Sodium Balance

Sodium consumption varies widely, ranging from 3 g to 7 g (7.5–17.5 g of salt), far more than is required. Most of the sodium consumed is absorbed from the gastrointestinal tract. Balance is maintained through kidney excretion. The amount excreted is regulated by the hormone aldosterone, which is secreted by the

Table 11-4. Effect of Food Processing on the Sodium Content of Foods

Food	Amount	Sodium (mg)
Salmon		
Broiled with butter	3 oz	99
Canned, salt added	3 oz	443
Canned, without added salt	3 oz	41
Cream of wheat		
Regular	¾ cup	2
Quick-cooking	¾ cup	126
Mix'n eat	¾ cup	350
Peanuts		
Unsalted	½ cup	4
Dry roasted, salted	½ cup	493
Peas		
Fresh, cooked	½ cup	1
Frozen, regular, cooked	½ cup	100
Canned, regular	½ cup	247
Canned, low sodium	½ cup	8
Meat		
Beef, lean, cooked	3 oz	55
Pork, fresh, lean, cooked	3 oz	59
Corned beef	3 oz	802
Ham	3 oz	1114
Frankfurters (1½)	3 oz	958
Beef salami	3 oz	1020
Olive loaf	3 oz	1248
Fast foods		
Fish sandwich	1	882
Jumbo hamburger	1	990
Pizza, cheese	¼ pie	599
French fries	2½ oz	146

(The Sodium Content of your Food. USDA Home and Garden Bulletin 233, 1980)

adrenal gland. When sodium intake is high, urinary excretion increases; when intake is low, excretion decreases. Aldosterone is secreted in response to low sodium levels and promotes reabsorption of sodium by the kidney.

Sources

Many foods in their natural state contain sodium. Animal sources, such as meat, fish, poultry, eggs, and milk are high in sodium, whereas fruits and most vegetables are low. In some areas, the water supply is a significant source of sodium. Some medications also contain significant amounts of sodium.

However, it is the salt and other sodium compounds added to food that account for the highest intake. Processed foods contribute large quantities of sodium to the diet (Table 11-4).

Recommended Allowances

According to the Food and Nutrition Board, a range of 1100 mg to 3300 mg of sodium daily is recommended for adults. This is about half the amount usually consumed. The U.S. Dietary Goals recommend a dietary salt intake of 5 g (approximately 1 tsp) per day. This is 2000 mg (2 g) of sodium since table salt is 40% sodium. Approximately 1 g (1000 mg) of sodium occurs naturally in food, for a recommended daily total of 3 g (3000 mg).

Potassium

The long-term use of diuretics in the treatment of cardiac disease has focused attention on the body's potassium requirement. Although diuretics are prescribed to prevent the accumulation of sodium and water, the kidneys excrete potassium along with the sodium and water. Potassium lost in this way must be replaced either by a potassium supplement or, preferably, by an increase in dietary potassium.

Functions and Clinical Effects

Water Balance and Acid–Base Balance. Potassium is the principal cation of the fluid within the cell. It maintains osmotic pressure, water balance, and acid–base balance.

Transmission of Nerve Impulses and Contraction of Muscles. A small amount of potassium in extracellular fluid, together with other ions, influences the transmission of nerve impulses and the contraction of muscles, including the heart.

Energy Metabolism. Potassium is a catalyst for reactions taking place in the cell.

Glycogen Synthesis. Potassium bound to phosphate is required for the conversion of glucose to glycogen.

Protein Synthesis. Potassium is needed for the synthesis of muscle protein.

Deficiency and Excess

Circumstances other than the use of diuretics can cause a potassium deficiency: severe vomiting, diarrhea, diabetic acidosis, severe protein–calorie malnutrition, and adrenal gland abnormalities. Symptoms include nausea, vomiting, muscular weakness, rapid heart rhythm, and heart failure.

Very high potassium levels in the blood (hyperkalemia) are also a threat to health. Cardiac arrhythmias (irregular heartbeats), muscular weakness, and numbness of the face, tongue, and extremities are symptoms of hyperkalemia. Death may result from heart failure. Toxic blood levels usually result from abnormal conditions such as kidney failure, abnormal adrenal function, and severe dehydration (see Chap. 24). Hyperkalemia may also be caused by a sudden increase in potassium intake to levels of about 18 g (18,000 mg) per day in an adult, as may occur when potassium supplements are used excessively.

Factors Affecting Potassium Balance

Potassium is readily absorbed from the gastrointestinal tract. The kidneys maintain potassium balance by excreting excessive amounts. However, the kidney's ability to conserve potas-

sium when a deficiency occurs is poor. Conditions that decrease potassium excretion include low potassium intake, low sodium intake, acute acidosis, and decreased aldosterone secretion. Conditions that promote potassium excretion include a high sodium intake, increased secretion of aldosterone, and alkalosis.

Sources

Potassium is found in liberal amounts in meat, fish, and poultry; whole-grain breads and cereals; fruits, especially oranges and grapefruits and their juices, dried fruits, and bananas; and vegetables, especially potatoes, winter squash, tomatoes, and legumes.

Recommended Allowances

The estimated safe and adequate intake for adults is 1875 mg to 5625 mg daily. Because potassium is found in many foods, a deficiency is not likely to occur under normal circumstances.

Magnesium

Magnesium occurs in the bones and teeth and in soft tissues and body fluids. It activates many enzyme systems involved in energy metabolism and in the metabolism of other minerals, such as calcium, potassium, phosphorus, and sodium. Together with other minerals, magnesium regulates nerve stimulation and muscle contractions. A deficiency leads to nervous irritability and, if untreated, can lead to convulsive seizures. Deficiency occurs in conditions in which magnesium intake or absorption is decreased or excretion is increased (such as chronic alcoholism, diabetes, malabsorption syndrome, kwashiorkor, kidney disease, and glandular disorders).

Magnesium plays an essential role in plant life. It is a component of the green pigment chlorophyll and is found abundantly in green leafy vegetables. It is also found in cocoa, nuts, whole-grain cereals, meat, milk, and seafood. The recommended daily allowances for magnesium are 350 mg for adult men, 300 mg for adult women, and 450 mg for pregnant and lactating women.

Chlorine

Chlorine occurs in the body mainly in the form of chloride, which is the chief anion (negatively charged ion) in extracellular fluid. Chloride helps maintain osmotic pressure, water balance, and acid–base balance. It is a constituent of hydrochloric acid, which is essential to protein digestion within the stomach. Chloride enhances the carbon-dioxide-carrying function of the blood. Table salt (sodium chloride) is the main dietary source of chloride. The safe range for adults is estimated to be 1700 mg to 5100 mg a day.

Sulfur

Sulfur is part of the protein in every cell. It is a component of several amino acids, several B vitamins, insulin, and other vital body compounds. No recommended allowance has been set for sulfur. Protein foods are sources of sulfur.

See Table 11-5 for a summary of macrominerals.

Microminerals

Iron

That the required quantity of a nutrient does not indicate its relative importance is well demonstrated by the mineral iron. The body contains less than 5 g of iron, but this small amount performs extraordinarily important functions. About two thirds of the iron is in the blood, and about one third is in the liver, spleen, and bone marrow (as ferritin and hemosiderin). Small amounts of iron are found in muscle myoglobin (an oxygen-carrying protein occurring only in the muscle tissue), in the blood serum, and in every cell as a component of enzymes.

Absorbed iron combines with protein to

Table 11-5. Summary of Minerals

Mineral	Function	Deficiency	Sources
Calcium	Bone and tooth formation; blood clotting; cell permeability; nerve stimulation; muscle contraction; enzyme activation	Stunted growth; rickets; osteomalacia; osteoporosis (porous bones); tetany ((low serum calcium)	Milk; hard cheese; salmon and small fish eaten with bones; some dark green vegetables; legumes (tofu)
Phosphorus	Bone and tooth formation; energy metabolism—component of ATP and ADP; protein synthesis—component of DNA and RNA; fat transport; acid–base balance; enzyme formation	Stunted growth; rickets (due to excessive excretion rather than to dietary deficiency)	Distributed widely in foods: milk; meats, poultry, fish, eggs; cheese; nuts; legumes; whole grains; processed foods
Sodium	Osmotic pressure; water balance; acid–base balance; nerve stimulation; muscle contraction; cell permeability	Rare: nausea; vomiting; giddiness; exhaustion; cramps	Table salt, salted foods, MSG and other sodium additives; milk; meat, fish, poultry, eggs
Potassium	Osmotic pressure; water balance; acid–base balance; nerve stimulation; muscle contraction; synthesis of protein; glycogen formation	Nausea; vomiting; muscular weakness; rapid heart beat; heart failure	Widely distributed in food: meats, fish, poultry; whole grains; fruits, vegetables, legumes
Magnesium	Component of bones and teeth; activates many enzymes, including those involved in energy metabolism; nerve stimulation; muscle contraction	Seen in alcoholism or renal disease: tremors leading to convulsive seizures	Green leafy vegetables; nuts; whole grains; meat; milk; seafood
Iron	Hemoglobin and myoglobin formation; cellular enzymes	Anemia	Liver, lean meats; legumes, dried fruits, green leafy vegetables; whole grain and fortified cereals
Iodine	Synthesis of thyroid hormones that regulate basal metabolic rate	Goiter; cretinism, if deficiency is severe	Iodized salt; seafood; food grown near the sea
Fluorine	Resists dental decay	Tooth decay in young children	Fluoridated water (1 ppm)

(continued)

Table 11-5.   (continued)

Mineral	Function	Deficiency	Sources
Zinc	Constituent of many enzyme systems, including those involved in protein digestion and synthesis, carbon dioxide transport, and vitamin A utilization	Delayed wound healing; impaired taste sensitivity. Severe deficiency (rare in U.S.): retarded growth and sexual development; dwarfism	Oysters, herring; meat, liver, fish; milk; whole grains; nuts; legumes

ppm = part per million

form transferrin, a transport form of iron in the blood serum. In this form, iron is carried to the bone marrow for hemoglobin synthesis, to the liver or spleen for storage, or to other tissues for their needs.

Functions and Clinical Effects

Component of Hemoglobin. Iron is a component of hemoglobin, the compound that carries oxygen from the lungs to the cells. Some of the carbon dioxide that is produced in the cell is carried back by the hemoglobin to the lungs, where it is exhaled. The hemoglobin molecule is composed of two parts: globin (a protein), and heme (the iron-containing pigment of the blood that is responsible for its characteristic color). Adequate protein and traces of copper are necessary for hemoglobin synthesis. Other nutrients, including certain vitamins, also promote hemoglobin formation. A red blood cell disintegrates after about 120 days. Its iron is used by the body over and over again for hemoglobin synthesis.

Cellular Enzymes. In every cell, iron is a constituent of certain enzymes that are important in energy production.

Deficiency

Iron deficiency anemia occurs when the iron supply is not sufficient to support the adequate formation of red blood cells and the oxygen needs of the tissues are not met. Although the number of red blood cells is sufficient, their size is inadequate because there is not enough hemoglobin to fill them. In infants and children, symptoms of iron deficiency anemia include irritability, apathy, lethargy, and pallor. Adults are pale and tire easily. Pallor of mucous membranes, especially on the underside of the eyelid and in the interior of the mouth, is a clinical sign of possible anemia. A deficiency of other nutrients, such as protein, can also cause nutritional anemia. Since there are several types of anemia, both nutritional and nonnutritional, a careful diagnosis by a physician is necessary to determine the kind and cause.

Iron intake is frequently inadequate during infancy and other periods of rapid growth when there is an increase in blood volume. In the United States, iron deficiency anemia is the most prevalent deficiency disease of early childhood. Milk, the infant's main food, is a poor source of iron, and the newborn's own iron stores are sufficient for only about 6 months. Iron-fortified commercial formula, fortified infant cereals, vegetable and meat purees, and other sources of iron are necessary to avoid deficiency.

If sufficient iron-rich foods are not provided, the shortage that begins in infancy usually peaks during the second year of life. The incidence of anemia decreases during later childhood but increases again in adolescence, especially among girls. It is also high among menstruating women and among pregnant women, in whom iron intake must meet the

needs of the fetus and must replace the iron in the blood that is lost during childbirth.

Poor selection of food, insufficient money to buy adequate food, or lack of appetite during illness may result in deficient iron intake.

Poor absorption of iron from the intestinal tract may also produce anemia. In malabsorption syndromes, there is usually poor absorption of several nutrients, including iron. Iron absorption is also reduced in diseases in which there is low gastric acidity. Acid increases the solubility of iron and thus promotes absorption. Both hydrochloric acid and iron supplements may be given in cases of malabsorption.

Excess

Hemochromatosis is a disease characterized by excessive iron absorption. It is due to an inability to regulate iron absorption from the intestinal lining. It is a serious condition that gives rise to an accumulation of iron in the liver, spleen, bone marrow, heart, and other tissues.

Factors Affecting Iron Balance

The intestinal mucosa regulates iron absorption. Except for very small amounts lost in the urine and through the skin, approximately 1 mg per day, iron absorbed from the gastrointestinal tract cannot be excreted. Therefore, iron absorption must be regulated so that dangerously high levels of the mineral do not accumulate. Iron is lost mainly through the loss of blood in hemorrhage, menstruation, blood donations, and parasitic infestations. How much dietary iron is absorbed depends upon the source and the composition of the meal in which the iron is contained. In the past, the RDA were based on the belief that only 10% of the iron in the diet was absorbed; however, more recent knowledge makes it feasible, by careful planning, to increase or decrease the amount of iron absorbed. Although we are mainly concerned with increasing the amount of iron absorbed, a small number of persons in whom iron stores accumulate excessively would benefit from a diet low in available iron.

The iron in food is divided into two categories: heme and nonheme iron. Heme iron accounts for 40% of the iron in meat, fish, and poultry. A high percentage (23%) of heme iron is absorbed, and absorption is not affected by other factors in the diet. Nonheme iron accounts for the remaining 60% percent of the iron in meat, fish, and poultry; for all the iron in other foods; for the iron in compounds added to enrich foods (such as cereals); and for the iron in iron supplements. Only a small amount of nonheme iron is absorbed (as little as 3%).

The absorption of nonheme iron can be increased to 8% if the mineral is ingested in a meal that includes ascorbic acid and/or meat, fish, or poultry. The maximum possible amount of nonheme iron is available in a meal that contains more than 90 g (3 oz) of meat, fish, or poultry; more than 75 mg of ascorbic acid (the amount provided by 8 oz of orange or grapefruit juice); or 30 g to 90 g (1–3 oz) of meat, fish, or poultry plus 25 mg to 75 mg of ascorbic acid (the amount in 4 oz of orange or grapefruit juice). Thus, meals can be planned so that the amount of available iron is increased or decreased according to individual needs.

Some substances in the diet and in medications decrease iron absorption. These include calcium and phosphate salts, edetate (EDTA), phytates, fiber, tannic acid (in tea), phosvitin in egg yolk, and antacid medications.

Sources

Liver is the richest source of iron. Although the iron contents of various types of liver differ considerably, even liver with the lowest iron value far outranks other foods as a source of this mineral.

For persons who do not like liver, iron can be provided by lean meat, fish, and poultry; cooked dried peas, beans, and lentils; dark green leafy vegetables; dried fruit and potatoes; whole-grain and enriched bread; fortified cereals; and nuts and nut butters. The iron content of whole grain, enriched cereals, and legumes is particularly important for vegetarians and persons who must limit purchases of more costly sources of iron, such as meat.

Foods such as oysters, clams, shrimp, sardines, and dark molasses, although good

Table 11-6. Iron Content of Selected Foods

Food	Amount	Iron (mg)*
Liver, beef	3 oz	7.5
Liverwurst	3 oz	5.1
Beef patty (10% fat)	3 oz	3
Shrimp, canned	3 oz	2.6
Chicken	3 oz	1.3
Frankfurter	3 oz	1.2
Bluefish	3 oz	0.6
Infant cereal†	½ oz (6 tbsp)	14.2
Bran flakes, fortified	1 cup	12.4
Oatmeal	1 cup	1.4
Puffed rice	1 cup	0.3
Whole-wheat bread	1 slice	0.8
White bread, enriched	1 slice	0.7
Split peas, cooked	1 cup	3.4
Peanut butter	2 tbsp	0.6
Spinach, leaf frozen, cooked	½ cup	2.4
Peas, frozen, cooked	½ cup	1.5
Potato, baked	large	1.1
Snap beans, cooked	½ cup	0.4
Prunes, dried	5	1.7
Raisins	3 tbsp	1.0
Orange	1	0.5

(Nutritive Value of Foods. USDA Home and Garden Bulletin 72, 1981)
* The iron in meat, fish, and poultry is more available to the body than the iron in plant sources.
† Infant cereal data from Pennington J, Church HN: Food Values of Portions Commonly Used. JB Lippincott, 1980.

sources of iron, are not eaten frequently enough or in large enough quantities to be considered important iron sources. The iron in egg yolk, although rich in quantity, is poorly absorbed.

The iron in fibrous vegetable foods, such as cereals with bran and leafy vegetables, is not as available to the body as that in meats. For this reason, vegetarians may need to consume considerably more iron in order to obtain the same amount as would be furnished by animal foods. Table 11-6 gives the iron content of selected foods.

The use of iron pots and pans can considerably increase the iron content of foods. The

increase is greatest when acidic foods (such as tomatoes) are prepared in iron containers.

Recommended Allowances

The recommended iron allowance for men throughout adult life and for women after menopause is 10 mg per day; for women of childbearing age, it is 18 mg per day. The high allowance for premenopausal women reflects the need for additional iron during menstruation, pregnancy, and lactation. (The loss of iron in menstrual blood flow ranges from 15 mg to 30 mg or more per month). These allowances are based on the assumption that approximately 10% of the iron consumed is available for absorption.

A standard diet that meets nutritional requirements in all other respects contains about 9 mg to 12 mg of iron. The typical American diet does not readily provide the 18 mg of iron needed by menstruating women. If food is consumed under conditions that increase the absorption of iron (discussed above), the amount absorbed will be greater than 10%. In this way, the amount of iron absorbed may meet desired amounts even though the total iron intake is below recommended amounts.

Iodine

Normal function of the thyroid gland depends upon the availability of adequate amounts of iodine. The thyroid produces hormones that regulate energy metabolism in the body tissues and are essential for normal tissue growth and development. An adequate supply of iodine is necessary for the production of the hormones thyroxine (T_4) and triiodothyronine (T_3). These hormones are transported in the blood bound to protein and are referred to as *protein-bound iodine* (PBI). Some T_4 and T_3 circulates freely. Iodine is easily absorbed from the intestinal tract. About 30% is used by the throid gland, and the remainder is excreted in the urine. Thyroid hormone production is controlled by thyroid-stimulating hormone (TSH) secreted by the pituitary gland. When the level of thyroid hormones in the bloodstream decrease, TSH stimulates the thyroid to produce more hormones.

Thyroid hormones regulate metabolic rate. Excessive production of thyroid hormones (hyperthyroidism) increases the metabolic rate above normal; low production (hypothyroidism) reduces the metabolic rate. Measurement of the serum T_3 and T_4 levels and of PBI is used to evaluate thyroid function. When thyroid production is low, increased quantities of TSH are found in the bloodstream as the pituitary attempts to stimulate the thyroid to increase hormone production. However, without iodine, the hormones cannot be produced.

Deficiency and Excess

When the thyroid gland cannot manufacture sufficient hormones, it responds by producing more and larger cells. *Goiter,* an enlargement of the thyroid that produces a swelling of the neck, results. Simple goiter is sometimes called *endemic goiter,* meaning that it is common to the inhabitants of a particular region where there is little iodine in the soil. If a goiter goes untreated during pregnancy and if the iodine deficiency is severe, the fetus will not receive enough iodine and is likely to be a cretin—a child with arrested physical and mental development.

Persons who live near seacoasts and eat enough seafood probably receive sufficient iodine. The iodine content of plant foods varies according to the iodine content of the soil in which the plants are grown. Plant foods grown near seacoasts or in the southern states contain more iodine than those grown in the Great Lakes area or in other areas where the surface soil is low in iodine. The use of iodized salt is the most practical way to obtain an adequate amount of iodine.

Concern has been expressed that we may be consuming too much iodine. Iodine is contained in some drugs and it is also used in food processing. Although the amount of iodine in the American diet has increased in recent years, there has been no increase in adverse reactions. Nevertheless, the Food and Nutrition Board recommends that iodine-containing compounds in food processing be reduced or eliminated. The recommended intake for both males

and females from the age 11 through adulthood is 150 μg (micrograms).

Fluorine

Fluorine is a component of bones and teeth that is especially abundant in dental enamel. The incidence of dental caries is reduced by 50% to 60% percent in communities in which the water supply has been fluoridated.

Fluoride is found in small amounts in all soils, water, plants, and animals. Consequently, a deficiency severe enough to affect normal growth has not been identified in humans. The Food and Nutrition Board recommends the fluoridation of the water supply where necessary to bring the fluoride level to a concentration of 1 mg/liter (or 1 part per million). Where fluoridated water supplies are not available, fluoride levels may be increased by the use of sodium fluoride tablets, fluoride toothpastes, and bottled fluoridated water, and by the application of fluoride to the teeth.

Zinc

Zinc is a constituent of many enzyme systems, including those involved in protein synthesis, carbon dioxide transport, and vitamin A utilization. It also occurs in insulin.

A condition that responds to zinc therapy has been identified in the Middle East. It occurs in children and adolescent boys and is characterized by dwarfism, enlarged liver and spleen, delayed sexual development, and anemia. Intestinal parasites, phytates in food, excessive sweating, and clay eating—all of which interfere with zinc absorption—are factors involved in the development of these deficiencies.

Zinc deficiency in adults occurs mainly as a result of diseases either that hinder absorption of zinc or that result in excessive excretion of

zinc in the urine. Poor taste sensitivity and impaired wound healing have been shown to improve with zinc supplementation.

The zinc in meats and seafood is much more readily available than that in vegetable products. Phytates (phosphorus-containing compounds in cereal products) and dietary fiber hinder zinc absorption. Oysters and herring are the richest sources of zinc. Meat, liver, milk, and fish are also good sources. The zinc in whole-grain cereals, legumes, and nuts is in a form that is less available to the body.

The recommended daily zinc allowance for persons over 11 years of age is 15 mg; 20 mg during pregnancy; and 25 mg during lactation. This is based on the assumption that 40% of the zinc in food is absorbed. The zinc intake of vegetarians should be higher, since the zinc in vegetable products is less well absorbed.

See Table 11-5 for a summary of microminerals.

Other Essential Trace Minerals

See Table 11-1 for estimated safe and adequate daily dietary intakes of trace minerals, with the exception of cobalt.

Manganese is an important mineral in enzyme systems; it functions in blood formation and tendon and bone structure.

Cobalt, a component of vitamin B_{12}, is necessary for the formation of red blood cells.

Copper is necessary for the utilization of iron in the formation of hemoglobin and is a constituent of many enzymes.

Molybdenum, a constituent of enzymes, may be involved in the metabolism of fats.

Selenium is a part of an enzyme that prevents oxidative damage to tissues.

Chromium is associated with the body's ability to use glucose and is necessary for normal insulin activity.

KEYS TO PRACTICAL APPLICATION

The assumption that if "a little is good,
    more is better" is risky when applied to

minerals. All minerals are toxic when taken in excessive amounts.

Calcium is needed throughout life. Encourage the consumption of milk at all age levels. Remember that nonfat and low-fat milks have just as much calcium as whole milk.

Avoid too much sodium. Add only a little salt in cooking and little or none at the table, and limit your intake of salty foods.

Increase your intake of potassium-rich foods. The sodium – potassium relationship is important, and the two should be consumed in approximately equal amounts. However, too much potassium is as bad as too little. Discourage the use of potassium supplements or potassium-containing salt substitutes without a physician's approval.

Discourage the frequent use of antacid preparations without a doctor's supervision. Reducing the acidity of the stomach reduces the absorption of calcium and iron.

The iron in meat, fish, and poultry is more efficiently absorbed than the iron from other sources, including iron supplements.

Use vitamin-C-rich foods at every meal. Vitamin C increases the absorption of nonheme iron.

Cooking in uncoated iron cookware significantly increases iron intake.

Encourage the use of iodized salt in noncoastal states. Sea salt should not be used as a substitute, since its iodine is lost during the drying process.

Support community efforts to fluoridate water. Dental decay is reduced 50% to 60% among children in fluoridated communities.

Encourage the use of legumes (dried peas, beans, lentils, and soybeans). They are excellent, inexpensive sources of many essential minerals.

KEY IDEAS

The difference between beneficial amounts and harmful amounts of trace elements may be very small.

The roles of minerals in the body are interrelated; in some cases they complement and in other cases they hinder one another's activities.

Minerals are most abundant in unrefined foods; increased use of synthetic foods may create deficiencies of trace minerals.

See Table 11-5 for a summary of minerals.

KEYS TO LEARNING: STUDY – DISCUSSION QUESTIONS

1. Using your food record for one day, compare your consumption of iron and calcium with the RDA for your sex and age group given in Chapter 4. Which items on your record provide the greatest amount of calcium? Which provide the greatest amount of iron?

2. Plan meals (including snacks) for two days that meet the RDA for adults of 800 mg of calcium. Plan one day's meals with milk and one day's meals without fluid milk. What foods account for most of the calcium in the meals that do not include fluid milk?

3. Rank the following foods according to calcium content, with the richest source of calcium first:

3 ounces	Ground beef, cooked
½ cup	Collards, fresh, cooked

1 ounce	Cheddar cheese
1 cup	Milk
½ cup	Carrots, cooked
3 ounces	Sardines, canned, Atlantic type

Check your answers with the calcium content listed for each of the above in Table 11-2.

4. The body has many checks and balances to maintain a state of dynamic equilibrium. Explain the bodily mechanisms that maintain calcium balance.

5. What factors promote the absorption of iron? How would you use this information to help a client who has iron deficiency anemia?

6. What is the benefit of a fluoridated water supply? Is the water in your community fluoridated? If not, why not? What is the status of efforts to fluoridate water in your area (check with your local health department)?

7. What is the importance of iodine? Where in the United States is there a lack of iodine in the soil and water? What is the most practical means of obtaining an adequate amount of iodine?

8. Discuss in class the importance of a varied diet and how it relates to an adequate intake of minerals. Some authorities have expressed concern about the excessive use of highly processed and synthetic foods. How does this trend threaten the adequate intake of minerals, especially trace minerals?

Bibliography is found at the end of Part Two.

Vitamins

KEY TERMS

anticoagulant   A substance that prevents clotting of blood.

antioxidant   A substance that hinders oxidation in other substances; oxidation is the combination of a substance with oxygen causing a breakdown or a change in the substance.

antivitamin   Any substance that interferes with the absorption or functioning of a vitamin. Some drugs are antivitamins.

avitaminosis   A deficiency of a vitamin.

carotene   A yellow pigment in plants that can be converted to vitamin A in the intestinal wall.

cheilosis   A condition in which lesions appear on the lips and cracks at the angles of the mouth.

coenzyme   A substance such as a vitamin that attaches to the inactive form of an enzyme, thus forming an active compound or complete enzyme.

collagen   A gelatinlike protein substance found in connective tissue and bones; a cementing material between body cells.

dementia   A deteriorated mental state.

dermatitis   Inflammation of the skin.

glossitis   Inflammation of the tongue.

hemolysis   Destruction of red blood cells resulting in the appearance of hemoglobin in surrounding fluid.

hypervitaminosis   A toxic condition due to excessive accumulation of a vitamin in the body.

megadose   A very large dose of a vitamin, 100 times or even 1000 times the recommended allowance.

myelin   A fatlike substance that forms a covering for some nerve fibers.

provitamin or precursor   A substance that precedes and is converted into a vitamin. For example, carotene is the precursor of vitamin A, tryptophan the precursor of niacin.

The vitamin story began hundreds of years ago with the recognition of a connection between food habits and certain diseases. Beriberi was described in the 7th century and scurvy in the 13th. Later, certain foods were identified as cures for specific diseases. Eventually, the specific chemical compounds in these foods that had produced the cures were identified.

In the early 1900s, Casimer Funk, a Polish scientist, discovered a group of substances for which he proposed the term *"vitamine,"* or vital amine. An amine is a nitrogen-containing com-

pound. When it was later learned that some vitamins could not be classified chemically as amines, the "e" was dropped and the accepted term became *vitamin.*

Vitamins are organic substances needed in small amounts for growth and for the maintenance of life. Some vitamins have hormonelike activity, whereas others are components of enzymes. Many enzymes can function only when combined with certain vitamins and minerals. A main function of many vitamins, especially the B-complex vitamins, is to act as coenzymes in metabolic reactions. A coenzyme is an organic substance that attaches to the inactive form of an enzyme. This combination makes the enzyme an active compound capable of bringing about chemical reactions. The body cannot manufacture vitamins; they must be supplied by foods or by vitamin supplements. A serious lack of one or more vitamins will result in one or more deficiency diseases.

Some vitamins exist in more than one form. These are chemically related substances that have similar activities in the body. One such vitamin, vitamin D, occurs in two forms, D_2 and D_3.

Terminology and Measurements

Before their exact chemical nature was known, vitamins were identified by letters of the alphabet. Later, chemical names replaced the letters. Letter names continue to be used to some extent. When what was thought to be one vitamin turned out to be many, each with a different function, numbers were added to the letter name, as in vitamin B_1, B_2, and B_{12}. Sometimes numbers indicate various forms of the same vitamin, such as D_2 and D_3 (which have similar functions).

A *provitamin,* or *precursor,* is a substance the structure of which is similar to that of a vitamin and which is transformed into the active vitamin in the body. *Avitaminosis* is a deficiency of a vitamin. *Hypervitaminosis* is the excessive accumulation of a vitamin in the body. An *antivitamin* is any substance that interferes with the absorption or the functioning of a vitamin. Vitamins are potent substances. Very little of a vitamin is needed to induce a chemical reaction in the body.

Vitamins occur in very small amounts in food. Quantities of most vitamins are measured in either milligrams (mg, 0.001 g) or micrograms (μg, 0.000001 g). Quantities of some vitamins may also be expressed in international units (IU), a specific measurable amount of vitamin activity. Vitamins A, D, and E used to be expressed in international units in the RDA. However, other units of measure are now used. Vitamin A is now expressed in retinol equivalents (RE); vitamin D, in micrograms cholecalciferol; and vitamin E, in milligrams of alpha-tocopherol.

Classification by Solubility

Vitamins are classified according to solubility into two groups: fat-soluble, and water-soluble. The fat-soluble vitamins are found in the fat parts of cells and foods; vitamins A, D, E, and K are fat-soluble. Water-soluble vitamins are found in the watery parts of cells and foods; vitamin C and the vitamin B-complex vitamins are water-soluble.

The fat-soluble vitamins are more stable than the water-soluble vitamins and are not easily lost in cooking and storage of food. The water-soluble vitamins are more readily lost in cooking water or destroyed by heat.

Recommended Allowances Versus Megadoses

The quantity of vitamins recommended by the Food and Nutrition Board is sufficient to provide a margin of safety—at least several times the quantity needed to prevent deficiency diseases. You should become familiar with the recommended allowances for each of the vitamins in the various age–sex categories.

Sufficient quantities of all the essential vitamins are supplied by a varied diet containing adequate amounts of fruits and vegetables, milk, bread, and meat and meat substitutes. Fresh or lightly processed foods are better sources of vitamins than refined, highly processed ones. During critical periods in life, as in infancy, early childhood, and pregnancy, vitamin supplements in amounts equal to the RDA may be prescribed. Larger doses are prescribed for persons with deficiency diseases or disease conditions that interfere with the adequate consumption of food or with the proper digestion, absorption, or utilization of nutrients.

Many persons take enormous doses (megadoses) of specific vitamins without medical supervision. These doses may be 50, 100, or even thousands of times greater than the amount needed to prevent deficiency diseases. Here again is an example of the mistaken belief that "if a little is good, more is better." These persons are swayed by false claims that large doses of vitamins will prevent or cure a wide range of physical and emotional ills. The wisdom of such a practice is very questionable on the following grounds:

Fat-soluble vitamins are stored in the body. Excess vitamin A and D can be highly toxic, even fatal. Excess water-soluble vitamins cannot be stored and are rapidly excreted in the urine once the tissues become saturated; however, the long-term effects of this supersaturation of tissues is unknown. Vitamins taken in quantities over and above nutritional needs act like drugs and should be treated as such. It should also be remembered that, at present, they are "untested" drugs. This point is illustrated by evidence of side-effects due to megadoses of vitamin C, to be discussed later in this chapter.

Fat-Soluble Vitamins

Vitamins A, D, E, and K are absorbed from the intestinal tract in the same manner as fats. Therefore, any disease condition that interferes with the absorption of fats may also inhibit the absorption of these vitamins. Including mineral oil in food preparaton for reducing diets or as a laxative also interferes with absorption of these vitamins. Mineral oil, a nonfood substance, is not digested, but instead passes through the gastrointestinal tract, carrying the fat-soluble vitamins with it.

Fat-soluble vitamins are all stored to some extent in the body, mainly in the liver. For example, the liver of a well-nourished person has several months' supply of vitamin A. Thus, signs of deficiency develop more slowly in the case of fat-soluble vitamins than in the case of water-soluble vitamins.

Vitamin A (Retinol)

Vitamin A is found in animal foods as the vitamin and in green and yellow plant foods as the provitamin carotene. What is called vitamin A as found in animal products is actually a group of similar compounds. Carotene, an orange yellow pigment in plants, is converted in the body to vitamin A. In many green, leafy vegetables, the color of chlorophyll conceals the yellow of carotene. Carotene also occurs in

forms that produce different amounts of vitamin A in the body. About one sixth or less of the carotene in food is actually converted to vitamin A in the body. Adequate protein is needed for the proper absorption, transport, and metabolism of carotene.

Functions and Clinical Effects

Adaptation to Changes in Light. Vitamin A is necessary for the formation of a pigment, visual purple, in the rods of the retina. This pigment is responsible for vision in dim light. Light bleaches the visual purple, and the ability of the eye to remake this pigment in darkness depends on the availability of vitamin A. When vitamin A is lacking, the formation of visual purple is slowed, and the eye has difficulty adjusting to dim light (night blindness). The cones of the retina also contain a light-sensitive vitamin-A-containing violet pigment that is responsible for vision in bright light; a vitamin A deficiency causes glare blindness. Poor adaptation to changes in light, such as temporary blindness caused by the glare of headlights or entering a darkened theater, is one of the first signs of vitamin A deficiency (Fig. 12-1).

Maintenance of Epithelial Tissue. Vitamin A is essential for the maintenance of normal epithelial tissue: the skin and mucous membranes, such as the epithelial layer of the eye; and the linings of the respiratory, gastrointestinal, and genitourinary tracts. When vitamin A is lacking, the epithelial cells keratinize (become dry and scaly). The mucus secretions diminish, and the mucous membranes lose their soft, moist characteristics that protect the body from bacterial infection. The senses of taste and smell may be affected. The skin becomes rough, dry, and scaly, especially on the arms and thighs, and has a "gooseflesh" appearance. Adverse changes in the epithelial cells of the genitourinary tract interfere with normal reproductive function.

In the eye, the epithelial tissue becomes dry and thick, the tear ducts fail to secrete, and eventually, in severe vitamin A deficiency, the cells of the cornea become opaque and slough

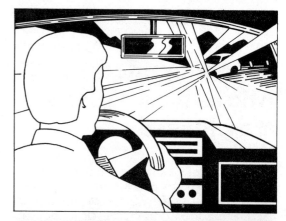

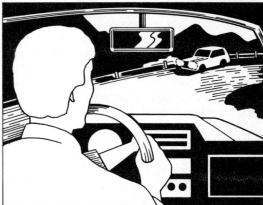

Fig. 12-1. (*Top*) "Glare blindness" often is a symptom of vitamin A deficiency. Headlights dazzle the eyes and cause discomfort. The driver is blinded temporarily by oncoming headlights, and the edge of the road is seen with difficulty. (*Bottom*) An adequate intake of vitamin A protects against "glare blindness" or remedies it. Properly focused headlights no longer dazzle so blindingly, and the road edge can be seen almost immediately after the headlight glare has passed. (Anderson L, Turkki P, Mitchell H et al: Nutrition in Health and Disease, 17th ed. Philadelphia, JB Lippincott, 1982)

off. This condition, called *xerophthalmia,* leads to blindness if untreated.

Formation of Bones and Teeth. Vitamin A is necessary for the normal growth and development of bones and teeth.

Excess

Vitamin A toxicity, or hypervitaminosis A, results from the ingestion of huge doses of the vitamin in pills or fish liver oils. Symptoms include nausea, headache, dry skin, dizziness, loss of hair, pain in the long bones, and increased bone fragility.

Sources

Fish liver oils are the richest natural source of vitamin A. These oils are dietary supplements rather than foods. (They are also rich in vitamin D; both A and D are stored in the body and can be toxic.) Fish liver oils should be measured carefully and taken only in recommended amounts.

Liver is an excellent source of vitamin A. Whole milk and food containing milk fat (butter, cream, and whole-milk cheeses), egg yolk, and margarine are good sources. All margarines are fortified with vitamin A and are nutritionally equal to butter in vitamin A content. Many skim and low-fat milks are vitamin-A-fortified.

Carotene occurs in deep yellow and dark green vegetables and in some yellow fruits. Good sources of carotene are apricots, broccoli,

Table 12-1. Vitamin A Content of Average Servings of Selected Foods

Food	Serving Size	International Units*	Retinol Equivalents†
Whole milk	1 cup	310	93
Nonfat or low-fat milk fortified with vitamin A	1 cup	500	150
Butter	1 pat	150	45
Margarine fortified with vitamin A	1 pat	170	51
Liver, beef, fried in margarine	3 oz	45,390	13,630
Liverwurst	2 oz	3,700	1,111
Egg, hard-cooked	1	260	78
Ground beef	3 oz	20	6
Carrots, cooked	½ cup	8,140	814
Sweet potatoes, baked in skin	1	9,230	923
Spinach, cooked from fresh	½ cup	7,290	729
Collards, cooked from fresh	½ cup	7,410	741
Broccoli, chopped, cooked	½ cup	2,405	241
Cantaloupe	¼ melon	4,620	462
Peach	1	1,330	133
Apricots	3	2,890	289
Apple	1	120	12
Orange	1	260	26

* Source of values in international units: Nutritive Value of Foods. USDA Home and Garden Bulletin 72, 1981.

† $\dfrac{\text{IU of retinol}}{3.33}$ or $\dfrac{\text{IU of B carotene}}{10}$ = retinol equivalents

cantaloupe, carrots, chard, collards, cress, kale, mango, persimmon, pumpkin, spinach, sweet potatoes, turnip greens and other dark green leaves, and winter squash (Table 12-1).

There is little loss of vitamin A or carotene in the processing or cooking of food; in fact, cooking increases the availability of carotene in vegetables.

Recommended Allowances

The expression of vitamin A in international units (IU) has been dropped in the 1980 RDA. Instead, the unit RE (retinol equivalent) is used. The recommended daily intake for ages 11 years to adult is 1000 RE (5000 IU) for males and 800 RE (4000 IU) for females.

Vitamin D (Calciferol)

Calciferol is the general name given to vitamin D, which includes several compounds. From the standpoint of humans, the two most important vitamin D compounds are ergocalciferol (D_2) and cholecalciferol (D_3). These substances are formed from precursors in plants and in the skin and are converted to vitamin D by the ultraviolet rays of the sun.

How much vitamin D is produced in the body is influenced by several factors: distance the person lives from the equator; how much sunlight he is exposed to; environmental conditions, such as fog and smoke; and whether the sunlight he receives is filtered through window glass. In some climates, there is not enough sunlight to provide for the needs of infants and children.

Vitamin D is stored mainly in the liver, and some is stored in the brain, bones, and skin. It undergoes changes in the liver and the kidney that convert it to its active, hormonelike form. The kidney plays an especially important role in vitamin D metabolism.

Functions and Clinical Effects

Vitamin D regulates the absorption and metabolism of calcium and phosphorus so that normal calcification of bone can take place and normal serum levels of calcium and phosphorus

are maintained. Vitamin D promotes bone formation by providing high levels of calcium and phosphorus. Direct involvement of vitamin D in bone calcification has not been proved.

Absorption of Calcium and Phosphorus. Vitamin D is necessary for the absorption of calcium and phosphorus from the small intestine. Without it, the amount of calcium absorbed would not meet requirements. Vitamin D activity is directed toward promoting the absorption of calcium; phosphorus absorption follows as an accompanying anion (negatively charged particle).

Removal of Calcium and Phosphorus from Bone. The presence of vitamin D is essential to the activity of the parathyroid hormone in removing calcium and phosphorus from the bone in order to maintain normal serum levels of these minerals.

Reabsorption of Calcium by the Kidney. Vitamin D stimulates the reabsorption of calcium by the kidney when serum calcium levels are low.

Hormonal Controls. Vitamin D metabolism is linked to the endocrine systems that control calcium–phosphorus balance. The parathyroid hormone stimulates the conversion of vitamin D to its active hormonal form in the kidneys when serum calcium levels fall. Calcitonin, secreted by the thyroid gland when serum calcium levels rise, depresses the production of vitamin D hormone.

Calcium loss from bones is typically seen in late stages of chronic kidney failure owing in part to the inability of the kidney to convert vitamin D to its hormonal form.

Deficiency

A deficiency of vitamin D causes rickets. This disease was formerly quite common among infants and children but is rarely seen today because practically all milk and infant formulas are vitamin-D-fortified. In rickets, calcium and phosphorus are lacking in the bones, causing them to become soft and pliable; the long bones bend under the body's weight. All the bones are

affected. Knock knees and bowed legs are seen, the wrists and ankles are thickened, and the teeth erupt late and are of poor quality.

In adults, a severe deficiency of vitamin D, calcium, and phosphorus can lead to osteomalacia, sometimes called *adult rickets.* The bones become soft, flexible, and deformed, giving rise to rheumatic pain. The disease is rare in western countries but is seen in the Middle East and the Orient.

Excess

Hypervitaminosis D generally results from the excessive intake of vitamin supplements, usually in the form of fish liver oils. Symptoms of hypervitaminosis D include weakness, weight loss, nausea, growth failure, and calcium deposits in the soft tissue, including the blood vessels, heart, and kidney.

Sources

Fish liver oils are very rich sources of vitamin D. Foods in their natural state are not good sources of vitamin D, so that fortified foods, vitamin concentrates, and fish liver oils are needed to supply the vitamin if circumstances warrant it. Almost all whole milk is fortified with 400 IU of vitamin D per quart; evaporated milk is similarly fortified.

Vitamin D in foods and supplements is stable to heat and storage.

Recommended Allowances

Vitamin D is now expressed in micrograms cholecalciferol rather than international units (2.5 μg = 100 IU). The RDA is 10 μg (400 IU) of vitamin D from birth through 18 years of age; for adults, it is 5 μg (200 IU), an amount that usually can be obtained by normal exposure to sunlight. Environmental conditions and clothing can block the sun's ultraviolet rays, making it necessary to obtain vitamin D from fortified foods or a vitamin supplement. Persons who are rarely exposed to sunlight, such as invalids and persons who work nights and sleep during the day, may also require a supplement.

Vitamin E (Tocopherols)

A group of closely related compounds exhibit vitamin E activity. Alpha-tocopherol is the most important form. Although vitamin E is known to be essential, its function is poorly understood. A very important characteristic is its ability to accept oxygen and thus prevent oxygen from destroying other substances. Such a substance is called an *antioxidant.*

Functions and Clinical Effects

Vitamin E in the tissue is thought to have a protective action, in that it prevents molecules from combining with oxygen to produce toxic substances that damage cell membranes. Vitamin E protects against hemolysis (destruction of red blood cells). It also protects essential fatty acids. The requirement for vitamin E increases with the amount of polyunsaturated fats in the diet.

Vitamin E protects vitamin A from oxidation in the intestinal tract and for this reason is added to vitamin A supplements. Its antioxidant properties make it useful in commercial foods as a means of retarding spoilage.

Deficiency

Vitamin E deficiency is rare. It may occur in premature infants, because vitamin E is poorly transferred across the placenta and the immature intestinal tract does not adequately absorb dietary vitamin E. It may also occur in clients with poor fat absorption over long periods of time. Symptoms include anemia resulting from a breakdown of red blood cells (hemolysis).

A host of vitamin E deficiency diseases have been identified in animals, including muscular dystrophy in rabbits; heart failure in calves; loss of fetuses in female rats, hamsters, mice, and guinea pigs; and brain damage in chickens. However, attempts to prevent or cure corresponding diseases in humans by administration of vitamin E have met with failure. There is no sound scientific evidence at present to support claims that vitamin E supplements delay the aging process or prevent or cure sterility, miscarriages, heart disease, muscle weakness, or cancer.

Excess

There is no strong evidence that large doses of vitamin E are harmful. However, it is advisable to use vitamin E cautiously, since it is established that high doses of other fat-soluble vitamins are toxic. Vitamin E appears to have anti-vitamin-K activity, reducing the body's blood clotting ability. Persons taking anticoagulant drugs should not take large doses of vitamin E because of the danger of hemorrhage.

Sources

Wheat germ and wheat germ oil are the richest sources of vitamin E, which occurs in many foods. Vegetable oils, shortening, margarine, whole-grain cereals, legumes (including peanuts), corn, nuts, and green, leafy vegetables are good sources. Except for liver and egg yolk, animal foods are relatively poor sources of vitamin E.

Vitamin E is not affected by heat but deteriorates when exposed to light or put into contact with iron or lead.

Recommended Allowances

The recommended allowance for vitamin E is expressed as alpha-tocopherol equivalents (α-TE). The recommendation is 8 mg α-TE for adult females and 10 mg α-TE for adult males.

There appears to be a greater need than normal for vitamin E when the diet is high in polyunsaturated fats. Because the polyunsaturated fats in the American diet are mostly vegetable oils, which are rich sources of vitamin E, a diet that is high in polyunsaturates is automatically high in vitamin E.

Vitamin K

There are a number of compounds with vitamin K activity. One form, menaquinone, is produced by bacteria in the intestinal tract. Bacterial synthesis is an important source of this vitamin. Another form, phylloquinone, is found naturally in foods. Some forms are made synthetically, menadione being the most potent.

Functions and Clinical Effects

Vitamin K has an essential role in the blood clotting process, being needed for the synthesis of prothrombin and other blood clotting factors in the liver.

It is probable that vitamin K has other physiological functions, but these have not been identified. Vitamin K appears to be closely associated with calcium metabolism.

Deficiency

Newborn infants are prone to vitamin K deficiency because during fetal life, little vitamin K crosses the placenta, and during the early postnatal period, the intestinal tract is sterile, so that vitamin K cannot be synthesized from bacteria. Prothrombin and other clotting factors are low for about one week after birth. A vitamin K supplement is usually given to newborn infants to prevent hemorrhage.

Impaired coagulation due to vitamin K deficiency is rare in adults. It may occur when there is poor absorption of fats or when certain drugs are used. Any condition that interferes with fat absorption affects vitamin K absorption and may produce a deficiency that makes the affected person prone to hemorrhage. Gallbladder disease, celiac disease, and ulcerative colitis are examples of such conditions. Intravenous vitamin K may be necessary. The use of sulfonamides and antibiotics can depress the production of intestinal bacteria, thereby causing a deficiency of vitamin K requiring supplementation.

The coumarin drugs and the salicylates are anticoagulants, which interfere with vitamin K production and thus prevent prothrombin synthesis. Therefore, in a patient who has been given too large a dose of one of these drugs during therapy for certain heart conditions, vitamin K is given to correct the problem.

Excess

Large doses of synthetic vitamin K (menadione) given over long periods of time are toxic. For this reason, menadione has been removed from over-the-counter drug preparations.

Symptoms of toxicity are lowered prothrombin levels, kidney tubule degeneration, and, in infants, jaundice and a type of anemia.

Sources

Synthesis by normal bacteria in the intestinal tract is an important source of vitamin K. Green, leafy vegetables are the best food source. Vitamin K is also found in cauliflower, alfalfa, liver, egg yolk, soybean oil and other vegetable oils, and, to a lesser extent, in wheat and oats. Vitamin K is destroyed by strong acids, alkalis, and certain oxidizing agents.

Recommended Allowances

No recommended allowance for vitamin K has been made by the Food and Nutrition Board. A deficiency is unlikely, because vitamin K is synthesized by intestinal bacteria and has a fairly wide distribution in food. An estimated adequate and safe daily intake for adults is 70 μg to 140 μg Unlike other fat-soluble vitamins, vitamin K is not stored by the body in any significant amount.

Fat-soluble vitamins are summarized in Table 12-2.

Water-Soluble Vitamins

Ascorbic Acid (Vitamin C)

A lack of ascorbic acid causes scurvy, which is probably the oldest recognized deficiency disease. It has been known for centuries that scurvy is caused by a limited food supply and that it

Table 12-2. Summary: Fat-Soluble Vitamins

Vitamin	Function	Deficiency	Sources
A (retinol); precursor: carotenes	Formation of visual purple; normal growth of epithelial tissue, especially skin and mucous membranes; normal bone and tooth structure	Night and glare blindness; deterioration of epithelial tissue leading to decreased resistance to infection; dry, scaly skin; eye changes; xerophthalmia leading to blindness	Liver; whole milk and foods containing milk fat, such as butter, cream, cheese; margarine; as carotene in dark green leafy vegetables and some fruits
D (calciferol)	Promotion of absorption of calcium and phosphorus; normal utilization of these minerals in skeleton and soft tissue	Faulty bone and tooth development; rickets; osteomalacia	Fortified milk; direct exposure of skin to sunlight; fish liver oils
E (tocopherols)	Antioxidation—protection of substances that oxidize readily, such as vitamin A and essential fatty acids; thus, prevention of damage to cell membranes	Destruction of red blood cells (hemolysis); deficiency is rare	Vegetable oils and shortening; margarine; green leafy vegetables; whole grains, legumes, nuts
K (menadione)	Normal blood clotting	Prolonged clotting time; hemorrhagic disease in newborns	Synthesis by intestinal bacteria; green leafy vegetables

can be prevented by the inclusion of fresh foods in the diet. The disease used to be especially threatening to sailors, who existed for long periods of time on a diet of salted meats and fish and breadstuffs. In the mid-1700s, as prevention against scurvy, limes and lemons were added to the rations of British sailors, who then became known as *limeys.*

Functions and Clinical Effects

Collagen Formation. Ascorbic acid plays a vital role in collagen formation; collagen is the protein "glue" that holds the tissue cells together. Collagen consists of insoluble protein fibers, which provide firmness and support to the tissues of the skin, cartilage, tendons, ligaments, blood vessels, bones, and teeth. Collagen is a major component of scar tissue formed during the healing of wounds and bone fractures.

Hemoglobin Formation. Vitamin C increases the absorption of iron from the intestinal tract and promotes its use in the body. It is also needed to convert the inactive form of the vitamin folic acid (another blood-building nutrient) to the active form.

Other Functions. Vitamin C appears to have numerous other roles in regulating body processes, many of which have not been clearly defined. It is involved in the metabolism of fats and protein. High concentrations of ascorbic acid in the adrenal gland and its depletion when the gland is stimulated suggest a need for vitamin C during periods of stress. Blood levels of vitamin C decrease during fever, also suggesting the body's increased need during this condition.

Deficiency

When vitamin C is deficient, the fibers of connective tissue are not properly formed. This results in skin abnormalities, fragile blood vessels, and poor wound healing (Fig. 12-2).

Skin abnormalities such as adult acne may be the earliest sign of scurvy. Hardening and

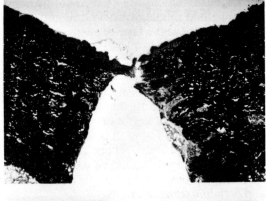
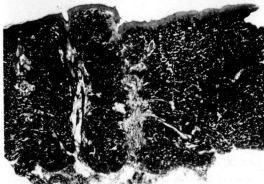

Fig. 12-2. Role of vitamin C in wound healing. (*Top*) Biopsy 10 days after an experimental wound was made in the back of Dr. John Crandon, who had not consumed any vitamin C for 6 months. No healing is evident except of the epithelium (a gap in tissues was filled with a blood clot). (*Bottom*) After 10 days of treatment with vitamin C, another biopsy of the wound shows healing with abundant collagen formation. (*The Vitamin Manual.* Kalamazoo, MI, Upjohn Co)

scaling of the skin surrounding the hair follicle and hemorrhages surrounding the hair follicle also point to scurvy. The hair may be broken and coiled, and some hairs may have a swanneck deformity. The skin of the forearms, legs, and thighs is most apt to be affected. Other symptoms of scurvy include weakness, fatigue, restlessness, and neurotic behavior; aching bones, joints, and muscles; sensitivity to touch; sore mouth and gums, with bleeding and loosening of the teeth and bruising and hemorrhag-

ing of the skin. Anemia may also occur. Death results if the deficiency is not corrected.

Scurvy is rare in the United States. It may still be found among the elderly, who may be eating poorly, or in persons on severely restricted diets, such as certain stages of the Zen macrobiotic diet.

Excess

Claims that large doses of vitamin C can prevent or cure the common cold have not been supported by carefully controlled research studies, though colds seen in these studies appeared to be less severe when large doses of vitamin C were taken.

Large doses of vitamin C have generally been considered harmless; however, the safety of megadoses has not been established. In fact, evidence is accumulating indicating that serious harm can result from large doses of vitamin C. Increased risk of kidney stones, destruction of vitamin B_{12}, and interference with anticoagulant drugs are among the harmful effects reported.

Because there is no strong evidence that large doses of vitamin C are useful, and because the possibility of harmful effects remains, large doses of vitamin C are not recommended without medical advice.

Sources

Citrus fruits and their juices, whether fresh, frozen, or canned, are excellent sources of vitamin C. Broccoli is another excellent source, as are strawberries, cantaloupe, guava, mango, papaya, and peppers. Other significant sources are tomatoes and tomato juice, cabbage, greens (such as collards, garden cress, kale, mustard, and turnip greens), and potatoes and sweet potatoes cooked in their jackets. Table 12-3 lists the vitamin C content of selected foods.

Vitamin C is the most unstable of all the vitamins. Care must be taken to conserve the vitamin by properly storing and cooking food. Vitamin loss from fruits and vegetables is reduced when these foods are stored in the refrigerator. Vitamin C is readily destroyed by alkali, therefore, baking soda should never be added to

vegetables in cooking. Excessive cutting and chopping should be avoided. Vegetables should be steamed, if possible, or cooked in very little water as briefly as possible. Adding vegetables to boiling water shortens the cooking time. Potatoes have a higher vitamin C content if cooked in their skins.

Recommended Allowances

The RDA for ascorbic acid is 60 mg from age 15 through adulthood; 80 mg during pregnancy; and 100 mg during lactation. From infancy through 14 years of age, the recommendation ranges from 35 mg to 50 mg.

Thiamine (Vitamin B_1)

The enrichment of cereal products has almost completely eliminated beriberi, a thiamine deficiency disease. Although rare, however, this disorder is still sometimes seen among alcoholics. Beriberi developed among rice-eating peoples when refined, polished rice began to replace brown rice. The bran layer that is removed during the milling process is rich in thiamine. The disease continues to be a problem in areas of the world where enrichment is not a standard practice.

Functions and Clinical Effects

Energy Metabolism. Thiamine is needed for the formation of a coenzyme involved in energy metabolism. Thiamine works with the coenzymes of other B vitamins in key reactions that convert glucose to energy. Their roles are interrelated.

Synthesis of DNA and RNA. Thiamine is also required for the conversion of some glucose to ribose, an essential component of deoxyribonucleic acid (DNA) and ribonucleic acid (RNA), carriers of the genetic code.

Deficiency and Excess

Thiamine deficiency affects the gastrointestinal, cardiovascular, and nervous systems, causing

Table 12-3. Ascorbic Acid Content of Average Servings of Selected Foods

Food	Serving size	Milligrams of ascorbic acid
Milk, whole or skim	1 cup	2
Cheddar cheese	1 oz	0
Egg	1	0
Beef liver	3 oz	23
Other meat, fish, poultry		0
Broccoli, cooked	$\frac{1}{2}$ cup	70
Collards, from fresh, cooked	$\frac{1}{2}$ cup	72
Turnip green, from fresh, cooked	$\frac{1}{2}$ cup	34
Cauliflower, from fresh, cooked	$\frac{1}{2}$ cup	35
Tomato, raw	1	28
Potato, boiled	1	22
Cabbage, cooked	$\frac{1}{2}$ cup	24
Carrots, cooked	$\frac{1}{2}$ cup	4.5
Peas, frozen, cooked	$\frac{1}{2}$ cup	10.5
Orange	1	66
Orange juice, frozen, diluted	$\frac{1}{2}$ cup	60
Strawberries, whole, fresh	$\frac{1}{2}$ cup	44
Grapefruit, fresh	$\frac{1}{2}$	44
Grapefruit juice, frozen, diluted	$\frac{1}{2}$ cup	48
Banana	1	12
Apple	1	6

(Nutritive Value of Foods. USDA Home and Garden Bulletin 72, 1981)

symptoms such as loss of appetite, constipation, fatigue, irritability, neuritis, and headaches. However, these same symptoms can be attributed to many other causes.

A serious B_1 deficiency has a devastating effect on the nervous system. The neurological symptoms are very evident in beriberi. In older children and adults, the disease occurs in two forms, dry beriberi and wet beriberi. The dry type is seen mainly among elderly adults and is often associated with long-standing alcoholism. There is a wasting of body tissue and various nervous disorders, including paralysis of the legs. Edema caused by heart failure is the most characteristic symptom of wet beriberi. In both types, there is irritablity, confusion, and nausea. Infantile beriberi occurs in infants consuming breast milk low in thiamine. The onset of symptoms is sudden, and the disease is fatal if not treated promptly.

Excessive intake of thiamine has no known effect.

Sources

Thiamine is found in meats, especially pork and organ meats, wheat germ, whole-grain and enriched breads and cereals, dry peas and beans, peanuts and peanut butter, and nuts.

If care is not taken in cooking, the thiamine

in food may be lost. Since thiamine is water-soluble, thiamine-containing foods should be cooked in as little water as possible, at low temperatures, and for as short a time as possible. Whenever practical, water remaining from cooked foods and meat drippings should be used. Alkaline substances, such as baking soda and antacid medications, destroy thiamine.

Recommended Allowances

A thiamine intake of 0.5 mg per 1000 kcal is recommended for infants, children, and adults. Therefore, a man consuming 2700 kcal daily would require 0.5 mg $\times$ 2.7, or 1.4 mg. Because there is evidence that elderly persons may not utilize thiamine as efficiently as younger adults, they should take in at least 1 mg/day, even when their caloric intake is below 2000 kcal.

Riboflavin (Vitamin B₂)

Functions and Clinical Effects

Energy Metabolism. Riboflavin is a component of enzyme systems necessary for the release of energy within the cell. This involves the metabolism of carbohydrates, proteins, and fats.

Tissue Growth and Maintenance. Riboflavin forms enzymes involved in protein metabolism.

Deficiency and Excess

Sensitivity to light and dimness of vision may be one of the first signs of ariboflavinosis (riboflavin deficiency). Later, the eyes become irritated and water readily. Lesions appear around the mouth and nose. The lips become cracked and sore, and fissures develop at the corners of the mouth (cheilosis). The tongue becomes abnormally smooth and purplish, a condition called *glossitis.* Riboflavin deficiency is rarely fatal, possibly because small amounts of the vitamin are synthesized by intestinal bacteria. Ariboflavinosis usually occurs with deficiences of other B-complex vitamins.

Riboflavin deficiency is a relatively common disorder in the United States as well as in other countries. The deficiency is most likely to occur when physical demands are high, as in periods of growth (childhood, pregnancy, lactation) and physical stress (surgery, burns, malabsorption disorders, chronic disease).

Excess riboflavin intake has no known effect.

Sources

Milk is an outstanding source of riboflavin, and persons who do not drink milk are likely to have a low riboflavin intake. Meats, especially liver and other organ meats, green, leafy vegetables, fish, eggs, and enriched breads and cereals are good sources.

Riboflavin is destroyed by ultraviolet light and sunlight, which is why cartons and opaque plastic containers are used for packaging milk.

Recommended Allowances

An intake of 0.6 mg per 1000 kcal is recommended for infants, children, and adults. The recommendation for the average woman is 1.2 mg; for the average man, it is 1.6 mg. For adults whose energy intake is less than 2000 kcal, a minimum of 1.2 mg per day is advised. Women using birth control pills may have an increased need for riboflavin.

Niacin

Early in efforts to discover a cure for pellagra (a disease affecting the skin, gastrointestinal tract, and nervous system), protein foods such as milk, eggs, and meat were found to have a positive effect. Later, it was discovered that niacin is the pellagra-preventive factor. However, milk, although curative in pellegra, is low in niacin. The connection among these facts became evident when it was learned that niacin can be synthesized from tryptophan, an essential amino acid (basic unit of protein).

Functions and Clinical Effects

Niacin occurs in two forms, nicotinic acid and niacinamide. Niacin affects a number of important metabolic activities needed for the maintenance of healthy skin and for the proper functioning of the nervous and digestive systems.

Energy Metabolism. Niacin is a coenzyme in energy metabolism along with the other B-complex vitamins.

Production of Fatty Acids, Cholesterol, and Steroid Hormones. Niacin-containing hormones are involved in the synthesis of fatty acids, cholesterol, and steroid hormones.

Deficiency

Early signs of niacin deiciency include fatigue, lack of appetite, weakness, mild digestive disturbances, anxiety, and irritability.

A prolonged niacin deficiency causes *pellagra,* an Italian word meaning "rough skin." The disease is characterized by the "4 Ds": diarrhea, dermatitis, dementia (deteriorated mental state), and finally death if the disease goes untreated. The skin is dry, scaly, and cracked, and the condition is aggravated by exposure to heat or light. In the acute stages, pellagra resembles severe sunburn; in later stages, the affected areas become darkly pigmented. The lesions occur in the same places on both sides of the body. Intestinal symptoms include soreness of the mouth, swelling of the tongue, and diarrhea. There are effects of mental irritability, anxiety, depression, and confusion.

At one time, pellagra was of great concern in the United States, especially in certain regions of the South. In these areas, the diet consisted mostly of corn, which is deficient in both niacin and protein. The enrichment of breads and cereals has eradicated the disease in the United States. It is now usually seen only in connection with chronic alcoholism.

Excess

Niacin is not stored to any significant extent in the body, and any excess is excreted in the urine. Large doses have been administered to lower serum cholesterol and other blood lipids and to treat schizophrenia. However, there is evidence that massive doses of niacin can cause heartbeat irregularities, gastrointestinal and liver disorders, and other health problems.

Sources

Niacin is found in meat (especially liver), fish, poultry, peanut butter, peas, beans, and whole-grain bread and cereal products. Milk, eggs, and cheese are poor sources of preformed niacin; however, as complete protein foods, they are good sources of tryptophan, which is converted in the body to niacin. Niacin is not readily destroyed by light, heat, acid, or alkali, but it does dissolve in water and thus may be lost in cooking. To preserve niacin, it is advisable to cook meats at low temperatures to avoid excessive loss of juices and to utilize the meat juices.

Recommended Allowances

The requirement for niacin is met by both the preformed vitamin and its synthesis from the amino acid tryptophan. For this reason, the recommended niacin allowance is expressed in niacin equivalents. One niacin equivalent is equal to 1 mg of niacin or 60 mg of tryptophan. This amount of tryptophan is supplied by approximately 6 g of protein. Because the typical American diet is high is protein, tryptophan contributes substantially to niacin in the diet. The recommended allowance for adults is 6.6 niacin equivalents for every 1000 kcal consumed, but not less than 13 niacin equivalents for caloric intakes below 2000 kcal.

Pyridoxine (Vitamin B_6)

Vitamin B_6 activity is demonstrated by three closely related compounds: pyridoxine, pyridoxal, and pyridoxamine. These substances form coenzymes that function in many reactions involving amino acids, some of which are described below.

Functions and Clinical Effects

Protein Synthesis. Vitamin B_6 is needed for the synthesis of nonessential amino acids.

Synthesis of Regulatory Substances. B_6 is involved in producing other compounds from amino acids, such as serotonin from tryptophan. Serotonin causes blood vessels to constrict and is involved in the regulation of brain and other tissue.

Niacin Production. B_6 is a catalyst in the conversion of tryptophan to niacin.

Hemoglobin Synthesis. B_6 is required for the synthesis of a substance involved in the production of heme. It is also required for the metabolism of folic acid.

Deficiency and Excess

Severe deficiency of vitamin B_6 is rare. Symptoms include anemia, nausea, soreness of mouth, smooth red tongue, dermatitis around the eyes and at the angles of the mouth, formation of kidney stones, and disturbances of the central nervous system. Infants fed a formula deficient in vitamin B_6 became irritable and experienced convulsions. The vitamin B_6 in the formula had been destroyed by overprocessing. A deficiency of B_6 occurs in 20% to 30% of alcoholics.

Excess vitamin B_6 produces no known effects.

Sources

The best sources of vitamin B_6 are liver, kidney, red meats, fish, whole-grain cereals, legumes, bananas, potatoes, green vegetables, and yellow corn.

Recommended Allowances

The need for vitamin B_6 increases with increased consumption of protein. The RDA for B_6 is 2.2 mg for men and 2 mg for women.

Certain drugs may interact with B_6. Isoniazid (INH), used in tuberculosis therapy, and penicillamine, used in the treatment of Wilson's disease (copper storage disease), inactivate B_6. Oral contraceptives may increase the B_6 requirement.

Folacin (Folic Acid)

Folic acid deficiency is a common disorder in the United States and throughout the world, especially in the tropics. It occurs most frequently in infancy, during pregnancy, and in conditions in which absorption is impaired. Folic acid has been very useful in the treatment of sprue, a malabsorption disease characterized by diarrhea, anemia, and general malnutrition.

Functions and Clinical Effects

Protein Metabolism. Folic acid is necessary for protein metabolism and the synthesis of DNA and RNA. Effects of a deficiency are most evident in rapidly growing tissues or tissues with rapid cell turnover.

Formation of Hemoglobin. The formation of heme, the iron-containing substance in the blood, is dependent upon folacin. Folic acid function is interwoven with vitamins B_{12} and B_6. Vitamin C plays a role in the conversion of folacin to its coenzyme form.

Deficiency

The outstanding symptom of folacin deficiency is macrocytic anemia, a condition in which the red blood cells become enlarged and are reduced in number. Glossitis, stomatitis (sore mouth), and gastrointestinal disturbances, including diarrhea, may also be present. Because of the interrelationships of folacin, ascorbic acid, B_6, and B_{12} in the formation of blood, the anemia of different vitamin deficiency diseases may be similar and may respond to treatment with one or several of these vitamins. However, all B vitamins are needed and cannot substitute for one another. Although folic acid can relieve the anemia of pernicious anemia, it does not cure the neurological symptoms.

Sources

Folacin is found in green leafy vegetables, liver, kidney, other meat, fish, nuts, legumes, and whole-grain cereals. It is easily destroyed by poor cooking or storage procedures and by food processing.

Recommended Allowances

The RDA for adolescents and adults is 400 μg. The need for folacin is substantially increased during pregnancy and lactation owing to the role of folic acid in cell multiplication. The RDA during pregnancy is 800 μg. Folic acid supplements are usually given during pregnancy.

Alcohol and some drugs decrease the absorption of this vitamin. Antimalaria drugs and the antitumor drug methotrexate inactivate folic acid. The use of oral contraceptives appears to increase the need for folic acid.

Cobalamin (Vitamin B_{12})

Vitamin B_{12} is present in all cells and is necessary for their normal functioning. The trace element cobalt is part of the B_{12} molecule. For this reason, the vitamin was named *cobalamin.*

Functions and Clinical Effects

Protein Metabolism. The synthesis of DNA depends upon B_{12}-containing enzymes. B_{12} is also necessary for the synthesis of one or more amino acids.

Production of Red Blood Cells. The role of B_{12} in DNA synthesis is of particular importance in bone marrow, where blood cells are formed. If B_{12} is lacking, red blood cells do not develop normally. Instead, they become larger than normal and fewer in number. Vitamin B_{12} appears to influence this blood-building process by promoting the functioning of folic acid.

Normal Functioning of the Nervous System. The exact role of B_{12} in the health of the nervous system is unknown but appears to be related to carbohydrate metabolism and to myelin formation.

B_{12} absorption from the intestinal tract and its transfer to the bloodstream is a slow and complex process that takes place over a period of hours, in contrast to the seconds required for the absorption of most of the other water-soluble vitamins. Absorption of vitamin B_{12} is dependent upon a protein in gastric juice called *intrinsic factor.* The B_{12} attaches to intrinsic factor and is carried to the ileum, where it is absorbed.

Deficiency and Excess

A deficiency of vitamin B_{12} usually results from absorption problems rather than from a dietary deficiency. Pernicious anemia, the B_{12} deficiency disease, is due to a lack of intrinsic factor in gastric juice. In this type of anemia, the red blood cells are abnormally large and reduced in number. Other symptoms include a sore mouth, lack of appetite, neurological difficulties, such as poor coordination in walking, and mental disturbances. A deficiency of B_{12} may also follow surgery of the stomach or small intestine and diseases that affect nutrient absorption. Injections of B_{12} must be given throughout the affected person's life. Maintenance dialysis in cases of renal failure may also cause low serum levels of vitamin B_{12} with symptoms of deficiency.

Since B_{12} is found only in animal foods, a deficiency may develop in persons who follow strict vegetarian diets. Children on vegetarian diets are at greatest risk, since they have not accumulated stores of the vitamin.

There are no known effects of excess vitamin B_{12} intake.

Sources

Vitamin B_{12} is found only in animal products such as meat, fish, poultry, eggs, milk, and cheese. Soybean milk substitutes, useful in strict vegetarian diets, are frequently fortified with B_{12}.

It is strongly recommended that children on vegetarian diet be permitted eggs and milk. B_{12} supplements or B_{12}-fortified foods are neces-

Table 12-4.   Summary: Water-Soluble Vitamins

Vitamin	Function	Deficiency	Sources
Ascorbic acid (vitamin C)	Collagen formation: strong blood vessels, healthy skin, healthy gums, wound healing; formation of red blood cells: absorption of iron, conversion of folacin to its active form	Adult acne; easy bruising; poor wound healing; swan-neck hair deformity; sore gums; hemorrhages around bones; scurvy	Citrus fruit; broccoli; strawberries; cantaloupe; guava, mango, papaya; peppers; tomatoes; greens; potatoes
Thiamine (B_1)	Energy metabolism; synthesis of DNA, RNA	Poor appetite; fatigue; constipation; neuritis of legs; beriberi: wasting, paralysis of legs, heart failure, mental confusion	Meats, especially pork; wheat germ; whole-grain and enriched bread; legumes; peanuts, peanut butter; nuts
Riboflavin (B_2)	Energy metabolism; protein metabolism	Sensitivity to light; eye irritation; cheilosis; glossitis	Milk; organ meats; meat, fish, eggs; green leafy vegetables; enriched breads and cereals
Niacin (precursor: tryptophan)	Energy metabolism; production of fatty acids, cholesterol, steroid hormones	Fatigue; poor appetite; weakness; anxiety; pellagra: diarrhea, dermatitis, deteriorated mental state	Liver; meat, fish, poultry; peanuts; legumes; whole-grain breads and cereals; sources of tryptophan: complete protein foods
Pyridoxine (B_6)	Amino acid metabolism involving protein synthesis; synthesis of regulatory substances such as serotonin; niacin production; hemoglobin synthesis	Anemia; sore mouth; nausea; dermatitis; irritability; convulsions	Liver, kidney; red meats; corn; whole-grain cereals; legumes; bananas; potatoes; green vegetables
Folacin (folic acid)	Protein metabolism: synthesis of DNA and RNA, red blood cell formation	Macrocytic anemia	Green leafy vegetables; liver, kidney, meats, fish; nuts; legumes; whole grains
Cobalamin (B_{12})	Protein metabolism: synthesis of DNA, production of red blood cells; healthy nervous system: carbohydrate metabolism, myelin formation (Intrinsic factor of gastric secretions is required for absorption)	Pernicious anemia: macrocytic anemia, sore mouth, poor appetite, poor coordination in walking, mental disturbances	Found only in animal products: meat, fish, poultry, eggs, milk, cheese
Pantothenic acid	Energy metabolism; synthesis of amino acids, fatty acids, cholesterol, steroid hormones, hemoglobin	Unlikely unless part of a deficiency of all B vitamins	Organ meats; salmon; eggs; broccoli; mushrooms; pork; whole grains; legumes; (synthesized by intestinal bacteria)

sary for both adults and children who are on strict vegetarian diets (those that exclude milk and eggs as well as meat, fish, and poultry).

Recommended Allowances

The RDA for vitamin B_{12} is 3 μg from age 7 through adulthood. Excess B_{12} is stored in the liver in relatively large amounts.

Pantothenic Acid

Functions and Clinical Effects

Pantothenic acid is part of coenzyme A (active acetate), which is essential for many chemical reactions, including the release of energy from protein, fats, and carbohydrates. This vitamin is also involved in the synthesis of amino acids, fatty acids, cholesterol, steroid hormones, and hemoglobin.

Deficiency and Excess

A deficiency is not likely except in cases of a deficiency of all the B vitamins. A deficiency might result from a diet consisting of highly processed foods, since processing causes large losses of pantothenic acid. Experimental deficiency has produced such symptoms as insom-

nia, leg cramps, numbness and tingling of the hands and feet, and personality changes.

Excess intake of pantothenic acid has no known effects.

Sources

The vitamin is distributed widely in foods. Yeast, organ meats, salmon, and eggs are the best sources. Other good sources are broccoli, mushrooms, pork, whole-grain cereals and breads, and legumes. Grains lose 50% of their pantothenic acid in milling.

Recommended Allowances

The requirement for pantothenic acid has not been established. The Food and Nutrition Board states that an intake of 4 mg to 7 mg/day is probably adequate for adults; a higher intake may be needed for pregnant and lactating women.

Biotin

Biotin is involved in the metabolism of proteins, fats, and carbohydrates. Deficiency is very rare. Avidin, a protein found in raw egg white, combines with biotin and prevents its absorption. Intestinal bacteria synthesize a considerable amount.

Water-soluble vitamins are summarized in Table 12-4.

KEYS TO PRACTICAL APPLICATION

When disease conditions interfere with the digestion or absorption of fats, expect fat-soluble vitamins to be poorly absorbed, increasing the risk of deficiency.

Beware of advertisements or articles that promote the benefits of a particular nutrient, such as vitamin C or vitamin E. All of the 50 or more nutrients work together. Adding large amounts of some nutrients may interfere with the functioning of others.

Remember that, in normal amounts, vitamins are food; in amounts 5, 10, 20 or more times the RDA levels, they are drugs and should be treated as such.

Instruct parents to measure supplements containing vitamins A and/or D very carefully and use them only in recommended amounts. These vitamins are stored in the body and are toxic in excessive amounts.

Encourage the use of vegetables in both raw and cooked forms. Raw vegetables are

not always the better source of vitamins. Cooking reduces the vitamin C content of vegetables, such as tomatoes. However, cooked carrots have more available carotene (provitamin A) than raw carrots.

Steaming vegetables for as short a period as possible is the best way to preserve water-soluble vitamins. Cooking in large quantities of water, overcooking, excessive cutting and chopping, and the addition of alkali (such as baking soda) increase the loss of water-soluble vitamins.

To preserve the vitamin content of meats, cook them at low temperatures and do not overcook. Utilize meat drippings (after removing fat).

KEY IDEAS

Vitamins are involved in regulating body processes. Many vitamins function as parts of enzymes; others have hormonelike activity.

Vitamins do not provide energy, but many are involved in enzyme systems needed to convert protein, fat, and carbohydrate to energy.

The body cannot manufacture vitamins; they must be obtained in the diet. A serious lack of one or more vitamins results in one or more deficiency diseases.

Vitamins are needed in very minute amounts, measured in either milligrams or micrograms.

Vitamins are classified as fat-soluble and water-soluble.

The fat-soluble group, vitamins A, D, E, and K, are absorbed in the same manner as fats. Because they are stored in the body, deficiencies of them develop slowly. These vitamins are not readily lost in cooking.

The water-soluble group, vitamins C and B-complex, are not stored to any great extent and are usually readily destroyed by heat and in cooking.

The safety of taking large doses of vitamins without medical supervision is questionable; vitamins taken in doses in excess of nutritional needs function as drugs and should be treated as such.

See Tables 12-2 and 12-4 for a summary of vitamins.

KEYS TO LEARNING: STUDY–DISCUSSION QUESTIONS

1. Using your food record for one day, compare your intake of vitamin A, vitamin C, and thiamine with the Recommended Daily Allowance for your sex and age group given in Chapter 4.
2. Rank the following foods in order of their vitamin content, with the richest source of the specified vitamin listed first:

Vitamin A

1 cup of milk
½ cup of cooked, chopped broccoli

1 cup of chopped or shredded lettuce
3 ounces of beef liver
1 peach
1 tablespoon of butter
1 tablespoon of margarine
½ cup of cooked carrots

Vitamin C

½ fresh grapefruit
½ cup of orange juice (from concentrate)
1 orange
½ cup of cooked collards (from raw)
1 baked potato

½ fresh cantaloupe
½ cup of tomato juice
1 cup of whole milk

Niacin

3 ounces of ground beef patty
1 cup of cooked lentils
1 cup of 40% bran flakes
3 slices of whole-wheat bread (18 slices per loaf)
1 chicken breast (approx. 3 ounces)
3 ounces of beef liver
3 slices of enriched white bread (18 slices per loaf)

Check your answers by recording the vitamin content listed for each of the foods above in Table A-1 in the Appendix.

3. Define the following: hypervitaminosis, antivitamin, avitaminosis, provitamin. Give examples of each.

4. Identify the vitamin involved and explain its relationship to each of the following: night blindness, intrinsic factor, scurvy, delayed blood clotting, sunshine, raw egg white, beriberi, isoniazid, cheilosis, pellegra, tryptophan.

5. Describe ways in which the consumer can conserve the vitamin content of food.

Bibliography is found at the end of Part Two.

Bibliography

Part Two. The Role of Nutrients in the Maintenance of Normal Health

General References

Anderson L, Turkki P, Mitchell H: Nutrition in Health and Disease, 17th ed. Philadelphia, JB Lippincott, 1982

Arlin M: The Science of Nutrition. New York, Macmillan, 1977

Burton, BT: Human Nutrition. New York, published for HJ Heinz by McGraw-Hill, 1976.

Food and Nutrition Board, National Research Council: Recommended Dietary Allowances, 9th ed. Washington, DC, National Academy of Sciences, 1980

Guthrie HA: Introductory Nutrition. St. Louis, CV Mosby, 1981

Mayer J: A Diet for Living. New York, David McKay, 1975

Nutritive Value of Foods. Science and Education Administration. USDA Home and Garden Bulletin 72. Washington, DC, US Government Printing Office, 1981

Pennington JAT, Church HN: Bowes and Church's Food Values of Portions Commonly Used, 13th ed. Philadelphia, JB Lippincott, 1980

Suitor CW, Hunter M: Nutrition: Principles and Application in Health Promotion. Philadelphia, JB Lippincott, 1980

Wurtman JJ: Eating Your Way Through Life. New York, Raven Press, 1979

Chapter 4. Food and Its Functions

Books and Pamphlets

Rozovski SJ, Winick M: Nutrition and cellular growth. In Winick M (ed): Nutrition: Pre- and Postnatal Development. New York, Plenum Press, 1979

United States Senate Select Committee on Nutrition and Human Needs: Dietary Goals for the United States. Washington, DC, U.S. Government Printing Office, 1977

Periodicals

Clydesdale FM: Nutritional realities—Where does technology fit? J Am Diet Assoc 74:17, 1979

Graham DM, Hertzler, AA: Why enrich or fortify foods? J Nutr Ed 9:4:166, 1977

Guthrie HA: Concept of a nutritious food. J Am Diet Assoc 71:14, 1977

Mertz W: The new RDAs: Estimated adequate and safe intake of trace elements and calculations of available iron. J Am Diet Assoc 76:2:128, 1980

Chapter 5. Digestion and Absorption

Books and Pamphlets

Iber FL: The gastrointestinal tract. An overview of function. In Goodhart RS, Shils ME (eds): Modern Nutrition in Health and Disease. Philadelphia, Lea & Febiger, 1980

Memmler RL, Wood DM: The Human Body in

Health and Disease, 5th ed. Philadelphia, JB Lippincott, 1983

Periodicals

Almy TP: Gastrointestinal illness and emotions. Carrier Foundation Letter 73, 1981

Friedman HI, Nylund, B: Intestinal fat digestion, absorption and transport: A review. Am J Clin Nutr 33:1108, 1980

Gray GM: Carbohydrate digestion and absorption: Role of the small intestine. N Engl J Med 292:1225, 1975

Sleisenger MH, Kim YS: Protein digestion and absorption. N Engl J Med 300:659, 1979

Chapter 6. Energy Metabolism

Books and Pamphlets

Brownell KD: Behavior Therapy for Weight Control —A Treatment Manual. Philadelphia, KD Brownell, 1979

Taylor TG: Principles of Human Nutrition. London, Edward Arnold, 1978

Periodicals

Boeker EA: Metabolism of ethanol. J Am Diet Assoc 16:550, 1980

Guthrie HA: Junk foods—A scientific evaluation. Nutr MD 7:2:2, 1981

Newsholme EA: A possible metabolic basis for the control of body weight. N Engl J Med 302:400, 1980

Webb P: The measurement of energy exchange in man: An analysis. Am J Clin Nutr 33:129, 1980

Webb P, Annis JF, Troutman SJ: Energy balance in man measured by direct and indirect calorimetry. Am J Clin Nutr 33:1287, 1980

Chapter 7. Carbohydrates

Periodicals

Bing FC: Dietary fiber—An historical perspective. J Am Diet Assoc 69:498, 1976

Bocker EA: Metabolism of ethanol. J Am Diet Assoc 76:550, 1980

Bohannon NV, Karam JH, Forsham PH: Endocrine responses to sugar ingestion in man. J Am Diet Assoc 76:6:550, 1980

Brown AT: The role of dietary carbohydrate in plaque formation and oral disease. Nutr Rev 33:353, 1975

Burkitt DP: The role of dietary fiber. Nutr Today 11:6, 1976

Graham DM, Hertzler AA: Why enrich or fortify foods? J Nutr Ed 9:4:166, 1977

Johnson CK, Kolasa K, Chenoweth W, Bennink M: Health, laxation and food habit influences on fiber intake of older women. J Am Diet Assoc 77:5:551, 1980

Kelsay JL: A review of effects of fiber intake on man. Am J Clin Nutr 31:142, 1978

Mandel ID: Dental caries. Am Sci 67:680, 1979

Symposium on Role of Dietary Fiber in Health. Am J Clin Nutr (Suppl) 31:1–255, 1978

Chapter 8. Fats

Books and Pamphlets

Committee on Nutrition: Diet and Coronary Heart Disease. Dallas, American Heart Association, 1978

Hodges R: Nutrition in Medical Practice. Philadelphia, WB Saunders, 1980

Periodicals

Eaters' Almanac, Vol I, numbers 4, 9, 14, 1979 (produced as part of a nutrition education program by Giant Food and the National Heart, Lung, and Blood Institute)

Hirono H, Hiroshi S, Igarashi Y: Essential fatty acid

deficiency induced by total parenteral nutrition and by medium-chain triglyceride feeding. Am J Clin Nutr 30:1670, 1977

Vergroesen AJ: Physiological effects of dietary linoleic acid. Nutr Rev 35:1, 1977

Chapter 9. Proteins

Books and Pamphlets
Brewster L, Jacobson MF: The Changing American Diet. Washington, DC, Center for Science in the Public Interest, 1978
Gamon PM, Sherrington KB: The Science of Food. New York, Pergamon Press, 1977
Jelliffe DB, Jelliffe P: Prevention is possible: The unnecessary story of two sad children. In The Neglected Years: Early Childhood. New York, United Nations Children's Fund, 1973
Lowenberg ME, Todhunter EN, Savage JR: Food and People. New York, John Wiley & Son, 1979
Robertson F, Flinders C, Godfrey B: Laurel's Kitchen. Petaluma, CA, Nilgiri Press, 1977

Periodicals
Broquist HP: Amino acid metabolism. Nutr Rev 34:289, 1976
Chopra JG, Forbes AL, Habicht J: Protein in the US diet. J Am Diet Assoc 72:253, 1978
Hegsted DM: Assessment of nitrogen requirements. Am J Clin Nutr 31:1669, 1978
Review: Immune deficiency in malnutrition. Nutr Rev 33:334, 1976
Spencer H, Kramer L, Osis D: Effect of high protein intake on calcium metabolism in man. Am J Clin Nutr 32:2167, 1978

Chapter 10. Water and Mineral Elements

Books and Pamphlets
Hargrave M: Nutritional Care of the Physically Handicapped. Minneapolis, Sister Kenny Institute, 1979

Periodicals
Harland BF, Johnson RD, Blendermann EM: Cal-
cium, phosphorus, iron, iodine and zinc labels in the "total diet." J Am Diet Assoc 77:16, 1980
Mertz W: Mineral elements: New perspectives. J Am Diet Assoc 77:258, 1980

Chapter 11. Minerals: Macro and Micro

Books and Pamphlets
The Sodium Content of your Food. USDA Home and Garden Bulletin 233. Washington, DC, US Government Printing Office, 1980.

Periodicals
Crosby WH: Who needs iron. N Engl J Med 297:543, 1977
Freeland-Graves JH, Ebangit ML, Bodzy PW: Zinc
and copper content of foods used in vegetarian diets. J Am Diet Assoc 77:648, 1980
Gallagher JC: Nutrition and bone disease. N Engl J Med 298:193, 1978
Harland BF, Johnson RD, Blendermann EM: Calcium, phosphorus, iron, iodine and zinc levels in the "total diet." J Am Diet Assoc 77:16, 1980
Massey LK, Strang MM: Soft drink consumption, phosphorus intake, and osteoporosis. J Am Diet Assoc 80:581, 1982

Mertz W: The new RDAs: Estimated adequate and safe intake and calculation of available iron. J Am Diet Assoc 76:128, 1980

Mertz W: Mineral elements: New perspectives. J Am Diet Assoc 77:258, 1980

Solomons NW: Factors affecting the bioavailability of zinc. J Am Diet Assoc 80:115, 1982

Swanson CA, King JC: Human zinc nutrition. J Nutr Ed 11:181, 1979

Ulmer DD: Trace elements. N Engl J Med 297:318, 1977

Chapter 12. Vitamins

Books and Pamphlets

Hodges RE: Nutrition in Medical Practice. Philadelphia, WB Saunders, 1980

Periodicals

Bieri JG: An overview of the RDAs for vitamins. J Am Diet Assoc 76:134, 1980

Bieri JG: Interactions among the fat-soluble vitamins. Nutr MD 8:3:1, 1982

De Luca HF: Some new concepts emanating from a study of the metabolism and function of vitamin D. Nutr Rev 38:169, 1980

Gallagher JC, Riggs BL: Nutrition and bone disease. N Engl J Med 298:193, 1978

Hecht A: Vitamins over the counter: Take only when needed. FDA Consumer 13:3:17, 1979

Lakdawala DR, Widdowson EM: Vitamin D in human milk. Lancet 1:167, 1977

Massry SG: Requirements of vitamin D metabolites in patients with renal disease. Am J Clin Nutr 33:1530, 1980

Solomons NW, Russell RM: The interaction of vitamin A and zinc—Implications for human nutrition. Am J Clin Nutr 33:2031, 1980

Thorp VJ: Effect of oral contraceptive agents on vitamin and mineral requirements. J Am Diet Assoc 76:581, 1980

Nutrition in the Life Cycle

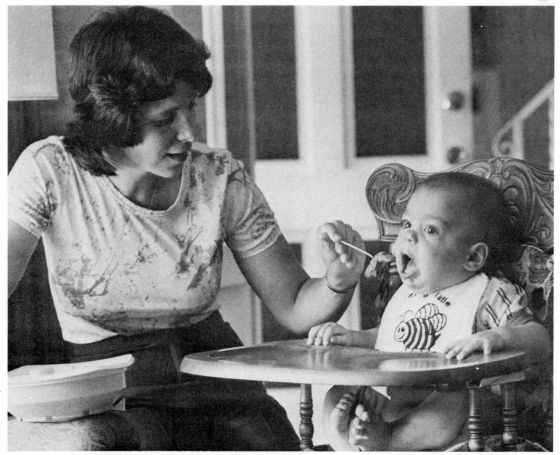

Meeting Nutritional Needs in Daily Meals

A good diet is one that supplies sufficient energy and all the essential nutrients in adequate amounts. In the preceding chapters, we studied the essentials of an adequate diet. In this chapter, we will "put it all together" by discussing how daily foods can be selected so that an adequate diet is achieved, even for those whose eating habits are somewhat unusual.

Obtaining an Adequate Diet

How do I know if I am eating a nutritious diet? is a question frequently posed. Two guidelines stand out: eat a wide variety of foods; and eat foods that have a high nutrient density.

Variety

A diet that includes a wide variety of foods is more likely to contain all the essential nutrients than one that includes a limited number of foods.

Nutrients are widely distributed in food, and no one food contains all the required nutrients. Nutrients differ in their concentration in food. For example, milk is high in calcium, so that adequate calcium intake can be obtained from consuming milk alone. In contrast, some nutrients, such as iron and B vitamins, are not highly concentrated in any one food, so that a wide variety of foods must be eaten to ensure adequate intake.

Variety is important for other reasons, too. As we have seen, nutrients frequently interact with other nutrients or with nonnutrient substances, sometimes creating a negative effect. For example, too much dietary zinc blocks the absorption of copper, high protein intake causes excessive calcium excretion, and fiber hinders the absorption of zinc and iron. Variety reduces the likelihood that too much of a single nutrient or other food component will be consumed.

Many substances in food, including nutrients, can be toxic when consumed in excess amounts. Some toxic substances occur naturally in foods, some are added in cooking or

processing, and some are introduced by a contaminated environment. Variety protects against the accumulation of toxic levels of these substances.

Nutrient Density

Nutrient density means the quantity of specific nutrients in relation to the caloric content of a food. A food of high nutrient density is one that provides the most nutrients for the fewest calories. This is especially important for persons who must limit their caloric intake because of their sedentary lifestyle. Fats, sugars, and alcohol provide mainly calories and contribute few, if any, nutrients. Refined, highly processed foodstuffs are less nutritious than those that are unrefined and lightly processed. A diet made up primarily of such foods is not desirable.

The USDA Daily Food Guide

To be of practical value, the scientific information contained in the Recommended Dietary Allowances (see Table 4-1) must be translated into terms of food. To accomplish this, food guides have been developed that indicate what kinds of foods and how much of them are needed daily to meet the recommendations. The USDA Daily Food Guide emphasizes four food groups: milk, meat, vegetable–fruit, and bread–cereal (Fig. 13-1). The foods in the groups have similar nutrient compositions. The fifth group, fats–sweets–alcohol, provides mainly calories.

Milk Group

The milk group includes milk (fluid whole, evaporated, low-fat, skim, nonfat dry, buttermilk), cottage cheese, cheddar-type natural or processed cheese, ice cream, ice milk, and yogurt. One cup (8 ounces) of milk counts as 1 serving.

Recommended Amounts. The recommended amounts vary because the need for calcium differs for various age groups. The following is

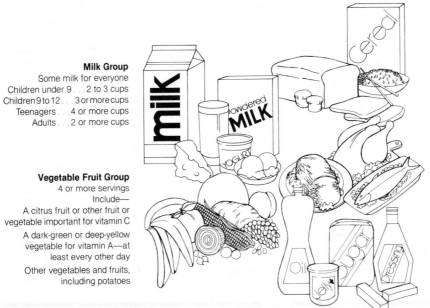

Milk Group
Some milk for everyone
Children under 9 . . .2 to 3 cups
Children 9 to 12 . . . 3 or more cups
Teenagers . . . 4 or more cups
Adults . . . 2 or more cups

Vegetable Fruit Group
4 or more servings
Include—
A citrus fruit or other fruit or vegetable important for vitamin C
A dark-green or deep-yellow vegetable for vitamin A—at least every other day
Other vegetables and fruits, including potatoes

Bread Cereal Group
4 or more servings
Whole grain, enriched, or restored

Meat Group
2 or more servings
Beef, veal, pork, lamb, poultry, fish, eggs
As alternatives—dry beans, dry peas, nuts

Other Foods
To round out meals and meet energy needs, most everyone will use some foods not specified in the Four Food Groups. Such foods include breads, cereals, flours, sugars, butter, margarine, other fats. These often are ingredients in a recipe or added to other foods during preparation or at table. Try to include some vegetable oils among the fats used.

Fig. 13-1.   Food for fitness: a daily food guide. (After Leaflet 424, U.S. Department of Agriculture, Insitute of Home Economics)

recommended: for children under 9 years, 2 to 3 8-ounce cups daily, children 9 to 12, 3 8-ounce cups daily; teenagers, 4 8-ounce cups daily; adults, 2 8-ounce cups daily; pregnant women, 3 8-ounce cups daily; and nursing mothers, 4 8-ounce cups daily.

Other milk products, such as cheese, ice cream, and yogurt, may replace some of the milk. Ice cream, ice milk, and sweetened and flavored milk beverages provide more kilocalories than milk. For example, 12 ounces of ice cream provide the calcium equivalent of 8 ounces of milk but add 3 times as many kilocalories.

Nutritional Contribution. The milk group supplies about three fourths of the daily calcium recommended, as well as significant amounts of riboflavin and high-quality protein. Milk is also a good source of phosphorus, thiamine, and vitamin B_{12}. Vitamin A occurs naturally in whole milk and is added to low-fat and skim milk. Most commercial milks are also fortified with vitamin D. Since an adequate amount of vitamin D is not found naturally in foods, D-fortified milk is the main source of the vitamin.

If weight control or reduced fat content is desired, whole milk can be replaced by fortified low-fat or nonfat milk. These milks have the same calcium, protein, and vitamin value as whole milk.

Meat Group

The meat group includes beef, veal, lamb, pork, wild game, poultry, fish, shellfish, organ meats (liver, kidney, heart, and others), dry peas or beans, soybeans, lentils, eggs, seeds, nuts, peanuts, and peanut butter.

Recommended Amounts. Two servings of meat a day for a total of 4 to 6 ounces, not including bone, is the recommendation. The following are equivalent to 1 ounce of meat: one egg; ½ to ¾ cup of cooked dry beans, dry peas, soybeans, or lentils; 2 tablespoons of peanut butter; ½ cup of tofu (soybean curd); and ¼ to ½ cup of nuts, sesame seeds, or sunflower seeds.

Nutritional Contribution. The meat group provides protein, iron, and B vitamins: thiamine, riboflavin, niacin, and B_6. Only the foods of animal origin in this group provide vitamin B_{12}.

It is wise to use a variety of foods from this group, since the contributions of nutrients in addition to those given above differ considerably. Red meats and oysters are rich sources of zinc; liver is an excellent source of vitamin A, and legumes are a good source of magnesium. Fish and poultry are relatively low in calories and saturated fat.

All meat, fish, and poultry contain cholesterol and varying degrees of saturated fat. Organ meats and egg yolks contain the most cholesterol. Shrimp is moderately high in cholesterol, and fish is relatively low.

The iron in meat, fish, and poultry is more readily absorbed than that in plant products. Liver is an excellent source of iron. Lean meat, heart, kidney, shellfish, and dried peas and beans are good sources of iron.

Cereals, especially whole-grain, in combination with dry peas, dry beans, lentils, and other legumes, provide significant amounts of protein, iron, and B vitamins.

Vegetable – Fruit Group

The vegetable–fruit group includes all fruits and vegetables. (The only exceptions are dry beans, dry peas, and lentils, which are in the meat group because of their protein content.)

Recommended Amounts. Four or more servings a day of vegetables or fruit are recommended, including one serving of a good source of vitamin C or two servings of a fair source of vitamin C; frequent use of deep yellow or dark green vegetables (for vitamin A); and unpeeled fruits and vegetables and those with edible seeds, such as berries (for fiber). Table 13-1 gives sources of vitamin A and vitamin C from this group.

One serving consists of the following: ½ cup of vegetable or fruit; one portion as ordinarily served, such as one medium orange, peach, pear, or potato; ½ of a medium grapefruit or cantaloupe; the juice of one lemon; a wedge of lettuce; or a bowl of salad.

Table 13-1. Sources of Vitamins A and C in Vegetables and Fruits

Vitamin A	Vitamin C	
	Good Sources	Fair Sources
Broccoli	Grapefruit or grapefruit juice	Honeydew melon
Carrots		Lemon
Chard	Orange or orange juice	Tangerine or tangerine juice
Collards	Cantaloupe	
Kale	Guava	Watermelon
Cress	Mango	Asparagus tips
Pumpkin	Papaya	Raw cabbage
Spinach	Fresh strawberries	Collards
Sweet Potatoes	Broccoli	Cress
Turnip Greens	Brussels sprouts	Kale
Other dark green leafy vegetables	Green pepper	Kohlrabi
Apricots	Sweet red pepper	Mustard greens
Cantaloupe		Potatoes and sweet potatoes cooked in jacket
Mango		Spinach
Persimmon		Tomato or tomato juice
		Turnip greens

Nutritional Contribution. The vegetable–fruit group supplies most of the vitamin C and a large portion of the vitamin A and fiber in the diet. However, the nutritional values of the individual foods in this group vary widely. You should know which are good sources of vitamins A and C (see Table 13-1).

Dark green vegetables provide vitamin C (if they are not overcooked), riboflavin, folacin, iron, and magnesium. Some greens—collards, kale, mustard, turnips, and dandelion—provide calcium. All fruits and vegetables (except olives and avocado) have only traces of fat, and none contains cholesterol. The fruit and vegetable group also contributes fiber to the diet.

Bread–Cereal Group

The bread–cereal group includes all breads and cereals that are whole-grain, enriched, or re-stored. Specific foods included are breads, crackers, cooked and ready-to-eat cereals, cornmeal, grits, flour, macaroni, spaghetti, noodles, rice, rolled oats, bulgur, barley, and quick breads and other baked goods made with whole-grain or enriched flour.

Recommended Amounts. Four or more servings a day of food from this group are recommended. Some whole-grain bread or cereal should be included.

The following are considered to constitute one serving: one slice of bread, ½ English muffin or hamburger roll; 1 ounce of ready-to-eat cereal; ½ to ¾ cup of cooked cereal, cornmeal, grits, pasta, noodles, or rice.

Nutritional Contribution. The bread–cereal group provides mainly B vitamins and iron. If these foods are eaten in large quantities, as

in vegetarian diets, they provide generous amounts of protein. Whole-grain breads and cereals also contribute magnesium, folacin, and fiber.

The nutritional contribution of this group is dependent on the use of whole-grain, enriched, or fortified products. Refined breads and cereals that are not enriched provide few vitamins and minerals. Because some products on the market are made with unenriched flour, the consumer should be cautioned to read labels carefully.

Fats – Sweets – Alcohol Group

The fats–sweets–alcohol group includes butter, margarine, mayonnaise and other salad dressings, and other fats and oils; candy, sugar, jam, jellies, syrups, sweet toppings, and other sweets; soft drinks and other highly sugared beverages; and alcoholic beverages, such as wine, beer, and liquor. Cereal products made from unenriched refined flour are also included.

Foods in this group have a low nutrient density. They are low in vitamins, minerals, and protein in relation to calories. One exception is vegetable oils, which provide vitamin E and essential fatty acids. Polyunsaturated oils, such as corn, safflower, sunflower, sesame, soybean, and cottonseed oils, and wheat germ supply linoleic acid, an essential fatty acid. These oils are used in making commercial mayonnaise, salad dressings, and margarines.

There are no specific recommendations for intake from this group. Foods from the other four groups should form the basis of the daily diet, with foods added from this group on the basis of individual needs.

Using the Daily Food Guide in Planning Meals and Snacks

The Daily Food Guide provides the foundation of an adequate diet. That is, foods from the first four groups in the amounts recommended provide about 1200 kilocalories and most, but not all, of the nutrients needed for good nutrition. How much of a person's energy requirements will be met by the Food Guide depends on his individual needs. A middle-aged woman with a sedentary life-style would need only a few additional foods to balance her energy needs with the caloric value of her diet, whereas a young man engaging in heavy physical activity might require 3 times the calories represented by the four food groups.

An attractive feature of the Daily Food Guide is its flexibility. It can be adapted to the eating habits of most cultural and religious groups and to different life-styles. Tables 13-2 and 13-3 show how to use the Daily Food Guide in planning and evaluating daily meals. Food choices that might be considered typical of the average American adult and of an ovolacto vegetarian (one who includes eggs and dairy products in his diet) are represented in these examples. However, if a family's food pattern does not conform to the four food groups, it should not be prejudged as being inadequate. Such a pattern must first be evaluated in terms of each essential nutrient according to tables of food composition such as Table A-1 (see Appendix).

The flexible nature of the food groups does have its pitfalls. There is a wide choice of foods within most of the food groups, and the nutritional values of the various foods differ. Knowledge of the nutritional composition of food will help you make the best choices within each group. This is especially important for persons whose life-style involves an eating pattern of "snacking" or eating a number of small meals rather than the traditional three meals a day. Such a person can have a nutritious diet if he uses the Food Guide in making choices. If the small meals include mostly so-called snack foods, the individual should be encouraged to investigate the nutrient and caloric value of these foods.

Spacing of Meals

Distribution of food throughout the day is important. The body needs a steady supply of nutrients, and it is unwise to overload the mechanisms for digesting, absorbing, and metabolizing the day's food.

A common pattern of eating in the United States is to have a small breakfast or none, a

Table 13-2. Using the Daily Food Guide in Meal Planning

A Typical Day's Menu for an Adult

Morning	Half grapefruit
	Oatmeal
	Peanut butter
	Whole-wheat toast
	Low-fat milk
Midday	Split pea soup
	Tossed salad with French dressing
	Enriched hard roll with margarine
	Pear
	Low-fat milk
Evening	Roast chicken
	Baked potato
	Broccoli
	Cole slaw
	Whole-wheat bread with margarine
	Sponge cake
	Coffee
Evening snack	Corn flakes with low-fat milk

Foods from the Menu Forming the Foundation of the Diet

Milk Group— 2 Cups	Veg.–Fruit Group— 4 Servings	Meat or Alternate— 2 Servings	Bread–Cereal Group— 4 Servings
2 Cups milk	Half grapefruit	Split pea soup	Oatmeal
	Tossed salad	Roast chicken	2 Slices whole-wheat bread
	Pear		Roll (enriched)
	Broccoli		

Foods Providing Additional Nutrients and Energy

From first four food groups	From fifth group
Peanut butter	French dressing
Cole slaw	Margarine
Sponge cake (enriched)	Slaw dressing
Corn flakes	Sugar for coffee
Milk — ½ cup	

(After U.S. Department of Agriculture: Yearbook of Agriculture. Washington, DC, U.S. Government Printing Office, p. 11, 1974)

Table 13-3.   Using the Daily Food Guide in Meal Planning

A Day's Meals for an Ovolacto Vegetarian Diet

Morning	Orange–grapefruit sections
	French toast
	Syrup
	Milk
Midday	Vegetable soup
	Cottage-cheese-stuffed tomato
	Whole-wheat bread with margarine
	Sherbet
	Milk
Evening	Meatless chili
	Rice
	Creamed spinach
	Cornbread with margarine
	Baked apple
	Tea
Evening snack	Peanut butter and crackers
	Milk

Foods from the Menu Forming the Foundation of the Diet

Milk Group— 2 Cups	Veg.–Fruit Group— 4 Servings	Meat or Alternate— 2 Servings	Bread–Cereal; Enriched Whole-wheat Grain— 4 servings
2 Cups milk	Orange–grapefruit sections	Cottage cheese	1 Slice toast (enriched)
	Tomato	Meatless chili (kidney beans)	1 Slice whole-wheat bread
	Spinach		1 Cube cornbread
	Baked apple		½ Cup rice (enriched)

Foods Providing Additional Nutrients and Energy

From First Four Food Groups	From Fifth Group
French toast (egg, bread)	Syrup
Vegetable soup	Margarine
Sherbet	Sugar for tea
Milk—1 cup	
Peanut butter	
Crackers (enriched)	

(After U.S. Department of Agriculture: Yearbook of Agriculture. Washington, DC, U.S. Government Printing Office, p. 11, 1974)

light to medium lunch, and a heavy dinner. Eating a more substantial breakfast and lunch and a lighter dinner would be a much healthier pattern. It makes little sense to eat very little after 10 or 12 hours without food and during the period of the day when one is most active, and to eat heavily when the day's activity is done.

Fast Foods

Changing lifestyles—especially the increased employment of women and the increase in single-person households—have been important factors in the popularity of fast-food restaurants. There are now more than 100,000 fast-food outlets across the country.

Because fast foods appear to be an ever-increasing part of the American diet, it is important to consider their nutritional impact. This depends upon several factors: how often fast foods are eaten, the nutritional content of the food, and the consumer's choices.

Occasional fast-food meals (once a week or so) have little impact on the nutritive value of a week's diet. However, many persons eat fast foods every day or almost every day. The expansion of fast foods into schools and colleges may make persons dependent on fast foods for one or more meals a day. This is contrary to one of the most important principles of nutrition: variety. Relying on such a limited selection of food increases the risk of nutrient deficiency.

Fast foods generally do not deserve the "junk food" label sometimes given them. Many fast-food main dishes supply substantial amounts of nutrients. However, they also tend to have high levels of kilocalories, sodium, and fat, problem areas in the American diet.

Fast-food meals provide 50% to 100% of the protein recommended for young adults. The energy they supply, ranging from 900 kcal to 1800 kcal, is 45% to 90% of the total daily energy intake recommended for young women (Table 13-4). The beverage selected has a considerable influence on the energy value of the meal. A milkshake adds about 400 kcal, and a large malt may add more than 800 kcal. The sodium content of fast-food meals is also very high, ranging from 1000 mg to 2525 mg of sodium. (Table 13-5 gives the approximate sodium content of various fast foods.) Some fast-food meals derive as much as 51% of their kilocalories from fat, in contrast to the maximum of 35% of kilocalories from fat recommended for the average American.

Beef patty or roast beef sandwich meals contain substantial amounts of iron. Adequate calcium is supplied by pizza or by milk or a milkshake. Typical fast-food meals are good sources of thiamine, riboflavin, niacin, vitamin B_{12}, phosphorus, and zinc. They are poor sources of vitamins A and B_6, folacin, pantothenic acid, vitamin C, and fiber. Foods in other meals must be chosen carefully to supply adequate amounts of the nutrients and fibers that are lacking in fast food. Emphasis should be placed on yellow and green leafy vegetables, fruits, nuts, and occasionally liver.

Table 13-4. Energy Content of Typical Fast-Food Meals

Food	Total Kcal
Large hamburger (661 kcal), regular order of French fries (250 kcal), vanilla milkshake (380 kcal)	1291
Fried fish sandwich (547 kcal), regular order of French fries (250 kcal), chocolate milkshake (403 kcal)	1200
Two slices of 13″ pizza with thin crust (520 kcal), 12-ounce cola (150 kcal)	670
Fried chicken dinner: 2 pieces of chicken, roll, cole slaw, mashed potato, gravy (1082 kcal); 12-ounce cola (150 kcal)	1232
Large hot dog with cheese (593 kcal), large chocolate malt (840 kcal)	1433

(Young EA, Brennan EH, Irving GL: Update: Nutritional analysis of fast foods. Dietetic Currents 8(2), 1981)

Table 13-5.   Approximate Sodium Content of Selected Fast Foods

Food	Sodium (Mg)
Large hamburger	1083
Fish sandwich	613
Roast beef sandwich	610
Fried chicken (2 pieces)	728
10″ Pizza, one-half	1281
Chili (10 oz)	1190
Tacos (two 2¾ oz)	926
Chocolate milkshake	300
French fries, small order (2½ oz)*	146

(Fast food chains. Consumer Reports, September, 1979)

* Data on French fries from The Sodium Content of your Food. USDA Home and Garden Bulletin 233, 1980.

Dietary Goals for the United States

Overconsumption of food in general, combined with a sedentary life-style, has become a major public health problem in the United States. Too much fat (especially saturated fat in the United States), cholesterol, refined and processed sugars, and/or alcohol are being linked to the development of major chronic diseases.

In 1977, in an effort to alert the public to this growing problem, the Select Committee on Nutrition and Human Needs of the United States Senate issued *Dietary Goals for the United States* (Table 13-6). The Goals provide guidance for the selection of foods for the individual consumer. They include basic dietary goals and guides for helping the consumer attain these goals. The Goals emphasize prevention of obesity as the best protection against heart disease.

Putting the U.S. Dietary Goals into Practice

A diet that embodies many of the recommendations of the U.S. Dietary Goals is the "prudent diet." This diet was developed in 1957 by the Bureau of Nutrition of the New York City Department of Health and has since been updated, most recently in 1981 (Table 13-7).

The U.S. Dietary Goals focus on weight control and on changes in the consumption of sugar, fat, sodium, and fiber. The following suggestions can help to achieve the goals.

Avoidance of Overweight

To lose weight, eat less sweets and fatty foods, avoid too much alcohol, reduce portion sizes, and increase physical activity.

Decrease in Sugar Consumption

Reduce the amount of sugar used at the table and in recipes. Much of the sugar consumed, however, is that found in processed foods. In addition to the word *sugar*, words on food labels that mean sugar are *sucrose, dextrose, glucose, fructose, corn syrup, corn sweetener, maple syrup, natural sweeteners, invert sugar, honey, molasses, dextrins, maltose,* and *brown sugar.* Look for foods without added sweeteners and avoid those that are predominantly sugar.

Use regular instead of sugar-coated cereals; substitute fruit juices or plain water for soft drinks, fruit drinks, ades, and punches, which contain considerable amounts of sugar; buy fresh fruit or fruit canned in water or juice rather than in heavy syrup; avoid heavily sugared foods, such as candies, pies, and cookies.

Decrease in Fat and Cholesterol Consumption

Limit use of eggs to 3 to 4 per week and of organ meats to not more than twice a month. Reduce fats by cutting down on fatty meats, such as regular ground hamburger, corned beef, spare ribs, sausage, luncheon meats, and heavily marbled meats such as prime rib. Trim fat from lean

Table 13-6. U.S. Dietary Goals

1. To avoid overweight, consume only as much energy (calories) as is expended; if overweight, decrease energy intake and increase energy expenditure.
2. Increase the consumption of complex carbohydrates and "naturally occurring" sugars from about 28% of energy intake to about 48% of energy intake.
3. Reduce the consumption of refined and processed sugars by about 45% to account for about 10% of total energy intake.
4. Reduce overall fat consumption from approximately 40% to about 30% of energy intake.
5. Reduce saturated fat consumption to account for about 10% of total energy intake; and balance that with polyunsaturated and monounsaturated fats, which should each account for about 10% of energy intake.
6. Reduce cholesterol consumption to about 300 mg a day.
7. Limit the intake of sodium by reducing the intake of salt to about 5 g a day.

The Goals Suggest the Following Changes in Food Selection and Preparation

1. Increase consumption of fruits and vegetables and whole grains.
2. Decrease consumption of refined and other processed sugars and foods high in such sugars.
3. Decrease consumption of foods high in total fat, and partially replace saturated fats, whether obtained from animal or vegetable sources, with polyunsaturated fats.
4. Decrease consumption of animal fat, and choose meats, poultry, and fish, which will reduce saturated fat intake.
5. Except for young children, substitute low-fat and nonfat milk for whole milk, and low-fat dairy products for high-fat dairy products.
6. Decrease consumption of butterfat, eggs, and other high-cholesterol sources. Some consideration should be given to easing the cholesterol goal for premenopausal women, young children, and the elderly in order to obtain the nutritional benefits of eggs in the diet.
7. Decrease consumption of salt and foods high in salt content.

(Staff of the Select Committee on Nutrition and Human Needs of the United States Senate: Dietary Goals for the United States, 2nd ed. Washington, DC, U.S. Government Printing Office, 1977)

meats. Eat more fish, shellfish, chicken, and turkey. Use dry peas and beans in place of meat at some meals. Limit consumption of nuts, peanuts, and peanut butter (although they contain no cholesterol, they are high in fat). Limit use of fats at table and in cooking; avoid frying. Reduce use of whole milk and whole-milk products, such as most cheeses and ice cream. Use skim milk or low-fat milk and low-fat cottage cheese. Increase use of fruits and vegetables. Avoid fatty snack foods, rich cakes, pastries, cookies.

Decrease in Sodium Consumption

Reduce sodium intake by using salt sparingly in cooking; don't salt food at the table. Cut down on salty foods, including foods prepared in brine, such as pickles, olives, and sauerkraut; salty or smoked meats and fish, such as luncheon meats, chipped beef, frankfurters, bacon, sausage, anchovies, herring, and smoked salmon; snack foods, such as salted potato chips, pretzels, crackers, and nuts; commercial soups, including canned, instant, and bouillon

Table 13-7. The Prudent Diet

Fruits

High-vitamin-C fruits daily: orange, grapefruit, tangerine, tomato, cantaloupe, strawberries, mango, papaya

Other fruits in season

Raw fruits for fiber

Vegetables

High-vitamin-A vegetables—dark green leafy and deep yellow—3 to 4 times a week: spinach, collards, kale, turnip and similar greens, broccoli, watercress, carrots, pumpkin, sweet potato, winter squash

Other vegetables, cooked and raw, for variety and assorted nutrients

Raw vegetables for fiber

Whole-Grain and Enriched Products

Include one or more of these at each meal: breads, cereals, rice, cornmeal, pasta, grits, buckwheat

Whole-grain cereals are preferred for the natural fiber they provide

Eggs

Not to exceed 4 a week for adults, 4 to 6 a week for children

Milk

2 to 4 cups for children (2 cups of whole milk daily are recommended for young children; milk in excess of 2 cups should be of a low-fat variety.

2 cups low-fat milk (1%) or skim milk daily for adults

Low-fat plain yogurt may be substituted for milk

1 oz hard cheese may occasionally be substituted for 2 oz lean meat

Fish, Poultry, Lean Meat

2 servings every day—choose from these with about equal frequency:

Limit portion sizes to 2 to 3 oz cooked

Liver may occasionally be substituted for meat (1–2 times a month)

Limit salty varieties (ham, smoked meat, and smoked fish) to small amounts

Dried legumes, peanut butter, and unsalted nuts, may be used to supplement small portions of meat, fish, and poultry, or they may be combined with grains to enhance protein value

Fats

1 to 2 tablespoons liquid vegetable oil every day

Corn, cottonseed, safflower, soybean, or sunflower oil for salads and cooking

Choose margarines that list liquid vegetable oil as the first ingredient on the label

Note

*Use fruit for daily snack.

*Low-fat milk should not exceed 1% fat.

*Modest portions of 2 to 3 oz of cooked fish, poultry, and lean meat are sufficient.

*Use liquid vegetable oil for salad dressings and cooking.

*A margarine that predominates in liquid vegetable oil may be used sparingly as a spread.

*Adjust amounts of breads, cereals, and other grain products and of fruits and vegetables to meet caloric needs.

*Limit use of refined sugar and salt.

(Bureau of Nutrition, New York City Dept. of Health, 1981. Printed with permission)

cubes; condiments, such as prepared mustard, prepared horseradish, catsup, seasoned salts, barbecue sauces, steak sauces, and soy sauce; and cheese, especially processed cheese.

Increase in Fiber Consumption

Increase use of whole-grain breads and cereals, bran, dry peas and beans, and fruits and vegetables, especially those that are unpeeled or have edible seeds, such as berries.

Food Assistance Programs

You will undoubtedly encounter situations in which an individual or family does not have enough money to purchase food for an adequate diet. You should be acquainted with your community resources.

The Food Stamp Program enables eligible households to purchase food stamps, which give the family more purchasing power than the stamp's cost.

For information about the Supplemental Food Program for Women, Infants, and Children (WIC), school feeding programs, and child care food programs, see Chapter 16.

Nutrition Programs for the Elderly provide at least one hot meal a day, 5 days a week, to persons 60 years old and over and their spouses of any age.

Home-Delivered Meals or "Meals-On-Wheels" is a community service that brings meals to ill, disabled, or elderly persons who are unable to obtain or prepare meals for themselves.

The Expanded Food and Nutrition Education Program (EFNEP) of the Cooperative Extension Service employs program aides to work directly with low-income families to help them improve their diets. (Contact local Cooperative Extension Service.)

Churches and other community organizations often help families or individuals with food purchases on a short-term basis.

KEYS TO PRACTICAL APPLICATION

Each day, make wise and varied choices of food to eat from the milk, meat and meat substitute, fruit–vegetable, and bread–cereal groups. This is the best way to achieve a balanced diet.

Because the fats–sweets–alcohol group contains mostly calories and few nutrients, use these foods sparingly.

Learn the vegetable–fruit sources of vitamins A and C.

Distribute your food intake into meals spread throughout the day. The body needs a steady supply of nutrients.

Enjoy fast foods without abusing them. Make fast-food choices with an awareness of the energy and nutrient value of these foods; choose appropriate foods at other meals to provide nutrients that are lacking in fast foods; use fast foods only on an occasional basis. (Remember the importance of variety!)

Reducing fat, cholesterol, salt, and sugar as recommended by the U.S. Dietary Goals appears to be prudent. Most Americans would benefit from these changes.

KEY IDEAS

A good diet is one that controls energy needs and supplies all essential nutrients in adequate amounts.

Selecting a wide variety of foods and foods of high nutrient density will best assure an adequate diet.

Food guides translate scientific information into practical terms of everyday eating.

The USDA Daily Food Guide emphasizes the selection of food from four groups: milk, meat and meat substitutes, vegetable – fruit, and bread – cereal; foods from a fifth group, fats – sweets – alcohol, should be used cautiously.

Fats yield the most calories; alcohol ranks next in caloric value.

The excessive use of fast food limits variety, creating the risk of nutritional deficiencies; the high energy, fat, and sodium contents of fast foods increase the risk of nutritional excess.

Fast foods tend to provide adequate amounts of protein, thiamine, niacin, riboflavin, vitamin B_{12}, phosphorus, and zinc; calcium and iron contents vary with the food.

Fast foods tend to lack vitamins A and B_6, folacin, pantothenic acid, vitamin C, calcium, and fiber.

The U.S. Dietary Goals recommend that Americans avoid overweight, increase use of complex carbohydrates and "naturally occurring" sugars, and reduce use of refined and processed sugars, total fat, saturated fat, cholesterol, and salt. The "prudent diet" embodies many of the principles of the U.S. Dietary Goals.

Various resources are available in the community to assist persons who do not have the financial or physical means to obtain a nutritious diet.

KEYS TO LEARNING: STUDY – DISCUSSION QUESTIONS

1. Record your food intake for 3 consecutive days. Include 1 weekend day in your record. Using the format in Table 13-2, evaluate your daily food intake. Have you eaten foods from all the food groups in the amounts recommended? Have you included sources of vitamins A and C?

2. In addition to the Daily Food Guide, what other factors are important in meal planning?

3. Why is the spacing of meals important? Overconsumption of food at the evening meal and excessive snacking in the evening are common problems in the United States. Discuss ways of controlling these habits.

4. Read the report *Dietary Goals for the United States, 2nd edition*, prepared by

the Senate Select Committee on Nutrition and Human Needs.* Discuss in class the pros and cons of the Goals.

5. Plan a week's menus for a *"prudent diet."*

6. Investigate the food assistance programs in your community. Give a report to the class on one program. Include eligibility requirements, benefits, and location of enrollment office (if it applies) of the program you have selected.

7. In light of this chapter's discussion of fast foods, what changes, if any, will you make in your use of fast foods?

Bibliography is found at the end of Part Three.

* May be obtained at a library or from U.S. Government Printing Office, Washington, DC.

Meeting Nutritional Needs in Various Cultures and Lifestyles

KEY TERMS

food fad Any diet concept that is unproved scientifically and claims exaggerated health benefits.

Hala'l Food lawful for the Muslim to eat.

kosher Food selected and prepared according to the Jewish Kashruth Dietary Laws; derived from a word meaning *right* or *fit*.

ovolacto vegetarian diet A diet of milk, cheese, and eggs, in addition to plant products.

vegan diet A diet including only foods of plant origin; all animal products, including dairy products and eggs, are avoided.

A person's food habits, with its elements of regional, religious, and cultural factors, in many ways express his way of life and must be respected. The health worker must not prejudge food habits with which she is unfamiliar, even when those habits do not seem to fit any acceptable pattern. Analysis may show the diet is perfectly adequate.

In the pages that follow, some food preferences of various ethnic groups are described. However, it should not be assumed that an individual of a particular ethnic group makes all his food choices or even any of them according to these traditional food habits. The health worker must find out what the individual is actually eating. Frequently, there is a blending of traditional ethnic food preferences and those of the general population.

Regional Food Patterns in the United States

Food habits are determined mainly by the variety of foods available in a particular area. Cul-

tural factors such as nationality and religious beliefs come into play, too. Near the sea, fish is an important source of protein, whereas inland, it is used less frequently. Agricultural conditions in the southern states favor the growth of a wheat suited to the preparation of hot breads rather than yeast breads. In the northern central states, the German, Polish, and Scandinavian influences are felt; in the far west, the influence of the Oriental culture; and so on. Fried chicken, hot breads, and fat-seasoned greens are associated with the South; tortillas, chili con carne, and enchiladas with the Southwest.

Regional differences are not as pronounced as they once were, owing to advertising in magazines, newspapers, and television; to the popularity of fast-food chains serving ethnic and regional foods; and to the mobility of the American family. Also, foods from all over the world are available throughout the year. Perhaps the greatest influence of ethnicity in food is seen in large cities, where entire sections are mainly inhabited by persons of similar backgrounds.

Cultural and Religious Food Patterns

Black American Food Habits

The food habits of the black American are usually identified with food customs that originated in the South. However, a person's food habits usually reflect the part of the country from which he comes. Many blacks have food preferences that are the same as those of white families who have always lived in the North.

The term *soul food* is associated with foods of the South that were eaten by both poor blacks and poor whites. The term connotes not only the food itself, but also an atmosphere of warmth, acceptance, and love.

Pork, fish, and chicken are popular among black Americans. Meat from every part of the pig is used, including chops, spareribs, sausage, country ham, bacon, salt pork, hog jowls, neck bones, ham hocks, chitterlings (lining of the pig's stomach, which is boiled and then fried), and feet, tail, and ears. Fresh vegetables are eaten in large quantity. Greens—mustard, turnip, collard, and kale—are widely eaten, usually cooked in a pot liquor with some form of pork. Stewed okra, corn, tomatoes, and cabbage are also well liked. Sweet potatoes and squash are popular pie ingredients. Oranges, melons, bananas, and peaches are favored fruits. Grits, rice, and white and sweet potatoes are the chief sources of carbohydrate. Hot breads, such as cornbread, biscuits, and muffins, take the place of yeast bread at meals. Black-eyed peas and other dried beans provide both carbohydrate and protein.

The intake of sweets in the form of syrups, cakes, pies, candy, soft drinks, and sweetened beverages is high.

Milk and milk products are used in limited amounts. The prevalence of lactose intolerance among the black population may be partially responsible for this. Buttermilk, evaporated milk, and ice cream are popular forms of milk.

Frying is the preferred method of cooking meat, fish, and poultry. Stewing is used for some meat–vegetable combinations. Vegetables are usually boiled for a long time with fat meat. Both the vegetable and the cooking liquid are consumed.

A reduction in sweets, soft drinks, fats, and foods high in sodium should be encouraged, and use of vitamin-D-enriched milk encouraged for children, especially when greens are not eaten frequently. However, the health worker should be aware of the possibility of milk intolerance. A person who does not take milk may be lacking in calcium and vitamin D.

Hypertension is prevalent among blacks; reducing sodium can serve as a preventive measure. The use of salty meats such as salt pork, ham hocks, bacon, and sausage should be reduced. Fish, poultry, and dried beans should replace fat meats, and baking and broiling rather than frying should be encouraged. These

practices will reduce the high fat level of the diet, which is also associated with cardiovascular disease.

Puerto Rican Food Habits

Puerto Ricans living in the United States tend to maintain a Spanish way of life. They often hold onto Puerto Rican food habits while adopting some of the eating habits of the American culture.

Foods frequently eaten on a daily basis by Puerto Ricans are rice, red kidney beans, and viandas. Viandas are a group of 14 or more starchy root vegetables and unripe starchy fruits with a nutritional value similar to that of potatoes. The flavors and textures of these starchy vegetables vary. Dried salted codfish, lard, and coffee with milk are also part of the daily fare. Other beans such as garbanzo beans (chick peas) and pigeon peas may be used, although red kidney beans are more popular.

A beverage called *malta* is a popular drink. It is made from caramel, malt extract, and sugar. Because it is thought to be very nutritious, it is frequently provided for pregnant women and for children; however, it actually has little nutritional value.

Sofrito, a sauce made with tomatoes, pepper, onions, garlic, herbs and spices, anato seeds, and lard, is used with many foods. It serves as a basis for most cooking.

A typical day's meal pattern begins with a breakfast of bread and coffee with milk (half coffee, half milk). Lunch consists of rice, beans, meat, and salad. Supper is similar, usually consisting of leftovers from lunch. If rice and beans are not served, the meal usually consists of viandas served with codfish and oil, or of a hearty soup. In addition to liberal amounts of sugar in coffee, sweets in the form of fruit preserves are popular. Fruit is usually eaten between meals as a snack. In the United States, there is heavy consumption of carbonated beverages, fried snacks, and sweets.

The basic Puerto Rican diet provides almost all the essential nutrients. Greater variety in food selection should be encouraged, including the use of deep yellow and deep green leafy vegetables. More frequent use of cheese will improve the calcium level. Using milk liberally in coffee and cooking cereals in milk should be encouraged.

Many Puerto Ricans buy food every day in the Spanish stores, which carry familiar foods. Using canned tomatoes and canned or frozen fruits and juices when fresh fruits and vegetables are out of season, using inexpensive cuts of meat, and buying all but the special Puerto Rican foods at the supermarket help to stretch the food budget.

Mexican–American Food Habits

Dry beans, chili peppers, and tortillas made from corn or wheat are staple items in the diet of Mexican–Americans. Pinto, calico, and garbanzos are the varieties of beans most commonly eaten. Chili peppers from mild to very hot are used as both vegetable and seasoning. Mexican–Americans of limited income use meat, fish, and poultry sparingly, combined with peppers and other foods in main dishes. Stewed tomatoes and tomato puree are common ingredients. Most foods are fried. Lard, the preferred fat, is used liberally.

Corn has been the basic cereal. Mexicans make a stiff dough, called *masa,* from dried corn that has been soaked in lime water. This dough is used to make tortillas — thin, flat, unleavened bread cooked on a hot griddle. The lime-treated dough has been a source of appreciable amounts of calcium. This is an especially important aspect of the diet, since Mexican–Americans drink very little milk. Wheat is gradually replacing corn in the making of tortillas, thus reducing the calcium intake.

Enchiladas, tamales, tacos, and chili-con-carne are popular Mexican–American dishes. Enchiladas are made by rolling tortillas with a filling of cheese, onion, and shredded lettuce. Tacos are tortillas folded with a filling of ground meat in a highly seasoned sauce and shredded lettuce. Tamales are made of corn dough and ground meat wrapped in corn husks and steamed. Chili-con-carne consists of beef seasoned with garlic, beans, and chili peppers.

Vegetables such as potatoes, pumpkin, greens, onions, and carrots are sometimes used. Bananas, melons, peaches, and canned fruit cocktail are the most commonly used fruit.

Sugar and sweets are used liberally. Candy, soda, and sweet rolls are popular. French fries and other deep-fat-fried foods add additional fat to a diet already high in fat.

The basic pattern of beans, chili peppers, and breads made of corn is nutritionally good and forms a good foundation on which to build. Increased use of economical cuts of meat should be encouraged. Tortillas should be retained in preference to sweet rolls.

More milk and cheese would greatly improve the protein quality and the calcium content of the diet. The latter is especially important if wheat is used in making tortillas. The addition of green and yellow vegetables and increased use of tomatoes, potatoes, and inexpensive sources of vitamin C, such as canned and frozen citrus fruits and juices, should be encouraged.

The American diet along the Mexican border has been greatly influenced by the Mexican culture.

Chinese Food Habits

The food habits of the Chinese differ according to the part of the country from which they come. Rice is the staple cereal in southern China, whereas wheat, corn, and millet seed are used in the north. These grains and, in some areas, sweet potatoes provide the chief source of calories.

Meat is eaten in small quantities and is usually mixed with vegetables. Pork, lamb, chicken, duck, fish, and shellfish are favored. Almost every part of the animal is used, including the brain, spinal cord, internal organs, skin, and blood. Blood pudding (coagulated blood) is inexpensive and eaten frequently. Beef is not commonly eaten. Soybeans are plentiful and an important source of protein.

In China, soybean milk, soybean cheese, and in some areas water buffalo milk are used. Chinese–Americans readily accept cow's milk and milk products. Eggs are well liked.

A large variety of vegetables are eaten, including cabbage, cucumbers, greens, bamboo shoots, bean sprouts, mushrooms, and sweet potatoes. Vegetables are prepared in a manner that preserves their nutritional value. They are cooked for a short time in a little oil, and then a bit of water is added. The cooking liquid is served with the vegetable.

Lard, soybean, sesame, and peanut oil are used in cooking. Soy sauce, which is highly salted, accompanies almost every meal. Tea is the most popular beverage.

There is prevalence of lactose intolerance among the Chinese. If milk is not drunk, soybean curd (tofu), soybeans, and greens should be eaten to increase calcium intake. A vitamin D supplement may be needed for pregnant women, infants, and children.

Some Chinese and other cultural groups with roots in Eastern religion or philosophy believe in a yin–yang theory that is similar to the hot–cold theory of the Puerto Ricans. (See Chap. 2.) The yin–yang theory holds that a proper balance between two opposing forces, the yin, or female, force and the yang, or male, force is necessary for good health. Whether a food belongs to the yin or yang classification depends upon the effects the food is believed to have on the body.

Jewish Food Habits and Dietary Laws

The dietary laws of the Jewish religion, called the *Rules of Kashruth,* are based on tradition and the Bible. Foods prepared and selected in accordance with these rules are called *kosher foods.* The degree to which these regulations are followed by American Jews depends on whether they belong to Orthodox, Conservative, or Reform groups. Orthodox Jews greatly value these practices and follow them under all conditions. Conservative Jews usually observe the laws in their own homes but accept changes outside the home. Reform Jews place less importance on the dietary laws.

Jewish dietary regulations require that dairy products not be eaten at a meal that contains meat or meat products. Usually, two

meals a day are dairy meals and one is a meat meal. Milk, sour cream, and cottage cheese are used in dairy meals. Fish, egg, vegetables, fruits, cereals, and bread may be eaten with both meat and dairy products. However, no milk, butter, or other dairy product can be used with these foods if they are included in a meat meal. Utensils and dishes used for dairy meals cannot be used for meat. A separate set is maintained for meat.

Legumes, fish, and dairy products are well liked. Many favorite foods, such as corned beef, smoked meats, herring, lox (salted, smoked salmon), and relishes, are highly salted. The Jewish diet may be rich in fats and in pastries, cake, and preserves. The use of more green vegetables and fruits should be stressed. In homes in which the dietary laws are strictly observed, children may lack the recommended amount of milk. In these cases, the use of more milk should be encouraged.

Muslim Dietary Laws

The dietary laws of the Muslims apply mainly to meat, pork products, and alcoholic beverages. These laws require that meat be slaughtered in the name of Allah or God in a prescribed manner. Muslims may choose to eat kosher meat, eliminate the use of meat entirely and possibly substitute fish, or do their own slaughtering. Some Muslims eat meat slaughtered by Jews or Christians and invoke the name of Allah before eating it.

Pork and all pork products and alcohol and any product containing alcohol are strictly forbidden. This includes flavoring extracts such as vanilla, which contains alcohol, and any drugs and cosmetics containing either alcohol or any product derived from pigs.

Foods that are lawful for the Muslim to eat are termed *Hala'l.*

Dietary Regulations of Religious Cults

Most religious cults have dietary regulations that are believed by their followers to promote spiritual and physical well-being. However, some of these dietary regulations are very inadequate and have been responsible for serious illness and even death due to malnutrition. An example of such a system is the Zen macrobiotic diet.

Zen macrobiotics centers on a rigid nutritional system in which only organically grown foods are eaten. Foods are classified into yang (the male principle) and yin (the female principle), and a certain ratio of one group of foods to the other in the diet is considered important.

There are 10 stages to the diet, progressing from inclusion to exclusion of animal products, fruits, vegetables, and cereals. Fluid is restricted at all levels. At the highest level, whole-grain cereal, usually brown rice, is the only food permitted. Some people have died as a result of following this diet.

The followers of Zen macrobiotics should be informed about the essential nutrients needed in a balanced diet and should be encouraged to select their macrobiotic foods so as to meet these nutritional requirements.

Vegetarian Diets

In recent years, an increasing number of people in the United States have chosen to become vegetarians.

Vegetarian diets can be nutritionally adequate, but careful planning and choice of foods is necessary. Vegetarian diets that are poorly planned can cause serious nutritional deficiencies. The health worker can help the client make better food choices and, when necessary, can obtain the services of a dietitian. As always, the attitude of the health worker is important in gaining the client's cooperation. The client's food habits should not be criticized, nor should his motives be judged.

There are various types of vegetarian diets, and food choices vary widely (Fig. 14-1). The most common ones are the following: vegetarians eat dairy products, eggs, fish, and poultry but no red meat (beef, lamb, or pork); ovolacto

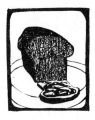

Grains, Legumes, Nuts, & Seeds

Six servings or more. Include several slices of yeast-raised, whole-grain bread, a serving of beans, and a few nuts or seeds.

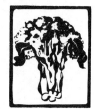

Vegetables

Three servings or more. Include one or more servings of dark leafy greens, like romaine, spinach, or chard.

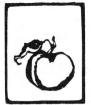

Fruit

One to four pieces. Include a raw source of vitamin C, like citrus fruits, strawberries, or cantaloupe.

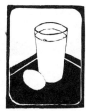

Milk & Eggs

Two or more glasses of fresh milk for adults, three or more for children. (Children under nine use smaller glasses.) Other dairy products or an egg may be used to meet part of the milk requirement. Eggs are optional—up to four per week.

Fig. 14-1. A reliable, easy-to-use daily guide to balanced vegetarian meals. (Robertson L, Flinders C, Godfrey B: *Laurel's Kitchen: A Handbook for Vegetarian Cookery and Nutrition.* Petaluma, CA, Nilgiri Press, 1976. Reprinted by permission)

vegetarians consume milk, cheese, and eggs but avoid all other animal products; lactovegetarians eat dairy products but avoid eggs and other animal products; and vegans are strict vegetarians who eat no food of animal origin, including dairy products, eggs, meat, fish, and poultry.

Adequate amounts of high-quality protein are not difficult to obtain in diets that contain dairy products and eggs. However, achieving adequate protein and other nutrients in a strict vegetarian diet requires considerable knowledge of the nutritional composition of food.

The strict vegetarian needs to know how to combine vegetable proteins so that all the essential amino acids are provided in adequate amounts. The following four food groups are presented as a daily guide for the vegan: grains, legumes, vegetables, and fruit. Legumes are a necessary food in the diet of the strict vegetarian. Legume protein is needed to balance the protein in grains so that all the essential amino acids are provided (see Chap. 9). Some vegetarians use meat analogs. These are products made from textured vegetable protein that resemble and taste like various meat, poultry, and fish products.

Vitamin B_{12} is found only in animal foods, so strict vegetarians require a B_{12} supplement, or they may obtain B_{12} from foods fortified with it, such as some brands of soybean milk. Because milk and cheese are excluded from the diet, careful planning is necessary to obtain adequate amounts of calcium and riboflavin from vegetable sources. If they do not use fortified soybean milk, pregnant women, infants, and children need a vitamin D supplement.

The feeding of infants in strict vegetarian families is of particular concern to the health worker. If breast feeding is not possible, a nutritionally adequate soybean formula should be provided. The soybean formula or soybean milk fortified with vitamin B_{12} should continue to be given by cup after the child is weaned. A wide variety of foods should be chosen, with emphasis on those that are high in iron and in vitamins A, B complex, and C. In addition to soybean milk, mixtures of legumes and cereals are needed to supply sufficient protein.

Fashions in Food Habits

In recent years, there has been increased awareness about and interest in nutrition and its relationship to health. One effect of this has been the acceptance of nontraditional or unusual eating habits by an increasing number of persons. Although unusual eating patterns are not new, many factors, including better communi-

cation, are attracting more and more people to them.

Psychological and emotional factors are frequently involved in these choices. Persons attracted to food faddism have been described as miracle seekers, antiestablishmentarians, fashion followers, and so on. Fear makes many persons susceptible to faddism — fear of death, fear of mental or physical problems, or fear of the loss of physical strength. Underlying these motives are such needs as stability, acceptance, independence, and self-worth. To work effectively with this group, the health worker needs to understand and respect these needs.

Food Fads

Despite remarkable advances in nutrition and medicine, food faddism is a strong force involving expenditures of close to 1 billion dollars yearly.

Food fads fall into four general categories: those claiming that specific foods can prevent or cure disease, those that omit certain foods because of their supposed harmful properties, those emphasizing "natural" foods, and those involving diets for certain conditions such as obesity and arthritis. The most acute problem created by food fads is that the false promises of superior health and cures for disease may cause persons with serious disorders to delay seeking competent medical care.

Knowing the facts about nutrition can help all health personnel recognize food misinformation. Food fallacies are often formulated by the pseudoscientist, who takes bits of information from scientific papers and puts them in a context that suits his purposes but changes their original meaning. The health worker should be suspicious of material that presents nutrition as a cure-all for serious disease or makes exaggerated claims for certain nutrients taken in high doses.

Organically Grown Foods

By *organically grown foods* is meant foods that are produced without the use of agricultural chemicals, such as pesticides, or other chemicals and that are free of additives and preservatives.

There is no scientific evidence that organically grown plants or meat from animals fed organically grown feed is nutritionally superior to or safer than foods produced under usual conditions. Plant roots absorb nutrient elements from the soil only in an inorganic form. Therefore, when organic fertilizers are used, they are broken down in the soil to basic chemical elements before they can be used by the plant. How the plant uses the elements in the soil is determined by its genetic make-up. If the soil is deficient in the nutrients the plant needs, the yield and not the quality of the plant is affected. However, despite the lack of evidence of any clear difference between organically and normally produced food, the consumer pays 30% to 100% more for organically grown food.

There are no federal labeling regulations governing organically grown foods, nor is there an agency certifying that the food is, in fact, organically grown.

Natural Foods

The term *natural foods* usually refers to foods in their original state or those that have undergone minimal refinement or processing. No artificial substances are added. Raw sugar, honey, brown rice, and stone-ground wheat are examples of so-called natural foods. These foods are good sources of trace minerals. However, they do not possess the "miracle" or curative properties sometimes attributed to them.

The so-called natural food movement has led to an increased demand for certified raw milk, but this milk may not be absolutely safe from disease-causing organisms.

Many of the so-called natural vitamin preparations are made in part of synthetic vitamins. Synthetic B vitamins may be added to yeast, or synthetic ascorbic acid may be added to preparations made from natural rose hips. You need to read labels carefully.

The term *health foods* usually refers to specific foods thought to have special health-giving properties. These foods are often purchased in health food stores and may be promoted as preventing or curing disease. Blackstrap molas-

ses, lecithin, kelp, and sea salt are examples of so-called health foods.

Evidence indicates that there is no significant difference in the nutritional qualities or safety of natural and organically grown foods and foods produced by the usual methods. An adequate diet can be obtained from food bought from either the so-called organic food store or the supermarket. The individual has a choice, and this choice should be respected. However, the public should be protected from claims that natural and organically grown foods or so-called health foods are cure-alls for the dreaded diseases of our time.

Sources of Reliable Nutrition Information

True and false information can be so skillfully mixed together as to make it impossible to judge what is valid. Food faddists may quote respected scientific journals but may slant the information or omit important aspects of scientific reports to suit their own purposes.

Where does one find reliable nutrition information? Nutritionists and dietitians, including those in state and local health departments and welfare agencies, nurse associations, diet counseling services, hospital clinics, and health centers can all help. Nutrition and medical faculty members in universities and colleges can also provide assistance, as can state and local chapters of professional associations such as the American Dietetic Association, the American Home Economics Association, and the American Public Health Association.

Nationally, the following are sources of reliable nutrition information:

U.S. Department of Health and Human Services, 5600 Fishers Lane, Rockville, MD 20857
　　Health Services Administration/Bureau of Community Health Services
　　Food and Drug Administration

U.S. Department of Agriculture, Washington, DC 20250
　　Agricultural Research Service
　　Consumer and Food Economics, Research Division
　　Food and Nutrition Service
　　Federal Extension Service

Superintendent of Documents, U.S. Government Printing Office, Washington, DC 20402 (Ask to have your name placed on their mailing list for publications related to food, nutrition, and health.)

American Dietetic Association, 430 North Michigan Avenue, Chicago, IL 60611

The American Home Economics Association, 2010 Massachusetts Avenue, N.W., Washington, DC 20036

American Institute of Nutrition, 9639 Rockville Pike, Bethesda, MD 20014

American Medical Association, 535 N. Dearborn Street, Chicago, IL 60610

American Public Health Association, Food and Nutrition Section, 1015 Eighteenth Street, N.W., Washington, DC 20036

Society for Nutrition Education, 2140 Shattuck Avenue, Suite 1110, Berkeley, CA 94704

KEYS TO PRACTICAL APPLICATION

There are many good reasons why people eat the way they do. The foods available in a particular region are an important factor.

Be respectful of your client's eating habits; in many ways, they express his way of life.

Accentuate the positive; emphasize the good points in an individual's eating habits.

Find out what the client is actually eating; do not assume that he is eating the traditional foods of his ethnic group.

Avoid judging as inadequate ethnic food habits that are not familiar to you. There may be hidden factors that improve the nutritional quality of the diet. Seek assistance from the dietitian in analyzing the diet.

Avoid attacking the value system underlying unusual eating habits.

Be aware that vegetarian diets can be nutritionally adequate but that careful planning is important.

Try to understand the psychological and emotional factors involved in food faddism.

Be suspicious of claims that specific foods or nutrient supplements taken in high doses can prevent or cure serious disease.

Learn to identify agencies where you can obtain reliable nutrition information.

KEY IDEAS

The availability of foods in a particular region, together with nationality and religious factors, are strong influences on food habits.

Vegetarian diets can be nutritionally adequate, but careful planning and choice of food is necessary.

Nutritional needs are readily met in vegetarian diets that include dairy products and eggs.

Achieving adequate amounts of nutrients in vegetarian diets that contain no animal products requires considerable knowledge of the nutritional composition of food.

Health workers must respect the beliefs of those following nontraditional eating habits if their nutrition education efforts are to be successful.

The most serious problem created by food faddism is that false promises may delay persons with serious health problems from seeking competent advice.

Sometimes food faddists distort scientific information to suit their own purposes.

Diets that severely limit variety and eliminate complete food groups can be extremely dangerous.

KEYS TO LEARNING: STUDY–DISCUSSION QUESTIONS

1. Prepare a report on the food habits of a particular ethnic or nationality group. If possible, select the one represented by your own family background. Discuss your report with the class. Include one or two favorite recipes illustrating the food habits of the group. Compile the recipes of all participants in a booklet for distribution to the class members.

The class might consider having a potluck party in which students singly or in groups of two or three are responsible for preparing and bringing to class a food representative of a particular cultural group. A variety of foods should be encouraged so that all the components of a meal are covered (i.e., entrees, vegetables, salads, breads, and desserts). The amount of money to be spent by each student should be set

beforehand and limited to a moderate amount, perhaps the cost of a cafeteria meal.

2. Why is it important to consider a client's regional or cultural food habits when providing advice on nutrition? Is it wise to assume that a person of a particular ethnic background is following a traditional diet?

3. Can the strict vegetarian diet be made nutritionally adequate? What aspects of the diet require special consideration?

4. Collect newspaper or magazine advertisements or articles that represent food misinformation. Discuss the fallacy involved. How is this fallacy psychologically or emotionally appealing? Keep these clippings in a class scrapbook.

5. If you were uncertain about the validity of nutrition books or other types of nutrition information, where would you seek reliable information? What are some clues to food misinformation?

6. Make a directory of nutrition resources in your community. As a class project, obtain the information for the directory by contacting various health and welfare agencies, organizations, and professional associations to determine what nutrition information services are provided.

Bibliography is found at the end of Part Three.

Nutrition During Pregnancy and Lactation

KEY TERMS

immature   Not fully developed.
interstitial   Refers to spaces between the functioning tissues of any part or organ.
maturity   Period of full growth or development.
placenta   An organ attached to the wall of

the uterus through which the fetus receives nourishment and eliminates waste products.
pubescence   Period of emergence of sexual maturity.

Physical growth occurs in several ways: by an increase in the number of cells; by an increase in the size of cells; and by an increase in intercellular matrix (the substance between cells). Most tissues, such as bone tissue, grow by increases in cell number and size.

Although growth is a continuous process, its rate is not uniform. There is rapid growth during prenatal life, early infancy, and adolescence. Slower and more uniform growth takes place between infancy and adolescence. There are critical stages of growth for some organs. For example, the number of brain cells increases rapidly prenatally, falls off at birth, and reaches its maximum at approximately 10 months of age.

The period of greatest risk of cellular dam-

age is when the number of cells is increasing. If cell division is disrupted because of a lack of nutrients, the desirable number of cells may never be achieved. Thus, nutritional deficiencies occurring during critical periods may result in permanent damage to a particular organ. The *critical periods of development* are those stages at which tissues and organs are at risk of permanent damage if the essential nutrients are not provided.

Overnutrition as well as undernutrition may play a role. There is evidence that infants who are overnourished at the stage at which the number of fat cells is rapidly increasing accumulate more fat cells than infants whose weight is normal. This overabundance of cells is permanent and may promote obesity in adulthood.

Importance of Good Nutrition During Pregnancy

Nutritional status exerts its greatest influence during prenatal life and infancy. Within 2 months of conception, all of the major body systems are formed. Embryonic growth is slow, and the quantity of food required is small; however, the *quality* of the food supply is critical.

In the next 7 months, the fetal period, the fetus undergoes phenomenal growth, from a weight of 6 g at 9 weeks to a weight of 3500 g at birth—an increase of 500 times. Skeletal development begins the second month (continuing to the end of puberty). Fatty tissue begins to develop about the sixth month. Throughout pregnancy, there is growth of maternal tissue in the uterus and the breasts and development of the placenta.

If maternal nutrition is poor, blood volume will not increase and fat will not be deposited normally. A malnourished woman is more likely than normal to have a very small baby, and a baby weighing under 5.5 lb is more likely than normal to have a birth defect and to have difficulty surviving the first year of life. There is also evidence that adequate nutrition during pregnancy is a factor in mental development. A malnourished baby will have fewer brain cells than a normal infant. Finally, a dangerous condition called *toxemia* of pregnancy is seen more frequently in poorly nourished than in well-nourished women. Toxemia is discussed later in this chapter.

Some pregnant women have been identified as being at high risk for developing nutritional deficiencies. This group includes pregnant adolescents and women who were underweight before pregnancy; who gained too little weight during pregnancy; who have insufficient money to purchase food; who have had frequent pregnancies; who have had previous low-birth-weight babies; who have diseases that affect nutritional status, such as diabetes, alcoholism, and anemia; who eat according to food fads; and who have pica (the abnormal craving during pregnancy of nonfood substances such as clay, dirt, starch, and chalk).

The health worker can help the pregnant woman avoid or correct at least some of these situations through counseling and by setting an example of good nutritional practices.

Normal Weight Gain During Pregnancy

The average weight gain during pregnancy is 24 lb. The range is 22 lb to 28 lb (Table 15-1).

Women who are underweight at the time of conception may be encouraged to gain additional weight. Teenagers are expected to experience the normal pregnancy weight gain in addi-

Table 15-1.   Weight Gain During Pregnancy

Body Part	Weight (lb)
Full-term baby	7.7
Placenta	1.4
Amniotic and body fluids	1.8
Uterus	2.0
Breasts	0.9
Blood volume	4.0
Interstitial body fluids	2.7
Maternal storage fat	3.5
Total	24

tion to the expected weight gain for nonpregnant girls of the same maturity. Women whose weight gain is less than normal are more susceptible than normal to complications and are more likely to have low-birth-weight babies. Women who are of ideal weight should avoid excessive weight gain during pregnancy. Women who are overweight at the time of conception should gain a normal amount of weight during pregnancy but, of course, should avoid excessive weight gain and should not attempt to lose weight during pregnancy. Severe calorie restriction during pregnancy can be harmful to both fetus and mother, depriving them of essential nutrients. Also, when calories are severely restricted, a condition known as *ketosis* develops. Ketosis is due to the excessive breakdown of fat and can cause neurological damage to the fetus.

If a pregnant woman is gaining too much weight, sweets and fatty foods, including cake, pie, rich desserts, candy, sugar, jelly, carbonated beverages, fried foods, and fatty meats, should be limited or eliminated from her diet, if necessary. Skim milk may be substituted for whole milk, and starches such as bread and potatoes may need to be limited.

In some cases, a diet moderately restricted in calories may be ordered, but calories should not be so few that protein is used for energy rather than for growth. It is recommended that the energy intake of healthy pregnant women not be reduced below 36 kcal per kg (about 16 kcal per lb) of pregnant body weight. For example, a pregnant woman weighing 130 lb should consume no fewer than 2080 kcal per day.

Recommended Daily Allowances

Metabolism undergoes tremendous changes during pregnancy. The tasks of the body are threefold: it must adapt to the pregnancy, which involves changes in the respiratory and circulatory systems and changes in hormonal secretions; it must prepare for lactation; and it must provide for fetal growth and development. Table 15-2 shows the added allowances recommended during pregnancy for selected nutrients.

The caloric increase of approximately 300 kcal per day during the second and third trimesters is relatively small when compared to the increases in nutrients that are necessary. Foods must be carefully chosen to supply the needed nutrients without excessive calories.

Food guides are available to assist pregnant and lactating women in making wise food choices. A typical guide is shown in Table 15-3. Most food guides for pregnancy meet the RDA for all nutrients except iron and folic acid, the need for which is so high that supplements are usually provided. The Food Stamp Program and WIC Program (Special Supplemental Food Program for Women, Infants, and Children) are available for women who need financial aid.

Selecting Foods to Meet the RDA

An additional 30 g per day of protein is recommended. Meat, fish, poultry, milk, eggs, and cheese are of high biological value and should be used liberally. An additional 2 cups of milk in the diet provide 16 g of protein, half of the recommended 30-g increase. Milk also provides calcium and phosphorus, needed for the development of the fetal bony structure and teeth as well as for the mother. Fortified milk also supplies 400 IU of vitamin D per quart.

Milk may be flavored with decaffeinated coffee, fruit purees, or molasses or may be taken in the form of cream soups, puddings, and custards. A 1½-ounce serving of cheddar cheese supplies the same amount of protein and calcium as 1 cup of milk.

The volume of milk consumed can be reduced by the addition of ⅓ cup of powdered skim milk to every 8 ounces of regular milk for a nutritive value of 2 glasses of milk.

Beef or pork liver, or chicken liver should be eaten at least once a week. Liverwurst or liver

Table 15-2. Recommended Amounts of Selected Nutrients During Pregnancy and Lactation

Nutrients	Needs of Nonpregnant Woman 25 yr old, 120 lb, 64" tall	Added Needs in Pregnancy	Added Needs in Lactation
Calories	2000 kcal	+300 kcal	+500 kcal
Protein	44 g	+30 g	+20 g
Calcium	800 mg	+400 mg	+400 mg
Iron	18 mg	*	*
Vitamin A	800 μg RE	+200 μg RE	+400 μg RE
Vitamin C	60 mg	+20 mg	+40 mg
Vitamin B_6	2 mg	+0.6 mg	+0.5 mg
Folacin	400 μg	+400 μg	+100 μg
Vitamin D	5 μg	+5 μg	+5 μg

Data are based on Recommended Dietary Allowances, 9th ed, 1980. The increases shown have been added to the RDA for nonpregnant women and girls at various age levels.

* Supplements of 30–60 mg of iron are recommended, since the usual American diet does not meet increased need. Supplementation should continue for 2 to 3 months after delivery to replenish the mother's iron stores.

RE = retinol equivalents.

spread can be substituted. Kidneys, lean meat, prune juice, dried peas, dried beans, lentils, green leafy vegetables, and whole-grain cereals are good sources of iron.

The recommendation for folacin, a B vitamin, doubles during pregnancy. It is found in leafy green vegetables, organ meats, dried peas and beans, nuts, fresh oranges, green vegetables such as asparagus and broccoli, and whole-grain cereals and breads.

Moderate use of salt is recommended, since the tissues of both mother and fetus require salt. Iodized salt should be used because of the increased need for iodine in pregnancy.

The need for water is also increased. The diet should include 6 to 8 cups of fluid, which can be obtained from a variety of beverages. Several glasses of water should be drunk each day.

Toxemia of Pregnancy

Toxemia is a condition of unknown cause that occurs after the 20th week of pregnancy. Symptoms include an elevated blood pressure, protein in the urine, edema of the hands, face, and ankles, and eventually convulsions and coma. The lives of the mother and child are threatened.

Poverty and lack of prenatal care are associated with the occurrence of toxemia. The influence of nutrition on the development of this disorder is uncertain. However, it appears to

Table 15-3. Choosing Foods Wisely

All members of the family need the same kinds of food. Only the amounts needed differ. If a woman's diet has been nutritious and balanced, few changes will be necessary during pregnancy.

Include in Family Meals	During Pregnancy
Milk (whole, low fat, skim or buttermilk)	
Children—3 or more cups	
Teenagers—4 or more cups	
Adults—2 or more cups.....................	Increase to 3 cups or more. Skim or 1%-fat milk is preferable.
Meat, Fish, Poultry (includes beef, veal, lamb, pork, poultry, eggs; as substitutes, cheese, dry beans, dry peas, peanut butter)	
2 or more servings......................... (a total of 4 oz or more)	Increase to 3 or more 2-oz servings (a total of 6 oz). Include liver and other foods high in iron frequently.
3–4 eggs weekly...........................	Increase to 1 egg each day.
Vegetables and Fruits	
4 or more servings........................	Increase to 5 or more servings.
Include:	
A food rich in vitamin C each day...........	Increase to 2 servings a day.
A food rich in vitamin A at least 3–4 times a week	Increase to 1 serving daily.
Other vegetables and fruits, including potato ...	Other vegetables and fruits including potato.
Bread and Cereals	
4 servings of whole-grain or enriched cereals......	4 servings of whole-grain or enriched cereal and bread.
Other Foods	
Eat additional quantities of the foods listed above and add other foods not listed, such as margarine, oil, and salad dressings, to meet energy needs.	Eat additional foods as your weight gain permits.

(Prepared by the Nutrition Department, Mercer Regional Medical Group, Trenton, NJ. Reprinted with permission.)

occur most frequently in poorly nourished women, especially those on low-protein diets.

Low serum protein levels, not sodium retention, is the cause of the edema. Salt restriction and the use of diuretics are not recommended to treat the edema, because sodium requirements are increased during pregnancy. Normal amounts of salt are recommended.

Diet counseling during pregnancy is extremely important, especially for women with poor food habits. A diet containing optimum amounts of high-quality protein, sufficient calories to achieve desired weight gain, and ample amounts of vitamins and minerals appear to be the best means we have of decreasing the risk of toxemia.

Anemia

Anemia is very common in pregnancy. The pregnant woman requires an adequate iron supply for her own needs and for the developing fetus, which is building its own blood supply. If iron is inadequate, the hemoglobin level of both mother and fetus will be adversely affected. Under normal conditions, the newborn has a reserve supply of iron that meets its needs for the first few months of life when milk is its main food (milk provides little iron). Most physicians prescribe iron supplements for pregnant women, since it is difficult to get enough iron from the diet alone.

Folacin is needed for optimal growth of tissues. A diet low in folacin will cause megaloblastic anemia, a condition in which the red blood cells are large and immature. Supplements of folic acid are also recommended.

Discomforts That May Be Aided by Dietary Measures

Nausea

Mild nausea may occur in the first trimester of pregnancy. Fats and fluids appear to aggravate the condition. Dry toast or a few unsalted crackers eaten before arising from bed are frequently helpful. Fluids should be taken between meals rather than with solid foods. Fatty foods should be avoided. The nausea frequently disappears by the middle of the day.

Constipation

Diminished peristalsis may give rise to constipation. Eating more raw fruits and vegetables, whole-grain cereals including bran, and prunes and prune juice may correct the problem. The liberal intake of fluids should also be encouraged.

Dietary Practices That the Pregnant Woman Should Avoid

Pica

Pica is most prevalent among low-income groups, especially in the South. The practice of eating nonfood substances may reduce the intake of nutritious food and interfere with iron absorption. As a result, the health of mother and infant may suffer. Pregnant women with pica are considered to be at risk of developing a nutritional deficiency.

Skipping Meals

The developing fetus requires a continual supply of energy and nutrients. The pregnant woman should avoid long intervals between meals. Breakfast is especially important, since it follows a long period without food.

Vitamin–Mineral Excess

Although most essential nutrients can be obtained in recommended amounts with a good diet, most obstetricians prescribe a vitamin and mineral supplement once pregnancy is diagnosed. The pregnant woman should take only the amounts prescribed and should avoid overdosage. Malformation of the fetal cardiovascular system has been attributed to high doses of vitamin D.

Alcohol

The risk of birth defects is also associated with the use of alcohol, which enters both the maternal and the fetal bloodstream. Babies born to alcoholic mothers may develop the fetal alcohol syndrome. This disorder is characterized by low birth weight, slow growth and development, and in some cases permanent mental retardation.

Saccharin

It may be wise to avoid use of saccharin, since questions have been raised concerning its relationship to cancer.

Caffeine

Caffeine, a central nervous system stimulant, crosses the placenta and enters the fetal bloodstream. It is considered wise, during pregnancy, to avoid substances that have a druglike effect and can cross the placenta. In 1980, the Food and Drug Administration issued a statement advising pregnant women to avoid or to use only sparingly foods and drugs containing caffeine.

The Lactating Woman

A lactating woman needs more calories; more of vitamins A, E, C, thiamine, riboflavin, and niacin; and more of the minerals zinc and iodine than she did during pregnancy.

An additional 500 kcal per day ensures production of 850 ml of milk daily during the first 3 months after delivery. Calories may have to be increased if the mother's weight gain during pregnancy was below normal, if she is underweight, or if she continues to nurse beyond 3 months.

A nursing mother can follow the food guide she used when pregnant, with the addition of 1 to 2 cups of milk a day. One to two servings of leafy green and deep yellow vegetables and two servings of a good source of vitamin C (or one good source and one fair source) should be included daily, and iodized salt should continue to be used.

The lactating woman's need for iron is the same as that of the nonpregnant woman, because breast milk is naturally low in iron. An iron supplement for 2 to 3 months after delivery is recommended, however, to rebuild iron stores.

The Problem of Teenage Pregnancies

Teenage pregnancies in the United States are increasing in number at a high rate. Teenagers are more vulnerable than other age groups to toxemia of pregnancy, and their pregnancies are more likely to end in stillbirths or in infants with serious defects. Nutritional status at the time of conception is of the utmost importance. The frequently inadequate diets of adolescents pose a particularly serious problem for pregnant teenagers.

The teenager herself is in a critical stage of growth, so pregnancy may seriously retard her own growth as well as that of her baby. This is especially true if the pregnant teenager is less than 14 years old or within 24 months of her first menstrual cycle.

The diet of the pregnant teenager should be evaluated as early as possible and diet counseling provided at frequent intervals. The most common nutritional deficiencies are of vitamin A, calcium, iron, and total calories.

Nutrition Education

The pregnant woman, especially one having her first child, is highly motivated to correct poor eating habits. Nutrition counseling during pregnancy is far-reaching if both the normal needs of family members and the additional needs imposed by pregnancy are considered. Parents-to-be should be helped to become aware of the influence of their eating habits on their children. Their many questions afford the nutrition counselor good opportunities for discussion.

The pregnant teenager presents the greatest challenge and may involve the efforts of the entire medical team. The teenager needs to know the relationship between her weight and that of the baby and the importance of quality versus quantity in her diet. Underweight teenagers should be encouraged to gain more than the average during pregnancy.

KEYS TO PRACTICAL APPLICATION

Avoid reducing diets during pregnancy. Gaining approximately 24 pounds is essential, even when overweight.

Careful planning of meals is essential to include all the nutrients needed during pregnancy without excessive calories. Using a food guide for pregnancy is helpful.

Pregnant women should avoid alcohol, caffeine, and excess vitamin and mineral supplements (use only the amounts prescribed).

Pregnant women should be encouraged to space meals throughout the day and not go for long periods without eating.

If mild nausea occurs in pregnancy, eat dry toast or a few unsalted crackers before getting out of bed; also, avoid fluids with meals, taking them between meals instead.

To avoid constipation during pregnancy, increase roughage in the diet; use prunes and prune juice, which contain a natural laxative; increase fluids; and increase exercise.

Encourage the nursing mother to continue the high-quality diet she consumed during pregnancy, only in greater quantities. Increased amounts of milk, green leafy and yellow vegetables, and vitamin-C-rich foods are needed to meet recommended levels of nutrients.

Give priority to helping pregnant teenagers improve their food habits.

Take advantage of the client's high motivation during pregnancy to provide nutrition education for the family as well as for the pregnant woman.

KEY IDEAS

Physical growth occurs by an increase in cell number, in cell size, and in the amount of material between cells.

The rate of growth is not uniform; rapid growth occurs in prenatal life, early infancy, and adolescence.

There are critical stages of development when certain tissues and organs of the body are at risk of permanent damage if the essential nutrients are not provided.

Major body systems of the embryo are formed in the first 2 months after

conception; therefore, the nutritional status of the mother at the time of conception is extremely important.

Adequate nutrition is an important factor in the successful outcome of pregnancy; nutrition has its greatest effect on physical and mental growth during prenatal life and infancy.

Low-birth-weight infants are more likely to have birth defects and have a higher death rate than normal-weight babies.

The pregnant teenager has growth needs of her own as well as those of the fetus, and complications of pregnancy are higher than normal among teenagers. High priority should be given to helping pregnant teenagers meet their nutritional needs.

Women with pica are also prone to the development of nutritional deficiencies.

The recommended weight gain during pregnancy is approximately 24 pounds; even women who are overweight should gain normal amounts of weight during pregnancy.

Energy needs during pregnancy increase relatively little when compared to increased needs for other nutrients; the diet must be carefully chosen to include all necessary nutrients without excessive calories.

The use of a food guide during pregnancy should be encouraged; most guides meet all RDA except for iron and folacin, for which supplements are given.

Long intervals between meals should be avoided during pregnancy; the fetus requires a continual supply of energy and nutrients.

Birth defects are associated with overdosage of vitamin supplements and the use of alcohol. The use of alcoholic beverages of any type is not recommended during pregnancy. The Food and Drug Administration also recommends the avoidance of caffeine.

The use of salt-restricted diets and diuretics is not recommended during pregnancy.

Nutritional needs continue to be high during lactation. For many nutrients, the need is even higher than during pregnancy.

Nutrition education directed toward the pregnant woman may influence the entire family; motivation is usually high at this time.

KEYS TO LEARNING: STUDY–DISCUSSION QUESTIONS

1. Why is the nutritional status of the woman at the beginning of pregnancy so important? What nutrition problems are involved in teenage pregnancies? What suggestions do you have for "reaching" the teenager so that her eating habits will improve? What approach would you use? Discuss in class.

2. What is meant by the phrase *critical stages of growth?* How does this apply to brain development? Overnutrition as well as undernutrition may affect the number of cells in certain tissue. Explain.

3. Why would it be unwise for an obese woman to attempt to lose weight or to severely limit her weight gain during pregnancy? What would you suggest to a woman who is gaining excessive amounts of weight during pregnancy?

4. Plan a day's menu for a pregnant teenager using the food guide in Table 15-3.

5. Priority should be given to providing nutrition education to parents-to-be. Why?

Bibliography is found at the end of Part Three.

16

Nutrition in the Various Stages of Life

KEY TERMS

atherosclerosis Accumulation of lipid-containing materials, especially in arterial walls.

colostrum A thin, yellow fluid secreted from the breast before the secretion of milk begins 2 or 3 days after childbirth. Colostrum contains mainly serum and white blood corpuscles.

homogenized Of uniform quality and consistency throughout.

obesity An increase in body weight beyond requirements resulting from the excess accumulation of fat in the body.

osteoporosis An abnormal decrease in bone mass, with decreased density and enlargement of bone spaces.

puberty The period during which the secondary sex characteristics begin to develop and the capability of sexual reproduction is attained.

Nutrition During Infancy

Growth during the early months of life is more rapid than at any other time. The infant's birth weight has doubled by the time he is about 5 to 6 months old. After that, weight gain slows down somewhat, but by the time he is 10 to 12 months old, the infant's birth weight has tripled and he has grown in length approximately 10 inches.

At birth, the head is large in proportion to the rest of the body. The brain and nervous system are developing rapidly. This is a critical stage of development for brain and nerve tissue, so adequate nutrition is extremely important.

Protein, emulsified fat, and simple carbohydrates can be readily digested by the newborn's gastrointestinal tract. As the infant's body increases its production of digestive enzymes, his ability to digest other fats and starches improves. The infant's skeleton is soft; it becomes hard during childhood and adolescence. Teeth begin to appear at 5 to 6 months, and by the end of the first year, the baby has 5 to 10 teeth.

The body of the newborn infant contains more water than that of an older child; however, the amount of subcutaneous fat increases during the first year. The full-term infant is born with a store of iron in the liver and with a high hemoglobin level. This is nature's way of providing an iron supply for the first few months of life, when iron intake is low; milk, the infant's

207

main food during this period, is a poor source of iron. The infant's iron store gradually becomes depleted unless iron supplements or iron-fortified foods are given.

Nutritional Needs

Because of the infant's extremely rapid growth rate, the requirements for energy and nutrients per unit of body weight are higher in infancy than at any other time of life. The caloric requirement during the first 6 months is 3 times the adult requirement *per unit of body weight.* The infant's growth rate gradually decreases, and so does the caloric requirement. Both breast milk and infant formulas supply about 20 kcal/ounce.

The infant's need for fluid is satisfied by breast milk or formula. When there is an unusual loss of water due to hot weather, fever, or diarrhea, additional water should be given. Additional water may also be necessary when supplemental foods are given, especially if these foods are high in protein, sodium, or potassium. The body needs extra water to excrete the endproducts that result from the metabolism of these nutrients.

It is not surprising that the protein requirement per unit of body weight is higher in infancy than at any other time of life. The recommendation is 2.2 g per kg during the first 6 months of life, decreasing to 2 g per kg during the latter half of the first year.

Meeting Nutritional Needs

Breast milk or infant formula supplies all the nutrients needed by the infant for the first 5 to 6 months of life, with the exceptions of ascorbic acid, vitamin D, iron, and fluoride.

Human milk contains adequate amounts of vitamin C, and most commercially prepared formulas have vitamin C added to them. Infants fed home-prepared formulas receive a vitamin C supplement or orange juice (or other juice fortified with vitamin C). The use of orange juice may be avoided because of possible allergic reactions.

The breast-fed infant should receive a supplement of vitamin D each day. Commercial formulas are already fortified with vitamin D. Evaporated whole milk used in home-prepared formulas contains 400 IU of vitamin D per quart. When either formula is used, no other supplementation of vitamin D is necessary.

Infants are at risk of developing a low hemoglobin level by 6 months of age if no source of iron is provided in the diet. The RDA are 10 mg per day during the first 6 months and 15 mg per day during the second 6 months of life. These recommendations are hard to meet without the use of a supplement or iron-fortified foods. Iron can be supplied in several ways: iron-fortified dry infant cereals (good sources of a form of iron that is well absorbed), iron-fortified commercial formulas, and iron supplements in drop form.

It is recommended that infants who are breast-fed or who receive a home-prepared milk formula should be given iron-fortified cereal or an iron supplement. Iron-fortified commercial infant formulas contain adequate amounts of iron. The iron-fortified infant cereals or iron-fortified formula should be used until the child is 18 months old.

Adequate amounts of fluoride increase resistance to dental decay. A fluoride supplement is recommended for fully breast-fed infants. Bottle-fed babies do not receive fluoride supplements for the first 6 months of life. After 6 months, fluoride supplements are recommended in areas where the public water supply has less than 0.3 part per million (ppm) of fluoride.

Breast Feeding

The Committee on Nutrition of the American Academy of Pediatrics has endorsed breast feeding as the best means of feeding the human infant. The composition of human milk is specifically suited to the infant's nutritional needs. The forms of protein and sugar in breast milk are more easily digested and absorbed than those supplied by cow's milk. Breast milk is higher in cholesterol than the commercial infant formulas made with vegetable oils. Breast milk contains more vitamin C than cow's milk,

which loses much of its vitamin C content during processing and storage.

Colostrum, a watery, yellowish fluid, is the first secretion to come from the breast a day or so after delivery. It is rich in body-building proteins. Both colostrum and the breast milk that follows provide the infant with antibodies and other factors that protect against infectious disease. Breast feeding appears to provide immunity against gastroenteritis, certain kinds of diarrhea, and respiratory infections.

Breast feeding is often recommended when there is a strong family history of allergy. Early exposure to cow's milk and to other foods is believed to be related to allergic conditions that develop later. Protection against obesity is another advantage of breast feeding; there is a tendency to overfeed when infants are bottle-fed, and this may result in early childhood obesity.

One major benefit of breast feeding is that it promotes a "bond of love" between mother and baby. Close physical contact with the mother gives the infant a sense of warmth and security. The mother feels a special closeness and a sense of accomplishment in fulfilling the infant's needs.

Most drugs taken by the mother pass from her blood to her milk. The use of medications, even over-the-counter varieties, must be restricted by the lactating woman. Drugs should be taken only under medical supervision. Also, the mother's body may concentrate toxic chemicals from the environment. These, too, may appear in the breast milk and may present a risk to the infant.

Although breast feeding offers many benefits, it is not always practical, and a mother should not be pressured to breast-feed or made to feel guilty if she decides against it.

Formula Feeding

Commercially prepared formulas are the most widely used type of infant feeding in the United States. In these formulas, cow's milk is modified so as to resemble breast milk. The changes made may include the treatment of protein to produce a more digestible curd and the replace-

ment of butterfat with vegetable oil. Several brands are available with or without iron fortification, and all are fortified with vitamins.

Home-prepared formula, made by diluting evaporated milk with water and adding corn syrup or sugar, is used in some parts of the United States but is far less common today than in the past.

Goat's milk is occasionally given to infants who are allergic to cow's milk. It is low in folic acid, so that infants receiving goat's milk as their main source of nourishment should receive a folic acid supplement.

Milk substitutes are available for feeding infants who are sensitive to the protein in all types of milk. The most popular are soybean preparations.

Skim milk is not recommended for infant feeding. It is deficient in calories and in essential fatty acids. Its use increases protein intake, and under certain conditions, excess protein may stress the infant's kidneys.

The physician usually determines the type of formula to be given the infant. Commercial formulas are available in powdered, concentrated liquid, ready-to-use, and ready-to-feed forms. Directions for use should be carefully followed, and the caretaker should be instructed in preparation. For sanitary reasons, the preparation of one feeding at a time rather than a 24-hour advance supply is favored.

The infant should be held as though he were being breast-fed. This physical closeness helps meet the infant's need for love and physical contact.

Formula stored in the refrigerator should stand out long enough to reach room temperature or be warmed to body temperature.

The infant should be fed whenever he is hungry, regardless of the time span since the last feeding. This might be as often as every 2 hours during the first few weeks. By 2 to 3 months of age, most infants fall into a schedule of feedings every 4 hours.

Supplemental Foods

Expert opinion seems to favor a delay in the addition to the infant's diet of food other than

breast milk or formula until the baby is at least 3 months of age and preferably until he is 5 or 6 months old. During the first 3 to 4 months, the infant is able to swallow liquids, and his intestinal tract and kidneys are not equipped to handle food other than milk. Furthermore, early introduction of solid food is likely to encourage overfeeding and to establish a habit of overeating. It is also thought to promote the occurrence of allergic conditions in later childhood.

The first supplementary food to be introduced is usually infant cereal. Infant cereal is more expensive than most regular cereals, having been enriched with iron in a form that is easily absorbed. Fruits and vegetables are usually added next, followed by hard-cooked egg yolk. The feeding of egg white is postponed until the tenth to 12th month because of possible allergic reactions. Strained meats are added at 6 to 7 months. If the feeding of supplemental foods is delayed until the infant is 5 or 6 months old, the order in which the various foods are introduced is not important.

New foods are added gradually beginning with very small amounts. One or two new foods may be added each week. A new food is given for 4 to 5 days before another new food is added. This gives the infant a chance to become accustomed to the food and allows time for the caretaker to observe any allergic reactions to it.

The three major baby food manufacturers stopped adding salt or other sodium compounds to their products in 1977. They have also reduced the addition of sugar to their products. Parents should be instructed to read labels carefully and to select those baby foods that have the least amount of unnecessary ingredients added.

Baby foods made at home are just as acceptable as commercial infant foods as long as high-quality ingredients are used and sanitary practices are observed when the foods are prepared and stored. All equipment, including blender jars, should be scrubbed in hot water and soap and rinsed well. Foods should be freshly prepared and then blended or pureed. Food that is not used immediately may be frozen in serving-size portions in ice-cube trays or paper cupcake liners. Fresh or frozen foods that do not have salt, sugar, or other unnecessary ingredients added should be used. Foods prepared from salted canned food or in salted water are higher in sodium than commercial baby foods.

Commercial baby foods containing substantial amounts of protein should not be heated in a microwave oven. Protein foods include plain meats and poultry, high-meat dinners, egg yolks, and meat sticks. These foods heat unevenly in the microwave oven, causing the danger of explosion. Other baby foods may be heated in the microwave oven, but extreme caution is advised. Follow the manufacturer's directions at all times.

Progression to Cup and Table Foods

When the infant is ready to progress from strained to more coarsely textured foods, table foods or commercial junior foods may be used. The latter are quite costly and basically unnecessary. When table foods are used, no fat or seasoning should be added to the infant's portion. When the infant begins reaching for things and putting them in his mouth, finger foods should be encouraged. In addition to cooked vegetables, such finger foods as melba toast, soda or graham crackers, and peeled and thinly sliced fruit, such as ripe apple, pear, or peach, may be offered.

Strained meats should be replaced by finely chopped meats without fat or gristle. Strips of chicken, tender lean meat, liver, or ground meat patties may be given the baby to suck or chew. Cooked fish from which all bones have been removed can be offered.

The infant can be fed pasteurized homogenized milk when he is between 6 and 9 months of age. Until 6 months of age, the infant may have difficulty digesting and absorbing the butterfat in whole milk. Undigested fat is excreted in the stool. The transition from breast or bottle is made slowly, starting with a small amount by cup and increasing gradually. By 9 to 12 months, all milk is usually taken by cup. If the infant still shows a desire to suck, one bottle a day may be given.

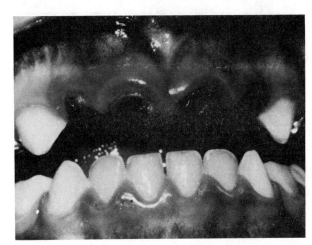

Fig. 16-1. A child with tooth loss (upper incisors) resulting from "nursing bottle syndrome." The lower teeth are as yet relatively unaffected. (Fomon SJ: Infant Nutrition. Philadelphia, WB Saunders, 1974. Reprinted by permission)

Foods That Should Be Avoided

The following foods should be avoided because the infant may choke on them: berries, corn, small candies, nuts, raw peas, raw carrots, and popcorn.

Foods that are highly sweetened should also be avoided. They have little nutritive value and take the place of more nourishing food. Also, sweet foods encourage a "sweet tooth," which is detrimental to the child's general state of health and promotes tooth decay and obesity. Foods high in fat should also be avoided.

Nursing bottle caries is decay of the upper front teeth resulting from the ingestion of sugary liquids from a nursing bottle (Fig. 16-1). This occurs when the sugar-containing fluid remains in contact with the teeth for long periods of time, such as at bedtime or naptime. Putting an infant to bed or nap with a bottle as a pacifier should be discouraged.

Feeding the Toddler

During the second year of life, the child's growth rate slows down. The average weight gain for the year is 8 to 10 pounds. The child's weight is approximately 4 times his birth weight at 2 years and 2 times his birth length at 4 years of age.

Foods must be carefully selected to provide all the essential nutrients. A pint of milk and 1 to 2 ounces of meat will meet the toddler's needs for protein, calcium, phosphorus, and magnesium. Table 16-1 gives a food guide for preschool children.

The recommendation of 15 mg of iron is not easily met. Iron-fortified foods (iron-fortified infant cereals and iron-fortified formula) or an iron supplement in drop form is recommended for children up to 18 months of age. In areas where the iodine content of the soil is low, small amounts of iodized salt are recommended.

The toddler should be offered as wide a variety of food as possible. Care must be taken to avoid the overuse of milk at the expense of other foods higher in iron. A pint to 3 cups of milk a day is adequate at this age. Vegetables and fruits that are good sources of vitamin C and vitamin A should be served each day (see Chapter 13). A vitamin D supplement may be necessary if the amount consumed in fortified milk and other fortified foods (such as cereal) does not meet the RDA.

In children between 6 and 12 months of age, the appetite begins to lessen, reaching a low point at about 3 to 4 years. This is to be expected

Table 16-1. Food Pattern for Preschool Children*

Food	Portion size	Number of portions advised	
		2- to 4-year-olds	4- to 6-year-olds
Milk and Dairy Products			
Milk†	4 oz	3 to 6	3 to 4
Cheese	½ to ¾ oz	May be substituted for 1 portion of liquid milk	
Yogurt	¼ to ½ cup	May be substituted for 1 portion of liquid milk	
Powdered skim milk	2 tbsp	May be substituted for 1 portion of liquid milk	
Meat and Meat Equivalents			
Meat,‡ fish,§ poultry	1 to 2 oz	2	2
Egg	1	1	1
Peanut butter	1 to 2 tbsp		
Legumes—dried peas and beans	¼ to ⅓ cup, cooked		
Vegetables and Fruits			
Vegetables		4 to 5—to include 1 green leafy or yellow ‖	4 to 5—to include 1 green leafy or yellow
Cooked	2 to 4 tbsp		
Raw	Few Pieces		
Fruit		1 citrus fruit or other vegetable or fruit rich in vitamin C	1 citrus fruit or otner vegetable or fruit rich in vitamin C
Canned	4 to 8 tbsp		
Raw	½ to 1 small		
Fruit juice	3 to 4 oz		
Bread and Cereal Grains			
Whole-grain or enriched white bread	½ to 1 slice	3	3
Cooked cereal	¼ to ½ cup	May be substituted for 1 serving of bread	
Ready-to-serve dry cereal	½ to 1 cup		
Spaghetti, macaroni, noodles, rice	¼ to ½ cup		
Crackers	2 to 3		
Fat			
Bacon	1 slice	Not to be substituted for meat	
Butter or vitamin-A-fortified margarine	1 tsp	3	3 to 4
Desserts	¼ to ½ cup	As demanded by calorie needs	
Sugars	½ to 1 tsp	2	2

(Lowenberg ME: The development of food patterns in young children. In Pipes PL: Nutrition in Infancy and Childhood, 2nd ed. St. Louis, CV Mosby, 1977)

* Diets should be monitored for adequacy of iron and vitamin D intake.
† Approximately ⅔ cup can easily be incorporated in a child's food during cooking.
‡ Liver once a week can be used as liver sausage or cooked liver.
§ Should be served once or twice a week to substitute for meat.
‖ If child's preferences are limited, use double portions of preferred vegetables until appetite for other vegetables develops.

Table 16-2. Examples of Nutritious Snacks

For toddlers and preschoolers

Small pieces of cheese with apple slices or whole-wheat crackers

Hard-cooked egg (quartered)

Cooked green beans (whole)

Peanut butter or toasted cheese sandwich on whole-wheat bread (quartered)

Oranges cut in wedges (this shape is preferred by most children)

Plain yogurt with unsweetened fruit and wheat germ

For older children and adolescents

Unsweetened fruit juices

A variety of fresh and dried fruit (it's best if some of these are preprepared, such as pineapple wedges or orange sections)

Cherry tomatoes or precut raw vegetables, such as carrot, green pepper, celery, or cucumber sticks

Plain yogurt with unsweetened fruit

Mixtures of whole-grain cereals with dried fruits and nuts

Small strips of meat, chicken, turkey, or cheese

Peanut butter or other nut butters

Homemade sandwich spreads, such as bean, cottage cheese, egg, or tuna

Whole-grain crackers and whole-grain breadstuffs

(Adapted from White A, Society for Nutrition Education: The Family Health Cookbook. New York, David Mckay Co, Inc, 1980. Copyright 1980 by the Society for Nutrition Education. Reprinted with permission)

urging or forcing the child to eat or bribing him with sweets as a reward for eating, more serious appetite problems may result. The child will become tense and may tend to eat less or to overeat. Parents may have unrealistic expectations as to the amount of food a toddler should eat. Table 16-1 provides a guide to portion sizes for a small child. Young children have a small capacity, and may not be able to eat all the food they need in three meals a day. Supplements of nutritious between-meal snacks may be necessary (Table 16-2).

Nutrition During Childhood and Adolescence

Between 4 and 10 years of age, there is a gradual increase in physical growth. However, motor coordination and intellectual development increase rapidly. The rate of physical growth is roughly equal for boys and girls. An annual gain of about 5 pounds in weight and 2½ inches in height is average. Muscles increase in size, bones harden, legs lengthen, and the body acquires proportions more like those of the adult. The recommended allowances are the same for both girls and boys.

The tremendous growth spurt of adolescence usually occurs in girls between the ages of 10½ and 13 years and in boys between the ages of 13 and 16 years. The age of sexual maturity varies widely, and at 10 years of age, some girls may have already entered puberty, the period of sexual maturity. Growth rate and therefore nutritional needs are related to sexual maturity and not to chronological age.

Girls gain more fat tissue than boys in specific areas. Boys gain mostly lean muscle tissue. The growth in height is approximately 3 inches a year for girls and 4 inches a year for boys.

as the growth rate slows down and the child becomes increasingly interested in his surroundings. Parents must be helped to understand that these changes in appetite are normal. If they become overly concerned and react by

From 13 to 16 years, the growth rate for girls decreases considerably, while boys continue to grow until their late teens.

The nutritional needs of boys are undoubtedly greater than those of girls, especially the requirements for protein, iron, zinc, and calcium.

Nutritional Needs

The RDA are given separately for boys and girls starting at age 11 (see Table 4-1).

RDA for calories represent average amounts for groups of children. The caloric requirement for an individual child depends on his size, activity, and rate of growth. A child's individual growth pattern is the most important consideration. Growth charts are constructed for different age levels and are separate for boys and girls.

If calorie intake is not adequate, protein will be used for energy rather than for tissue building. As the growth rate increases, additional amounts of protein foods—meat, fish, poultry, eggs, milk, cheese, dried peas and beans, and peanut butter—are necessary.

Milk in the amounts listed in the Daily Food Guide in Chapter 13 together with other calcium-containing foods will meet the requirements for calcium.

The iron requirements of children between the ages of 2 and 10 years can be met by a well-chosen diet. When there is an excessive use of milk and other dairy products, or when a high percentage of the calories in the diet are provided by unenriched bakery goods, candies, and soft drinks, the iron content of the diet is likely to be low. Adolescent boys may be able to meet the RDA for iron of 18 mg because of the large quantity of food needed to meet their energy requirements. For girls between 12 and 17 years of age, diet alone is not likely to provide adequate amounts of iron. Iron supplements are recommended for most girls in this age group. When a wide variety of foods are used, vitamin needs are likely to be met. Good food choices between meals are encouraged if nutritious snack foods are on hand (see Table 16-2).

Preventing Nutrition-Related Health Problems in Infants and Children

Preventive health care is the greatest challenge to the health professional.

Obesity

Obesity, the excessive deposit of fat in the body, is the most serious nutritional problem in the United States. It is difficult to treat, especially when it has its beginnings in childhood. Educating parents to the dangers of overfeeding deserves high priority. The encouragement of breast feeding and the delayed use of solid foods (discussed earlier) are useful in preventing overfeeding. Lack of sufficient physical activity is frequently a contributing factor in the development of obesity. Intense physical activity should be encouraged. Sports the child can continue to enjoy as an adult, such as hiking, swimming, and tennis, should be emphasized (see Chap. 20).

Dental Caries

Dental caries is the progressive decay of teeth caused by destruction of the outer tooth surface. It is the most prevalent disease for all age levels after infancy. Carbohydrates, especially sugars, promote caries by helping the growth of the harmful bacteria that produce the tooth-eroding acids (see Chap. 7).

The finding that fluoride can protect the teeth from decay has been one of the most important discoveries in nutrition. A person who consumes fluoridated water throughout his

lifetime reduces his risk of dental caries by 50% to 60% in permanent teeth (see Chap. 11).

Anemia

Iron deficiency anemia occurs most commonly among infants of low birth weight, full-sized infants between the ages of 6 and 24 months, and children and adolescents from low-income families. Preventive measures have been discussed previously in this chapter.

Atherosclerosis

Atherosclerosis, the progressive deposition of fatty substances on the inner walls of the arteries, has its beginnings in infancy and childhood. High levels of saturated fat and cholesterol in the diet are believed to promote atherosclerosis and coronary heart disease. Whether saturated fat and cholesterol should be restricted in the diets of children is a controversial issue (see Chaps. 8 and 22). It is generally agreed that children with high cholesterol levels and those with a positive family history should receive a fat-modified diet. It is also generally agreed that there should not be any fat modification during infancy.

Food Programs That Affect Children

Community programs can improve the nutritional status of children. Some are designed specifically for children, whereas others reach children by providing food assistance and nutrition education to entire families. The Food and Nutrition Service of the U.S. Department of Agriculture, with the cooperation of state agencies, administers most of these programs.

The health worker should know about these programs, keep abreast of changes in them, and promote their use by eligible persons. Family-oriented programs are listed in Chapter 13. Those geared specifically to children are discussed below.

The Special Supplemental Food Program for Women, Infants, and Children, known as *WIC*, provides monthly food packages of baby formula, milk, cereal, eggs, cheese, and juice for pregnant and lactating women and for infants and children up to 5 years of age. Eligible applicants must be at nutritional risk because of a poor or inadequate diet and low income. Nutrition education is included in this program.

The National School Lunch Program provides a federal subsidy toward lunches served to all children and a larger subsidy for meals served to needy children. Children from low-income families may receive the lunches free of charge or at reduced prices. The school lunch is designed to provide about one third of the RDA for children. It must provide the foods in the "school lunch pattern," which includes the following components:

½ pint of low-fat milk, skim milk, or buttermilk. Whole milk or chocolate milk may also be offered.

2 ounces of meat or a food from the meat alternative group. This includes meat, fish, poultry, or equivalent amounts of protein in the form of egg, cheese, dried peas or beans, and peanut butter. An equivalent combination of these foods may also be served.

2 servings or more (at least ¾ cup) of vegetables and fruit.

Whole-grain or enriched bread or alternative (muffin, roll), or ½ cup of enriched pasta, rice, or noodles.

The child may choose 3 to 5 of these components.

The School Breakfast Program is available in some schools. The breakfasts are available to all children and are free or reduced in cost for needy children. The breakfast pattern must include, as a minimum, ½ pint of fluid milk; ½

cup of fruit, fruit juice, or vegetable juice; and 1 slice of whole-grain or enriched bread or substitute or whole-grain, enriched, or fortified cereal. The addition of a protein food, such as egg, meat, fish, poultry, cheese, or peanut butter, is encouraged.

Child care food programs assist public and nonprofit child care facilities in providing nutritionally adequate meals. The school lunch pattern is followed, but portion sizes are smaller.

Nutritional Needs of the Adult

Adulthood spans ages 18 to 65. Early adulthood spans the years 18 to 30, and middle adulthood 30 to 65. With the cessation of physical growth in early adulthood, nutritional needs decrease to a maintenance level, the amount needed to maintain and repair body tissue. These needs remain the same throughout adulthood, except for calories and iron in women. After age 21, energy needed for metabolism slowly decreases with age. Iron requirements in women decrease after menopause. Nutritional needs during adulthood have been emphasized throughout this book. Meal planning for adults is described in Chapter 13.

During this stage in the life cycle, a number of nutrition-related health problems surface. Obesity, hypertension, and atherosclerosis are serious health problems that are especially prevalent in middle adulthood. Osteoporosis, which occurs mostly in women, shows up in the 50 through 70 age group.

Birth control measures may also pose nutritional problems for women. An intrauterine device (IUD), which is inserted in the uterus to prevent pregnancy, tends to increase menstrual blood loss, thus increasing the need for iron. Birth control pills affect body metabolism of certain nutrients. Although obvious nutritional deficiencies due to birth control pills are rare, studies suggest that the woman's requirement for riboflavin, vitamin B_6, folic acid, vitamin B_{12}, and vitamin C increases while she is using these pills. Requirements for vitamin A and iron are reduced. If pregnancy occurs within 6 months after the woman has taken birth control pills, the possibility of nutritional deficiencies also poses a threat to the unborn child.

Nutrition During the Later Years of Life

The nutritional well-being of the elderly adult is influenced by many factors, among them the person's general state of health, established food habits, ability to obtain and prepare food, financial situation, level of physical activity, emotional state, and mental health. Because these factors differ widely from one person to another, nutritional care must be individualized. A careful nutrition history is needed to determine how each of the factors mentioned influences dietary needs.

Lost teeth that are not replaced with properly fitting dentures, a diminished sense of smell and taste, and reduced secretion of saliva all influence food choices. Soft, sweet, high-carbohydrate convenience foods are frequently selected because they are easy to prepare and eat, satisfy hunger, and are pleasing to the taste. Nutrients are less well absorbed because of reduced secretion of digestive juices and enzymes. The motility of the digestive tract decreases, causing constipation. Added to these are other

nutrition problems created by physical handicaps and chronic diseases.

Psychological factors exert a great influence on nutritional well-being. Loneliness, worry about health and finances, frustration at one's inability to accomplish tasks previously taken for granted, and fear of hospitalization and death are common. Many elderly persons living alone lack the motivation to prepare meals that are eaten alone.

Drugs may give rise to anorexia, mouth dryness, and alterations in the sense of taste which depress appetite. Some drugs interfere with the digestion or absorption of food or cause constipation.

With the exception of recommendations for calories, recommendations for nutrients are mostly the same for elderly persons as for younger adults. Because needs for thiamine, riboflavin, and niacin are related to caloric intake, RDA for these vitamins are slightly lower.

A protein intake of 1 g per kg of body weight is advised. Some high-quality protein should be taken at each meal. Low-fat milk and cheese, peanut butter, legumes, and eggs are suitable and inexpensive. Hearty soups and stew-type meals with a protein base such as meat, fish, poultry, or milk and vegetables added are excellent one-dish meals. Dishes of this type also provide moisture, which makes swallowing easier. Mouth dryness due to reduced saliva is a frequent problem.

Persons over 50 require fewer calories than younger adults because of a decrease in the number of functioning cells. Physical activity also usually falls off after 50. Calories should be consumed in the form of milk, cheese, meat, fish, poultry, whole-grain cereals, and fruits and vegetables. Intake of sugar, fat, and unenriched baked goods should be reduced.

Common Nutrition-Related Problems of Elderly Persons

Constipation, caused by a decrease in both intestinal motility and physical activity, is a serious problem among the elderly. Foods that are high in fiber and have natural laxative properties, such as prunes, and increased fluids should be encouraged. Persons who eat large quantities of bran cereals should be cautioned to increase their fluid intake. Also, persons who have been consuming low-fiber diets for long periods should be advised to increase their fiber intake gradually rather than abruptly.

Iron deficiency anemia may result both from a diet low in iron and from decreased absorption of iron due to changes in the digestive tract. Pernicious anemia commonly occurs, usually due not to a dietary deficiency but rather to decreased production of a substance required for absorption of vitamin B_{12}.

Dental problems interfere with the enjoyment of food and limit the variety of food that can be eaten. If only very soft foods can be tolerated, the health worker should investigate to see what is being eaten. A nutritionally adequate diet can be built around baby foods if they are carefully selected. The health worker should also try to determine whether the baby food is necessary or is being used for other reasons, such as lack of interest in cooking and eating.

Because many elderly persons suffer from chronic diseases for which there is no cure, they are easy targets for the false and exaggerated claims of food faddists. Money that could be used for better purposes is thus diverted to foods and vitamin and mineral supplements that are falsely promoted as "miracle foods" and cure-alls.

Community Nutrition Programs

Many communities sponsor programs that improve the nutritional status of the elderly. Group meals, home-delivered meals, and food stamps are examples (see Chap. 13). The health worker should be informed of the services available in her locality.

Home health or neighborhood aides are made available by certain community agencies to help the elderly. The aides are trained and supervised by nurses, nutritionists, or home economists.

KEYS TO PRACTICAL APPLICATION

Advise parents to avoid overfeeding from the very first. A "good eater" is a child who eats moderately, not excessively.

Encourage parents to follow their pediatrician's advice about introducing supplementary foods.

Don't feed cereal or other semisolid food from a bottle.

Avoid giving infants and small children foods that are high in sugar, salt, and fat and those that may cause choking.

Make parents aware of the effects of overtiredness, excitement, and strange surroundings on a child's appetite. Don't bribe, force, or coax a child to eat.

Provide nutritious between-meal snacks such as fruit, vegetables, cheese, cereal, cold meat, whole-wheat bread, pudding, and custard.

Encourage active play by the small child and intense physical activity by the older child. Monitor the child's T.V. viewing.

Encourage food choices from the Daily Food Guide in persons of all ages, children, adolescents, and the elderly included.

Discourage putting an infant to bed or to nap with a bottle as a pacifier. This practice promotes decay of the upper front teeth.

Be alert to the possible effects of birth control measures on the nutritional needs of women.

Be aware of the impact of emotional factors and drugs on the nutritional well-being of elderly persons.

Remember that, except for energy, the nutritional needs of the elderly are just as high as, if not higher than, those of the younger adult.

Encourage the use of foods with a high moisture content, such as hearty high-protein soups and stews, by elderly persons with swallowing difficulties.

Become aware of the programs in your community that promote the nutritional well-being of infants, children, and the elderly.

KEY IDEAS

Requirements for energy and nutrients per unit of body weight are higher during infancy than at any other time of life.

Breast feeding provides better nutrition than bottle feeding, psychological advantages, immunity against infection, and protection against allergy and obesity.

Breast milk or infant formula provides all the nutritional needs of the infant for 5 to 6 months with the exceptions of fluoride, iron, vitamin D for breast-fed infants, and vitamin C for infants on home-prepared formula.

The infant is at risk of having a low hemoglobin level by the age of 6

months unless an iron supplement or an iron-fortified food is used.

Fluoride supplements are recommended for fully breast-fed infants, for bottle-fed infants over 6 months of age, and for children living in areas in which the public water supply has a low fluoride level.

Early introduction of solid foods may promote overeating and allergies.

New foods should be added gradually, one at a time, and in small amounts.

Later in the first year of life, the infant progresses from strained to chopped food and from breast or bottle to cup.

To feed the older infant or toddler excessive

amounts of milk is unwise, as this milk tends to be given at the expense of iron-rich foods.

Changes in appetite are normal during the toddler stage.

During the ages 4 to 10, growth slows down and becomes more uniform; RDA are the same for both boys and girls.

During adolescence, growth is very rapid; nutritional needs are related to sexual maturity, not chronological age.

Prevention of obesity in childhood deserves high priority; both eating habits and physical activity should be considered.

Making available nutritious snacks for children and adolescents can do much to improve their nutritional intake.

Carbohydrates, especially sticky sweets, promote the development of dental caries; the use of fluoridated water reduces the incidence of caries by 50% to 60%.

Iron deficiency anemia is a common problem in childhood and adolescence; especially in low-birth-weight infants, in normal-weight infants between 6 and 24 months, and in adolescent girls.

Birth control measures can affect a woman's nutritional status.

Obesity, atherosclerosis, hypertension, osteoporosis, constipation, iron deficiency anemia, pernicious anemia, and dental problems are among the nutrition-related health problems of elderly persons.

Nutritional care of elderly persons must be individualized.

Physical factors affecting the nutritional status of the elderly include loss of teeth, reduced sense of smell and taste, diminished secretion of saliva and other digestive juices and enzymes, decreased peristalsis, physical handicaps, and chronic diseases.

Emotions such as worry, loneliness, and fear greatly influence the nutritional well-being of elderly persons.

Drugs taken by elderly persons may seriously affect their nutritional status.

With the exception of the need for calories, the need for nutrients is about the same for the elderly as for younger adults.

Meals with a high moisture content, such as soups and stews, help to overcome mouth dryness.

Group meals, home-delivered meals, food stamps, and home health aide services are among the community programs available to promote the nutritional status of the elderly.

KEYS TO LEARNING: STUDY-DISCUSSION QUESTIONS

1. What are the benefits of breast feeding? What factors may hinder successful breast feeding?
2. What advice would you give parents who favor the early feeding of supplemental foods because it helps their infant sleep through the night?
3. What instruction should be given parents about the use of commercial formula? Why should the propping of a nursing bottle be discouraged?
4. During the second half of the first year and during the toddler stage, there is a tendency for parents to give their children a lot of milk. Why should this practice be discouraged?
5. It is recommended that fruit juice be fed by cup and not in a nursing bottle. Why?
6. A mother is concerned about her toddler's lack of interest in food and his occasional refusal to eat at mealtime. What advice would you give her?
7. Discuss the importance of active play and its relationship to a child's nutritional well-being.
8. What measures should be taken during infancy, childhood, and adolescence to prevent iron deficiency anemia?

9. Make posters comparing the nutritional value of commonly used snack foods. Compare the costs of what you would consider "good snacks" and "poor snacks."

10. Discuss the role of nutrition in the prevention of dental caries.

11. What feeding or nutrition education programs are available in your community? Investigate one of these progams and report to the class. Include in your description such points as benefits, eligibility requirements or target population, and acceptance by the community. (Assign programs so that all community agencies will be covered.)

12. Discuss the psychological factors affecting the nutritional well-being of elderly persons.

13. In your experience of feeding the elderly, what types of food have you found to be most readily eaten and swallowed?

14. Why do the elderly differ more from each other than younger adults? How does this affect nutritional care?

15. With the help of your instructor, make a list of medications commonly used by elderly persons that have an adverse effect on nutritional status. List the drugs, their harmful effect, and ways of counteracting them so that their effects on nutrition will be minimized.

Bibliography is found at the end of Part Three.

17

Food Management

KEY TERMS

leader nutrients   Term applied to the first eight nutrients listed on nutrition labeling under the heading "Percentage of U.S. RDA." Called *leader nutrients* because it is assumed that if intake of these nutrients is adequate, intake of other micronutrients should also be adequate.

standard of identity   Regulations that specify the ingredients and amounts that must be included in certain food products, including milk, ice cream, margarine, and catsup. Specified ingredients do not have to appear on the labels of these products; optional ingredients must appear on the labels.

By *food management* is meant meal planning, food buying, safe storage and handling of food, and food preparation. You can apply all the information given in this chapter in both your personal food management and your professional interaction with clients. As the cost of food and meal preparation rises, people want to eat well at the lowest possible cost. Health workers can play an active role in educating consumers. For example, a young pregnant woman may need guidance in food purchasing and preparation, or a client on a fat-restricted diet may need help interpreting diet instructions that list pan broiling as a method of cooking.

standpoint of nutritional quality and economy. Haphazard meals are usually unbalanced and costly.

A guide such as the Daily Food Guide (see Chap. 13) can assist the homemaker in planning nourishing meals.

The "specials" that local markets offer and foods that are plentiful should be incorporated in the menu. The family that enjoys a variety of food has the widest choices and is likely to be well nourished.

Most Americans could lower their food bills without sacrificing nutritional quality by buying more milk and milk products, vegetables and fruit, and whole-grain and enriched bread and by buying less food in the meat group and other foods such as fats, oils, sugars, sweets, coffee, tea, soft drinks, and snack foods.

Planning Ahead

Planning what the family will eat for a few days or a week in advance is important from the

Purchasing Food from a Shopping List

The purpose of a shopping list is to reduce the impulse to buy "extras"—those items that are

not planned and not needed. This also avoids the need to make several trips to market every week, and encourages buying on the basis of menus planned for a specific period of time.

Large markets usually offer better value than small local stores. Families that purchase food at the "corner store" because of a need for credit may accept help in managing their finances so they can eventually buy food where they receive the greatest value.

Unit Pricing

Unit pricing is a method of displaying the price per weight or measure of a particular product, such as the price per ounce or per quart. It enables the shopper to compare the costs of a product on the basis of size and brand and hence find the "best buy." Of course, personal preference and quantity or amount needed enter the picture, too.

Open Dating

Open dating is another helpful guide in making food purchasing decisions. It has existed for some products for years. Recently, many food processors have begun open dating programs. There are four types of dating: pack date ("Packed Dec. 1984"); pull date ("Sell by January 3"); quality assurance or freshness date ("Best if used before August 30, 1984"); and expiration date ("Do not use after Sept. 15, 1984").

Open dating is helpful in making food selections and in can rotation at home. However, its usefulness is limited, since the handling and storage of food have a greater bearing on freshness than time.

Grade Shields

U.S. Department of Agriculture (USDA) grade shields provide another aid for the consumer. Foods that carry these shields have been graded according to federal quality grade standards. Grading is not required by law.

The shopper who understands the meaning of USDA grades is equipped to choose food items that are most suitable for their intended use.

USDA grade shields are most likely to be found on beef, lamb, turkey, chicken, duck, eggs, instant nonfat dry milk, and butter.

Information on grading standards can be obtained from the U.S. Department of Agriculture, Office of Communication, Washington, DC 20250.

Brands

A brand is a company name or a product identified with a specific company. Some supermarkets also offer products carrying their own labels. These private-label goods are usually well-established products of reliable quality and are cheaper than name-brand items. Some chains offer store-brand labels that reflect grades; for example, tomatoes may be packed under three labels comparable to grades A, B, and C.

In recent years, food retailers have introduced generic labeling as a means of offering the consumer a wider choice in price and quality. These generic or "no-frills" products carrying no brand name or trademark can save the consumer an average of 25% over national brands and 15% over store brands. Most generic food items are USDA grade C, and some are grade B. Name brands and top-label store brands are primarily grade A, with a few grade B.

The health worker should keep in mind that grading does not indicate nutritional value. A low grade does not mean that the nutritional quality is inferior to higher grades.

Choosing Food Wisely

Cost per Serving. One can determine cost per serving by dividing the cost per market unit

(pound, can, package) by the number of servings the unit affords. It may be more economical to pay more per pound for meat that is well trimmed of fat and waste than to select meat on the basis of price alone. A pound of boneless meat yields 4 servings per pound, whereas a pound of meat with bone yields 2 to 3 servings.

The number of servings per market unit varies; for example, fresh green snap beans yield 5 to 6 servings per pound, frozen green beans yield 3 to 4 servings per 10-ounce package, and canned green beans provide 3 to 4 servings per 16-ounce can.

Milk and Dairy Products

As has been stated, nonfat dry milk provides excellent nutritional value at a very low price. Both nonfat dry milk and evaporated milk are money savers. Half a cup of evaporated milk diluted with half a cup of water can be substituted for 1 cup of whole milk in recipes.

Less expensive types of cheese are as good a source of protein and calcium as more expensive types. Sharp cheddar costs more than mild cheese. Processed cheese is less expensive than natural cheese. Grated cheese and individually wrapped slices are more expensive.

Meat and Meat Substitutes

Many people have become accustomed to overly generous portions of meat, fish, and poultry — more than the recommended 4 to 6 ounces a day. Eating large quantities of meat is not in keeping with recommendations to reduce saturated fat and cholesterol in the diet. A family may be able to reduce the size of their portions of meat, fish, and poultry without sacrificing nutritional well-being. Substitutes for meat can be planned for some of the week's meals. Macaroni products, rice, and corn make nutritious main dishes when combined with eggs, milk, cheese, dried peas, beans, nuts, or small amounts of meat, poultry, or fish.

The purple stamp of the USDA on meat indicates that the meat is safe and wholesome. The USDA grades for beef are Prime, Choice, Good, Standard, and Commercial. They are a guide to tenderness and flavor but not to nutritiousness or protein content. Less expensive cuts of meat are just as nutritious as more expensive ones but require longer cooking.

Planning for two or three meals from one cut of meat can also save money. One large chuck roast can provide beef stew, a pot roast, and Swiss steaks. Preparing cold cuts at home in the form of roast beef, turkey, ham, and meat loaf can save considerable money over delicatessan prices.

Organ meats, especially beef, pork, and chicken liver, give excellent nutritional value for the money.

Frozen fish is usually less expensive than fresh fish. Large chickens and turkeys have more meat in relation to bone and are generally a better buy.

The quality and size of eggs determine their price. Grade AA or A eggs are best for poaching and frying, and grade B eggs are suitable for general cooking and baking. Brown eggs and white eggs have the same nutritional value.

Comparing Protein Cost. One way to identify "good buys" among various protein foods is to compare costs in terms of the quantity of protein provided. Price per pound or other unit of measure does not necessarily indicate the cost of protein, since the amount of protein in meats and meat substitutes varies. One pound of frankfurters, for example, provides only half the protein of 1 pound of ground beef. Although the frankfurters may cost less per pound, they are actually a more expensive source of protein than ground beef.

Foods that provide the protein equivalent of 1 ounce of meat and cost considerably less are 1 egg, 1 ounce of domestic cheddar-type cheese, ¼ cup of cottage cheese, 2 tablespoons of peanut butter, and ½ cup of cooked dried peas, beans, or lentils.

Vegetables and Fruits

Compare prices of fresh, frozen, and canned fruit and vegetables to determine "best buys."

Fresh fruit should be purchased in season when there is a plentiful supply, not when it first appears on the market. Large plastic bags of frozen fruits and vegetables cost less per serving than smaller packages.

The USDA grades for canned and frozen fruits and vegetables are grade A or Fancy, grade B or Choice, and grade C or Standard. The nutritive value of lower grades of canned fruits and vegetables is the same as that of the more expensive grades.

Breads and Cereal Products

Home-cooked hot cereals are less expensive than ready-to-eat cereals. Presugared cereals, "natural" cereals, and multipack individual boxes of cereal are especially costly. One may be able to save money by buying large loaves of bread, large boxes of cereal, and day-old bakery products.

Convenience Foods

In general, fully or partially prepared food items cost more than unprocessed food items, but there are some, such as frozen concentrated orange juice, canned orange juice, canned and frozen out-of-season vegetables and fruits, pancake and waffle mixes, and pudding mixes, that cost less.

Though frozen dinners and casseroles are sometimes sold at what appear to be bargain prices, the amount of meat, fish, or poultry in these products is small. You have to decide how much you are willing to pay for convenience.

Coffee and Tea

Instant coffee is less expensive per cup than regular coffee. An 8-ounce jar of instant or freeze-dried coffee yields the same number of cups (120 6-oz cups) as 2 pounds of fresh-roasted coffee. Instant teas, however, are more expensive per cup than tea leaves. A pound of loose tea yields about 200 cups and costs less than the equivalent in tea bags.

Food Labeling

The food labeling regulations of the Food and Drug Administration (FDA) were originally established to assure that the labeling and packaging of foods were not false or misleading. In 1973, a nutrition labeling program became effective, adding force to the FDA's efforts to protect the consumer.

FDA regulations require that the following information appear on food labels: the common name of the product, with any appropriate descriptions, such as whole, sliced, pieces, condensed, cream-style; the name and address of the manufacturer, packer, or distributor; the net weight in ounces, including both liquid and solid contents, and the number and size of servings; and a list of ingredients (except for standardized foods) in descending order by weight of the amounts used in production—for example, if sugar is the ingredient used in the largest amount and oats in the next largest amount in a ready-to-eat oat cereal, sugar must be listed first and oats second. Unfortunately, there is no way of knowing what percentage of the total is represented by the first-named ingredient or any others. Chemical terms listed as ingredients refer to additives (Fig. 17-1).

Standard of Identity

Some food products come under a standard of identity. These foods must be made according to standard recipes established by FDA. The mandatory ingredients, the minimum and maximum amounts of each, and optional ingredients are established. Standards of identity have been formulated for milk, cream, cheese, cheese products, margarine, mayonnaise, jellies, preserves, French dressing, and frozen desserts, among others. Under the current regulations, only optional ingredients must be listed; the standard ingredients need not be.

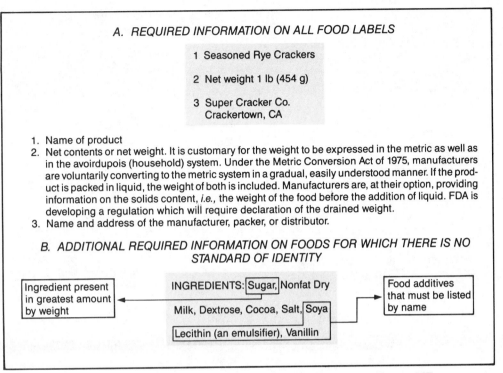

Fig. 17-1. Mandatory general information on food labels. (Suitor CW, Hunter MF: Nutrition: Principles and Application in Health Promotion. Philadelphia, JB Lippincott, 1980)

Nutrition Labeling

FDA regulations require nutrition labeling for all foods to which a nutrient is added, such as restored, fortified, or enriched foods, and for foods for which a nutritional claim is made. For example, nutrition labeling is required for enriched bread and milk fortified with vitamin D. Nutrition labeling is also required for low-fat yogurt, since a claim involving a nutrient has been made. For all other products, nutrition labeling is optional. Many processors are voluntarily including nutrition labeling on their product packages.

Formats for the nutrition label have been standardized on the basis of 1 serving. The information must include serving size; number of servings per container; calorie content per serving; protein content per serving in grams; fat content per serving in grams; carbohydrate content per serving in grams; and percentages per serving of the U.S. RDA of protein, vitamin A, vitamin C, thiamine, riboflavin, niacin, calcium, and iron.

If any nutrient content is given, all eight of the nutrients listed under "percentage of U.S. RDA" must also be listed. The first eight nutrients are called the *leader nutrients*. It is assumed that if these nutrients are provided in adequate amounts, the quantities of other essential nutrients will also be adequate.

Twelve other vitamins and minerals must be listed if they have been added or may be listed on an optional basis if naturally present in

the food. Cholesterol, polyunsaturated and saturated fat, and sodium content may also be listed on the label and must be listed if a claim is made about them. The sodium content of a food may appear on a label that does not carry nutrition labeling. Table 19-5 gives an example of a nutrition label.

United States Recommended Daily Allowances (U.S. RDA)

The United States Recommended Daily Allowances (U.S. RDA) provide a standard to which the nutrient content of the product is compared. The nutrient content of the product is expressed as a percentage of the U.S. RDA. The U.S. RDA are derived from the Recommended Dietary Allowances (RDA) of the National Research Council. For practical purposes, the RDA of the National Research Council are condensed into four categories for use in the U.S. RDA. These categories are infants, children under four years of age, adults and children over four, and pregnant and lactating women. Generally, the highest values for the ages combined in the U.S. RDA are used. For example, the U.S. RDA for adults and children over four are generally representative of the dietary allowances recommended for the teenage boy. This category appears on most nutrition labels. The categories for infants and for children under four years are used on infant formulas, baby foods, and other foods appropriate for these age levels. As you can see, the U.S. RDA standards are used as a frame of reference and not as a guide for planning adequate diets for individuals.

U.S. RDA for protein have been established on the basis of the quality of the total protein in a food product. The U.S. RDA for protein of high biological value (animal protein) is 45 g, and for protein of lower quality (plant protein) 65 g. When protein is of high biological value, less is needed to meet needs.

For the most up-to-date information on food labeling, write to the Food and Drug Administration, 5600 Fisher Lane, Rockville, MD 20852, or contact the consumer affairs officer of the FDA office nearest you.

Importance of Labeling in Nutrition Education

Nutrition labeling is an important tool in nutrition education. It heightens the consumer's awareness of the nutrients his body needs while giving information about the nutritional contributions of various foods and of various brands of the same food. Labeling helps you answer such questions as whether a canned stew provides sufficient protein to qualify as a main dish. It also helps identify foods that are good sources of specific nutrients. A food that provides at least 10% of the U.S. RDA for a particular nutrient is an important source of that nutrient; if it contains 25% to 35% of the daily required amount, it is an excellent source of the nutrient. Labeling can help persons on certain types of modified diets determine whether a food is appropriate for them.

Pitfalls of Nutrition Labeling

The U.S. RDA are not suitable for planning an adequate diet or for verifying the adequacy of a diet. They are very high for some nutrients and omit the lesser known essential nutrients. Even if the leader nutrients are provided in adequate amounts in a diet, the other essential nutrients may be inadequate.

Nutrition labeling may be misleading when applied to highly fortified processed foods compared to unfortified conventional products that are in their natural state or only lightly processed. Although fortified processed foods may have impressive amounts of the eight key nutrients listed on the label, they may contain little or none of the lesser known but equally important nutrients that are present in lightly processed foods. Nutrients such as magnesium, zinc, potassium, pantothenic acid, and folic acid, which are not listed on labels, may be very scanty, especially in a food made from highly refined ingredients. Thus, when comparing synthetic foods with conventional foods (*e.g.,* nondairy creamer or orange-flavored instant breakfast drink), one should look at the ingredient label as well as the nutrition label. If the product is made from refined ingredients, it probably

has few nutrients other than those listed on the nutrition label.

Portion sizes may also be misleading. Sometimes the portion given is larger than what a person would normally consume. Therefore, one needs to adjust for the true portion size. Also, when comparing products, one should check portion sizes to make sure to compare equal portions of similar products.

Regulating Health Claims

FDA regulations prohibit manufacturers from making certain claims about products on labels. Prohibited are statements that claim or suggest that a product can prevent, cure, treat, or lessen any disease or symptom; that a balanced diet of ordinary foods cannot supply adequate nutrients; that poor diets are a result of the soil in which the foods are grown; that transportation, storage, or cooking of food may be responsible for an inadequate diet; that a food has nutritional properties due to the presence of certain substances if these substances have no known significant value; and that a "natural" vitamin is superior to a "synthetic" vitamin or that there is any difference between natural and synthetic vitamins.

Unfortunately, unfounded claims for foods continue to be made through various avenues of advertising, though they are not included on labels.

Storing Foods Safely

The consumer's responsibility for proper storage and handling of food begins in the store. Unrefrigerated foods should be selected first and meat, dairy, and frozen items last. Thirty or 40 minutes of shopping time can cause a loss of quality in perishable items. Also, keeping foods in a warm car for an extended period encourages the growth of bacteria and molds; perishable items should be placed in an insulated picnic chest if necessary.

Chilled or frozen items should be unpacked quickly and refrigerated or frozen. Meat to be frozen should be wrapped tightly in freezer paper and dated (Table 17-1). Vegetables to be stored covered in the refrigerator (Table 17-2) should be placed in plastic bags in the crisper and should not be washed until they are to be used.

Staples

Staples should be stored in a clean, dry place, preferably not above 70°F, away from drains, stoves, and heating pipes. They should not be stored under the sink or next to the stove. Pipes under the sink can leak, the moisture causing rust and encouraging the growth of molds and insects. Heat from the stove can dry up mixes, bread, and flour and promote the growth of insects.

Both canned and dry foods should be rotated. The date of purchase on the labels of packages should be noted. Cans should be opened within 60 days of purchase. The quality of some canned foods deteriorates after a long period. Berries, cherries, onions, pumpkin, sauerkraut, and tomato products are among the foods that may be affected. The lining of the can may become badly discolored, and the food may develop a metallic taste. Canned goods should be kept no more than 1 year. A can that is rusted or swollen or that shows any signs of leakage should be discarded without being opened.

Nonfat dry milk should be stored in a cool, dark place, and the package should stay closed tightly. It should be used within 2 to 3 months after the package is opened.

Food should be purchased in quantities that can be used up within a reasonable length of time. The large economy package or the case of sauerkraut purchased on sale isn't a bargain if it is wasted.

Table 17-1. Recommendations for Maximum Storage Time of Meat, Fish, and Poultry

Food	Refrigerator (36°–40°F)	Freezer (0°F or Lower)
Ground Meat		
Beef, veal, lamb	1–2 days	3–4 months
Pork	1–2 days	2–3 months
Steaks and Chops		
Beef	3–5 days	6–9 months
Veal, lamb	3 days	6–9 months
Pork	3 days	3–6 months
Roasts		
Beef, veal, lamb	3–5 days	6–9 months
Pork	3–5 days	3–6 months
Organ Meats	1–2 days	3–4 months
Smoked Ham		
Whole	1 week	2 months
Half or slice	3–5 days	2 months
Luncheon Meats	1 week	Not recommended
Sausage		
Fresh pork	1 week	2 months
Smoked	3–7 days	Not recommended
Dry and semidry, unsliced	2–3 weeks	Not recommended
Frankfurters, Bacon	7 days	Not recommended
Leftover Cooked Meat	3–4 days	2–3 months
Fish		
Fresh	1–2 days	4–6 months
Cooked	3–4 days	2–3 months
Chicken, Turkey		
Fresh	1–2 days	1 year
Cooked	3–4 days	6 months

Perishable Foods

Perishable foods that must be kept cold should be stored in the refrigerator at a temperature below 40°F or in the freezer at 0°F or below. A thermometer should be used to check the temperature at various places in the refrigerator and freezer (Fig. 17-2; see also Tables 17-1 and 17-2).

Dairy Products

All fresh milk should be kept under refrigeration; if properly stored, it will keep at least a

Table 17-2. Storage Guide for Fruits and Vegetables

Hold at room temperature until ripe; then refrigerate, uncovered

Apples	Cherries	Peaches
Apricots	Melons, except watermelons	Pears
Avocados	Nectarines	Plums
Berries		Tomatoes

Store in cool room or refrigerate, uncovered

Grapefruit	Limes
Lemons	Oranges

Store in cool room, away from bright light

Onions, mature	Rutabagas	Sweet potatoes
Potatoes	Squash, winter	

Refrigerate, covered

Asparagus	Cauliflower	Parsnips
Beans, snap or wax	Celery	Peas, shelled
Beets	Corn, husked	Peppers, green
Broccoli	Cucumbers	Radishes
Cabbage	Greens	Squash, summer
Carrots	Onions, green	Turnips

Refrigerate, uncovered

Beans, lima, in pods	Grapes	Pineapples
Corn, in husks	Peas, in pods	Watermelons

(Family Fare, USDA Home and Garden Bulletin 1, 1978)

week after the pull date. Reliquefied dry milk should be used and stored in the same manner as fresh milk.

Cottage cheese and other uncured cheeses such as ricotta or farmer's cheese should be kept covered in the refrigerator. Eating directly from the container contaminates the product and causes it to spoil more quickly. If handled carefully, cottage cheese should keep for 5 days after the pull date on the container.

Eggs

Eggs should be stored in the refrigerator. Flavor and cooking quality are best if eggs are used within 1 week. Cracked or soiled eggs may contain harmful bacteria that cause food poisoning. These organisms are destroyed only if the eggs are thoroughly cooked.

Meat, Fish, Poultry

Fresh meat, fish, and poultry should be stored promptly in the coldest part of the refrigerator. Ground meat, fish, poultry, and organ meats are most likely to spoil and should therefore be used within 1 or 2 days. Steaks and roasts may be stored in the refrigerator for 3 to 5 days. Cured and smoked meats, such as ham, frankfurters, bacon, and sausage, may be stored for a period of 3 to 7 days, depending on the type (see Table 17-1).

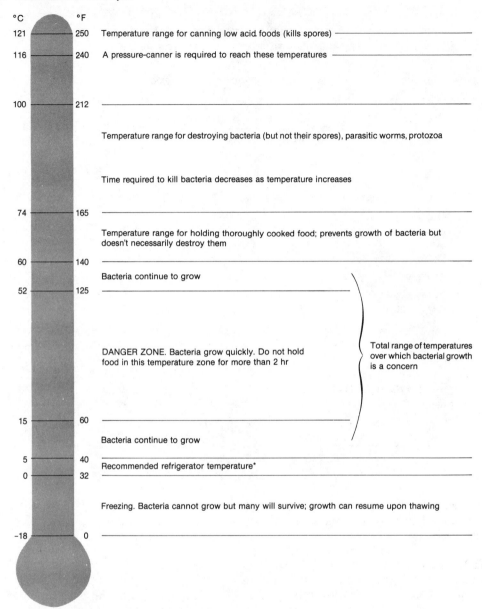

°C 121 250 °F — Temperature range for canning low acid foods (kills spores)

116 240 — A pressure-canner is required to reach these temperatures

100 212

Temperature range for destroying bacteria (but not their spores), parasitic worms, protozoa

Time required to kill bacteria decreases as temperature increases

74 165

Temperature range for holding thoroughly cooked food; prevents growth of bacteria but doesn't necessarily destroy them

60 140

Bacteria continue to grow

52 125

DANGER ZONE. Bacteria grow quickly. Do not hold food in this temperature zone for more than 2 hr

Total range of temperatures over which bacterial growth is a concern

15 60

Bacteria continue to grow

5 40 — Recommended refrigerator temperature*

0 32

Freezing. Bacteria cannot grow but many will survive; growth can resume upon thawing

−18 0

*Store raw meats for no more than 5 days and poultry, fish, and ground meat for no more than 2 days at refrigerator temperature

Fig. 17-2. Effects of temperature on organisms that cause food-borne illness. (After Temperature guide to food safety. USDA Food and Home Notes, No. 25. June 20, 1977)

Other Foods

Proper storage of fruits and vegetables is indicated in Table 17-2. Fats such as lard, drippings, butter, margarine, and opened jars of salad dressing should be refrigerated. Nuts, dried fruit, and whole-wheat flour should be refrigerated to prevent insect infestation in hot weather. Frozen foods should be kept at a temperature of 0°F if stored for more than 1 week.

Preparing Food Economically

There are many ways to save food dollars. For example, one can use leftovers in casseroles, soups, salads, sandwich spreads, and desserts. Leftover syrup from canned fruit can be used in a gelatin dessert or salad. Stale bread can be made into bread crumbs, French toast, or bread pudding.

One-pot meals and complete oven meals are energy savers, as is cooking double recipes and freezing one batch for later use. Other ways to save energy are to use a small burner for a small pan, cook with as little water as possible, and make sure that cooking pots have properly fitting lids.

Eating "out" is much more expensive than eating at home.

Conserving Nutrients in Fresh Vegetables

Fresh vegetables should be thoroughly washed before cutting to remove dirt and traces of insecticide spray. Root vegetables should be scrubbed. The dark outer leaves of greens are rich in iron, calcium, and vitamins, so they should be trimmed sparingly.

Peeling vegetables and fruit should be avoided whenever possible, because vitamins are concentrated just beneath the skin. Potatoes should be baked or cooked in their skins, even if one is making hashed browns or potato salad.

Vegetables should not be cut into small pieces but cooked whole or cut into large pieces to avoid exposing a large surface area. Leafy green vegetables should be torn rather than cut.

Vegetables should be cooked in very little or no water—the more water used, the greater the loss of vitamins and minerals. Thus, vegetables should be steamed whenever possible. The Chinese method of stir-frying preserves nutrients, because the vegetables are cooked quickly and with little water.

Whenever practical, any remaining cooking liquid should be served with the vegetable or used in a sauce, gravy, or soup. One should not use baking soda to preserve the green color; it destroys B vitamins and vitamin C.

Conserving Nutrients in Other Foods

To retain the nutrients in canned vegetables, one should pour the liquid from the can into a saucepan, and heat to reduce liquid; add vegetables to remaining liquid and heat before serving.

All protein foods are best cooked at low temperatures; this prevents the protein content from coagulating and causing the final product to be tough rather than tender. Low temperatures also reduce shrinkage and loss of nutrients.

To preserve the nutrients in rice, one should not wash it before cooking it or rinse it after cooking it.

KEYS TO PRACTICAL APPLICATION

Plan meals ahead — it's the key to nutritious and economical eating.

Use unit pricing to find the best buy among a variety of brands in a package size that is most practical for you.

Become familiar with the grading system involved in USDA grades, name brands, store brands, and generic labeling; buy the quality that suits your needs.

Remember that cost per serving, not cost per pound or package, is the key to finding the most economical buy.

Encourage the use of nonfat dry milk. It is the least expensive source of high-quality protein.

Discourage the use of excessive amounts of meat, fish, and poultry. It is too expensive to use for energy.

Learn to identify good buys among protein foods by comparing costs in terms of the amount of protein the foods provide.

Remember to check both the nutrition label and the ingredient panel when comparing a lightly processed food with a highly fortified refined product. The nutrition label does not always tell the whole story.

Cook vegetables by steaming, if possible; avoid cutting, soaking, peeling, and overcooking. In this way, nutrients will be conserved.

KEY IDEAS

Advance planning is the most important factor in obtaining nutritionally adequate and economical meals.

An understanding of unit pricing, open dating, and food grading can result in more efficient food purchasing.

Cost per serving, not cost per pound, can or package, is important in economical food buying, especially in meat buying.

Most Americans could lower their food bills without sacrificing nutritional quality by buying more milk, vegetables and fruit, and whole-grain and enriched cereals and bread and by buying less meat, fats, oils, sugar, coffee, tea, and snack foods.

Figuring the cost of protein will identify foods that are good buys among protein-rich foods.

One can reduce the cost of protein by using smaller portions of meat, fish, and poultry; by using lower grades and less expensive cuts of meat; and by using legumes, peanut butter, eggs, and cheese in place of meat for some meals.

Comparisons of the costs per serving of fresh, frozen, and canned fruits and vegetables should be made periodically to determine the best buy at a particular time of year.

Bakery foods and convenience foods usually cost more than those products made entirely at home.

FDA food labeling regulations aim to prohibit false or misleading labeling and packaging of food; nutrition labeling acknowledges the consumer's right to know the nutritional qualities of processed foods.

Nutrition labeling is required for all foods to which a nutrient is added or for which a nutrient claim is made; commercial pressure is causing manufacturers to use nutrition labeling voluntarily on all foods.

Nutrition labeling increases the consumer's awareness of the nutritional contributions of groups of foods and provides a means for comparing the nutritive values of similar foods and for identifying good sources of particular nutrients.

One should read both the nutrition labeling

and ingredient panels when comparing lightly processed conventional products with highly fortified refined products; nutrition labeling does not include the lesser known but equally important nutrients found in unprocessed food and can mislead the consumer into thinking the highly processed food is more nutritious.

Proper storage of both perishable and nonperishable food prevents loss of quality, waste, and food-borne illness.

Food should be purchased in quantities that can be used before quality deteriorates or spoilage occurs. Waste is thereby avoided.

Good food preparation and cooking techniques are needed to conserve nutrients, minimize shrinkage, and avoid waste.

Vegetables are especially prone to the loss of nutrients by poor food preparation practices; one should avoid cutting, peeling, and soaking of vegetables and should cook them as quickly as possible in as little liquid as possible; steaming is the best method for cooking vegetables.

Cooking protein foods at low temperatures produces a more tender product, reduces shrinkage, and preserves nutrients.

KEYS TO LEARNING: STUDY – DISCUSSION QUESTIONS

1. Why is the advance planning of meals and snacks an important factor in food management?

2. Plan what you consider to be a low-cost menu for 1 week for a family of four consisting of a mother, 30 years old; father, 32; girl, 9; and boy, 6. Include three meals a day and an after-school snack for the children. Calculate the cost based on current market prices.

    In class, compare the costs of the various plans. Are the four food groups adequately represented in all plans? What factors account for differences in cost?

3. Define the following, and explain their importance in food management: *unit pricing, open dating, USDA grade shields, supermarket private label grading system, cost per serving, brand name, generic labeling, cost of protein.*

4. Some food products come under what is known as a *standard of identity.* What does this mean, and how does it affect food labeling regulations? Of what special importance is the standard of identity to persons on restricted diets?

5. What are the advantages of nutrition labeling? Explain the meaning of U.S. RDA. In what ways may nutrition labeling mislead the consumer?

6. Compare the nutrition labeling on the following: homogenized whole milk, 2%-fat milk, 1%-fat milk, nonfat milk, commercial buttermilk, dry skim milk powder (reconstituted), regular yogurt, and low-fat yogurt. Compare the costs of an 8-ounce serving of each of these forms of milk.

7. Assume that you are attempting to encourage a mother of two school-age children to use more milk instead of sweetened fruit-flavored drinks at mealtime. How could you use nutrition labeling in your discussions with the mother?

8. What are the advantages of using low temperatures in cooking protein foods?

9. Discuss food preparation practices that conserve the nutritive value of vegetables.

Bibliography is found at the end of Part Three.

Food Safety

KEY TERMS

carcinogenic Tending to cause cancer.
germinate To cause to develop or produce.
interstate commerce Goods or services between states; business that crosses state boundaries.
mycotoxins Poisonous products produced by molds.

spore Reproductive cell produced by microorganisms; spores are very resistant to heat.
toxins Poisons excreted by disease-causing microorganisms.

It has been said that food represents the most complex aspect of the human chemical environment and is much less understood than the air we breathe and the water we drink. We rarely think of foods in their natural state as a group of chemicals. Nevertheless, a food as seemingly simple as potato is made up of well over a hundred chemicals.

Toxicity in Food

Some foods contain toxic substances as part of their chemical make-up. Potatoes contain solanine, a compound that can interfere with the transmission of nerve impulses. Spinach and rhubarb contain oxalates, which combine with calcium, making it unavailable for its functions. Cabbage and turnips contain goitrogens, sub-stances that may interfere with the proper functioning of the thyroid gland and cause it to enlarge. A cancer-causing substance in pollen has been found in honey. These are just a few examples of potentially harmful substances that occur naturally in foods. However, these substances do not automatically present a threat to health for several reasons. First, the quantity of toxic substances found in commonly eaten foods is very low, and extremely large amounts of a food containing a toxin would have to be ingested over a long period of time to do harm. Next, interactions between chemicals may block the toxic substances. Finally, methods of preparation may protect against toxic substances; for example, the toxins contained in certain legumes are destroyed by cooking. Here, too, variety is the key; when there is wide variety in the diet, there is little chance that the toxic properties of any one food will reach a harmful level.

The safety of food can also be adversely affected by bacterial toxins or mold; by contam-

235

Table 18-1. Bacterial Food-Borne Illness: Causes, Symptoms, and Prevention

Disease	Cause	Symptoms	Characteristics	Preventive Measures
Salmonellosis Examples of foods involved: poultry, red meats, eggs, dried foods, dairy products	*Salmonellae.* Bacteria widespread in nature, live and grow in intestinal tracts of human beings and animals	Severe headache followed by vomiting, diarrhea, abdominal cramps, and fever; infants, elderly, and persons with low resistance are most susceptible; severe infections cause high fever and may even cause death	Transmitted by eating contaminated food or by contact with infected persons or carriers of the infection; also transmitted by insects, rodents, and pets Onset: Usually within 12–36 hr Duration: 2–7 days	Salmonellae in food are destroyed by heating the food to 140°F and holding for 10 minutes or to higher temperatures for less time, *e.g.,* 155°F for a few seconds; refrigeration at 40°F inhibits the increase of salmonellae, but they remain alive in foods in the refrigerator or freezer, and even in dried foods
Perfringens poisoning Examples of foods involved: stews, soups, gravies made from poultry or red meat	*Clostridium perfringens.* Spore-forming bacteria that grow in the absence of oxygen; temperatures reached in thorough cooking of most foods are sufficient to destroy vegetative cells, but heat-resistant spores can survive	Nausea without vomiting, diarrhea, acute inflammation of stomach and intestine	Transmitted by eating food contaminated with abnormally large numbers of the bacteria Onset: Usually within 8–20 hr Duration: May persist for 24 hr	To prevent growth of surviving bacteria in cooked meats, gravies, and meat casseroles that are to be eaten later, cool foods rapidly and refrigerate promptly at 40°F or below, or hold them above 140°F
Staphylococcal poisoning (frequently called *staph*) Examples of foods involved: custards, egg salad, potato salad, chicken salad, macaroni salad, ham, salami, cheese	*Staphylococcus aureus.* Bacteria fairly resistant to heat; bacteria growing in food produce a toxin that is extremely resistant to heat	Vomiting, diarrhea, prostration, abdominal cramps; generally mild and often attributed to other causes	Transmitted by food handlers who carry the bacteria and by eating food containing the toxin Onset: Usually within 3–8 hr Duration: 1 to 2 days	Growth of bacteria that produce toxin is inhibited by keeping hot foods above 140°F and cold foods at or below 40°F; toxin is destroyed by boiling for several hours or heating the food in a pressure cooker at 240°F for 30 minutes

Table 18-1. *(continued)*

Disease	Cause	Symptoms	Characteristics	Preventive Measures
Botulism Examples of foods involved: canned low-acid foods, smoked fish	*Clostridium botulinum.* Spore-forming organisms that grow and produce toxin in the absence of oxygen, such as in a sealed container.	Double vision, inability to swallow, speech difficulty, progressive respiratory paralysis; fatality rate is high, in the United States about 65%	Transmitted by eating food containing the toxin Onset: Usually within 12–36 hr or longer Duration: 3 to 6 days	Bacterial spores in food are destroyed by high temperatures obtained only in the pressure canner*; more than 6 hr is needed to kill the spores at boiling temperature (212°F); the toxin is destroyed by boiling for 10–20 minutes; time required depends on kind of food

(Keeping Food Safe to Eat. USDA Home and Garden Bulletin 162, 1977)

  * For processing times in home canning, see Home and Garden Bulletins 8, "Home Canning of Fruits and Vegetables," and 106, "Home Canning of Meat and Poultry."

ination due to carelessness, accident, or ignorance; and by chemicals added during production and processing. Because the problem of food safety is so important, each of these topics is discussed individually.

Toxins Produced by Bacteria or Molds

The most common cause of illness related to food consumption is the contamination by pathogens (disease-causing organisms) or harmful toxins produced by them. The appearance, taste, or smell of the contaminated food may be unaffected, and the consumer often is completely unaware that the food is unsafe.

Pathogens enter food by several pathways. A food animal may itself be infested with salmonellae or trichinae. An infected food handler may introduce disease organisms into the food by hands soiled with feces or urine or by coughing or sneezing over the food as he prepares it. Contaminated equipment, such as butcher blocks and meat slicers, can be another source of infection. Working surfaces, such as counter

tops and cutting boards can become contaminated from infected food. If these surfaces are not properly cleaned, other foods prepared on them can become infected. Household pets, dust, and the feces and bodies of insects are other sources of contamination.

The most common type of food-borne disease in the United States is food poisoning caused by *Staphylococcus, Salmonella,* and *Clostridium perfringens* bacteria. Botulism, another type of food poisoning, is rare but usually fatal (Table 18-1).

Bacterial Toxins

Salmonellosis, a bacterial infection, can be extremely serious in infants, the elderly, and persons weakened by illness. Characteristics of the disease are described in Table 18-1. Fresh raw eggs should not be used in the preparation of soft custard and egg-nogs, especially if these foods are to be served to small children or persons with low resistance to disease. Pasteurized dried egg powder or egg-nog mix should be used instead of raw eggs, which may carry salmonellae. Heat destroys salmonellae; hence, cracked

eggs should not be used unless they can be hard cooked or used in baking.

Typhoid fever, caused by a species of *Salmonella,* is usually transmitted to food by a food handler who is a carrier. The disease affects the gastrointestinal tract, liver, gallbladder, spleen, and kidney.

Staphyloccoccal bacteria produce a toxin that can cause food poisoning if enough of it is present in the food (see Table 18-1). The organisms are found in the respiratory passages and on the skin. They enter food from boils or infected cuts, or when the person coughs or sneezes. If the contaminated food is kept at too high a temperature or is not reheated thoroughly, the toxin can accumulate and cause illness.

Clostridium perfringens is a spore-forming bacterium. Its spores are resistant to heat, ordinary cooking, and methods of food preservation such as freezing and drying. When the affected food is left at room temperature for long periods of time, the spores germinate and produce tremendous numbers of bacteria (see Table 18-1).

Food poisoning from *Clostridium perfringens* occurs most often when large amounts of food have been prepared and held for long periods of time on steam tables or at room temperature, such as in restaurants or other large feeding establishments.

Another bacterium, *Clostridium botulinum,* produces a toxin that is the cause of a serious, usually fatal illness, even in very small amounts. The spores grow only in anaerobic conditions (without oxygen) and are destroyed by high temperatures (see Table 18-1).

Botulism occurs most frequently from the use of home-canned foods low in acid that have not been adequately processed. The *Clostridium botulinum* organism may provide some clues about its presence in canned foods: a bulging can, an off-color, or a strange odor. Any food that looks spoiled, foams, or has an off-odor should be destroyed without being tasted.

Mycotoxins

Aflatoxin, a toxin produced by certain molds, is a cancer-causing substance that develops in spoiled peanuts, peanut butter, nuts, soybeans, grains, spices, and animal products. Apparently, aflatoxins cannot be completely eliminated from the food supply, but the FDA strictly limits the amount permitted to 15 ppb (parts per billion) in food for sale in interstate commerce.

Because the long-term effects of mold toxins is not known, it is advisable to avoid eating moldy foods and to avoid sniffing mold, which can enter the body through the respiratory tract. The mold that is seen is only the spore-bearing part, the rest of the mold being buried deep inside the food substance. For this reason, cutting away the moldy part of the food is not sufficient; the entire item should be discarded. Peanuts and other nuts should be examined carefully and any that are moldy, shriveled, or damaged discarded. Cooking does not destroy mold toxins. Mold-ripened cheese such as bleu cheese or Roquefort is apparently safe to use.

Parasitic Infestation

Trichinosis occurs when raw or undercooked pork that is infected with the parasite *Trichinella spiralis* is eaten. The causative organism is destroyed by very thorough cooking, preferably to an internal temperature of 170°F (77°C).

Accidental or Natural Food Contamination

There are many avenues by which harmful chemicals can enter food through either accident or carelessness. Foods can become contaminated when placed in containers made with toxic materials. Lead poisoning can occur from an earthenware pitcher used to store orange juice, copper poisoning from soft drinks dispensed through tubing that has eroded to its copper base.

Toxicity of Metals

Toxic metals such as mercury, lead, and cadmium contaminate the environment and may enter the food supply. The high levels of mer-

cury occurring in fish are in some cases due to pollution and in other cases simply to a high mercury concentration occurring naturally in some unpolluted waters. Industrial pollution is the main cause of contamination of freshwater fish. In contrast, such fish as swordfish, which have a relatively long life-span, tend to accumulate the mercury that is naturally present in the ocean. The federal government has set a limit of 5 ppm (parts per million) as an acceptable level of mercury in fish. Because mercury in swordfish exceeds this level, it has been removed from the market. Acceptable levels of lead and cadmium in earthenware products have also been established.

Radioactive Fallout

Radioactive fallout following nuclear testing has given rise to concern about the safety of the food supply, due to the possible presence in the environment of two radioactive substances, strontium 90 and iodine 131. Small amounts of ^{90}S may be deposited in the bones; the absorption of ^{131}I increases the possibility of thyroid cancer.

Accidents

Accidents in which poisonous substances are mistaken for food are another cause of illness and death. Rat poison has been mistaken for flour and boric acid for sugar. Deaths of infants in hospital nurseries have been caused by the use of a boric acid solution instead of distilled water in the preparation of a milk formula. And in one case, a teenager died after drinking a household chemical he mistook for soda because it had been stored in a soda bottle.

Chemical Toxins

The safety of foods to which chemicals have been added in production or processing is under question.

Additives

A food additive is any substance that becomes part of a food when added either intentionally or incidentally. Food additives are not new. Salt, herbs, and spices have been used for years as preservatives. However, in this century, the increase in food additives has been tremendous, a result of changes in life-style that have brought about mass production of food, transportation of food over long distances, storage of food for long periods, and increased demand for convenience foods.

Intentional food additives include food supplements (vitamins, minerals), preservatives, antioxidants, stabilizers, emulsifiers, and coloring and flavoring agents, all of which have some useful purpose in the food product. Some 2800 of these substances are used today. Another 10,000 are incidental additives that find their way into food although their presence is not desired: pesticides, fertilizers, hormones and tranquilizers given to animals used for meat, and chemicals used in packaging to preserve freshness.

Pesticides

Pesticides are an example of an incidental or indirect additive. The federal government has determined what pesticides may be used and what pesticide residue levels are permissible, and the Federal Drug Administration (FDA) monitors these levels. Various state agencies also play a role in regulating pesticide use.

Importance of a Varied Diet

A diet consisting of a wide variety of foods provides the best protection against potentially harmful chemicals in food. This is because the body tolerates very small quantities of many toxic substances but has only a limited ability to cope with large quantities of any single one.

Almost any chemical can have a harmful effect if taken in large enough quantity, even sodium and vitamin D. It is important to understand the difference between toxicity and hazard. Many foods contain toxic chemicals, but these chemicals do not present a hazard in the usual amounts consumed.

Regulating the Food Supply: Role of the Federal Government

As we have seen, the consumer has an important role in safeguarding his food supply. However, consumers obviously have only very limited powers, and many agencies, local, state, and federal, are also involved in this work.

The federal government regulates the shipment of foods over state lines, foods manufactured in territories of the United States and in the District of Columbia, and the import and export of foods. State governments control most foods manufactured and sold within state boundaries.

Food and Drug Administration

The FDA of the U.S. Department of Health and Human Services is responsible for protecting the consumer against unsafe, unsanitary, and improperly labeled products. Most of FDA's authority comes from the following four laws.

Fair Packaging and Labeling Act of 1966

This act requires that the label on a food can or package disclose the ingredients and state the weight of the package. Drugs, cosmetics, and medical devices come under this act.

Radiation Control for Health and Safety Act of 1968

This act protects the public from unnecessary exposure to radiation from electronic products, including microwave ovens.

Public Health Services Act of 1944

This act gives the FDA authority to regulate and control pasteurized milk and shellfish, sanitation of interstate restaurants, and sanitation of food, water, and toilet facilities on trains, planes, and buses.

Federal Food, Drug, and Cosmetic Act of 1938

The FDA was established under the terms of the Food, Drug, and Cosmetic Act of 1938, which gave it control over foods and medicines for man and animals, cosmetics, and medical devices. This law and its amendments give FDA far-reaching powers, as outlined below.

Adulterated and Misbranded Foods. The FDA prohibits the sale of adulterated or misbranded food. A food is considered adulterated if it contains spoiled or filthy products, meat from diseased animals, or noncertified colors; if the product is diluted, or if a substitute ingredient is used; if an essential ingredient is omitted; if the packaging material is made from hazardous substances; if it contains additives that conceal nutritional deficiencies; if it contains additives that have not been approved by FDA; and if it is produced or stored under unsanitary conditions.

A food is considered misbranded if the package label makes false claims; if the use of synthetic substances such as artificial colors and flavors is not clearly stated; if the statement of weight, measure, or count is incorrect; if the name of manufacturer, packer, or distributor is not listed on the label; if nutrition labeling is not provided for products about which a nutritional claim is made (see Chap. 17).

Standards have been established relating to identity, quality, and fill. Standards of identity established for certain foods specify which ingredients must be included, the minimum and maximum amount of each ingredient permitted, and optional ingredients. Standards of

quality, used chiefly for canned fruits, vegetables, and meats, relate to color, tenderness, flavor, and freedom from blemishes. If a food does not meet the minimum standards for quality, the container must be labeled "below standard in quality." Standards of fill relate to the volume of product in the container and were established to protect the consumer from deceptive packaging practices.

Labeling regulations on fats and oils are an aid to persons on fat-controlled diets and others who need to know what types of fats are used in producing the food in question. Fat- and oil-source labeling requires that the specific fat be identified (*e.g.*, "corn oil" or "lard," rather than simply "vegetable oil" or "shortening"). The term *hydrogenated* or *partially hydrogenated* must be used rather than *saturated* or *partially saturated*.

Additives. The amendments to the Food, Drug, and Cosmetic Act that cover additives require that the manufacturer prove that each proposed additive is safe for human consumption. The FDA is authorized to regulate only the safety of additives, not the number of additives or the necessity for them.

The steps required for approval of an additive may take several years, during which time the manufacturer must prove by various tests and procedures that the additive is not a cause of cancer or birth defects and has no other known harmful effects.

Two important categories of additives are exempt from the testing and approval process. One group consists of substances that were approved for use in food before 1958; the second consists of some 700 additives known as the *GRAS list.*

A GRAS additive is one that has been judged by experts to be "generally *recognized as* safe." GRAS additives did not undergo extensive testing to determine their safety and have not been strictly regulated. The reasoning behind the GRAS list is that it is unnecessary to prove the safety of substances that have been in use for long periods of time with no known harmful effects. However, prompted by uncertainty about the safety of cyclamates, the FDA recently reviewed the GRAS list. The review has been completed, and most of the additives have been approved. Others have been reclassified and further testing is recommended.

Bureau of Animal Husbandry

The Bureau of Animal Husbandry of the U.S. Department of Agriculture (USDA) is responsible for the inspection of all meats sold for human consumption anywhere in the United States. The USDA receives its authority from the Meat Inspection Act of 1906 and the amendments of 1967. Meats found to be wholesome are stamped "Inspected and passed"; those unfit for human consumption are stamped "Inspected and condemned." Condemned meats must be destroyed under the supervision of a federal inspector. Sanitation and operating procedures of meat processing plants also are supervised by federal inspectors.

The Poultry Inspection Act of 1957 provides for the compulsory inspection of poultry and poultry products.

Environmental Protection Agency

The Safe Drinking Water Act of 1974 under the Environmental Protection Agency (EPA) has established minimum standards for drinking water, including limitation of potentially harmful substances. States are responsible for enforcing the regulations. The FDA, however, has responsibility for regulating the purity of bottled water and water used in food and food processing.

Federal Trade Commission

The Federal Trade Commission regulates the advertising of foods, drugs, and cosmetics through media such as television and radio. Its responsibility is to protect the public against false and misleading advertising.

Role of State and Local Agencies

The pasteurization of milk and the inspection of cattle and goats are all under state control. State agencies are also responsible for regulating the production and the processing of certain food products that are sold within its boundaries.

Local governments may also have sanitary codes that regulate food production and processing and that provide for the inspection of public eating establishments.

KEYS TO PRACTICAL APPLICATION

Do not work with food if you have an infectious disease or infected cuts or other skin infections.

Always work with clean hands, clean fingernails, and clean hair, and wear clean clothing.

Wash hands thoroughly with soap and water after using the toilet or after assisting anyone using the toilet; after smoking; after sneezing, coughing, or blowing your nose; and after using the telephone.

Wash hands thoroughly after handling raw meat, poultry, or eggs and before working with other food.

Keep hands away from the mouth, nose, and hair.

Mix foods with clean utensils rather than hands.

Avoid using the same spoon more than once for tasting food while preparing, cooking, or serving.

Do not serve baby foods directly from the jar or can to avoid contaminating any remaining food.

Never store cleaning supplies, pesticides, and drugs with food or in food containers such as soda bottles and food jars.

Refrigerate perishable foods at 40°F or below. Store perishable and frozen foods in the refrigerator and freezer as soon after shopping as possible.

Keep hot foods hot — above 140°F — and cold foods cold — below 40°F. Foods that are held for more than 2 to 3 hours at a temperature between 60°F and 125°F may not be safe to eat.

Keep food that contains milk or egg products and little vinegar or other acids refrigerated. This includes cream, custard, and meringue pies; foods containing custard fillings, such as cakes, cream puffs, or eclairs; and salads and sandwich fillings. If taken on summer outings, these foods should be kept in a cooler with ice or reusable cold packs.

Cook commercially frozen stuffed poultry from the frozen state and keep it in the refrigerator until time to start cooking. If the stuffing is made in advance, store it separately in the refrigerator. Remove the stuffing from all leftover cooked meat, poultry, or fish before storing, and store it in the refrigerator in a separate container.

Refrigerate leftover meat, fish, poultry, broth, and gravy immediately after a meal. Freeze them if they are to be kept longer than a few days.

Clean all dishes, utensils, and work surfaces thoroughly with soap and water after each use. It is especially important to clean equipment and work surfaces that have been used for raw food, such as raw poultry or meat, before they are used for cooked food or foods such as salads that are eaten without cooking.

A chlorine solution prepared with chlorine laundry bleach in the proportion of 1 tablespoon of chlorine bleach in 1 quart of cold water will destroy bacteria. This solution can be used for rinsing utensils and work surfaces. Equipment such as cutting boards, meat grinders, blenders, and can openers particularly need to be sanitized in this way.

Serve foods immediately after cooking or refrigerate promptly. Hot foods can be placed in the refrigerator as long as they do not raise the temperature of the refrigerator above 45°F. Large quantities of food can be cooled more quickly if refrigerated in shallow containers.

Thaw frozen meat, fish, or poultry in the refrigerator. These meats may be cooked from the frozen state if cooked for at least 1½ times as long as required for the unfrozen product. Undercooked foods may be unsafe. Cook stuffing to a temperature of at least 165°F, even if you are cooking it separately. Use a meat thermometer.

Heat leftovers thoroughly; boil broths and gravies for several minutes before reusing.

Handle foods to be put in your home freezer as little as possible to keep bacteria at a minimum before freezing. Freezing does not kill bacteria but merely stops their growth; the bacteria then continue to multiply after the food is thawed. Can home-canned meat, poultry, and low-acid vegetables in a pressure canner at the proper temperature and for the time specified in the directions. The boiling-water-bath method is not safe for these foods.

Simmer all home-canned vegetables, meat, and poultry for 10 to 20 minutes before tasting.

Heating makes the odor of spoilage more noticeable. If a food looks spoiled, foams, or has an off-odor, destroy it without tasting.

Cook pork thoroughly to an internal temperature of 170°F.

Do not eat moldy foods. Discard the entire food, including those portions on which the mold is not apparent.

Do not use fresh raw eggs in egg-nog or soft custard, especially when serving the food to small children or persons in a weakened condition. Use pasteurized dried egg powder instead.

Use cracked eggs only if thoroughly cooked, as in hard-cooked eggs or baked dishes.

KEY IDEAS

A varied diet and the consumption of no single food in excessive amounts are the best protection against harmful chemicals in food. Such harmful chemicals may occur naturally in food or be added by humans.

Contamination of food by disease-causing organisms or harmful toxins produced by organisms is the most common cause of illness due to food consumption. *Salmonella* and *Clostridium perfringens* infection and staphylococcal poisoning are the most common food-borne diseases; botulism is a rare but usually fatal form of food poisoning.

Salmonellae are carried by raw meats, poultry, eggs, milk, fish, and household pets. They are destroyed by heat.

Clostridium perfringens infection usually occurs when food is left at room temperature for long periods of time.

Staphylococcal poisoning is caused by toxins from "staph" bacteria, which enter food from boils, infected cuts, and coughing and sneezing; the toxins accumulate when food is held at improper temperatures.

Botulism, a rare but deadly form of food poisoning, is caused most frequently by home-canned, low-acid foods.

Poisons produced by molds may have long-term harmful effects; it is advisable to discard moldy food.

Trichinosis is caused by eating raw or undercooked pork.

Food-borne illness is prevented by the protection of food from contamination and by temperature control (hot foods should be kept above 140°F and cold foods below 40°F).

The consumer's role in food safety involves good food-handling practices, such as good personal hygiene, proper food storage, and sanitary practices in preparing and cooking food.

Accidental contamination of food can result from food containers made with toxic materials, environmental pollution, the accumulation of toxic metals in animals and fish, radioactive fallout. Poisoning can also occur through ingestion of toxic substances mistaken for food.

Various government agencies protect the food supply in those aspects of food safety that are beyond the control of the individual. These agencies receive their authority from federal laws designed to protect the public from unsafe food and water and from deception or fraud in the sale of food products.

The presence of chemicals added either on purpose or indirectly in the production or processing of food (*e.g.,* pesticides, food additives, and drugs given to animals used as food) are monitored by the FDA. This agency also protects against unsanitary and improperly labeled products.

Manufacturers must prove by extensive tests that an additive is safe.

The GRAS list is a list of food additives that have been generally recognized as safe and are by law exempt from testing. A recent review of all of these substances has resulted in some additives being reclassified and recommended for further testing.

The Bureau of Animal Husbandry of the USDA is responsible for inspecting meat and poultry for wholesomeness, the sanitation of meat processing plants, and the safety of manufactured meat products.

The EPA is responsible for establishing safety regulations for drinking water.

The Federal Trade Commission protects against false and misleading advertising of foods.

State and local governments also have important roles in food safety.

KEYS TO LEARNING: STUDY–DISCUSSION QUESTIONS

1. The consumer can prevent food-borne disease by controlling the number of bacteria in food eaten at home. In what two basic ways is this control accomplished? Discuss the sanitary food-handling practices that promote the control of harmful bacteria.

2. What is the proper method for the home-canning of low-acid foods? Why is the use of this method so important? What precautions should be taken before home-canned, low-acid foods are eaten?

3. Discuss the importance of a varied diet from the standpoint of food safety.

4. Contact the Consumer Information Officer of the FDA office in your area. Become informed of the services this office provides for the consumer. Obtain the most recent FDA publications relating to food additives, nutrition labeling, or other related subjects of interest to the class. Discuss with the class the information you have obtained.

5. Visit your local health department or have a representative from the department speak to the class about the department's role in protecting the safety of the food supply.

Bibliography is found at the end of Part Three.

Bibliography

Part Three. Nutrition in the Life Cycle

General References
American Dietetic Association: Handbook of Clinical Dietetics. New Haven, Yale University Press, 1981
Anderson L, Dibble MV, Turkki PR et al: Nutrition in Health and Disease, 17th ed. Philadelphia, JB Lippincott, 1982
Food and Nutrition Board, National Research Council: Recommended Dietary Allowances, 9th ed. Washington, DC National Academy of Sciences, 1980
Suitor CW, Hunter MT: Nutrition: Principles and Application in Health Promotion. Philadelphia, JB Lippincott, 1980
White A and the Society for Nutrition Education: The Family Health Cookbook. New York, David McKay 1980

13. Meeting Nutritional Needs in Daily Meals

Books and Pamphlets
Dietary Goals for the United States, 2. U.S. Senate Select Committee on Nutrition and Human Needs. Washington, DC, U.S. Government Printing Office, 1977
Dosti R, Kidushim D, Wolke M: Light Style: The New American Cuisine. Hagerstown, MD, Harper & Row, 1979
Food. USDA Home and Garden Bulletin 228. Washington, DC, U.S. Government Printing Office, 1979
The Prudent Diet—Eating Today for a Healthier Tomorrow. New York, New York City Department of Health, 1981
The Sodium Content of Your Food. USDA Home and Garden Bulletin 233. Washington, DC, U.S. Government Printing Office, 1980

Periodicals
Bray GA: Dietary guidelines: The shape of things to come. J Nutr Ed 12(Suppl 1):97, 1980
Reaction Statement. Dietary goals for the U.S. *J Am Diet Assoc* 74:529, 1979
Fast Food Chains. Consumer Reports, Sept., 1979
Guthrie HA, Scheer JC: Validity of a dietary score for assessing nutrient adequacy. J Am Diet Assoc 78:240, 1981
Hegsted DM: Dietary guidelines: Where do we go from here? J Nutr Ed 12:100, 1981
Jansen GR, Harper JM, Kendall P et al: Menu evaluation—A nutrient approach for consumers. J Nutr Ed 9:162, 1977
Latham MC, Stephenson LS (For); Harper AE (Against): U.S. dietary goals—For and against. J Nutr Ed 9:152, 1977
Olson RE: Are professionals jumping the gun in the fight against chronic disease. J Am Diet Assoc 74:543, 1979
Shannon BM, Parks SC: Fast foods: A perspective on their nutritional impact. J Am Diet Assoc 80:242, 1982
Simopoulos AP: The scientific basis of the 'goals': What can be done now? J Am Diet Assoc 74:539, 1979
Welsh SO, Marston RM: Review of trends in food use in the U.S. 1909 to 1980. J Am Diet Assoc 81:120, 1982
Wittwer AJ, Sorenson AW, Wyse BW, Hansen RG: "Nutrient density—Evaluation of nutritional attributes of foods. J Nutr Ed 9:26, 1977

Young EA, Brennan EH, Irving GL: Perspectives on fast foods. Dietetic Currents 5:5, 1978

Young EA, Brennan EH, Irving GL: Update: Nutritional Analysis of Fast Foods. Dietetic Currents 8:2, 1981

14. Meeting Nutritional Needs in Various Cultures and Lifestyles

Books and Pamphlets

Herbert V: Nutrition Cultism. Philadelphia, George F Stickley, 1980

Lowenberg NE, Todhunter EN, Wilson ED et al: Food and People. New York, John Wiley & Sons, 1979

Robertson L et al: Laurel's Kitchen: A Handbook of Vegetarian Cookery and Nutrition. Petaluma, CA, Nilgiri Press, 1976

Periodicals

Baird PC, Schutz HG: Life style correlates of dietary and biochemical measures of nutrition. J Am Diet Assoc 76:228, 1980

Bell AC, Stewart AM, Radford AJ et al: A method for describing food beliefs which may predict personal food choice. J Nutr Ed 13:22, 1981

Bergan JG, Brown PT: Nutritional status of "new" vegetarians. J Am Diet Assoc 76:151, 1980

Bruch H: The allure of food cults and nutrition quackery. J Am Diet Assoc 57:316, 1977

Crane NT, Green NR: Food habits and food preferences of Vietnamese refugees living in northern Florida. J Am Diet Assoc 76:591, 1980

Day M, Lentner M, Jaquez S: Food acceptance patterns of Spanish-speaking New Mexicans. J Nutr Ed 10:121, 1978

Grivetti LE, Paquette MB: Nontraditional ethnic food choices among first generation Chinese in California. J Nutr Ed 10:109, 1978

Helmick SA: Family living patterns—Projections for the future. J Nutr Ed 10:155, 1978

Lekon BM, Kris-Etherton PM: Meal cost analysis: Health food store versus conventional food sources. J Am Diet Assoc 79:456, 1981

Norman RE: Ideas for teaching nutrition. J Home Economics 69:45, 1977

Position paper on the vegetarian approach to eating. J Am Diet Assoc 77:61, 1980

Schafer R, Yetley EA: Social psychology of food faddism. J Am Diet Assoc 66:127, 1975

Wheeler M, Haider SQ: Buying and food preparation patterns of ghetto blacks and hispanics in Brooklyn. J Am Diet Assoc 75:560, 1979

Yang GI, Fox HM: Food habit changes of Chinese persons living in Lincoln, Nebraska. J Am Diet Assoc 75:420, 1979

Yahai F: Dietary patterns of Spanish-speaking people living in the Boston area. J Am Diet Assoc 71:273, 1977

15. Nutrition During Pregnancy and Lactation

Books and Pamphlets

Committee on Maternal Nutrition: Supplementation and the Outcome of Pregnancy. Washington, DC, National Academy of Sciences, National Research Council, 1975

Durhring JL: Nutrition in comprehensive maternity care. In Proceedings of Nutrition Throughout the Life Cycle. Austin, Texas Department of Health, 1977

Food for Mothers-To-Be. Trenton, Mercer Regional Medical Group, 1979

Gibbs CE: Nutritional needs of the pregnant teenager—Successful management. In Proceedings of Nutrition Throughout the Life Cycle. Austin, Texas Department of Health, 1977

Luke B: Maternal Nutrition. Boston, Little, Brown & Co, 1979

Nutrition During Pregnancy and Lactation. Sacramento, Maternal and Child Health Unit, California Department of Health, 1975

Recipe for Healthy Babies. White Plains, NY, March of Dimes, Birth Defects Foundation, 1979

Worthington-Roberts BS, Vermeersch J, Williams SR: Nutrition in Pregnancy and Lactation. St. Louis, CV Mosby, 1981

Periodicals

Beagle WS: Fetal alcohol syndrome: A review. J Am Diet Assoc 79:274, 1981

Brennan RE, Caldwell M, Rickard KA et al: Assessment of maternal nutrition. J Am Diet Assoc 75:152, 1979

Edwards LE, Alton IR, Barrada MI et al: Pregnancy in the underweight woman: Course, outcome and growth patterns of the infant. Am J Obstet Gynecol 135:297, 1979

Endes JM, Sawicki M, Casper, JA: Dietary assessment of the pregnant woman in a supplemental food program. J Am Diet Assoc 79:121, 1981

Falkner F: Maternal nutrition and fetal growth. Am J Clin Nutr 34:769, 1981

Fielding JE: Adolescent pregnancy revisited. N Engl J Med 299:893, 1978

Hook EB: Dietary cravings and aversions during pregnancy. Am J Clin Nutr 31:1355, 1978

Jacobson HN: Diet in pregnancy. N Engl J Med 297:1051, 1978

Jacobson HN: Maternal nutrition in the 1980's. J Am Diet Assoc 80:216, 1982

Lind T: Nutrient requirements during pregnancy. Am J Clin Nutr 34:669, 1981

Metcoff J, Costiloe JP, Crosby W et al: Maternal nutrition and fetal outcome. Am J Clin Nutr 34:708, 1981

Pitkin RM: Nutrition in pregnancy. Dietetic Currents, 4:1, 1977

Singleton NC, Lewis H, Parker JJ: The diet of pregnant teenagers. J Am Home Ec Assoc 68:43, 1976

Special report: Second international caffeine workshop. Nutr Rev 38:196, 1980

Thenen SW: Folacin content of supplemental food for pregnancy. J Am Diet Assoc 80:237, 1982

16. Nutrition in the Various Stages of Life

Books and Pamphlets

Alford BB: Nutritional care of the elderly. In Proceedings of Nutrition Throughout the Life Cycle. Austin, Texas Department of Health, 1977

Beal VA: Nutrition in the Life Cycle. New York, John Wiley & Sons, 1980

Committee on Nutrition: Pediatric Nutrition Handbook. Evanston, American Academy of Pediatrics, 1979

Foman SJ: Nutritional Disorders of Children. Prevention, Screening, and Follow-up. DHEW Publication (HSA) 77-5104. Washington, DC, U.S. Government Printing Office, 1977

Pipes PL: Nutrition in Infancy and Childhood, 2nd ed. St. Louis, CV Mosby, 1977

Periodicals

Alfin-Slater RB, Jelliffe, DB: Nutritional requirements with special reference to infancy. Pediatr Clin North Am 24:3, 1977

Burt JV, Hertzler AA: Parenteral influence on the child's food preference. J Nutr Ed 10:127, 1978

Busse EW: How mind, body, and environment influence nutrition in the elderly. Postgrad Med 63:117, 1978

Caliendo MA, Sanjur D: The dietary status of preschool children: An ecological approach. J Nutr Ed 10:69, 1978

Combs KL: Preventive care in the elderly. Am J Nurs 78:1339, 1978

Fisk D: A successful program for changing children's eating habits. Nutr Today 14:6, 1979

Foman SJ, Filer LJ, Anderson TA et al: Recommendations for feeding normal infants. Pediatrics 63:52, 1979

Gotz BE, Gotz VP: Drugs and the elderly. Am J Nurs 78:1347, 1978

Grotkowski ML, Sims LS: Nutrition knowledge, attitudes and dietary practices of the elderly. J Am Diet Assoc 72:499, 1978

Jelliffe DB, Jelliffe EFP: Breast is best: Modern meanings. New Engl J Med 297:912, 1977

Krondl M, Lau D, Yurkiu MA et al: Food use and perceived food meanings of the elderly. J Am Diet Assoc 80:523, 1982

Marino DD, King JC: Nutritional concerns during

adolescence. Pediatr Clin North Am 27:125, 1980

Mata L: Breast feeding: Main promoter of infant health. Am J Clin Nutr 31:2058, 1978

Pipes P: When should semi-solid foods be fed to infants. J Nutr Educ 9:57, 1977

Pollitt E, Wirtz S: Mother–infant feeding interaction and weight gain in the first month of life. J Am Diet Assoc 78:596, 1981

Posner BM: Nutrition education for older Americans: National policy recommendations. J Am Diet Assoc 80:455, 1982

Read MH, Graney AS: Food supplement usage by the elderly. J Am Diet Assoc 80:250, 1982

Review: The development of adipose tissue in infancy. Nutr Rev 37:194, 1979

Review: Nutrition in adolescence. Nutr Rev 39:37, 1981

Todhunter EN, Darby WJ: Guidelines for maintaining adequate nutrition in old age. Geriatrics 33:49, 1978

Woodruff CW: The science of infant nutrition and the art of infant feeding. JAMA 240:657, 1978

17. Food Management

Books and Pamphlets

Black H (ed): The Berkeley Co-op Food Book. Palo Alto, Bull Publishing, 1980

Family Fare. USDA Home and Garden Bulletin 1. Washington, DC, U.S. Government Printing Office, 1978

Family Food Budgeting. USDA Home and Garden Bulletin 94. Washington, DC, U.S. Government Printing Office, 1980

How to Buy Dairy Products. USDA Home and Garden Bulletin 201. Washington, DC, U.S. Government Printing Office, 1978

Money-Saving Main Dishes. USDA Home and Garden Bulletin 43. Washington, DC, U.S. Government Printing Office, 1979

Nutrition Labeling: How It Can Work for You. Washington, DC, National Nutrition Consortium, 1975

White A and the Society for Nutrition Education: The Family Health Cookbook. New York, David McKay, 1980

Your Money's Worth in Foods. USDA Home and Garden Bulletin 183. Washington, DC, U.S. Government Printing Office, 1977

Periodicals

Handy C, Seigle N: Generic labeling. Nat Food Rev Sept., 1978

18. Food Safety

Keeping Food Safe to Eat. USDA Home and Garden Bulletin 162. Washington, DC, U.S. Government Printing Office, 1975

U.S. Department of Health and Human Services, Public Health Service, Food and Drug Administration: FDA Consumer Memo: Milestones in U.S. Food and Drug Law History. H.H.S. Publication (FDA)79-1063, 1979

Wood B: Please don't eat moldy foods. In Black H (ed): The Berkeley Co-Op Food Book. Palo Alto, Bull Publishing, 1980

Periodicals

Jukes TH: Food additives. New Engl J Med 297:427, 1977

Lehman P: More than you ever thought you would know about food additives. Part I. FDA Consumer 13:10, 1979

Plumlee C, Bjeldanes LF, Hatch FT: Priorities assessment for studies of mutagen production in cooked food. J Am Diet Assoc 79:446, 1981

Rodricks JW: Hazards from nature. Aflatoxins. FDA Consumer 12:16, 1978

Symposium: Risk versus benefits: The future of food safety. Nutr Rev 38:35, 1980

Wilson BJ: Naturally occurring toxicants in foods. Nutr Rev 37:305, 1979

Yesterday's additives—Generally safe. FDA Consumer, March, 1981

Zattola EA: "Food-borne disease I. Contemp Nutr 2:9, 1977

Zattola EA: Food-borne disease II. Contemp Nutr 3:1, 1978

PART FOUR

Diet Modifications During Illness

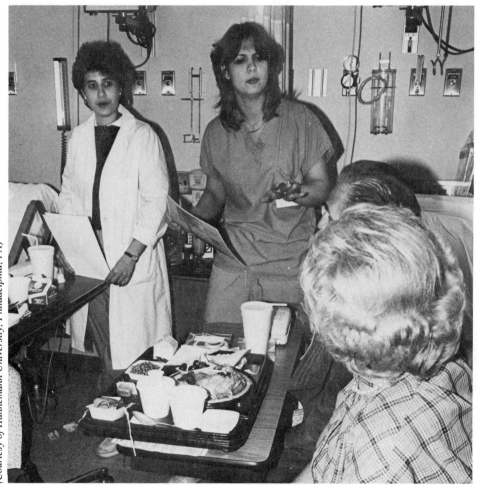

(Courtesy of Hahnemann University, Philadelphia, PA)

Providing Nutritional Counseling and Care

KEY TERMS

anorexic Having poor appetite.
coordinated Brought together with other aspects of care in an organized manner.
document To make a written record of important events, activities, and impressions as they occur in the course of providing health care.
goal Desired change necessary to solve a nutritional problem; aim or end result desired.

motivate To cause or stimulate to take action.
nomenclature A system of names or terms used in a particular science or art.
objective Statement of what is to be accomplished to meet goals.
rapport A trusting, respectful relationship.

The problem-solving approach is applied to nutritional care as to other health specialties. It consists of four elements: assessment, in which the client's problems are identified; planning, in which a plan is developed for correcting these problems; implementation, in which care is provided; and evaluation, in which progress toward the correction of the problems is determined.

identified. These data include the client's medical history, diet history, sociocultural history, physical examination, laboratory tests, and interviews with the client and his family. The data are analyzed and the client's problems identified. (See Chap. 2.)

Assessment

The first step in providing nutritional care is to collect data so that the client's problems may be

Planning

The next step is to formulate a plan for correcting or treating the problem. Goals, objectives, specific activities, priorities, and means for eval-

Table 19-1. Nutritional Care Plan (in a Nursing Home)

Nutritional problem:	Client is a 72-year-old woman with rheumatoid arthritis; she is approximately 25 pounds under normal weight owing to inadequate caloric intake.
Nutritional goal:	Gradual gain of weight until desirable weight is attained.
Objective:	Weight gain of 4 pounds in 1 month by the addition of 500 kcal per day to meals and snacks.

Action	Responsible Staff
Obtain diet history	Food service supervisor
List favorite foods in dietary Kardex	
Post caloric values for favorite foods and additional food supplements in kitchen and nursing station	Consultant dietitian
Determine time of day when client is most hungry and alert	Nursing assistant
Add sufficient food to increase intake by 200 kcal per day	Food service supervisor
Prepare client for mealtime and transport her to solarium in wheelchair so that she may have lunch and supper in company of other clients; record food intake	Nursing assistant
Add sufficient preferred foods to increase intake by 300 kcal between meals daily.	Charge nurse
Weigh client at same time on same day of each week	Nursing assistant

(After Hargrave M: Nutritional Care of the Physically Disabled. Minneapolis, Sister Kenny Institute, 1979)

uating progress are established. All members of the health team, especially the client, should have an opportunity to contribute to the planning process.

The goals and objectives should be realistic and should describe measurable results. *Goals* express the desired results or outcomes in general terms; *objectives* are specific, indicating what is to be accomplished and how.

The nutritional care plan is a written statement that outlines specific activities to meet the goals and objectives (Table 19-1). Staff members responsible for carrying out each activity are designated. The plan is coordinated with all other components of the client's overall plan of care and is usually developed with the guidance of a nutrition specialist (dietitian, nutritionist, or dietary consultant).

The plan may be shared among all members of the health team or may be intended for a particular group such as the nursing staff or dietary staff.

Implementation

The next step is to put the plan into action. Two functions are involved: providing an adequate normal or modified diet for a client in a hospital or other health care facility; providing nutrition education and counseling. In a health care facility, both components may be involved, whereas in the outpatient setting, only the educational and counseling component is needed.

Providing an Adequate Normal Diet

In the healthy adult, catabolism (breakdown) and anabolism (building) are balanced; in the sick person, especially one who is confined to bed, catabolism is greater than anabolism. The sick person thus has a greater need than normal for nutrients that promote tissue building: proteins, vitamins, and minerals.

Inactivity or immobilization for a long period of time causes alterations in body function, and these influence nutritional requirements. Digestion, metabolism, and elimination are all affected. As a result, nutritional requirements may increase or decrease.

When achieving an adequate food intake is a problem, specific measures need to be taken. For example, a client who is anorexic (has no appetite) because he is depressed may not be consuming adequate quantities of food. The objectives of nutritional care for this client are to increase the quality of his diet and to create an environment that promotes the appetite. Bulky, low-calorie foods such as salads, soups, and tea may be reduced and low-volume, high-calorie foods such as meats, starches, and fortified milk beverages may be emphasized. Small, frequent meals may be more appealing to the client than three large meals a day. Arranging for the client to eat with other persons may also be listed in the care plan.

Providing a Modified Diet

Medical treatment may require changes in the normal diet. Changes in diet are made necessary by the following conditions:

Caloric imbalance resulting in overweight or underweight

Poor or abnormal utilization of nutrients (*e.g.,* poor utilization of carbohydrates in diabetes mellitus, retention of sodium in congestive heart failure)

Abnormalities in digestion of food or absorption of nutrients; these occur in diseases of the gastrointestinal tract such as

gastric ulcer, colitis, and lactase deficiency disease

Nutritional deficiencies, including iron deficiency anemia, and severe malnutrition due to emotional disturbances

Rest required for the body or an organ (*e.g.,* in gallbladder disease, rest may be afforded the organ by a restriction of fat; in the acute phase of coronary heart disease, a liquid diet may be prescribed to conserve the client's strength)

Abnormal laboratory findings indicating an increased risk of development of health problems, such as abnormal cholesterol and triglyceride levels

The normal diet is the basis of most modified diets. Despite the seemingly large number of diets, changes are limited to four categories:

Texture. The consistency and fiber content may be altered; liquid diets, soft diets, and high-fiber diets are examples of this type of modification.

Certain nutrients may be increased or decreased in amount. A client suffering from renal failure may require a diet restricted in protein, whereas one recovering from extensive burns requires greatly increased amounts of protein.

Frequency of meals. The usual three meals a day may be replaced by six small meals to reduce stress to the body; clients with ulcers may receive food every 2 or 3 hours to dilute the acid contents of the stomach.

Products normally included in the diet may be eliminated; for example, wheat products are eliminated for clients who are allergic to wheat.

Every effort is made to adjust the diet to the client's needs. It is planned to be as similar as possible to the customary family diet, with as wide a range of choices as possible. Of course, the client's condition may require a drastically different diet from what he is used to, and it is up to the health team to help the client accept this.

Providing Nutrition Education

Education is an essential part of health care. Clients want to know, and have a right to know, how they themselves can help achieve and maintain good health.

A person does not learn by memorizing. Acquisition of information must be accompanied by a change in attitude and in behavior. If a person has learned something about nutrition, his attitude toward food will have changed, the way he eats will have changed, and he will have increased his understanding of how his diet influences his health.

Treat your client as an individual with personal eating habits, knowledge about nutrition, and the ability to learn. Be a good listener so you can learn about his food habits. Involve the client in the educational process. He should understand his problems and what he can do to correct them. Without his active participation, your efforts will be fruitless.

Help your client see how nutritional health can help him meet his goals and be useful to him. These goals may not necessarily be health-related, especially for a young person, who may be more interested in sports activities or in peer group acceptance.

Build on strengths of the client's food habits rather than emphasizing shortcomings. Set realistic goals. Suggestions for improving a diet or following a therapeutic diet should be within the client's reach.

Give careful attention to timing. Periods of stress may not be the best time for changing long-standing food habits. The client may be too upset to concentrate or to understand what is being taught. Return visits or referral to a community agency after discharge from the hospital may be necessary.

Avoid teaching too much at one time. Try to concentrate on one or two points during a 15- to 30-minute period rather than trying to cover the entire topic in 1 hour.

Help the client see the progress he is making no matter how small it may be.

Informal Teaching

There are many opportunities for informal teaching, which is usually carried out on-the-spot as the need arises. For example, a client may have questions regarding the food served on his tray or may need help making correct choices from a selective menu. You can encourage discussion by pointing out, for example, which foods on the tray are of particular importance to the client's health.

You aren't expected to know all the answers about nutrition. When confronted with a question you cannot answer, consult the nurse in charge or the dietitian.

Formal Teaching

Diet counseling and group instruction are examples of formal teaching situations.

Diet Counseling. Diet counseling is the process of helping a client develop the ability to manage his own nutritional care (through a trusting relationship). The counselor provides encouragement and support as the client gradually makes changes in his eating behavior. Counseling that involves behavioral change should be conducted by psychologists, nurses and dietitians who have been trained in behavior change skills.

Group Instruction. In hospitals and clinics and in group medical practice, it is often possible to bring together groups of people with common needs. Besides receiving information and guidance from the nutrition instructor, the members can help each other face common problems. The health worker assists by providing instruction, giving demonstrations, and preparing visual aids.

Communication Tools That Promote Nutritional Care

Clear, Precise Diet Orders and Terminology

The diet order is an important communication tool. It is usually written by the physician, but in certain situations may be written by dietitians, nurse practitioners, or clinical nurses working

Table 19-2. Diet History Questionnaires

Questionnaire I. Adult
(directed to client or primary caretaker)

Background Information:
  Name, age, sex, family and occupational roles, general health status, dietary restrictions (past or present)

Food Purchase and Preparation:
  Who purchases and prepares food?
  What factors influence kinds of foods purchased?
  Is budgeting a matter of concern when buying food?
  Where is food purchased?
  How often do you shop?
  What facilities are available for food storage and preparation?
  What foods are served most frequently?
  Do you participate in community food programs?

Relationship of Food to Lifestyle:
  Food likes and dislikes
  Favorite foods when growing up
  Special family foods for celebrations
  Atmosphere at mealtime
  Foods your body needs
  Food supplements (vitamins, minerals)
  Sources of information about nutrition

Questionnaire II. Infant/Toddler
(directed to parents or primary caretakers)

Who feeds? What foods does an infant need?
Breast or formula feeding—approximate amount and frequency?
If breast feeding—Pattern and duration of feeding?
If formula—Type? Iron-fortified? Preparation?
Supplemental feedings—Fluids, solids? Preparation? How liked?
Weaning? Teething? Self-feeding?

Questionnaire III. Young Child
(directed to parents or primary caretaker)

What foods does your child need? When does he eat?
Appetite? Likes, dislikes? Food jags?
Frequency of snacking? Types?
Vitamin and mineral supplements?
Method of rewarding and punishing child?
Whom does child eat with?
Arrangements for eating away from home (school)?

Questionnaire IV. Adolescent
(directed to adolescent)

What is nutritious? Foods body needs?
Where are meals eaten? When is food eaten?
How much snacking?
How does eating affect appearance?
What do you do when you're unhappy or upset?
Does anyone comment about your eating habits?

Questionnaire V. Elderly
(directed to client or primary caretaker)

Amount of income budgeted for food?
Where client lives? Where he eats?
Whom he eats with?
Who prepares meals? Purchases food?
Dentures or own teeth? Effect on eating?
Recent changes in food habits?
How does food taste?
Likes, dislikes?
Use of alcohol?
Dietary restrictions?
Amount of normal activity?

(Suitor CW, Hunter MF: Nutrition: Principles and Application in Health Promotion, p 227. Philadelphia, JB Lippincott, 1980)

closely with physicians. The diet ordered may be either normal or modified.

The term *therapeutic* or *modified* is preferred in reference to diets that deviate from normal, and the description of the diet should be specific and accurate. *Low-calorie diet* could refer to a 1200-kcal diet or to a 1700-kcal diet; *low-sodium diet* could apply to severe restriction (500 mg of sodium) or to moderate restriction (1500–2000 mg of sodium).

The Medical Record

All elements of the client's treatment, including nutritional care, are recorded in the medical record. The chart is a communication tool for all members of the health team—physician, nurse, dietitian, and others. These professionals write progress notes on the client's chart describing the care being given, the progress being made to solve the client's problems, and follow-up plans. Nutrition education activities are also documented in the client's medical record.

The Interview

An interview is a planned conversation aimed at obtaining specific information and ideas from a client. It is a component of the assessment phase of care. Its purpose is to help determine the client's nutritional needs or to determine what progress is being made toward goals. The interview may be formal or informal. Taking a diet history is an example of a formal interview. Table 19-2 gives examples of the type of information that may be obtained in a diet history and how the questionnaire may be adapted for clients of different ages. An informal interview is a meaningful conversation occurring in a hospital or clinic setting or on the telephone in which the health worker tries to learn how the client is getting along, what his needs are, and what progress he is making.

An exchange of information is promoted in an atmosphere of mutual trust and respect. Your attitude is important in establishing such an atmosphere. The successful interviewer displays interest, friendliness, kindness, and acceptance. Do not pass judgment on the information the client gives you. Accept the client as he is, and recognize that his behavior has meaning and purpose for him. Being aware of the factors that have influenced your own eating habits will help you to understand those of other people (see Chap. 2).

There are straightforward techniques that may encourage the client to talk freely. Open-ended questions such as "When do you eat or drink for the first time in the day?" require that the client respond clearly. In contrast, asking "Do you eat breakfast?" requires only a "yes" or "no" answer. Direct questions—how?, what?, where?, why?, and who?—elicit a clear response. Avoid asking questions that suggest answers ("You eat vegetables, don't you?").

Don't teach while conducting an interview. If you lecture the client or indicate that you disapprove of what he is saying, he will hesitate to answer your questions.

Be specific: "What kind of bread?" "How much margarine?" "What is added to vegetables in cooking?"

Evaluation

Evaluation is measurement of the client's progress. Has he gained or lost the appropriate amount of weight? If the client is diabetic, is his blood sugar under control? If he is hypertensive, has his sodium-restricted diet caused a reduction in blood pressure? Above all, is he learning to be in control of his nutritional status?

If progress has not been made, the cause is determined and the care plan revised. The client's needs may change, and a new plan may be required. In any case, once the reason for failure has been determined, a new plan aimed at correcting the problem is developed.

Tools for Diet Instruction

Diet Plans

A diet plan is a guide to the number and size of servings of recommended food groups and the dietary pattern for the day. Table 19-3 gives an example of a diet plan.

Table 19-3. 1800-kcal Diet Using Exchange Lists*

Daily Diet Plan

Nutritional Composition		Amount	Kind of Food	Choose from
Protein	95 g	3	Skim Milk Exchange	List 1
Carbohydrate	220 g	3	Vegetable Exchange	List 2
Fat	60 g	5	Fruit Exchanges	List 3
		8	Bread Exchanges	List 4
		7	Meat Exchanges (Lean-Medium Fat)	List 5
		5	Fat Exchanges (Polyunsaturated)	List 6

Meal Plan

Breakfast
1 fruit exchange
3 bread exchanges
1 meat exchange
2 fat exchanges
1 skim milk exchange

Lunch
2 meat exchanges (lean–medium-fat)
2 bread exchanges
1 vegetable exchange
1 fat exchange
2 fruit exchanges
1 skim milk exchange

Dinner
3 meat exchanges (lean–medium-fat)
2 bread exchanges
2 vegetable exchanges
2 fat exchanges
1 fruit exchange
1 skim milk exchange

Coffee or tea, if desired

Evening Snack
1 bread exchange
1 meat exchange
1 fruit exchange

Sample Menu

½ cup of frozen orange juice
¾ cup of cornflakes
1 slice (1 oz) of Canadian bacon
2 slices of whole-wheat toast
2 tsp of margarine
1 cup of skim milk

Turkey sandwich:
  2 slices of rye bread
  2 oz of turkey
  1 tsp of mayonnaise
  ½ sliced tomato
  2 peaches
  1 cup of skim milk

3 oz of pot roast
½ cup of mashed potato
½ cup of green beans
½ cup of pickled beets
1 slice of whole-wheat bread
2 tsp of margarine (for bread and vegetable)
¼ cantaloupe
1 cup of skim milk
Tea
Artificial sweetener

2 graham crackers
¼ cup of cottage cheese mixed with ½ cup of pineapple chunks

* Used with exchange lists in Table A-2.

Exchange Lists

If control of calories or of the quantities of one or more nutrients is required, exchange lists may be used. Exchange lists group foods of similar compositions with respect to the nutritional factors being controlled; for example, foods with similar protein, fat, and carbohydrate contents may be grouped together. Measured amounts of foods in a single exchange group are equal to each other with respect to the nutrient(s) being controlled and may be exchanged for one another. Exchange lists simplify meal planning for the client and make possible a wide choice of foods. The system was originally developed for planning diabetic diets. However, the basic idea has been adapted for use in other modified diets such as sodium-restricted and weight-reducing diets.

The health worker should be familiar with the most widely used exchange lists, the "Exchange Lists for Meal Planning" prepared jointly by the American Diabetes Association, the American Dietetic Association, and the National Institutes of Health (see Table A-2 in the Appendix).

The exchange lists are used in conjunction with a diet plan, which indicates the number of servings the client may choose from each exchange group. For example, if 2 bread exchanges are permitted for dinner, the client may choose 2 slices of bread, 1 slice of bread and ½ cup of mashed potato, or any two choices from the bread exchange list.

One exchange represents an average serving of each food with the exception of meat. One exchange of meat represents 1 ounce of meat or its equivalent. Whenever household measure is used to describe a serving such as 1 cup, 1 teaspoon, or 1 tablespoon, reference is to a standard 8-ounce measuring cup and standard measuring spoons.

It is essential that the client have an understanding of the amount of food being considered. "A bowl of cereal" or "a glass of milk" is not an accurate description. Each food should be described in terms of standard household measures, such as 3 ounces of meat, ½ cup of applesauce, or 1 teaspoon of margarine.

When calculating a diet for a certain calorie level or for a certain protein, fat, and carbohydrate composition, the dietitian takes into account the nutrient values of the exchanges given in Table 19-4. Anyone who has used food composition tables for the calculation of diets can readily see what a time-saver this method can be.

In the Exchange Lists for Meal Planning (see Table A-2), foods with a similar composition in respect to protein, fat, and carbohydrate are listed in 6 groups as follows:

List 1: Milk Exchanges

Nonfat milk is the basic milk exchange. If low-fat milk or whole milk is used, the client is instructed to deduct the fat value of that milk from the total amount of fat in the diet.

List 2: Vegetable Exchanges

Vegetable exchanges include all vegetables except starchy ones. The vegetables in list 2 average 25 kcal per ½-cup serving. Starchy vegetables appear in list 4, bread exchanges.

List 3: Fruit Exchanges

Fruit exchanges include fruit and fruit juices that are fresh, canned, or frozen without the addition of sugar. In the amounts listed, 1 exchange of fruit provides approximately 10 g of carbohydrate and 40 kcal.

List 4: Bread Exchanges

Bread exchanges include bread, rolls, crackers, cereals, rice, macaroni, starchy vegetables (potatoes, corn, lima beans, peas, pumpkin, parsnips, winter squash, dried peas, beans, lentils), and some prepared foods, such as muffins, biscuits, pancakes, and waffles. When prepared foods containing fat are used, fat exchanges in amounts indicated must be subtracted from the day's total.

List 5: Meat Exchanges

The meat exchange group is composed of three subgroups: lean meat, medium-fat meat, and

Table 19-4. Nutrient Values of the Exchange Lists

Food	Measure	Carbohydrate (g)	Protein (g)	Fat (g)	kcals
Milk Exchanges, list 1					
Nonfat	1 cup	12	8	Trace	80
1% fat	1 cup	12	8	2.5	105
2% fat	1 cup	12	8	5	125
Whole	1 cup	12	8	10	170
Vegetable Exchanges, list 2	½ cup	5	2	—	25
Fruit Exchanges, list 3	Varies	10	—	—	40
Bread Exchanges, list 4	Varies	15	2	—	70
Prepared foods	Varies	15	2	5–10	115–160
Meat Exchanges, list 5					
Lean	1 oz	—	7	3	55
Medium-fat	1 oz	—	7	5.5	80
High-fat	1 oz	—	7	8	100
Fat Exchanges, list 6	1 tsp	—	—	5	45

(After Exchange Lists for Meal Planning prepared by Committes of the American Diabetes Association and the American Dietetic Association in cooperation with the National Institute of Arthritis, Metabolism and Digestive Diseases and the National Heart and Lung Institute, National Institutes of Health, Public Health Service, U.S. Department of Health and Human Services)

high-fat meat. Lean meat is the basic exchange. If medium-fat or high-fat meat is used or if it is assumed that a variety of meats will be used, the dietitian makes adjustments when calculating the diet plan or instructs the client to subtract a certain quantity of fat exchanges when he eats a medium-fat or high-fat food from this group.

The meat exchanges also include fish and poultry, eggs, cheese, peanut butter, and dried peas and beans.

List 6: Fat Exchanges

Fat exchanges include butter, margarine, oil, cream, salad dressings, olives, bacon, nuts, and cream cheese. The list is separated into two groups: polyunsaturated and saturated fats.

Using Nutrition Labels with the Exchange Lists

Nutrition labels are especially helpful to persons on restricted calorie or diabetic diets. They indicate the amounts of calories, protein, fat, and carbohydrate in a serving of food. This information can be compared with the exchange lists used with diets; by estimating how many exchanges are represented in a serving of food, one may find that it is possible to include that food in the meal plan (Table 19-5).

Table 19-5.   Using Nutrition Labels with Food Exchange Lists

Macaroni and Cheese Casserole

Nutrition Information, per serving

Serving size	¾ cup
Servings per container	5
Calories	240
Protein	10 g
Carbohydrate	32 g
Fat	7 g

Percentage of U.S. Recommended Daily Allowance (U.S. RDA)

Protein	15
Vitamin A	10
Vitamin C	0
Thiamine	15
Riboflavin	15
Niacin	10
Calcium	15
Iron	8

The number of food exchanges in the serving amounts shown on the label can be estimated as follows:

Label Serving		Food Exchange Values			
	Amount	kcal	Protein (g)	Carbohydrate (g)	Fat (g)
¾ cup macaroni and cheese =	1 high-fat meat & 2 bread exchanges	100 140	7 4	— 30	8 —
Total exchange values		240	11	30	8
Total serving values (from nutrition label)		240	10	32	7

This chart shows that a serving provides about 1 high-fat meat and 2 bread exchanges.

Special Foods for Modified Diets

Some food package labels also list sodium, cholesterol, and fatty acids in grams per serving. In accordance with nutrition labeling regulations, foods for which a nutrition claim is made must provide full nutrition information about the product.

Care must be taken in the purchase of so-called dietetic foods. Some may be prepared without the addition of salt or other sodium-containing products; others may be lower in calories than comparable regular foods. Some clients mistakenly think that any food labeled "dietetic" is permissible on their diets. Inform your clients about the place, purpose, and suitability of dietetic foods in their diets.

KEYS TO PRACTICAL APPLICATION

Take advantage of opportunities to find out how your client is getting along as far as his diet is concerned. Is he eating well? If not, why not? Does he foresee any problems when he goes home from the hospital?

When gathering information, learn to ask questions that require more than a "yes" or "no" answer. How, what, why, where, and who questions encourage your client to give information.

Avoid being critical or showing disapproval of the information your client provides. Recognize that his eating behavior has meaning and purpose for him. Emphasize the good things he is doing.

When goals are not met, learn to ask "Why has this happened?" Then seek the answer.

Study the exchange lists for meal planning (Table A-2 in the Appendix) carefully. You will undoubtedly encounter the use of exchange lists many times. You may need to help a client make menu selections that fit into his diet pattern.

Be sure the client understands that a "dietetic" food is not necessarily permitted on his particular diet. He must learn to identify which ones, if any, are useful for him.

KEY IDEAS

Providing good nutritional care involves four basic elements: identifying the client's problems, developing a plan for correcting the problems, providing care as planned, and evaluating results.

The nutritional care plan is a written statement that describes the steps to be taken to meet the goals of nutritional care. All team members, including the client, should be involved in planning.

Goals and objectives should be realistic and should describe results that can be measured.

Nutritional care involves providing an adequate normal or modified diet for a client in a health care facility and providing nutrition education and counseling so that the client can manage his own nutritional needs.

All diets, whether normal or modified, contribute to the health care of the individual.

Breakdown (catabolic) body processes are increased in the ill person, especially one confined to bed; greater than normal amounts of nutrients that promote tissue building — protein, vitamins, and minerals — are required. The hospital diet usually exceeds recommended allowances of these nutrients.

Modified diets are those that are changed from normal because of one or more of the following conditions: caloric imbalance, poor use of nutrients by the cells or organs of the body, abnormal digestion or absorption, nutritional deficiency or excess, the need to rest an organ or conserve body strength, and abnormal laboratory findings indicating increased risk of developing chronic disease.

The normal diet forms the basis of most modified diets. Changes may be made in texture, amounts of certain nutrients, frequency of meals, and quantity of substances normally found in the diet.

The modified diet should be as similar as possible to the usual diet of the client

and his family; as wide a range of food choices as possible should be included.

Good communication among members of the health team is essential to good nutritional care. Accurate diet orders and the documentation of nutritional care on the client's medical record are tools that promote good communication.

The client has a right to know how to manage his own nutritional care. Education is an essential part of health care.

Learning is not simply the acquisition of facts; a change in attitude and behavior must also be accomplished.

Good listening skills help us to determine the individual needs of a client; each person has individual characteristics.

Success depends on the willingness of the client to accept change; he must be included in setting goals and in other aspects of the educational process.

Behavior change is difficult, especially when it involves long-standing food habits. What appear to be small changes in behavior may represent a great accomplishment.

Good interviewing techniques are important skills for the health worker.

There are many opportunities while providing health care to strengthen, reinforce, and support nutrition teaching the client has already received.

Diet counseling is the total process of helping a client manage his own nutritional care. Group instruction, another type of formal teaching, enables group members to help each other.

The exchange system simplifies meal planning and provides the client on a special diet with a wide choice of foods. Foods with similar contents in respect to the nutrients being controlled are grouped together into various lists. Any food within a list may be exchanged for any other food within the same list.

In the exchange system used in diabetic and calorie-controlled diets, foods with similar protein, fat, carbohydrate, and energy compositions are listed in 6 groups, or exchanges: milk, vegetable, fruit, bread, meat, and fat.

Reading food labels is very important for a person on a modified diet.

The client must learn to identify which "dietetic foods," if any, are appropriate for his particular modified diet.

KEYS TO LEARNING: STUDY–DISCUSSION QUESTIONS

1. With the help of your instructor, select a client who is on a modified diet. How would you evaluate the client's progress? Are the goals of nutritional care being met?
   Observe the client's reaction to the food served him. If he is considered a "feeding problem," try to determine the reason behind his behavior. Discuss your findings with the class. What are some possible solutions to this problem?
2. In what ways can the normal diet be changed to treat disease? Can you name a diet that is an example of each modification?

3. Why is it so important to involve the client in the educational process, including the setting of goals?
4. Using the diet history form used in your hospital, role-play a formal interview with a classmate. The class will evaluate the interview. What techniques encourage the client to provide information? What hinders the exchange of information?
5. The food exchanges given below represent the total amount of food permitted on a particular diet for one day. Using the food values given for the exchange lists in Table 19-4, find out

how much protein, fat, carbohydrate, and kilocalories the diet contains.

2 skim milk exchanges, list 1
2 vegetable exchanges, list 2
3 fruit exchanges, list 3
6 bread exchanges, list 4
7 meat exchanges, list 5 (lean meat)
6 fat exchanges, list 6

6. Divide the above exchanges into three meals. Using the exchange list in Table A-2 in the Appendix, provide a menu for each meal. Be sure to include the amount of each food permitted.

7. Bring to class a nutrition label from a packaged product. Show how a serving of this food compares with the exchange lists as in Table 19-5.

8. As a class, make a collection of "dietetic" foods. (The dietitian in your hospial can assist you in assembling your collection.) Identify the diet or diets in which each food could be used. Which "dietetic" foods do you think are most useful? Which are useless? Which are misleading?

Bibliography is found at the end of Part Four.

Weight Control

KEY TERMS

adipose tissue   Fatty tissue.
anorexia nervosa   A psychological disorder manifested by self-starvation.
behavior modification   A teaching technique in which learned behaviors (habits) are changed.
bulimia   Binge eating followed by self-induced vomiting or purging.

gross obesity   Extreme fatness up to 2 to 3 times ideal weight.
habitual   Occurring automatically, sometimes without thought; resulting from a frequently repeated behavior.

Probably no other aspect of health is as much the topic of conversation as weight. Although in the United States obesity is much more prevalent than underweight, both deviations are representative of malnutrition, and both can have serious and far-reaching effects on physical and mental health.

Height–weight tables measure desirable weights (Table 20-1). It is generally accepted that a weight appropriate for a person 25 years old is the weight that should be maintained throughout that person's adult life. Once a person has reached his full height, he should not gain additional weight.

Weight control is a matter of balancing the energy value of the foods eaten with the energy needs of the body (Fig. 20-1). When more kilocalories are provided than are needed, the extra energy is stored as fat (positive energy balance). When the caloric intake is less than is needed, the body uses up stored fat, and weight is lost (negative energy balance). When all fat deposits are used up, muscle and other body tissue are drawn upon for energy.

One pound of body fat represents approximately 3500 kcal. Consumption of an excess of only 100 kcal a day means an excess of 3000 kcal a month, or 10 pounds a year (and 20 or 30 lb in 2 or 3 years). This 100 kcal can be supplied by 2 tablespoons of sugar, one large "sandwich" cookie, 2 teaspoons of butter or margarine, or 2 tablespoons of jelly. Thus, many people become obese, not by eating huge amounts of food but by eating small amounts of extra food over a period of years.

Table 20-1.   1983 Metropolitan Height and Weight Tables

Men				Women				
Height	Small	Medium	Large	Height	Small	Medium	Large	
Feet Inches	Frame	Frame	Frame	Feet Inches	Frame	Frame	Frame	
5 2	128–134	131–141	138–150	4 10	102–111	109–121	118–131	
5 3	130–136	133–143	140–153	4 11	103–113	111–123	120–134	
5 4	132–138	135–145	142–156	5 0	104–115	113–126	122–137	
5 5	134–140	137–148	144–160	5 1	106–118	115–129	125–140	
5 6	136–142	139–151	146–164	5 2	108–121	118–132	128–143	
5 7	138–145	142–154	149–168	5 3	111–124	121–135	131–147	
5 8	140–148	145–157	152–172	5 4	114–127	124–138	134–151	
5 9	142–151	148–160	155–176	5 5	117–130	127–141	137–155	
5 10	144–154	151–163	158–180	5 6	120–133	130–144	140–159	
5 11	146–157	154–166	161–184	5 7	123–136	133–147	143–163	
6 0	149–160	157–170	164–188	5 8	126–139	136–150	146–167	
6 1	152–164	160–174	168–192	5 9	129–142	139–153	149–170	
6 2	155–168	164–178	172–197	5 10	132–145	142–156	152–173	
6 3	158–172	167–182	176–202	5 11	135–148	145–159	155–176	
6 4	162–176	171–187	181–207	6 0	138–151	148–162	158–179	

(Source of basic data 1979 Build Study, Society of Actuaries and Association of Life Insurance Medical Directors of America, 1980. Copyright 1983, Metropolitan Life Insurance Company)
Weights at ages 25–59 based on lowest mortality. Weight in pounds according to frame (in indoor clothing weighing 5 lb for men and 3 lb for women; shoes with 1″ heels).

Obesity

Types of Obesity

Obesity is the excessive accumulation of adipose (fatty) tissue. The term *overweight* means excessive heaviness and does not necessarily indicate overfatness. For example, an athlete with above-average muscular development may be overweight without being obese. The skinfold thickness test provides a useful means of distinguishing between overweight and obesity (see Chap. 2) and is a more accurate guide than height-weight tables in determining degree of fatness or leanness.

Obesity may be classified as follows: obesity resulting from another condition such as hypothyroidism (underactive thyroid)—this form of obesity is rare; childhood-onset obesity, characterized by overweight in infancy and early childhood or adolescence; adult-onset obesity; and situational obesity.

Childhood obesity is usually more difficult to deal with than adult obesity. Obese infants tend to become obese children, and obese children tend to become obese adults. Often, these persons become grossly obese, weighing 2 to 3 times their desirable weight.

Obesity can develop through an increase either in the size of fat cells or in their number; in contrast, weight reduction can occur only by a reduction in the size of the fat cells, since the number of fat cells remains unchanged. Mild or

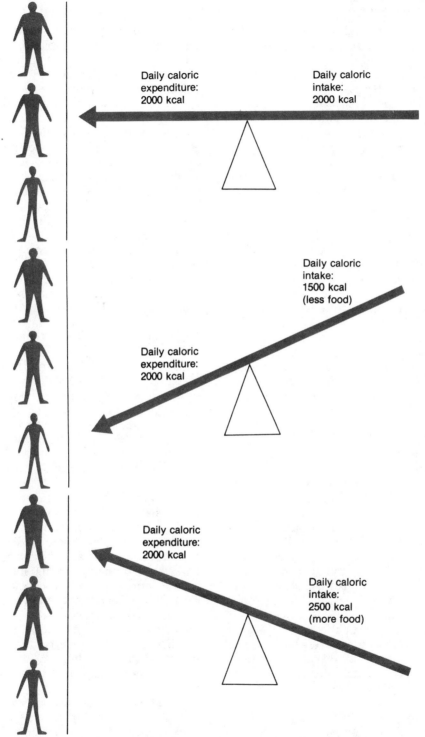

Fig. 20-1. Weight control is a matter of balance. (*Top*) Energy balance. (*Center*) Negative energy balance. (*Bottom*) Positive energy balance. (Suitor CW, Hunter MF: Nutrition: Principles and Application in Health Promotion. Philadelphia, JB Lippincott, 1980)

moderate adult obesity is believed to be the result of an increase in the size of fat cells only. When a mildly obese adult loses weight, the size of each fat cell is reduced, and the amount of fatty tissue becomes the same as that of a thin person. In childhood obesity, in contrast, there is an increase in the actual number of fat cells, with the size of the cells remaining level. For a person with childhood obesity to have a normal amount of fatty tissue, the size of his many fat cells must be reduced below normal. It is difficult for such a person to achieve and maintain normal weight.

Most obese adults were of normal weight until their late 20s or early 30s, when they gained weight slightly. They then continued to gain weight slowly into their 50s or early 60s. Traditional methods of weight control work reasonably well for this type of obesity.

Situational obesity may develop when a person is faced with a stressful situation or a traumatic emotional experience to which he responds by overeating. Early counseling, understanding and support, and help in dealing with the emotional problem may point the way to more healthful food habits.

A Many-Sided Problem

The complications of obesity shorten life. Obesity puts stress on the body, increases the risk that certain diseases will develop, and worsens existing illnesses. Bones and joints must support extra weight, and the heart and lungs must work harder. Fat tissue crowds the organs and reduces their efficiency. Grossly obese persons are poor risks for surgery because their reactions to anesthesia are impaired and they heal more slowly than normal. Often, obese persons have accompanying psychological and social problems, though it may be difficult to determine whether these are cause or effect.

Obese persons are more likely than normal to have hypertension and diabetes, and their triglyceride and cholesterol levels are more likely to be elevated. Weight reduction is usually of great benefit for these persons; for example, many obese hypertensives achieve normal blood pressure after losing weight.

Though obesity may appear to be rather easy to deal with, it is complex. Environmental, social, economic, hereditary, metabolic, and emotional factors and activity levels are all involved in its development.

Lack of physical activity contributes to the development of obesity. Modern technology has created many labor-saving devices that have greatly reduced energy expenditure. Riding replaces walking; the clothes washer replaces scrubbing by hand. With lessened activity, food intake has decreased, but not enough to compensate for the lowered activity level. Obese persons, especially children and adolescents, often do not eat more than "normals" but gain weight because they are inactive and slow-moving.

A genetic factor may be at work in obesity. It is believed that there may be an inherited tendency toward obesity, inasmuch as body type is inherited. However, this does not mean that a person is powerless to control his weight.

The basal metabolic rate (BMR) decreases with age. If a person does not adjust his food intake to the slower metabolic rate, he can gain unwanted weight. Moreover, in some persons, the metabolic process may be impaired. Even a minor metabolic defect can be a cause of overeating and thus of eventual obesity. Another contributing factor may be hypothyroidism, a rare condition that causes a reduced metabolic rate.

A family food pattern that emphasizes meats, starches, sweets, and fats to the exclusion of fruits and vegetables obviously encourages weight gain. Persons whose professions require that they frequently attend luncheons, cocktail parties, and dinners often find it difficult not to eat too much. Food has a social role in the celebration of happy occasions, as a manifestation of welcome and hospitality, and in mourning activities. Most of us have at one time or another eaten too much because we have felt frustrated, angry, or anxious. But some persons tend to "fall back" on food habitually as a release from their problems.

Parental attitudes also play a part in obesity. An overanxious mother may make a habit of overfeeding her child. A parent who uses food

as a reward may create an emotional dependence on food.

Some obese persons use their obesity as a defense mechanism — it becomes an excuse for failure to get a certain job or a way of avoiding contact with the opposite sex. In some cases, attempts to lose weight give rise to severe psychological problems. When this occurs, the person is advised to discontinue weight control efforts — the obesity is thought to be preferable to serious emotional problems.

Role of the Health Worker

What should the health worker's attitude toward the obese person be? Her attitude is important, because she may play a key role in resolving the problem. The obese person should never be made to feel that his obesity is his "fault." Nor should he be made to feel that he is wasting time and space in the health care facility just by being there. Most obese persons have at one time or another been the butt of ill-considered jibes or jokes. Don't add to these insults — the obese client has already suffered keenly. Accept the person as he is, and offer your sympathetic support to his efforts to lose weight. Be a good listener, too, so he comes to know that you are on his side. If he senses your support, he will be more receptive to the information you give him about diet and activity.

Undoubtedly the best way to treat obesity is to prevent it. The health worker can play a key role here in her interactions with families and individuals. She can help the family to see that physical activity, as appropriate to various ages and stages of development, is a good health habit. She can help parents to see that children benefit from being fed appropriate amounts of food, not from overeating. She may be able to help identify persons at risk of becoming obese — a baby who is gaining weight too rapidly, the child of obese parents, or the person who experiences an abrupt gain in appetite.

Treatment of Obesity

The obese person not only must attain the desirable weight but also must maintain that weight for the rest of his life. To accomplish these goals, a moderate reduction in caloric intake is necessary together with a moderate increase in physical activity. The client must be persuaded that weight loss is very important. Improvements in appearance and state of health are usually the strongest motivating factors.

The person may find it extremely difficult to resist food on his own, whereas being counseled or being a part of a small, self-help group may be a strong motivating force.

The physician and dietitian counselor can offer consistent assistance and encouragement. They see the client frequently, understand his problems, and involve him in his weight control program.

Self-help groups such as Overeaters' Anonymous (OA) and TOPS (Take Off Pounds Sensibly) also may be beneficial.

Physical Activity. The obese person benefits from increased physical activity for several reasons. First, exercising more is similar in effect to eating less. One need not reduce one's caloric intake to dangerously low levels to lose weight; a very low caloric intake may not provide all the required nutrients. Second, exercise improves muscle tone and blood circulation. Third, exercise diverts the mind from thoughts of food. Finally, exercise increases the BMR both during exercise and for many hours after exercise ceases. The latter effect is of considerable importance to the dieter because dieting reduces the BMR. This reduction in BMR is the body's natural response to a decreased energy intake and explains why the rate of weight loss frequently slows as a person continues to diet. Studies reveal that exercises such as jogging, swimming, and walking can increase metabolic rate by as much as 25% above basal level for 15 hours after strenuous exercise, and may continue to have some stimulating effect on the BMR for as long as 48 hours afterward.

To be effective, the exercise program must be carried out on a regular basis. The client should always check with his physician before beginning an exercise program. Brisk walking instead of driving whenever possible and climb-

ing a few flights of stairs instead of taking the elevator are very simple forms of exercise that most persons can follow even if they are not able to participate in active sports on a regular basis.

Setting Realistic Goals. The poor success rate for correcting obesity may be due in part to the setting of unrealistic goals. A woman weighing 200 pounds whose best weight is 130 pounds is consuming 2600 kcal or more every day. To put her on a 1200-kcal diet is to cut her food intake by more than half; this is setting a goal that is not likely to be achieved.

The calorie level of a reducing diet is frequently based on the person's normal weight; however, it is far more realistic to begin where the person is and calculate an appropriate calorie level from that point. A person who is maintaining his weight on 2600 kcal per day will lose approximately 1 pound per week on a 2100-kcal diet and approximately 2 pounds per week on a 1600-kcal diet. As he loses weight, his diet is adjusted.

The grossly obese person of 350 pounds who has been overweight from childhood is not likely to reach a weight of 160 pounds and maintain it for the rest of his life; his weight is more likely to fluctuate between 160 and 350 pounds. It may be healthier for him to reduce to 250 pounds and stay there.

The Diet

Balanced reducing diets are most successful when they are part of a planned program that includes exercise and behavior change; unless poor food habits and activity patterns are both corrected, the likelihood that weight loss will be long-lasting is small.

In a dietary interview, the dietitian obtains information on the basis of which the client's energy needs and caloric intake can be estimated. Then a caloric level designed to produce a gradual weight loss is determined. This level must be lower than the client's energy needs. A diet providing 500 kcal below energy needs should result in a weight loss of 1 pound per week; 1000 kcal below, approximately 2 pounds per week. A loss of more than 2 pounds

per week is not recommended unless the client is under a physician's close supervision. Diets of below 1000 kcal per day are appropriate only for hospitalized clients.

Providing Essential Nutrients

In a diet of less than 1800 kcal to 2000 kcal, there is little room for sugar and alcohol. Even when the diet is made up entirely of nutritious foods, levels of minerals, such as iron, zinc, and magnesium, and vitamins E and folacin are likely to be below recommended levels. A vitamin–mineral supplement may be prescribed to persons on such a diet.

Twenty percent of total calories in a reducing diet are usually from protein. On this basis, a 1500-kcal diet provides 75 g of protein. Fats and carbohydrates are restricted, but an appropriate balance between the two is maintained. A distribution of 30% to 35% of calories from fat and 45% to 50% of calories from carbohydrate is common. Water and other noncaloric fluids are not restricted unless there are complicating factors.

Table 20-2. Reducing Diets Based on Food Exchange Lists

	Number of Exchanges	
Food Exchanges	1200 kcal	1500 kcal
Milk, skim	2	2
Vegetable	2	2
Fruit	3	4
Bread	4	6
Meat	6	7
Fat	3	4
Nutrient Content		
Protein	70 g	81 g
Fat	45 g	55 g
Carbohydrate	124 g	164 g
kcal	1181	1475

Table 20-3.   1200-kcal Diet Plan and Sample Menu

Meal	Food Exchange	No. of Exchanges	Sample Menu
Breakfast	Fruit	1	¼ cantaloupe with
	Meat	1	¼ cup of low-fat cottage cheese
	Bread	1	1 slice of whole-wheat toast
	Fat	1	1 tsp of margarine
	Milk, skim	1	1 cup of skim milk
			Coffee
			Tuna salad plate:
Lunch	Meat	2	½ cup of water-packed tuna
	Vegetable	1	Cucumber slices marinated in herb vinegar
			Tomato wedges
			Salad greens
	Bread	1	6 rye rounds
	Fat	1	1 tbsp of diet mayonnaise
	Fruit	1	2 medium-sized fresh plums
			Tea
Dinner	Meat	3	3 oz of baked chicken
	Bread	1	½ cup of cooked rice boiled in chicken bouillon
	Vegetable	1	½ cup of broccoli with 1 tsp of margarine
			Green salad with
	Fat	2	1 tbsp of French dressing
	Fruit	1	Banana-gelatin dessert: ½ small banana in dietetic gelatin
			Seltzer water
Bedtime snack	Milk, skim	1	1 cup of skim milk
	Bread	1	3 arrowroot crackers

Meal Planning

Planning meals ahead is of great importance to the dieter. Haphazard eating habits, skipping meals, and impulse eating are the enemies of weight control. Persons living alone, whether in their 20s or their 70s, are especially likely to have irregular meal patterns. Merely a half hour or so a week devoted to planning meals and a market order based on these meals will reap many benefits. Planning ahead makes it easier to stick to a diet, results in more balanced meals, and reduces the impulse buying of snacks and sweet desserts, which sabotage weight control efforts as well as the food budget.

Using Exchange Lists

The exchange list system described in Chapter 19 is the basis of reducing diets (Table 20-2). The client is given a diet plan, a sample menu, and a set of exchange lists (see Table A-2 in the Appendix). A 1200-kcal diet plan and sample menu are shown in Table 20-3.

A few points should be kept in mind as follows.

Milk Exchanges. A diet of 1500 kcal or less will usually include nonfat milk or 1%-fat milk. The nonfat milk may be fresh fluid milk or milk made from nonfat dried milk powder. Buttermilk made from skim milk may also be used. One pint of milk provides adequate calcium and riboflavin for adults.

One cup (8 oz) of plain (unflavored) yogurt made from skim milk or 1%-fat milk may be substituted for 1 cup of skim milk.

Vegetable Exchanges. For only 25 kcal per ½-cup serving, the vegetables on the vegetable exchange list can add much variety to the diet. Raw or cooked, they can be used as appetizers, salads, garnishes, and between-meal snacks, as well as an accompaniment to the main course of a meal. Flavoring aids such as spices, herbs, low-calorie dressings, vinegar, and lemon can also be used.

The client must be cautioned about the addition of fats to vegetables other than the amounts specified in the diet plan. Extra amounts of fat in the form of butter, margarine, salt pork, oil, gravy, sour cream, and cream sauces can add many additional kilocalories to vegetables.

Fruit Exchanges. Fruit—fresh, canned, or frozen without the addition of sugar—in the amounts listed in the exchange list provides approximately 40 kcal. Some persons assume that they can have fruit or juice in unlimited quantities as long as it is unsweetened. This is not true. Many fruits have a relatively high concentration of natural sugar; for example, an 8-ounce glass of either apple or pineapple juice is equivalent to 3 fruit exchanges, or 120 kcal.

Bread Exchanges. Bread exchanges supply approximately 70 kcal per serving listed. It is a good practice to measure foods such as rice, pastas, cereals, and starchy vegetables for a while until portion sizes can be estimated accurately. The client should be reminded that he can't afford to add oil, butter, or other fats to these foods in excess of the amounts included in his diet.

Meat Exchanges. Lean meat, fish, or poultry should be selected as the meat exchange. Poultry and fish are frequently emphasized because they contain less fat than red meats. Fat should be trimmed from meat and skin removed from poultry before cooking. (A 3-oz portion of sirloin steak yields 300 kcal if both lean and fat are eaten, whereas a 3-oz portion of lean yields only 180 kcal.) Fried foods should be avoided or limited to rare occasions.

Meat and poultry juices can be used for soup or gravy if the fat in them is removed. If the drippings are refrigerated overnight, the fat will rise to the top and harden and can easily be removed. If it is inconvenient to refrigerate drippings, as much fat as possible should be removed by spoon after the liquid is allowed to set. One or two ice cubes should then be added to the drippings. The fat droplets that rise to the surface can then be removed by blotting with absorbent paper toweling.

Fat Exchanges. Fat exchanges are usually limited to 1 or 2 per meal on diets of 1500 kcal or below. This includes the amount used in cooking and at the table. One teaspoon of butter, margarine, oil, or mayonnaise represents 1 fat exchange.

Clients may need guidance in preparing flavorful foods without the use of fat. Meat, fish, and poultry are kept moist if they are baked in aluminum foil. Foods may be cooked with bouillon, tomato juice, lemon juice, or vinegar to which onion, garlic, spices, and herbs may be added. A mixture of tomato juice and flavorings such as grated onion, celery, garlic, horseradish, spices, and herbs to taste can be used hot or cold to add flavor and moisture.

Some General Information That is Useful to the Dieter

Mixed Dishes

Foods permitted in a diet pattern may be combined in mixed dishes. For example, skim milk, egg, and artificial sweetener can be combined in a baked custard. If a recipe for two custards

requires 1 cup of skim milk and 1 egg, each portion would be equivalent to ½ of a skim milk exchange and ½ of a meat exchange.

Adding fats or sugar in the preparation of a food can add considerably to the food's caloric value.

Convenience Foods

Most convenience foods, such as TV dinners and vegetables in sauces, cannot be included in calorie-restricted diets. An exception is the calorie-restricted TV dinner. Labeling regulations require that foods that make a diet claim give calorie and nutrient information on the label. By comparing this information with his diet plan, the dieter can determine whether the food is acceptable.

Dietetic and Low-Calorie Foods

The sweetening agent in dietetic desserts is commonly sorbitol, xylitol, or fructose, all of which have the same caloric content as table sugar. Furthermore, dietetic desserts may be high in fat. The client must know to read labels carefully.

Liquids

Clients need to know that fluids may be high in calories. An 8-ounce glass of canned fruit punch supplies 120 kcal, so three or four glasses contribute 300 kcal to 500 kcal (Table 20-4).

Fad Diets

Faddism has thrived on weight reduction diets. The search for a quick, easy way to lose weight appears to be endless. Also unending is the number of fad diets that come and go. Nevertheless, there is no food or combination of foods that causes a magical burning of body fat.

Fad diets severely limit food choices, emphasizing only one or two foods—the grapefruit diet, the boiled-egg diet, and the all-meat diet, to name a few. Although these foods are nutritious and wholesome in themselves, they

Table 20-4. Caloric Value of Selected Liquids

Fluid	Amount	kcal
Cola-type soda	12 oz	145
Fruit-flavored soda	12 oz	170
Club soda	12 oz	0
Sugar-free soda	12 oz	0–5
Beer	12 oz	150
Wine, dry	3½ oz	85
Wine, sweet	3½ oz	140
Gin, vodka, whiskey (80 proof)	1½ oz jigger	95
Manhattan cocktail	3½ oz	164
Tomato juice	8 oz	45
Grapefruit juice, unsweetened	8 oz	100
Lemonade	8 oz	105
Fruit punch, canned	8 oz	120
Fruit-flavored drink from mix	8 oz	100
Coffee, black	6 oz	5
Coffee with 1 heaping tsp of sugar	6 oz	30
Coffee with 1 heaping tsp of sugar plus 1 tbsp of Half'n Half or liquid creamer	6 oz	50
Water	8 oz	0

(USDA Home and Garden Bulletin 72, 1981; Pennington JA, Church HN: Food Values of Portions Commonly Used. Philadelphia, JB Lippincott, 1980)

do not contain all the needed nutrients in adequate amounts. Fortunately, these diets become so monotonous that they are rarely followed long enough to do harm. Weight loss can be as much as 5 pounds or more a week, but most of this loss is body water or body protein or both.

Behavior Modification

Behavior modification for weight control is a method of teaching that focuses on behavior change rather than on food or weight loss. A

habit is a persistent behavior that is automatic and not a result of thought. Behavior modification is based on the theory that bad eating habits are learned behaviors and that they can be replaced by other, better behaviors. Thus, if the problem is obesity and eating habits are changed, weight loss will follow.

Behavior modification programs for weight control are directed by health professionals specially trained in the techniques. They may be conducted on an individual or a group basis.

The client begins the program by collecting information about his food habits. He keeps a food diary that describes not only the foods and amounts eaten but also the circumstances: how long it takes him to eat, where he eats, with whom, what he does while eating, and so on. (See the sample food diary form in Chap. 2.) From this information, the person identifies those factors that promote excessive caloric intake. A diary may also be kept for physical activity. Once problem behaviors are identified, specific steps are taken to deal with them. Usually, no specific diet is recommended and no particular food is prohibited, but recommendations for food selection and preparation are presented. The client continues to maintain a record to monitor change.

Some practical approaches that help to build better eating habits include the following:

Eat slowly and concentrate on what you are eating—the smell, taste, and texture.

Plan a pause midway through the meal so you can assess what you have already eaten.

Celebrate or reward yourself with treats other than food—a movie, a manicure, some time for yourself, a new necktie.

Serve food directly on your plate. Don't place serving dishes of food on the table.

Choose food that requires some preparation and has to be eaten slowly, such as a whole orange rather than orange juice.

Ask family members to get their own snacks, especially desserts. Many calories are consumed over the course of a year in snacks.

Other Types of Treatment

Starvation

Starvation should be conducted only in a hospital setting; an obese client should never take this drastic measure on his own.

In a starvation diet, only water, bouillon, and tea, along with vitamin and mineral supplements, are ingested for up to 30 days or more. Fat stores and muscle protein provide energy. However, much lean body tissue is also lost in this way. Complications include gout, edema, renal failure, abnormal heart rhythm, and severe weakness. Many clients later regain the weight they have lost, because once the starvation period is over, they resume their earlier eating habits.

Surgery

Surgery is occasionally performed on persons who are grossly obese—2 or 3 times ideal weight—and whose obesity is seriously interfering with their health. There are two types of surgery: jejunoileal bypass (bypass of a part of the small intestine) and gastric bypass.

In intestinal bypass, the length of the functioning small intestine is reduced drastically to about 25 inches. Weight loss occurs by decreased intake of food because of extremely unpleasant gastrointestinal symptoms and the reduced absorption of food. Gastric bypass greatly reduces the size of the stomach; only a small pouch remains. Obviously, a change in eating habits results.

Both procedures cause substantial loss of weight, which is not likely to be regained. They are both very hazardous and may give rise to serious complications, including malnutrition, severe chronic diarrhea, electrolyte imbalances, and liver disease. Clients must be very carefully selected for this form of treatment.

Protein-Sparing Modified Fast (Liquid Protein Diet)

The theory behind the protein-sparing modified fast is that, by providing protein, the diet will

prevent the loss of lean body tissue that occurs in total fasting or with very-low-calorie diets. Although less body tissue loss occurs by this method than by total fasting, considerable loss of body protein does occur; some persons are still in negative nitrogen balance (losing body protein) on the 40th day of the diet.

A few years ago, diets that were composed of high-quality protein and that provided 300 kcal to 400 kcal per day were reported to be successful in obesity clinics under careful medical supervision. At the same time, liquid and powdered protein products became available to the public, and many persons used these products without medical supervision. In 1977, the Center for Disease Control reported 40 deaths due to cardiac irregularities among users of these products. Some of the protein products used by the public were of poor-quality protein; however, deaths due to cardiac irregularities also occurred among persons using high-quality protein products under medical supervision. Some authorities are of the opinion that liquid protein diets should not be taken under any circumstances until the cause of the cardiac problems is determined. Others believe that there is a place for the protein-sparing modified fast for extremely obese persons who are carefully monitored under medical supervision. All authorities are agreed that a person should never follow such a diet on his own.

Unacceptable Treatments

Starch Blockers. These are a relatively recent entry in an endless stream of weight control fads. These substances block or hinder starch digestion and thus help control weight by preventing the absorption of carbohydrates. Starch blockers are made from raw beans, such as kidney beans, and possibly other, unknown, substances.

Complaints of nausea, vomiting, diarrhea, and stomach pains have been reported by users. Because they interfere with digestion, starch blockers may affect the body's normal metabolism. For this reason, the Food and Drug Administration (FDA) considers the blockers to be a drug, not a food. The FDA is concerned about

the safety of long-term use, since the product has not been adequately tested. The agency has ordered the manufacturers to discontinue marketing the product, and the matter is now in the courts. Meanwhile, starch blockers continue to be sold.

Diuretics and Laxatives. Both diuretics and laxatives promote weight loss, but the weight lost is due to water loss, not to a decrease in fatty tissue. Physicians prescribe diuretics only for clients retaining abnormal amounts of water.

Persons who use laxatives habitually to decrease absorption of food will have problems, because the disruption of normal nutrient absorption leads to fluid and electrolyte imbalance.

Underweight

The plight of persons who are severely underweight can be just as desperate as that of grossly obese persons. This is especially true of persons whose extreme thinness is the result of heredity. They lack the normal number of adipose cells that can accumulate fat, and as a result they quickly feel "full" when they eat.

Underweight resulting from prolonged illness is a frequent problem. Such symptoms as lack of appetite, vomiting, diarrhea, and high fever can cause serious weight loss. An endocrine disorder such as hyperthyroidism is another cause of underweight.

Underweight is defined as 10 to 20 pounds under the desirable weight for height and bone structure. The underweight person is susceptible to infection, particularly tuberculosis. Underweight may also complicate pregnancy. Nevertheless, thin people are the least affected by so-called degenerative diseases—heart, liver, and kidney disease and diabetes.

Psychological harm may be a consequence of underweight. Young people who have inher-

ited their thinness may suffer from an inadequate self-image: a young man may feel that he looks weak and unimpressive to the opposite sex, whereas the extremely thin girl may feel that her flat body is unattractive.

Treatment

To treat underweight, a diet increased in calories is prescribed, as are supplements of vitamins and minerals. Regular exercise and plenty of rest are advised.

Persons who have inherited their thinness usually fail in their efforts to increase their caloric intake. Probably the best thing for them to do is to forget their thinness and keep physically fit, get plenty of outdoor activity, maintain good posture, and wear clothing and hairstyles that complement their slimness.

Diet Increased in Calories

Setting a goal for weight gain must take into consideration the individual's age, height, and previous weight status.

Some suggestions follow:

The Daily Food Guide should form the basis of the client's food intake.

Calories must be increased gradually to a level above the client's needs. This may be accomplished by increasing the amount of food eaten at each meal, increasing carbohydrate and fat intake, and providing more frequent feedings in the form of between-meal nourishments or a bedtime snack.

Because protein tissue as well as fat is lost, a liberal protein level of 1 g to 1.5 g per kg of body weight is recommended.

Vitamins and minerals must be adequate, especially thiamine.

There should be reduced consumption of foods that have little caloric value (e.g., broth, salads, coffee, tea) but that may reduce the appetite for other, more concentrated foods.

Foods rich in carbohydrate are easily digested and quickly converted to body fat. They should be eaten liberally. Although fatty foods offer the most calories, they must be eaten cautiously, since they may depress the appetite. Butter, cream, and salad oils are usually better tolerated than fats in fried foods.

The frequency of meals depends on the client. For some, it may mean concentrating on increased intake at regular meals and eating a substantial bedtime snack. For others, small, frequent feedings rather than large meals may work best.

The caloric level of the diet should be increased gradually. A sudden increase in food intake may discourage the client and further depress his appetite. Every effort should be made to prepare the foods the client likes appetizingly and serve them attractively.

Eating Disorders

The health worker should be aware of the symptoms of two eating disorders, anorexia nervosa and bulimia, that cause severe physical problems. Immediate medical and psychiatric attention is required for both.

Anorexia Nervosa

Anorexia nervosa is a life-threatening psychological disorder characterized by deliberate self-starvation. It is seen most often in adolescent girls and young women. The person is not anorexic in the true sense of the word (having a poor appetite). Rather, because of emotional problems, she refuses to permit herself to eat and/or engages in binge eating followed by self-induced vomiting or taking laxatives; she may also engage in excessive physical activity. The anorexic is preoccupied with food and is an expert at calorie counting, frequently limiting herself to 600 kcal to 900 kcal per day. This behavior

produces extreme weight loss, metabolic problems such as amenorrhea (absence of menstruation), and hair loss; death eventually follows if the condition is not treated. The physical symptoms are the body's way of adapting to starvation.

Treatment involves both medical and psychiatric care for the client and counseling for the family. Participation in a self-help group is often a useful aid in treatment.

The psychological disturbances of the anorexic are complex and usually require long-term psychotherapy. A poor mother–daughter relationship, a desire for control, a distorted body image, and fear of physical maturation may be among the problems. The person may have been overweight before the onset of the illness and may be highly sensitive about her tendency to gain weight.

The goal of medical treatment is to prevent the client from starving to death while psychiatric treatment is progressing. Hospitalization may be needed until a reasonable stable weight is achieved; this may be much below desirable weight but is at least compatible with life. If the client refuses to eat, food and medication are given by nasogastric tube or parenterally. Nursing and dietetic personnel usually need specific orientation to work effectively with anorexic clients.

The American Anorexia/Bulimia Association, Inc., 133 Cedar Lane, Teaneck, NJ 07666, provides information and services for clients and their families and for health personnel.

Bulimia

Bulimia, which means, literally, *ox hunger,* is binge eating—sudden, impulsive gorging in a short period of time. The term most often refers to recurrent episodes of gorging followed by self-induced vomiting or purging by laxatives or diuretics as a means of controlling weight. It usually appears as an aftermath of dieting. Bulimia is seen in about 50% of persons who have anorexia nervosa. Emotional tensions appear to induce the craving for food, and the tensions are temporarily quieted by the binging, even though the bulimic person fears that she will not be able to stop eating.

Bulimia is the cause of serious physical problems. The fasting, vomiting, and use of laxatives and diuretics may cause dehydration, electrolyte imbalances, and malnutrition. The frequent vomiting causes esophageal irritation, extensive erosion and decay of teeth, and glandular and metabolic disturbances.

Treatment calls for medical and psychiatric intervention, family counseling, and group therapy.

KEYS TO PRACTICAL APPLICATION

Do not focus entirely on food when attempting to control weight.
Maintaining a physically active life-style is also important.
Remember that obesity is a very complex problem. Accept the obese person as he is, apart from his ability to lose weight. Helping him develop a more positive self-image is probably the greatest contribution one can make toward helping him with his weight problem.
Help the dieter set realistic goals. Drastic reductions in food intake are self-defeating and rarely result in permanent weight loss.
Be assured that calories do count. Regardless of the type of diet or other method of treatment, a person loses weight only when caloric intake is lower than caloric expenditure.
Be suspicious of programs that offer quick solutions to obesity. Successful treatment is long-range and requires changes in eating habits and/or activity patterns.
Keep an eye on portion sizes, fatty foods and fats added to foods, and liquid

calories. They are frequently responsible for excessive calorie intake.

Emphasize planning ahead. Haphazard eating habits make caloric control difficult.

Evaluate carefully the client who needs to gain weight. The approach varies depending upon the cause of the underweight condition. A gradual increase in caloric intake usually works best for anorexic clients.

KEY IDEAS

Weight appropriate for a person 25 years old is that which should be maintained throughout life.

Skinfold thickness measurements are a more accurate means of determining fatness or leanness than height–weight tables.

Weight control is a matter of balance — when energy intake (food) is greater than energy output (energy used by the body), the excess food energy is stored as fat; 3500 kcal represent 1 pound of body fat.

Childhood obesity is more serious than adult obesity because the child will always carry extra fat cells with him.

The complications of obesity shorten life, put stress on the body, increase the risk of disease, and make already existing illness worse.

Grossly obese clients need to be accepted as they are, apart from their ability to lose weight.

Obesity is a complex problem that involves many factors; permanent weight reduction is difficult to achieve.

Prevention of obesity must begin in infancy and childhood; parents must be educated to the dangers of overfeeding and of inactivity.

Successful treatment of obesity involves not only losing weight, but also keeping the weight off for a lifetime; a moderate reduction in energy intake together with a moderate increase in physical activity is the best formula.

Retraining of eating habits is an essential part of weight control programs.

To achieve permanent weight loss, the client must be motivated; counseling and self-help groups provide outside motivation and are useful to many.

When exercise is part of a weight control program, the diet need not be so severely restricted, muscle tone and blood circulation are improved, the mind is diverted from food, and the BMR is increased.

Careful planning is necessary to include all the essential nutrients in diets of less than 1800 kcal to 2000 kcal per day; there is little room for foods such as fats, sugars and other sweets, and alcohol, which are high in calories for the nutrients they provide.

Planning meals ahead is a most useful technique for the dieter.

Behavior modification focuses on behavior change rather than on diet. It is based on the belief that weight loss will result if problem eating habits are changed.

In behavior modification, the client analyzes his eating habits and evaluates his progress by means of carefully kept records of his eating behavior.

Fad diets severely limit food choices, are frequently nutritionally inadequate, do not retrain eating habits, and can produce harmful effects if followed for extended periods of time.

Diets for the underweight require a gradual increase in calories to a level greater than the client's energy needs by an increase in the amount of food eaten at each meal, by emphasis on carbohydrate-rich foods with some increase in easily digested fats, and by more frequent feedings.

Liquid-protein diets may cause cardiac

irregularities; they should never be undertaken without medical supervision. Immediate professional attention should be obtained for persons exhibiting symptoms of anorexia nervosa or bulimia; both are psychological disturbances that result in serious physical deterioration.

KEYS TO LEARNING: STUDY-DISCUSSION QUESTIONS

1. Develop a 1500-kcal diet plan, based on the 1500-kcal reducing diet given in Table 20-2. Assume that you are planning this for yourself; make it as close to your own eating pattern as possible. Give a sample menu for one day.

2. Discuss the social problems the grossly obese client faces. How important is the attitude of health personnel toward the obese patient? Why? What approach do you think would be most helpful to the client?

3. What is your opinion of the statement, "Losing weight only takes will power." Why do you feel this way? Has your opinion changed recently?

4. Obtain a copy of a currently popular fad diet. In light of what you have learned about obesity, present to the class an evaluation of the diet.

5. Assume that you are a parent with three children, two between the ages of 6 and 10, and one teenager. What measures would you take to prevent the development of obesity in the entire family, parents included?

6. How would you go about increasing the caloric intake of an underweight person recovering from a severe illness?

Bibliography is found at the end of Part Four.

Diabetes Mellitus

KEY TERMS

gestational   Related to pregnancy.

glycosuria   An abnormal amount of glucose in the urine.

glycosylated hemoglobin (A$_{1c}$)   A type of red blood cell that has bonded with glucose. The quantity of this cell present in blood indicates how well blood sugar has been controlled over the previous weeks.

hyperglycemia   An abnormal increase in the amount of glucose in the blood.

hypoglycemia   An abnormal decrease in the amount of glucose in the blood.

insulin resistance   Failure of tissues to use insulin normally.

ketonuria   Ketone bodies in the urine.

nephropathy   Kidney disease.

polydipsia   Excessive thirst.

polyphagia   Excessive desire to eat.

polyuria   Excessive quantity of urine.

renal threshold   The concentration at which a substance in the blood normally not excreted by the kidney begins to appear in the urine.

retinopathy   Disease of the retina.

vascular   Relating to blood vessels.

Diabetes mellitus is a mysterious disease. Although it was recognized as early as 2000 B.C., there are still many unanswered questions about its cause and long-range effects. It is estimated that there are 10 million diabetics in the United States alone, 40% of whom do not know they have the disease.

The increased life span for diabetics made possible by insulin has also permitted the development of long-range complications of the cardiovascular, renal, and nervous systems.

Types

It appears that diabetes mellitus is not one but several diseases characterized by an abnormally high blood glucose (sugar) level. The classification currently in use is the following:

Type I, insulin-dependent diabetes mellitus (IDDM), formerly called *juvenile-onset diabetes.* Insulin is required to keep

the person with IDDM alive. This form of diabetes usually occurs during youth but can occur at any age.

Type II, noninsulin-dependent diabetes mellitus (NIDDM), formerly called *maturity-onset* or *adult-onset diabetes*. In this form of diabetes, insulin is not required to sustain life but may be required during periods of stress. NIDDM occurs most frequently in adults but can occur in persons of any age. Most persons in this category are obese and usually have a family history of diabetes.

Diabetes associated with other conditions and syndromes. This includes diabetes caused by drugs or chemicals or resulting from other diseases, such as pancreatic or endocrine disease.

Gestational Diabetes (GDM) is a kind of diabetes that develops in pregnant women, most of whom are obese. Blood sugar levels may return to normal after pregnancy or may continue to be abnormal.

The diagnosis of diabetes is made on the basis of blood sugar levels.

Nature

Glucose is the substance primarily used by the body for fuel. Carbohydrates (starches and sugars) in food are the main source of glucose. Protein and fat also yield some glucose.

Insulin has been described as the "spark" that the cells need to convert glucose to energy. The diabetic is unable to use or store glucose normally because of an insulin deficiency, a defect in the action of insulin, or a defect in the use of insulin by the cells. In some persons, more than one cause may be involved.

Glucose that cannot be stored or used accumulates in the bloodstream. When it reaches a certain level (usually 160–180 mg/dl), it spills into the urine and is excreted. The blood sugar level at which glucose spills into the urine is

called the *renal threshold.* Water and sodium are lost along with the excess sugar. (See Chapter 5 for discussion of insulin and other hormones.)

Type I Insulin-Dependent Diabetes

IDDM is caused by a deficiency of insulin. When carbohydrate cannot be used for fuel, the body looks for other sources of energy: protein and fat. The increased breakdown of protein and fat that results creates additional metabolic disorders. Urinary excretion of urea (waste products of protein metabolism) is increased. Ketone bodies, produced by the incomplete burning of fat, accumulate in the blood. Most ketones are acid, and their presence leads to a condition known as *diabetic acidosis* or *ketosis.* Severe acidosis can lead to diabetic coma and, if untreated, can cause death. The body's efforts to rid itself of urea and the ketones in the urine further increase the loss of water. This contributes to the dehydration that can occur in untreated diabetes. The insulin-dependent diabetic requires insulin injections to prevent ketosis and maintain life.

Symptoms usually associated with diabetes are found in insulin-dependent diabetics. The increase in blood sugar levels followed by the excretion of glucose and ketones in the urine (glycosuria, ketonuria) produce the most common symptoms, polyuria (excessive urination) and polydipsia (extreme thirst). Since the diabetic does not receive full benefit from the food he eats, he feels constant hunger (polyphagia) and experiences rapid weight loss.

Type II Noninsulin-Dependent Diabetes

NIDDM is believed to be caused in large part by insulin resistance due mainly to tissue defects. The problem is thought to be that the tissue cells have too few insulin receptors, the molecules that attract insulin. The surface of every normal cell has thousands of such receptors; if they are lacking, insulin builds up in the blood while the blood sugar level continues to rise. The result is

hyperinsulinism (excessive insulin), which may further depress receptors. The decrease in receptors may be the body's way of protecting itself from too much insulin.

Insulin resistance is also seen in obese persons. The number of receptors is increased when the person loses weight: in some persons, weight loss may totally correct the diabetic condition. Diabetics who are not obese may also manifest insulin resistance.

Other factors, such as a delayed release of insulin by the pancreas and a failure of the liver to store sugar, may also play a part in type II diabetes.

Eighty-five percent of diabetics have the noninsulin-dependent type of the disease, which is seen most often in obese persons 40 years or older. The disease develops so slowly that it may not be diagnosed until years after onset. It can be controlled by diet and exercise. Oral medication may be prescribed. During periods of physical or emotional stress, the type II diabetic may require insulin.

Laboratory Tests

The blood sugar level is a reliable indicator of how efficiently the body is using glucose. Blood sugar is the quantity of circulating glucose. Laboratory values vary according to whether plasma or whole blood is used in the tests.

If a person has the classic symptoms of diabetes and his blood sugar level is well above normal, a diagnosis of diabetes can be made without further testing. When the blood glucose level is suspect but not high enough to definitely establish the presence of diabetes, an oral glucose tolerance test is done. In this test, the client, who has been fasting for at least 10 hours, has a fasting blood sample taken and then is given a solution containing 75 g of glucose. After the client has drunk the solution, blood samples are collected at ½-, 1-, 1½-, 2-, and 3-hour intervals. In normal persons, the fasting plasma glucose level will be equal to or less than 115 mg/dl (100 mg/dl venous whole blood) at the 2-hour interval. Persons whose blood sugar levels fall between normal and diabetic have what is called *impaired glucose tolerance* and are not classified as diabetic. The terms *borderline diabetic, mild*

diabetic, and *chemical diabetes* are no longer used.

Hemoglobin A_{1c} is a blood test that is useful in evaluating the degree of control over his blood glucose level the diabetic has maintained during preceding weeks. Hemoglobin A_{1c}, also called *glycosylated hemoglobin,* is a red cell that has bonded (connected) with the circulating glucose. The higher the blood glucose level, the more bonding takes place, and the higher the level of A_{1c} hemoglobin. This bond remains for the life of the cell (approximately 90 days). A high A_{1c} level indicates that blood sugar levels have been abnormally high over an extended period of time. This test can be done at any time of day, and does not require fasting.

Complications

The diabetic is more susceptible than the nondiabetic to diseases of both the small and the large blood vessels. Small-blood-vessel disease may result in nephropathy (kidney disease), neuropathy (damage to nerves), and retinopathy (damage to the blood vessels of the retina).

Atherosclerosis, a disease of the large blood vessels, is the cause of death of approximately three fourths of American diabetics. Why diabetics are more susceptible than normal to cardiovascular disease is not completely understood. However, diabetics frequently have elevated blood lipid levels (cholesterol and triglycerides), which are a risk factor in cardiovascular disease. High blood sugar may be another risk factor. There is strong evidence that control of blood sugar will lessen these serious complications.

Treatment

The purposes of treatment is to help the diabetic maintain as nearly normal a blood sugar level as possible, to maintain good nutritional status,

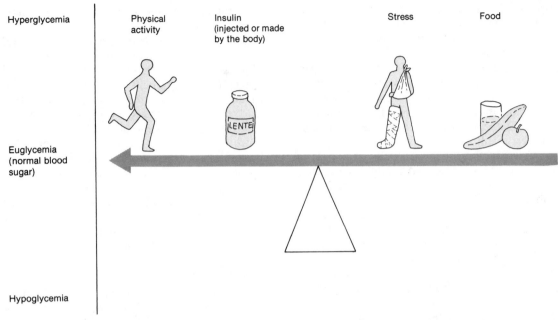

Fig. 21-1.   Factors that must be balanced to maintain normal blood sugar level. (Suitor CW, Hunter MF: Nutrition: Principles and Application in Health Promotion. Philadelphia, JB Lippincott, 1980)

and to be able to continue the normal activities of daily living. Therapy also aims at preventing or delaying complications. The diabetic client should be under the continual care of a physician. Diet is an extremely important aspect of treatment for all diabetics, so the services of a qualified dietitian should always be available.

A normal blood sugar level reflects a balance between factors that reduce blood sugar — physical activity and insulin — and factors that increase blood sugar — food intake and stress —(Fig. 21-1). In the insulin-dependent diabetic, careful management of these factors is necessary to prevent wide swings in blood sugar from dangerously high levels (hyperglycemia) to dangerously low levels (hypoglycemia). Physical stress such as an infection may substantially increase blood sugar levels. Increased insulin is required to restore the balance.

A small number of insulin-dependent diabetics have an unstable form of the disease called *brittle diabetes*. In these persons, wide changes in blood sugar from very high to very low occur for no obvious reason.

Noninsulin-dependent diabetics who are controlled by diet alone may experience a sharp rise in blood sugar when under psychological or physical stress. Depending on the cause of this rise, a balance can be achieved by an increase in activity, reduction of stress, better control of the diet, or use of insulin or oral hypoglycemic agents.

Insulin and Oral Hypoglycemic Agents

Persons with type I IDDM require daily injections of insulin to maintain life. The insulin cannot be taken by mouth because it is a protein and would be digested or broken down in the intestinal tract. The physician determines the kind and amount of insulin to be used.

There are various types of insulin. They

Table 21-1.   Insulin Action

Type	Onset of Action (hours)	Peak Action (hours)	Duration (hours)
Regular	½	1–2	5–10
Semilente	1	3–4	10–16
Globin	2	6–8	12–18
NPH	2	8–14	18–24
Lente	2	8–14	18–24
Protamine zinc	6	16–20	24–30
Ultralente	6	18–29	30–36
Combinations			
Regular + NPH	½	2–10	18–24
Regular + lente	1	2–10	18–24
Semilente + lente	1	4–10	18–24
Semilente + ultralente	1	2–24	30–36

(After Owen OE, Boden G, Shuman CR: Managing insulin dependent diabetic patients. Postgrad Med 59:127, 1976. Copyright © McGraw-Hill, Inc.)

differ in the length of time required to take effect, time of peak action (greatest sugar-lowering effect), and length of action (Table 21-1). Insulins are classified as rapid, intermediate, and slow-acting. The kinds most commonly used are short-acting insulins, such as regular insulin, and intermediate-acting insulins, such as NPH. Different types of insulin may be used by themselves or can be combined, depending on the needs of the client.

Most noninsulin-dependent diabetics can be controlled by the management of diet, exercise, and stress. Sometimes sulfonylurea compounds (oral hypoglycemic agents) are used to help control blood sugar. These drugs cause a faster release of insulin and increase the number of insulin receptors.

Exercise

In well-controlled diabetics, physical activity improves the body's ability to use glucose and lowers the insulin requirement. It also improves circulation and muscle tone and provides a sense of well-being. During strenuous exercise, persons taking insulin or glucose-lowering pills may need to take more food or reduce insulin or glucose-lowering medication or both.

Diet

The diabetic diet is designed to control both the disease and its complications and to meet nutritional needs. The dietitian plans the diet according to the physician's order, though in some situations, such as nursing homes, the nurse or nurse practitioner may need to assume this responsibility.

Dietary treatment aims to achieve the following: optimum nutritional status, desirable body weight, blood glucose levels as near the normal range as possible, prevention or delay of complications such as atherosclerosis, changes

in diet required by other conditions such as hypertension, and an individualized diet that is practical and realistic and that is presented in an individualized educational and follow-up program. Nutritional requirements for diabetics are the same as for nondiabetics of the same age, sex, and size. Normal growth and development in the child, nutritional needs of the pregnant woman, and weight reduction for the obese adult must be taken into account. The nutritional needs of the diabetic can be met by everyday foods prepared by common cooking methods. Special "dietetic" or "diabetic" foods are not necessary.

Because IDDM differs from NIDDM in a number of ways, the goals and priorities of dietary treatment also differ. When insulin is used, careful attention must be given to the timing of meals, the composition of the diet (amount of protein, fat, carbohydrate, and fiber), and the energy content of the diet, in that order. The diet must be carefully controlled from day to day.

For the obese noninsulin-dependent diabetic, weight reduction is the most important objective. With weight loss, blood sugar levels are reduced, and the individual may no longer require insulin or oral hypoglycemic drugs. High levels of cholesterol and triglycerides in the blood, as well as elevated blood pressure, may also be reduced with weight loss. Timing of meals is important if oral hypoglycemic agents are used.

Composition

Energy

The total caloric value of the diabetic diet is usually determined by the physician. The allowance may range from 1200 kcal per day for an obese adult to 3500 kcal for an active adolescent.

Carbohydrate

Diets relatively high in carbohydrate are well tolerated by diabetics as long as the total caloric intake is within the amount prescribed and is properly divided throughout the day. The carbohydrate level should represent 50% to 60% of total calories; at 50% of total calories, an 1800-kcal diet would contain 225 g of carbohydrate ($1800 \times 0.50 = 900 \div 4$ cal/g $= 225$ g).

Complex carbohydrates found in starches make up most of the carbohydrate in the diet. Breads, cereals, vegetables, pastas, and rice are rich sources. Sugars found naturally in milk and fruit are permitted, but other sugars, such as table sugar, honey, and corn syrup, are avoided.

The emphasis on complex carbohydrates and the avoidance of sugars has been based on the belief that sugars are immediately absorbed from the intestinal tract and cause a rapid rise in blood sugar, whereas complex carbohydrates (starches) take longer to digest and absorb and, therefore, cause a slower and more moderate rise in blood sugar. Recent research questions these traditional concepts and will undoubtedly bring about changes in the diabetic diet in the future. (See discussion below.)

Varying Effects of Complex Carbohydrates on Blood Sugar Level

Recent research has found that not all complex carbohydrates are digested and absorbed in the same way. The elevating effect of cooked potatoes on blood sugar has been found to be much greater than that of rice. In fact, potatoes cause as much of a rise in blood sugar as oral glucose.

In a study of four starches, foods that elevated blood sugar in increasing order were rice, bread, corn, and potatoes. Legumes have very little effect on blood sugar. Differences also exist among sugars. Glucose and maltose greatly influence blood sugar levels, while lactose and fructose have much less effect.

In the light of these findings, the wisdom of classifying all starches into a single group has been questioned. Presently, changes in the diabetic exchange lists are being considered.

Fiber

Certain types of fiber reduce the rise in blood sugar that occurs after a meal. Foods containing unrefined fiber, such as whole grains, legumes,

and vegetables, should be substituted for refined carbohydrates that are low in fiber.

Protein

The protein level of the diabetic diet is 12% to 20% of total calories.

Fat

A total fat level of 30% to 35% of total calories or less is recommended. Saturated fats should be decreased to less than 10% of total calories, and polyunsaturated fats should supply no more than 10% of total calories. A cholesterol level not exceeding 300 mg/day is preferred.

Timing of Meals

The timing and the number of daily meals are essential aspects of treatment. The client is strongly encouraged to follow a regular pattern of eating and physical activity.

The type of insulin used is an important factor in determining the spacing of meals. For example, an afternoon and an evening snack should be planned for a person receiving NPH insulin before breakfast. To avoid hypoglycemia during the peak hours of insulin activity (for NPH insulin, peak action occurs 8–14 hours after injection), each snack may provide one tenth of the day's carbohydrate and caloric intake. Protein should be included in the snack; it is converted to glucose more slowly than carbohydrate and affords longer protection against an insulin reaction, which is especially important during the night.

The unstable insulin-dependent diabetic has wide fluctuations in plasma glucose levels. This type of diabetic usually requires frequent snacks in addition to meals. Arrangements must be made with school authorities for diabetic children to eat snacks at established times during the day.

The diabetic who is taking an oral hypoglycemic agent should also maintain a regular eating and exercise pattern. For the obese diabetic who is being controlled by diet and exercise alone, regularity in meals is not absolutely essential but is usually helpful.

Planning

The diabetic diet is well balanced and nutritious and can serve as a model for the rest of the family. Since the diabetic's family is susceptible to the disease, it is wise for all members to take a good look at their eating habits. Skipping meals, "stuffing" at one large meal a day, and excessive snacking on foods with little nutritive value are examples of practices that need to be corrected.

Adapting the Diet to Individual Needs

The diet must be tailored to the person and not vice versa. It is an essential aspect of treatment that will be necessary for the rest of the client's life.

The dietary interview (see Chap. 19) plays an important role in establishing individualized care. What the client eats, with whom he eats, his occupation and after-work activities, and economic and ethnic factors all influence his dietary habits.

The Exchange List Method

The exchange list method is the most frequently used method for planning the diet and teaching the client. Occasionally, however, another method may be more suited to individual needs. For example, an elderly person might find the exchange lists confusing. As an alternative, a plastic plate divided into three sections might be used and the client taught what kind of food and how much to put into each section. Another client who resists following a specific diet pattern might be willing to keep a food diary. By means of the diary, he could then be shown where changes might be made to meet his requirements.

Usually, the menu pattern is developed according to the exchange list system. This simplifies menu planning and affords a wide variety of choices without the need for the client to calculate calories and nutrients.

Portions of food given in the exchange lists should be measured carefully with standard measuring cups and spoons. This can be done until the client is able to estimate portion sizes accurately.

Estimating portion sizes of meat, fish, and poultry presents the greatest difficulty to most clients. Clients might be advised to weigh portions of meat until they can estimate accurately or to use the following guide: 4 ounces of raw

Table 21-2. 1800-kcal Diabetic Diet — Meal Plan and Sample Menu

Your Meal Plan in Exchanges
Must Be Planned with the Assistance of Your Diet Counselor

Meal Plan for ___John Doe___

Carbohydrate ___220___ g Protein ___100___ g Fat ___59___ g Calories ___1800___

	1 Milk (Skim)	2 Vegetable	3 Fruit	4 Bread	5 Meat (Lean)	6 Fat (Polyunsaturated)	Approx. Carbohydrate Distribution
Breakfast Time __7:00 AM__	1/2 cup		1	2	1	1	2/10
Snack Time __							
Lunch or Dinner Time __12:00 noon__	1 cup		1	3	2	2	3/10
Snack Time __3:00 PM__	1/2 cup			1	1	2	1/10
Dinner or Supper Time __6:00 PM__		2	1	3	3	2	3/10
Bedtime Snack Time __9:30 PM__	1/2 cup			1	1		1/10

Menu Pattern   Sample Menu

Breakfast

½ milk exchange ———— ½ cup of skim milk

2 bread exchanges ———— 1 biscuit of shredded wheat
———— 1 slice of rye toast

1 fat exchange ———— 1 tsp of margarine

1 lean meat exchange ———— ¼ cup of low-fat cottage cheese mixed with

1 fruit exchange ———— ½ cup of unsweetened pineapple chunks

Free item ———— 1 cup of coffee

meat, 5 ounces of raw meat with bone, one small chicken leg and thigh, and half of a small chicken breast all equal approximately 3 ounces cooked.

The health worker should be thoroughly familiar with the exchange lists and how they are used in planning meals. Nurses are frequently called upon to help clients interpret their diets and may help them plan meals or make menu choices using the exchange lists. A

Menu Pattern	Sample Menu
Lunch	
	Turkey sandwich
2 lean meat exchanges	2 oz of turkey
2 fat exchanges	2 tsp of mayonnaise
3 bread exchanges	2 slices of rye bread
	3 arrowroot crackers
1 fruit exchange	1 orange
1 milk exchange	1 cup of skim milk
Free item	lettuce for sandwich
Snack	
1 bread exchange	1 slice of whole-wheat bread
1 lean meat exchange	2 tbsp of peanut butter
2 fat exchanges	
½ milk exchange	½ cup of skim milk
Dinner	
3 lean meat exchanges	3 oz of eye round roast
3 bread exchanges	1 cup of rice
	1 slice of whole-wheat bread
2 fat exchanges	2 tsp of margarine
	(for vegetables and bread)
2 vegetable exchanges	½ cup of green beans
	½ cup of beet–onion salad
	vinegar
Free items	1 cup of tea
1 fruit exchange	1 medium-sized pear, juice pack, drained
Snack	
1 bread exchange	4 (2½-inch square) soda crackers
1 lean meat exchange	1 oz of low-fat cheese
½ milk exchange	½ cup of skim milk

meal pattern and sample menu for a diabetic is given in Table 21-2.

Exchange lists for meal planning are found in the Appendix, and are discussed in Chapters 19 and 20 as well as in this chapter. There are some differences among various exchange lists, so the health worker should become familiar with the one being used by the client.

Fat Modification

Although it is not certain that a fat-modified diet will delay atherosclerosis, it seems reasonable to expect this result. Because diabetics are susceptible to premature cardiovascular disease, the trend is to reduce saturated fat and cholesterol and to replace some of the saturated fat with polyunsaturated fat. The use of skim-milk products, low-fat meat exchanges with emphasis on fish, poultry, and legumes, and polyunsaturated fats is encouraged.

Using Exchanges in Meals and Food Preparation

Skim milk or low-fat (1%-fat) milk is included in fat-modified diabetic diets and in calorie restriction for weight-reducing purposes. The quantity of milk specified in the diet plan includes that used in cereal, tea, and coffee, in cooking, and for drinking.

Vegetables may be used alone or in soups, casseroles, salads, and as appetizers. Vegetables cooked with fat meat or other fats average 1 fat exchange per ½-cup serving.

Fruit exchanges include unsweetened fruit in a variety of forms: fresh, dried, canned, frozen, cooked, and raw. Fruit can be included by itself, combined with other foods, or consumed in the form of fruit juice.

Due to the trend of increasing carbohydrate levels in the diabetic diet, more bread exchanges are included in the diabetic diet patterns than in the past. This may meet with some resistance from diabetics who have the idea that starches should be omitted from the diet or severely restricted. Not only bread, but also cereals, rice, pastas, crackers, starchy vegetables (such as corn, dried peas and beans, potatoes), and some snack foods are found in the bread exchange list.

Ingredients used in the cooking of meat must be included in the meal pattern. Visible fat should be trimmed from meat. If the diet is to be low in saturated fat and cholesterol, meat choices are limited to the lean meat exchanges (and peanut butter). Eggs and organ meats are omitted or limited.

Butter, margarine, bacon, cream, oil, salad dressings, and nuts are found in the fat exchange. The amount of fat permitted on the meal plan includes that used in cooking. The use of polyunsaturated fats rather than saturated fats is encouraged.

Mixed Dishes

Mixed dishes such as beef stew, French toast, and baked macaroni and cheese can be made by the combination of exchanges. *The American Diabetes Association/American Dietetic Association Family Cookbook** is a useful guide to mixed dishes.

Convenience Foods

If a food product lists the per-serving nutrition information on the label, the diabetic can determine its exchange value and then decide whether it fits into his meal plan. If the nutritional composition is not given on the label, the product cannot be used. (See Table 19-5.)

Alcohol

Only with the approval of the physician should alcohol be included in the diabetic diet. Alcohol lowers blood sugar levels. Diabetics taking insulin may experience a hypoglycemic reaction if they consume alcohol between or before meals. This can have tragic results if the person's strange behavior or loss of consciousness is confused with drunkenness.

Alcohol consumption may also cause a toxic reaction in persons taking oral hypoglycemic agents (sulfonylurea compounds).

---

* Englewood Cliffs, NJ, Prentice-Hall, 1980.

Sweeteners and Dietetic Foods

Aspartame (APM), a protein-based sweetener, became available in 1982. It is manufactured by Searle Laboratories under the brand names *Equal* and *NutraSweet*.* Equal is a table-top sweetener; NutraSweet is used in commercial food processing. APM is about 200 times sweeter than sugar. The amount of APM equal in sweetness to 1 teaspoon of sugar contains only $\frac{1}{10}$ kcal. However, because lactose is used as a filler in the product, 1 packet of Equal contains about 2 kcal. APM is said to be identical in taste to sugar and to leave no bitter aftertaste. Its use in products is limited because it is unstable in heat and acid and loses its sweetness when used in cooking or baking. The American diabetes Association has approved the moderate use of APM by diabetics. APM contains phenylalanine, an amino acid, so it cannot be used by phenylketonurics (see Chap. 28).

Saccharin is a noncaloric sweetener used by itself or as an ingredient in foods, such as diet sodas, to reduce their sugar or caloric content. The American Diabetes Association has taken the position that the evidence linking the use of saccharin with cancer of the lower urinary tract is not strong enough to warrant a ban on the product.

Fructose and sorbitol have the same caloric value as table sugar. However, in well-controlled diabetics, they do not cause a rapid rise in blood sugar and may be permitted in limited amounts.

So-called dietetic foods are not necessarily intended for use by diabetics. Clients should be taught to read labels carefully to see how these foods differ from regular foods. Those that are reduced in calories are usually the most useful.

Adapting Exchange Lists

The exchange lists can be adapted to various cultural food patterns. These lists are available from state and city health agencies, social welfare agencies, and visiting nurse services in large cities. Exchange lists can also be modified to

* Searle Food Resources, Inc., NutraSweet, P.O. Box 1045, Skokie, IL 60076

accommodate other diseases that may be present.

Circumstances Requiring Diet Changes

Delayed Meals

An unavoidable situation may occasionally result in a delayed meal. The diabetic who is taking insulin or an oral hypoglycemic agent may experience a serious hypoglycemic reaction if he does not eat, regardless of the circumstances. He should always carry a readily available source of carbohydrate, such as a lump of sugar, hard candy, or a tube of concentrated glucose. If he anticipates that a delay may occur, as when going to a dinner party or a restaurant, he should eat a snack beforehand.

Strenuous Exercise

When a diabetic taking insulin or glucose-lowering medication increases his physical activity, he may need extra food. If the activity is strenuous, such as running or swimming, the diabetic taking insulin will have to increase his carbohydrate intake or reduce his insulin intake or both. It may be easiest to eat food — at least 1 bread exchange and possibly 1 glass of milk before the activity, especially if it occurs during the time of peak insulin activity. Sugar-containing foods such as fruit, fruit juice, sweetened beverages, or candy may be needed during the activity to prevent hypoglycemia.

Illness

A decrease in appetite often accompanies illness or emotional upset. Sometimes the usual diet plan can be followed by the substitution of foods that are readily tolerated, such as cooked cereal, eggs, crackers, soups, and tender meats. If the client is too ill to eat solid foods, sugar-containing liquids may be sipped to make up for carbohydrate in the diet plan.

Insulin-dependent diabetics should not omit their insulin when they do not feel well, since illness usually causes a rise in blood sugar.

Carbohydrate Replacement for the Hospitalized Client

When a hospitalized insulin-dependent diabetic fails to eat a significant portion (usually 10 g or more) of the carbohydrate on his tray, a replacement should be given. The hospital usually has a policy indicating what replacements should be offered. If the client requires replacements repeatedly, the dietitian should be notified.

Diabetic Acidosis and Coma

Diabetic acidosis, sometimes called *ketosis* or *ketoacidosis,* is a critical condition that can lead to coma and even death. Immediate medical treatment is required, and the client is usually hospitalized. Insulin and intravenous fluids are given. Diabetic acidosis may result from failure to take insulin or from infection or another stress condition that requires increased insulin. Symptoms include nausea, vomiting, severe abdominal pain, deep and rapid breathing, drowsiness, and sometimes coma (unconsciousness). The symptoms appear gradually, over a period of days, in adults. Symptoms may develop more rapidly in young people but usually appear over a period of hours.

Hypoglycemia

Hypoglycemia, or insulin shock, results from too much insulin, which causes the blood glucose level to fall below normal (hypoglycemia). The underlying cause may be too large a dose of insulin or oral hypoglycemic medication, too little food or a delayed meal, or too much strenuous exercise without increases in food intake. The symptoms, which develop quickly, include hunger, trembling, sweating, nervousness, drowsiness, headache, and nausea. The client may give the appearance of being drunk or of having a stroke. If untreated, he will lapse into unconsciousness.

Sugar is required at once to treat hypoglycemia. If the client is unconscious, he is given a glucose solution intravenously or an injection of glucagon (a hormone that stimulates the release of glucose by the liver). The intravenous glucose solution must be administered by a member of the medical team; a family member can be taught to inject glucagon.

Diabetes in Children

An insulin-dependent diabetic child has changing nutritional needs. His diet must contain sufficient calories for normal growth and development and will have to be altered to suit his changing growth and energy needs.

Midmorning, midafternoon, and bedtime are appropriate times for snacks of milk, crackers, fruit, or a sandwich. The bedtime snack is extremely important, since bedtime begins an 8- to 10-hour period without food during which the child is not awake to experience the symptoms of an insulin reaction. The bedtime feeding should contain some protein food, such as milk, meat, cheese, or peanut butter, in addition to a carbohydrate food.

There is some controversy about the value of a specific diet with a fixed calorie level for young diabetics. It is felt by some that a specific diet leads to emotional and physical problems; that a rigid diet may give rise to psychological disturbances; and that a rigid diet may induce frequent hypoglycemic reactions, which can damage the nervous system. However, studies indicate that children with good blood sugar control have a lower incidence of diabetic complications than children with moderate control. The solution probably lies between the two positions: good control with as little interference in the child's life as possible; once good control is established and the child is developing normally, some flexibility may be more beneficial than an absolutely rigid diet.

When no specific diet is followed, the parents and child are shown how to include daily foods that meet the child's nutritional needs in regular meals of approximately the same amounts and nutritional compositions. Concentrated sweets are avoided. The parents and

child must be taught how to increase the child's food intake when he takes part in strenuous activity.

Educating the Client

Education is essential to the diabetic, because he is responsible to a great degree for his own treatment. Obviously, the more he understands about his disease, the better care he can provide for himself.

The physician, nurse, and dietitian work together to educate the client. The physician and nurse teach the client about the nature of his disease and how it can be controlled. The client is taught how to manage his daily care: insulin injection, blood testing, urine testing, treatment for insulin reaction and ketoacidosis,

personal hygiene, and so on. The dietitian, in consultation with the physician and nurse, provides dietary instruction.

A diet is planned that fits as much as possible with the client's earlier eating habits, lifestyle, and social activities. He is shown how and when to increase his food intake and how to alter his diet during illness when he cannot tolerate regular meals.

If the client is hospitalized, the hospital tray can serve as an effective teaching tool for demonstrating portion sizes, the variety of exchange foods, the total quantity of food at each meal, and so on. For a client who is not hospitalized, food models can be used to demonstrate portion sizes as well as exchanges.

The client often has questions after facing the reality of adhering to the diet on his own, and he should have the opportunity for follow-up visits to resolve these questions. The family should also be included in the teaching plan. The bimonthly magazine *Forecast**, written for diabetics, may be helpful.

* ADA Forecast, American Diabetes Association, 1 East 45th Street, New York, NY 10017

KEYS TO PRACTICAL APPLICATION

Encourage noninsulin-dependent diabetics to take care of themselves. Some tend to neglect their disorder because they mistakenly believe that they have a "mild" form of the disease.

Oral sugar-lowering drugs are not a substitute for diet and exercise. Inform your client of the importance of regular meals and physical activity.

The insulin-dependent diabetic should know when to expect the greatest sugar-lowering effect from the insulin he is using. Explain the relationship of insulin to the timing of meals and snacks and the importance of eating at the times specified on his diet plan.

Emphasize the importance of weight reduction for the obese diabetic. Losing weight can improve the body's ability to utilize glucose.

Check trays of diabetic clients after meals to see how well they are eating. If a client is taking insulin or a hypoglycemic drug and refuses food, a carbohydrate replacement is made according to the policy of the hospital.

Make sure that the hospitalized diabetic client receives the between-meal snacks included in his diet plan. Insulin-dependent diabetics usually have one or two such feedings.

Use the client's tray to reinforce diet instruction. Help him relate the food on his tray to the exchange lists. Encourage him to be aware of portion sizes.

Be alert to misconceptions the client may

have about "dietetic" foods. Special foods are not necessary. The diabetic should learn to identify "dietetic" foods he can use if he desires and how to exchange them for "regular" foods in the diet.

Emphasize that the diabetic diet is a well-balanced, nutritious diet that can be a model of good nutrition for nondiabetics.

KEY IDEAS

Diabetes mellitus is a group of diseases in which there is an abnormally high blood sugar level.

The diabetic is unable to use or store glucose normally because of a deficiency of insulin, a defect in the release or action of insulin, or a defect in the use of insulin by the cells.

Type I, insulin-dependent diabetes, is caused by a deficiency of insulin. Insulin injections are required to prevent ketosis and maintain life. This form of the disease is characterized by the classic symptoms of diabetes: excessive thirst, excessive urination, extreme hunger, and weight loss.

Type II, noninsulin-dependent diabetes, is the most common form and occurs most frequently in obese persons over 40 years of age. It is caused mainly by insulin resistance defects in the tissues that use insulin; insulin resistance fequently decreases when the obese person loses weight.

The terms *borderline* and *chemical diabetes* are not used today. Persons with blood sugar levels between normal and diabetic are said to have *impaired glucose tolerance* and are not considered to be diabetic.

Normal blood sugar levels reflect a balance between factors that reduce blood sugar — physical activity and insulin — and factors that increase blood sugar — food intake and stress.

The goals of treatment are to maintain as nearly normal a blood sugar level as possible, to maintain good nutritional status, and to enable client to lead a normal life.

One or more injections of insulin daily may be used by the insulin-dependent diabetic to control-blood sugar; the type of insulin used depends on individual needs.

Most noninsulin-dependent diabetics can be controlled by management of diet, exercise, and stress; sometimes oral hypoglycemic agents are used. Insulin may be necessary during periods of stress.

Physical activity improves the ability of the body to use glucose and lowers insulin requirements in well-controlled diabetics; improved circulation and muscle tone are additional benefits.

The goals of dietary treatment are to control blood sugar levels, achieve good nutritional status and desirable body weight, and prevent or delay the complications of diabetes.

Priorities of dietary treatment differ, depending on the type of diabetes: in insulin-dependent diabetes, the timing and composition of meals are of the greatest importance; in noninsulin-dependent diabetes, weight reduction is most important.

The caloric level of the diabetic diet depends on whether weight gain and growth, weight maintenance, or weight loss is desired. The diet is composed of 50% to 60% carbohydrate, 12% to 20% protein, and 30% to 35% fat.

The carbohydrate in the diet is mainly complex carbohydrate. Sugars are

restricted to those found naturally in fruit and milk; foods containing concentrated sugars, such as table sugar, honey, and corn syrup, are avoided.

Meals high in fiber reduce the rise in blood sugar that occurs after meals.

Saturated fats and cholesterol are restricted as a means of delaying the progress of atherosclerosis, a frequent complication of diabetes.

The type of insulin used is an important factor in determining the composition of meals and the intervals between them.

The diabetic diet must be adapted as much as possible to the food preferences and life-style of the client; in no other condition is individualized dietary treatment more important.

A diabetic diet based on the exchange list system is frequently followed, providing the client with a wide variety of foods; occasionally, however, other approaches are necessary. The diabetic exchange lists commonly used are fat-controlled.

Use of alcohol by diabetics should be discussed with the physician.

"Dietetic" foods are not necessary on a diabetic diet. If they are used, the package labels should be read to determine whether the foods are appropriate.

Fructose and sorbitol are sweeteners that have the same caloric value as table sugar but do not cause as rapid a rise in blood sugar. They may be useful in limited amounts for well-controlled diabetics but are not useful for overweight diabetics.

Insulin-dependent diabetics and diabetics taking glucose-lowering pills should always carry a readily available source of carbohydrate to eat in case a meal is delayed.

The diabetic taking insulin will have to eat extra food before engaging in a strenuous activity and possibly during the activity to prevent hypoglycemia.

When the diabetic taking insulin or glucose-lowering pills is too ill to take solid foods, sugar-containing liquids should be given; insulin or pills should not be omitted.

Diabetic coma results from uncontrolled diabetes and requires immediate medical treatment so that insulin and fluid therapy can be administered.

Insulin shock results from too much insulin caused by too large a dose of insulin or oral hypoglycemic agent, too little food or a delayed meal, or too much strenuous exercise without increases in food intake; a quick source of glucose is required treatment.

The diet for the insulin-dependent child must be changed as the child's growth and energy needs change; once good control is established, a diet with some flexibility rather than an absolutely rigid one may be more beneficial.

The diabetic client is responsible for managing the treatment of his own disease; a good educational program is necessary to prepare him for this task.

KEYS TO LEARNING: STUDY – DISCUSSION QUESTIONS

1. You are attempting to help an elderly woman understand what foods are included on each exchange list. Her eyesight is failing, and she has difficulty reading the printed lists. Prepare a chart or booklet to illustrate the most commonly used items in each exchange.

2. Make two different meal selections from the hospital selective menu given here. What choices could a diabetic patient make who is allowed the following exchanges for the meal: 3 lean meat exchanges, 2 bread exchanges, 1 fruit exchange, 1 vegetable exchange, 2 fat

exchanges, and 1 milk exchange? Be sure to give the quantity of each food that should be provided.

Beef bouillon
or
Cream of mushroom soup

Broiled flounder
or
Fried chicken
or
Cottage cheese (low-fat), fresh fruit salad plate

Tomato juice
Lima beans
Baked potato
Asparagus tips

Tossed salad
Lemon or french dressing

Dinner roll
Bread, white or whole-wheat
Margarine
Jelly

Apple pie
Graham crackers
Fresh grapes
Milk   Coffee   Tea

3. What factors determine how the total food for the day on a diabetic diet is divided into meals and between-meal snacks? What advice is often given for insulin-dependent diabetics who engage in strenuous activity? What procedure is followed in your hospital for replacing food not eaten by the diabetic patient taking insulin or oral hypoglycemic agents?

4. Check the "dietetic" foods in your supermarket or local health food store. Which products would be useful in a diabetic diet? Why? Compare the nutrient composition of "dietetic" cookies or "dietetic" ice cream with that of the same amount of a standard product.

5. Using the nutrition labeling on a convenience food product, determine the exchange value of one serving of the product.

6. An obese client with type II noninsulin-dependent diabetes tells you that he is a "mild" diabetic and does not have to watch what he eats. How would you answer him?

Bibliography is found at the end of Part Four.

Cardiovascular Disease: Atherosclerosis

KEY TERMS

angina pectoris A severe choking pain in the chest commonly due to a decrease in the blood supply to the heart muscle.

arteriosclerosis A hardening of the arteries caused by a number of related diseases.

atheromatous plaques Fatty deposits of cholesterol or other fatty substances on the inner wall of an artery.

atherosclerosis A disorder involving the lining of the arterial walls in which yellowed patches of fat and cholesterol are deposited, forming plaques that decrease the size of the lumen.

cerebral hemorrhage (*stroke*) Destruction of brain tissue due to rupture of a blood vessel or blockage of a blood vessel in the brain by an abnormal material, such as a clot or fat globules.

hyperlipidemia Elevation in the levels of one or more of the fatty substances that circulate in the bloodstream, such as cholesterol and triglycerides.

hyperlipoproteinemia Elevation in the levels of one or more of the lipoprotein groups in the blood.

lipoprotein A combination of fat and protein that makes possible the transport of fat in the bloodstream.

myocardial infarction Heart damage due to a lack of oxygen and nutrients in the heart muscle.

xanthelasma Cholesterol deposits in the soft tissues around the eyes.

In the United States, diseases of the heart and blood vessels are the leading cause of death in persons above the age of 35. Atherosclerosis and hypertension account for 90% of these deaths. Diet therapy in the treatment of atherosclerosis is discussed in this chapter, and diet therapy in the treatment of hypertension and congestive heart failure in Chapter 23.

Atherosclerosis is a form of arteriosclerosis, commonly called *hardening of the arteries.* Al-

though it may begin early in life, symptoms may not appear until middle age or beyond. By this time, the disease has usually progressed to an advanced stage.

The hallmark of atherosclerosis is a thickening of the inner wall of the artery. This thickening is due to the buildup of soft cellular fatty substances, especially cholesterol, on the artery wall. The deposits first take the form of streaks within the inner lining of the artery. They then

297

gradually enlarge to form plaques (patches). The passageway through which the blood flows becomes increasingly narrow, hindering or completely cutting off blood flow to the tissues (Fig. 22-1).

Both nutrition and the removal of waste products from the tissues supplied by the affected blood vessels are hampered. Eventually, the tissues and organs become damaged. When the arteries feeding the heart muscle itself are involved, the condition is called *coronary heart disease. Myocardial infarction, coronary thrombosis,* and *heart attack* are names given to the heart damage resulting from a blockage of the blood supply to the heart muscle. A cerebral hemorrhage (stroke) occurs when there is blockage of a blood vessel that supplies the brain. Atherosclerosis may also be involved in angina pectoris, chest pain due to an inadequate supply of oxygen to the heart muscle; aneurysm (dilation or ballooning) of the abdominal aorta; and gangrene of the extremities.

Certain factors predispose a person to atherosclerosis. These include a family history of atherosclerosis, high blood lipid levels (especially of cholesterol), high blood pressure, obesity, diabetes, cigarette smoking, lack of exercise, a diet high in saturated fat, and emotional stress.

Elevated Blood Lipids

Hyperlipidemia, or elevated blood lipids, is an abnormal rise in levels of serum cholesterol, triglycerides, or specific lipoproteins (Table 22-1). The elevation may be due to primary causes (inherited disorders), to secondary causes (conditions such as diabetes and obesity), or to food habits.

Cholesterol

Cholesterol is a fatlike waxy substance. The body both synthesizes it and obtains it from food. The higher the level of blood cholesterol, the greater the risk of coronary heart disease, though no "risk point", has been established. Age also has a bearing on risk. A man between 30 and 39 years of age who has a blood cholesterol level of less than 200 mg/dl is only one third as likely to develop early heart disease as a man of the same age who has a blood cholesterol level greater than 240 mg/dl. In general, elevated cholesterol levels become less important as a person grows older.

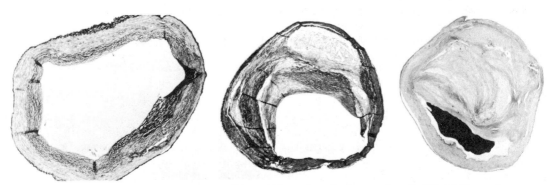

Fig. 22-1. *(Left)* Normal artery. *(Center)* Fatty deposits in vessel wall. *(Right)* Plugged artery with fatty deposits and clot. (Courtesy American Heart Association)

Table 22-1. Lipid Disorders Associated with Increased Incidence of Atherosclerosis*

Hyperlipidemia Type	Plasma Lipids		Age Range and Frequency	Characteristics
	Cholesterol (mg)	Triglycerides (mg)		
Normal (desirable)	220 or lower	150 or lower		
IIa	300–600	Normal	All ages; severe cases occur in early childhood	Tendon and tuberous xanthomas; corneal arcus; premature atherosclerosis
IIb	300–600	150–400	Usually adult; common	Xanthomas; premature atherosclerosis
III	350–800	400–800	Adult (vascular disease frequently evident before age 35 in males, 10–15 years later in females)	Tuberoeruptive lesions over elbows, knees, buttocks; orange yellow streaking of palmar creases; carbohydrate intolerance
IV	Normal or slightly high	200–1000	Adult; very common	Obesity; carbohydrate intolerance; often associated with diabetes mellitus and probably with premature atherosclerosis; usually no external signs

(Data from Dietary Management of Hyperlipoproteinemia. Bethesda, National Heart and Lung Institute, DHEW Publ. No. (NIH) 78-110, 1978)

* Types I and V hyperlipidemia are not associated with an increased incidence of atherosclerotic disease.

Triglyceride

Triglyceride is the fat in food and the main component of adipose tissue. It is also found in blood plasma. Triglyceride that circulates in the plasma comes from fats in the diet or from fats manufactured in the body from sources of energy such as carbohydrate. If calories consumed in a meal are greater than those needed immediately by the tissues, the excess is converted to triglyceride. It is then transported to fat cells for storage. Between meals, triglyceride is released from adipose tissue to meet energy needs. Hormones regulate the release of triglyceride from adipose tissue.

Triglyceride and Disease

Moderately elevated blood triglyceride levels are a risk factor for coronary disease in some individuals. In persons with elevated triglyceride levels, who are frequently obese, weight reduction often corrects the condition. Extremely high triglyceride levels (greater than 1000 mg/dl), which are associated with abdominal

pain and pancreatitis, are very serious conditions. Dietary treatment is essential.

Lipoprotein

Cholesterol and triglycerides are not soluble in water and are carried in the blood by protein. These combinations of lipids and protein circulating in the blood are called *lipoproteins*. The term *hyperlipoproteinemia* refers to an elevation of one or more lipoproteins. Four groups of lipoproteins have been identified: those composed mostly of fat from a recent meal (chylomicrons); those rich in fats synthesized by the body, called *very-low-density lipoproteins* (VLDL); those rich in cholesterol, called *low-density lipoproteins* (LDL); and those containing a high percentage of protein, called *high-density lipoproteins* (HDL). Normally, HDL carry almost one fourth of the blood cholesterol.

High-Density vs. Low-Density Lipoprotein Cholesterol

Most plasma cholesterol is carried by two lipoprotein groups: LDL and HDL. Persons with high amounts of HDL cholesterol have lower rates of coronary heart disease than those with low HDL, whereas persons with high levels of LDL cholesterol have a higher risk of heart disease than persons with low LDL. The protective action of HDL is thought to be due to its ability to transport cholesterol from the tissues to the liver. The cholesterol is then excreted in the bile. Determining the ratio of HDL cholesterol to LDL cholesterol is considered to be a more reliable guide than total cholesterol in determining heart disease risk. Even persons with relatively low total cholesterol levels may have a higher risk of coronary heart disease if their HDL levels are low.

Scientists do not completely understand the bodily processes that elevate HDL. Supervised exercise, weight loss, and cessation of cigarette smoking may have beneficial effects. Some studies have indicated that certain drugs and light alcohol consumption may increase HDL levels.

Dietary Treatment of Lipoprotein Disorders

Lipid disorders are characterized by an excessive amount of one or more of the lipoprotein groups described above. Six types of hyperlipoproteinemia have been identified, each one having a specific blood lipoprotein pattern. In each type, excessive cholesterol and/or triglycerides are involved, but in different proportions. Most but not all of the hyperlipoproteinemias are involved in the early development of coronary heart disease. Unsightly skin lesions called *xanthomas* and *xanthelasma* (Figs. 22-2 and 22-3) and abdominal pain are symptoms in some types of hyperlipidemia.

Diet is the basic treatment for hyperlipidemia. Even in those types for which drugs are available, diet is the treatment of choice and is continued even when drugs are used. The effects of drug and diet together are greater than those of either alone.

Goals

The aim of dietary treatment is to reduce blood cholesterol and triglycerides to desirable levels. The client must follow the diet closely in order to effect such a reduction. Permanent changes in eating habits are required; the diet must be followed for a lifetime. A careful, detailed food history is taken so that the client's life-style, food preferences, and food preparation techniques can be determined. Whenever possible, substitutes are suggested for favorite foods.

Dietary changes necessary to reduce serum cholesterol and triglyceride levels include calorie control, reduction in total fat, reduction in saturated fat, reduction in cholesterol, and partial replacement of saturated fat with polyunsaturated fat.

The basic diet in the more common lipid

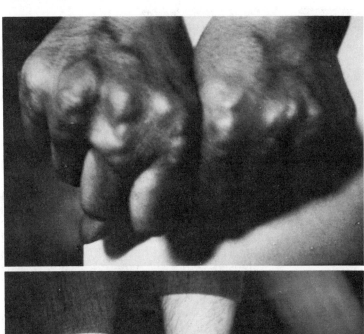

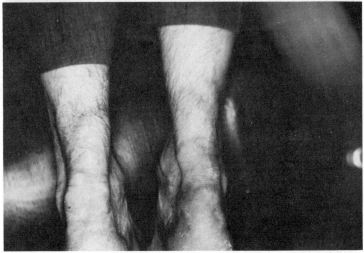

Fig. 22-2. Thickening of tendons (tendon xanthomas) occurs in patients with hyperlipidemia, especially type II. (Hodges RE: Nutrition in Medical Practice. Philadelphia, WB Saunders, 1980)

disorders is low in cholesterol (200 mg a day or less), low in total fat (20–25% of total kilocalories), and low in saturated fat (5–10% of total kilocalories). It is high in complex carbohydrates (starches). Moderate amounts of polyunsaturated fats are included; diets high in polyunsaturated fat are not recommended.

Table 22-2 lists foods allowed and foods prohibited in the basic diet. The amounts of meat, fish, poultry, and fats permitted depend upon the calorie, fat, and cholesterol levels ordered by the physician. The diet provides only enough calories to maintain ideal weight or may be reduced in calories if weight loss is desired.

Although each of the diet changes listed above is discussed separately in this chapter, one diet includes all of these modifications. All parts of the diet work together to bring about desired lowering of blood fats.

Table 22-3 summarizes the types of changes that are useful in reducing elevated blood cholesterol levels.

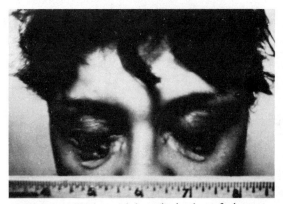

Fig. 22-3. Cholesterol deposits in the soft tissues around the eye are called *xanthelasma* and are an indication for lipid studies. (Hodges RE: Nutrition in Medical Practice. Philadelphia, WB Saunders, 1980)

Total Fat Reduction

Studies of population groups indicate that those with a low fat intake have lower blood lipid levels and a lower incidence of coronary heart disease than those with a high fat intake. In the average American diet, fat constitutes 42% of total calories. Reducing fat intake to 20% to 25% of total calories requires a considerable change in eating habits.

Restricted Fat Diet. Only lean, well-trimmed meats containing 15% fat or less are permitted. Table 22-4 lists the percentage of fat in various meat products. Meats that are well marbled (with fat distributed throughout the lean) must be carefully trimmed of fat before being cooked to meet the 15% fat limit. Poultry skin should be removed before the poultry is cooked. The

Table 22-2. Low-Cholesterol Fat-Controlled Diet for Hyperlipidemia

Food Group	Foods Allowed	Foods to Avoid
Beverages	Skim milk, buttermilk, coffee, tea, decaffeinated coffee, cereal beverages, cocoa made with skim milk, carbonated beverages	Whole, 2%, or 1% milk; cream; Half-and-Half
Breads	Enriched white and whole-grain breads, breadsticks, English muffins, melba toast, rusk, Syrian bread, tortillas, zwieback; hot breads, pancakes, and waffles made with egg substitute or egg white and allowed fats (count as part of daily fat allowance); crackers: graham, matzo, saltine, soda, other low-fat crackers	High-fat dinner rolls; egg or cheese breads; commercial biscuits, muffins, quick breads, doughnuts, sweet rolls, biscuit or quick-bread mixes; commercial pancakes or waffles; high-fat party crackers
Cereals	All except those to avoid	Granola, cereals with coconut or high levels of fat
Desserts	Fruits, fruit whips made with egg white, gelatin, fruit ices, ice pops, low-fat frozen desserts (1 g fat per serving), sherbet, commercial angel food cake, arrowroot cookies, ginger snaps, vanilla wafers, animal crackers, sugar or waffle ice cream cones, canned fruit pie fillings, pudding mixes prepared with skim milk The following are permitted if made with allowed ingredients and if fat is counted in daily allotment: cakes, pies, cookies, pastries	Most commercial cookies, cakes, pie, or pastries; ice cream; ice milk; nondairy ice cream; desserts containing chocolate, butter, cocoa butter, or coconut; pudding made with egg or milk other than skim; cookie and cake (except angel food cake) mixes

Table 22-2.   *(continued)*

Food Group	Foods Allowed	Foods to Avoid
Eggs	Egg whites, cholesterol-free egg substitutes (quantity limited because of fat content)	Egg yolk, whole egg, egg substitutes containing cholesterol
Fats	Margarine with a P/S ratio equal to or greater than 1; vegetable oils, including corn, soy, cottonseed, safflower, peanut; salad dressings: commercial or homemade French, Italian, Western, vinegar and oil, mayonnaise type, buttermilk and mayonnaise, thousand island; polyunsaturated-fat coffee creamers; peanut butter; nuts; olives *(amount of fat limited)**	Butter; margarine containing animal fat or with a P/S ratio less than 1; hydrogenated shortening or oil; oils: olive, coconut, palm, palm kernel, oils used for restaurant frying; lard; bacon fat; other animal fat; salad dressings: blue cheese, green goddess, other containing cheese, whole milk, or sour cream; creamers containing saturated fat; sour cream; cocoa butter
Fruits, fruit juices	All	None
Meat, fish, poultry	Lean (15% fat or less) beef, pork, veal, lamb; chicken and turkey with skin removed; fish, clams, scallops, oysters, lobster, water-packed tuna *(amount of meat, fish and poultry limited)** (All meat, fish, and poultry should be trimmed of visible fat before cooking, and baked, broiled, roasted, stewed, or steamed to eliminate excess fat)	All meat with more than 15% fat; duck; goose; poultry skin; shrimp; oil-packed fish; caviar; organ meats (liver, kidney, heart, sweetbreads); creamed or commercially fried meat, fish, or poultry; meat canned in gravy or sauce
Cheese	Rinsed cottage cheese, sapsago, special cheese containing no more than 1% fat	Whole or part skim-milk cheese (some may be substituted for allowed meat servings), cream cheese, filled cheese
Potatoes or substitutes	White and sweet potatoes, macaroni, spaghetti, rice, hominy, cornmeal, cholesterol-free egg noodles, homemade noodles if made with egg substitute or egg white	Egg noodles; potato chips, corn chips, or similar products
Soups	Broth-base canned or homemade soups if made with allowed ingredients and if fat is counted in daily fat allotment, tomato if made with skim milk or water	Commercial cream soups; chowder or other soups made with cream, whole milk, or butter
Sugar, sweets	Sugar, hard candy, gum drops, marshmallows, syrups (including chocolate), honey, jam, jelly, marshmallow creme	Chocolate candy, white chocolate, commercial fudge or other high-fat candies, chocolate or butterscotch sauce
Vegetables, vegetable juices	All if prepared with allowed foods	None except those prepared or packaged with foods to avoid
Miscellaneous	Mustard; catsup; steak sauces; gravy made with fat-free broth, skim milk, and margarine or made from dry mixes containing only allowed foods; cocoa powder	Conventional gravy, commercially prepared popcorn, whipped toppings

(After *Recent Advances in Therapeutic Nutrition,* pp 66–68. Ames, Iowa State University Press, 1979)
* Amount of meat, fish, poultry, and fat limited according to the calorie, fat, and cholesterol level desired.

Table 22-3. Dietary Goals in the Treatment of Elevated Serum Cholesterol

Weight control to achieve normal weight

Reduction of total fat intake to approximately 20% or 25% of calories; saturated fat reduced to 5% to 10% percent of total calories

Reduction of cholesterol to 200 mg/day or lower

Moderate increase in polyunsaturated fat to a level equal to that of saturated fat in the diet

amount of meat permitted is also limited to a specific amount, depending on the total caloric intake and degree of fat restriction. In some diets, fish, poultry, and veal may be emphasized while meats with a higher fat content—beef, lamb, ham, and pork—may be limited. Very fatty meats, such as frankfurters, luncheon meats, sausage, bacon, duck, and fish canned in oil, are avoided entirely. Meat should be baked or broiled on a rack to drain off fat. Barbecuing and pan broiling are also acceptable methods. In pan broiling, the meat fat should be drained off as it accumulates in the pan. Pan frying and deep fat frying must be avoided.

Table 22-4. Percentage of Fat in Meat Products

Recommended		Not Recommended	
Variety Meats			
(% fat)		(% fat)	
3.5	Cold cuts: low-fat, dried, or pressed meat or poultry (*special low-fat brands*)	16	Salami (kosher)
4	Venison, rabbit, squirrel, and other wild game	19.8	Vienna sausage
		22	Headcheese
4.1	Horsemeat	23.2	Sausage (knockwurst)
5.2	Guinea hen, pheasant, others with or without skin; wild duck, squab, and other wild game without skin	25.8	Polish sausage, bratwurst
		27.2	Frankfurters (average, cooked)
		27.4	Braunschweiger
14.5	Opossum, raccoon	27.5	Bologna, cooked salami, or similar cold cuts (nonkosher)
15	Turkey variety meats (*special low-fat brands*)	30	Frankfurters (cooked, all beef, kosher)
		38.1	Salami (dried, hard), pepperoni
		44.1	Sausage (link, cooked)
		44.2	Sausage (patty, cooked)
Fresh Pork			
(% fat)		(% fat)	
10	Leg (fresh ham), trimmed: rump, center, or shank	30	Leg (fresh ham), untrimmed: whole, rump, center, or shank
10	Leg, trimmed: cube steak	30	Loin, untrimmed: roast or chops (blade, rib, center, top loin, sirloin); tenderloin
15	Loin, trimmed: roast or chops (blade, rib, center, top loin, sirloin); tenderloin	30	Pork, ground
15	Shoulder, trimmed: arm picnic, roast or steak; blade Boston, roast or steak	30	Shoulder, untrimmed: arm picnic, roast or steak; blade Boston, roast or steak
		40	Spare ribs
		40	Loin back ribs, country style

Table 22-4. *(continued)*

Recommended		Not Recommended	
Beef			
(% fat)		(% fat)	
6	Beef, chipped or dried	20	Chuck, untrimmed: pot roast, steak, or ground
6	Flank steak, plain, cubed, or rolled	25	Ground beef
6	Round, trimmed: bottom round roast or steak	30	Brisket, fresh
6	Shank, center cut, trimmed	30	Corned beef brisket, canned corned beef
10	Chuck, trimmed: arm pot roast or steak	30	Pastrami
10	Loin, trimmed: porterhouse, sirloin, and T-bone steaks; tenderloin roast, steak, or tips	30	Regular hamburger
		30	Loin, untrimmed: porterhouse, sirloin, and T-bone steaks
10	Loin, trimmed: top loin (Kansas City, club) and top sirloin steaks	30	Loin, untrimmed: tenderloin, roast, steak, or tips; top loin steak (Kansas City, club); top sirloin steak
10	Plate ribs, short ribs, spare ribs, trimmed		
10	Plate skirt steak, boneless, cubed, rolled, trimmed	30	Plate ribs, short ribs, spare ribs, untrimmed
15	Ground round	30	Rib eye, untrimmed, roast or steak (Delmonico)
15	Round, untrimmed: bottom round roast or steak, corned beef	30	Rib roast or steak, untrimmed
15	Rib eye, trimmed: roast or steak (Delmonico)	30	Shank, center cut, untrimmed
15	Rib roast or steak, trimmed		
Pork, Smoked and Cured			
(% fat)		(% fat)	
10	Ham, trimmed: center slices, rump, shank	17	Canadian bacon, untrimmed
15	Canadian bacon, trimmed	20	Ham, untrimmed: center slices, rump, shank
15	Pickled pigs' feet	25	Shoulder picnic or roll, untrimmed
15	Loin, trimmed: roast or chops	30	Loin, untrimmed, roast or chops
15	Shoulder picnic or roll, trimmed	30	Ham, deviled, canned
		35	Ham, country style, dry cure, untrimmed
		35	Hock, jowl, neckbones
		40	Ribs, loin back or spare ribs
		50	Bacon, regular, sliced
		70	Salt pork, cooked
		85	Salt pork, raw

(Developed for the Coronary Primary Prevention Trial by the Iowa Lipid Research Clinic, Nutrition Section. Adapted from Recent Advances in Therapeutic Diets, pp 68–70. Ames, Iowa State University Press, 1979)

Milk fat in any form — whole milk, cream, butter, cheese, ice-cream — is avoided. Some low-fat dairy products may be substituted for small amounts of lean meat. Skim milk is used. Cheese is restricted to kinds that are very low in fat, such as rinsed cottage cheese, sapsago cheese, and specially prepared dietetic cheese containing up to 1% fat. Egg yolks are omitted entirely because of their high cholesterol content.

Separated polyunsaturate fats, such as vegetable oils, margarine, and mayonnaise, are permitted in small amounts. The quantity allowed depends upon the total fat content of the diet and includes the amount used in cooking as well as at the table. Suggestions for flavoring foods in the absence of fat are found in Chapter 20.

Fruits (except avocado); vegetables (except olives); cereals products such as bread, rice, macaroni, and breakfast cereals; and sugars are free of fat or contain only negligible amounts. These foods are allowed as desired unless calories are restricted or carbohydrate is controlled.

Baked goods made with permitted ingredients may be used if the fat in them is counted as part of the daily amount.

Decreased Saturated Fat - Molderately Increased Polyunsaturated Fat Diet

Saturated fatty acids tend to increase blood cholesterol levels, whereas polyunsaturated fatty acids tend to lower blood cholesterol levels. Monounsaturated fatty acids (neutral fats) have a neutral effect, neither raising nor lowering blood cholesterol levels.

Diets in which saturated fat is decreased and polyunsaturated fat is increased are called *fat-controlled* or *fat-modified diets.* The expression *P/S ratio* is frequently used in connection with these diets. It refers to the total amount of polyunsaturated fat in relation to the total amount of saturated fat in the diet. A ratio of 1 : 1 means that the amount of polyunsaturated fat is equal to the amount of saturated fat. Diets very high in polyunsaturated fats in which the P/S ratio is greater than 1.5 : 1, are not recommended.

Saturated fats are decreased by the use of only lean, well-trimmed meats and by the limitation of meat, fish, and poultry to specific amounts. Skim milk and skim milk products are substituted for whole milk and whole milk products such as cream, butter, ice cream, and cheese. Foods containing coconut oil, palm oil, or cocoa butter, which are highly saturated, are avoided. Coconut oil and palm oil are used in commercial products such as nondairy creamers, nondairy whipped toppings, and baked goods. Hydrogenated fats such as vegetable shortening and regular margarines are also omitted.

Polyunsaturated fats are increased by the use of polyunsaturated oils in cooking and in salad dressings and by the use of margarines with a P/S ratio equal to or greater than 1 : 1 (those containing at least as much polyunsaturated as saturated fat). Safflower oil is the highest in polyunsaturated fat. Corn, sunflower, soybean, and cottonseed oils also contain a high percentage. Peanut oil is acceptable in diets in which polyunsaturated fats are only moderately increased. Olive oil is avoided, since it adds fat without lowering cholesterol.

Cholesterol Reduction

A low-cholesterol diet is used in combination with a fat-controlled diet. Restriction of total fat and saturated fat, increased intake of polyunsaturated fat, and restriction of cholesterol work together to reduce blood cholesterol levels. *Cholesterol restriction* may be severe — less than 300 mg — or moderate — 300 mg to 500 mg. The customary diet in the United States contains 800 mg to 1000 mg or more of cholesterol per day.

Cholesterol is obtained from animal foods only. Egg yolks, organ meats such as liver, brains, and sweetbreads, are especially high. One egg yolk contains 250 mg of cholesterol; a 3-ounce portion of liver contains 370 mg. Meat, fish, poultry, and dairy products contain significant amounts.

On a cholesterol-restricted diet, lean muscle meats, poultry, fish, and shellfish (except shrimp) are permitted in limited amounts.

Skim milk and skim milk products replace whole milk products, and margarine is used in place of butter. Egg yolk, organ meats, and shrimp are omitted entirely or are severely limited, depending on the level of cholesterol restriction.

Calorie Restriction

Reducing to ideal weight or maintaining ideal weight is a priority in most lipoprotein disorders. Weight reduction in many cases reduces serum lipid levels.

Carbohydrate and Alcohol Restriction

Triglycerides are produced in the liver from carbohydrate and alcohol. In some persons, even moderate amounts of alcohol increase serum triglyceride levels. Alcohol is eliminated or strictly limited when serum triglycerides are elevated.

Even in diets in which carbohydrate constitutes 50% or more of total calories, triglycerides can usually be controlled as long as calories are not excessive and the carbohydrates are mostly complex. In some cases, carbohydrates are more severely restricted.

Implementation of the Diet

Exchange Lists for Fat-Controlled Diets

For clients for whom calories and/or carbohydrate is not restricted, a diet such as the low-cholesterol fat-controlled diet described in Table 22-2 may be followed. However, many clients with hyperlipidemia require calorie restriction to achieve or maintain ideal weight, and some require carbohydrate restriction. In these cases, the exchange list system is more suitable.

The Exchange Lists for Meal Planning (Table A-2 in the Appendix) may be used. Only skim milk, skim milk products, and lean meat exchanges are used. Choices on the fat exchange list are limited to those that are polyunsaturated; animal fats are omitted. Foods high in

cholesterol, such as egg yolks and organ meats, are limited or omitted.

Buying and Preparing Food for the Fat-Controlled Diet

Certain nutrition information must be provided on the labels of margarine about which a diet claim is made. If it is implied that a product is high in polyunsaturated fat, the ratio of polyunsaturated fat to saturated fat must be stated on the label. Margarine with a P/S ratio of 1 : 1 or more is readily available.

Commercial products containing fat should be used cautiously. Even those that state "vegetable fat," "containing no animal fat," or "nondairy" may have to be avoided. These products frequently contain coconut oil or hydrogenated vegetable fats, which are highly saturated. Most convenience foods cannot be used unless the cholesterol content, fat content, and fatty acid composition are listed on the label and are compatible with the client's diet.

Cholesterol-free egg substitutes and meat substitutes, low-cholesterol filled cheeses (skim milk cheese with added vegetable oil), and dietetic cheese products containing only 1% fat are available. The nutrition labels on these products must list the total fat, fatty acid composition, and cholesterol content per serving. Unfortunately, many of these products have a high sodium content and cannot be used by clients who must also restrict sodium. Cheeses high in polyunsaturated fat are not suitable for low-fat diets unless the fat is counted in the daily allotment. When in doubt as to the suitability of a particular food, consult the dietitian.

Mixed dishes and baked goods can be made at home with permitted ingredients. Egg whites or egg substitutes can be substituted for egg yolks in French toast, custard, and baked goods. Evaporated skim milk or triple-strength skim milk made from powdered skim milk can replace coffee cream. Fat-free buttermilk can be mixed with dry cottage cheese and flavored with spices and chopped vegetables and fruit to make dips and salad dressings. The use of wine marinades can improve the flavor and moistness of meat. The hospital dietitian, community diet counselor, or public health nutritionist can be

of assistance in recommending reliable cookbooks.

Client Education

Dietary treatment for the various types of hyperlipoproteinemias requires a considerable change in the client's food habits. Some types of hyperlipoproteinemia, such as type IIa (elevated cholesterol), may be inherited, so it is a common practice to screen the client's family. If the children are found to have abnormal lipoprotein patterns, the food habits of the entire family may have to be modified. For persons who are accustomed to home-cooked meals and are interested in cooking or have family members who are interested in cooking, the change is easier. In contrast, the change is difficult for persons who are used to convenience foods or who eat many meals in restaurants.

If the person who buys and/or prepares the food is someone other than the client, this person should be present for the diet history and all diet instruction. In most cases, changes will have to be made in food buying and food preparation practices. The media have made the term *polyunsaturates* familiar to Americans. However, the problem is often oversimplified, concentrating on isolated foods, such as butter vs. special margarine, while disregarding important aspects of the problem. Misconceptions gained from television, magazines, and so on have to be corrected.

KEYS TO PRACTICAL APPLICATION

There is much reason to believe that persons with high blood cholesterol levels are more likely than normal to develop coronary heart disease. The value of treatment is greatest in the age groups below 55 to 60 years of age. Help your client believe in the importance of reducing risk.

Emphasize the importance of weight loss. Weight reduction is the most important factor in reducing moderately elevated blood triglyceride levels.

Assure your client that, in most cases, cholesterol can be lowered by dietary treatment.

Remember that reducing cholesterol in the diet is not the only factor involved in lowering blood cholesterol. Reducing total fat and saturated fat levels and moderately increasing polyunsaturated fat levels are also important.

Be understanding of the objections of your client to the dietary changes required of him to correct hyperlipidemia. Reducing fat intake to 20% to 25% from approximately 42% of total calories in the average American diet requires a considerable change. However, emphasize that dietary treatment is preferable to drug treatment.

Concentrate on the positive aspects of the required diet change. Fat- and cholesterol-modified meals can be tasty and nutritious; acceptable substitutes can often be found for well-liked foods that must be omitted. Seek the help of a dietitian in assisting the client to become creative in meal planning and food preparation.

Remember that meat contains considerable amounts of fat. When reducing fat in the diet, give special attention to the selection of meat and preparation techniques that reduce the fat in meat, and to portion sizes.

Consult the dietitian about the suitability of low-cholesterol or dietetic foods for a particular cholesterol-lowering diet. A food may be low in cholesterol but high in saturated fat, excessively high in polyunsaturated fat (when total fat is limited), or high in sodium.

KEY IDEAS

Complications of atherosclerosis are the greatest cause of death in the United States.

Elevated blood lipid levels, elevated blood sugar, and obesity are diet-related risk factors in cardiovascular disease.

The higher the level of blood cholesterol, the greater the risk of coronary heart disease; moderately elevated triglyceride levels are a risk factor for some persons.

Elevated blood lipids may be an inherited disorder or may be due to other factors, such as diabetes, obesity, and food habits.

Cholesterol and triglycerides are insoluble in water. They are transported in the blood by protein. These combinations of protein and lipids are called *lipoproteins.* There are four types of lipoprotein.

Hyperlipoproteinemia (or hyperlipidemia) indicates that one or more of the lipoprotein groups are present at greater than normal levels.

Most of the cholesterol in the plasma is carried by two lipoprotein groups: low-density lipoprotein (LDL) and high-density lipoprotein (HDL). Persons with high amounts of HDL cholesterol have a lower risk of heart disease than those with low HDL levels.

Six types of lipoprotein disorders have been identified. Each is characterized by an excessive amount of one or more of the four lipoprotein groups. Four types are associated with increased risk of early coronary heart disease.

Diet can reduce elevated blood lipids, and is the basic treatment for hyperlipidemia.

It has not been proved that lowering cholesterol levels by diet or drugs prevents the development of cardiovascular disease; however, this result appears logical.

The basic diet for treating elevated serum cholesterol is reduced to a fat composition of 20% to 25% of total calories, to a cholesterol level of 100 mg to 200 mg, and to a saturated fat level of 5% to 10% of total calories. The diet is increased moderately in polyunsaturated fat to a level equal to the amount of saturated fat in the diet. Calories are controlled so as to reduce to ideal weight or maintain ideal weight.

Dietary treatment for hyperlipidemia requires considerable and permanent change in usual American eating habits.

Diet counseling is necessary to assist the client and his family in making the required changes in food habits. Substitutes are suggested for favorite foods whenever possible. Food preparation techniques that allow food to retain moisture and that provide flavor for the restricted fat diet are helpful.

KEYS TO LEARNING: STUDY–DISCUSSION QUESTIONS

1. The cholesterol in food is not the only source of cholesterol in the body. What is the other source? What dietary changes are made to lower blood cholesterol levels?
2. Write a menu for 2 days for a client on the low-cholesterol fat-controlled diet.

Assume the client is limited to 7 ounces of lean meat and 5 fat exchanges (use the polyunsaturated fat exchanges in the Exchange Lists for Meal Planning, Table A-2 in the Appendix).

In class, discuss any problems you encountered in completing this

assignment. In your opinion, what aspects of this diet would be most difficult for the client to accept?

3. Discuss food buying practices and food preparation techniques aimed at reducing saturated fat in meat and poultry.

4. Reducing fat from 42% of total calories (the approximate level of fat consumption in the United States) to the 20% to 25% of total calories required by the fat-controlled diet involves drastic changes in food preparation. Discuss ways of making food flavorful without the addition of fat.

5. What advice would you give a client who is on a low-fat, low-cholesterol, fat-controlled diet about the purchase of commercial products and convenience foods? Would all foods containing vegetable fat or labeled *low cholesterol* be acceptable? Explain your answer.

6. What changes are made to reduce the cholesterol content of the diet?

Bibliography is found at the end of Part Four.

23

Cardiovascular Disease: Hypertension, Congestive Heart Failure, Acute Illness

---

KEY TERMS

acute   Severe: occurring suddenly.
ascites   Excessive accumulation of fluid in the abdominal cavity.
congestive heart failure   Failure of the heart to maintain an adequate output causing reduced blood flow to the tissues; the result is a disproportionate amount of blood

accumulating in the lungs or the systemic circulation.
edema   Accumulation of fluid in the tissues.
hypertension   Abnormally high blood pressure.
pulmonary edema   Fluid accumulation in the lungs.

Clients with cardiovascular disease usually require some type of modified diet. The obese ones are placed on calorie-restricted diets. Achievement of ideal weight or somewhat below ideal weight is an essential part of treatment. Weight loss reduces the workload of the heart and also tends to reduce blood lipid levels. Clients with edema and hypertension may require sodium restriction, and those whose blood lipid levels are elevated are given fat-controlled diets (see Chap. 22). Any associated condition such as diabetes or kidney disease must also be considered. Frequently, the diet ordered is a combination of two or more modifications, such as a 1500-kcal, 2000-mg sodium diet.

Common Cardiovascular Disorders

Hypertension

Hypertension, or high blood pressure, places heavy stress on the heart and other organs, including brain, eye, and kidney. Undetected and uncontrolled hypertension contributes to the occurrence of heart attacks, heart failure, stroke, renal failure, and aortic aneurysm. In

about 85% of cases, the cause of the hypertension is unknown. In such cases, the disorder is referred to as *essential* or *primary hypertension.* In the remaining cases, the hypertension is secondary to another disorder such as disease of the kidney or adrenal glands.

Congestive Heart Failure

Congestive heart failure occurs when the heart loses a significant amount of its normal pumping power and is unable to pump blood efficiently. Congestive failure results from injury to the heart muscle due to atherosclerosis, infarction, hypertension, a birth defect, or rheumatic fever. The oxygen supply becomes inadequate because blood flow to the lungs is slowed. There is shortness of breath and chest pain with exertion.

The slowed circulation causes more fluid than normal to escape from the capillaries into the tissue spaces, where it is held rather than being returned to the circulation. Sodium excretion is reduced because blood flow to the kidney is diminished. Thus, sodium accumulates and causes further fluid retention.

Conditions Requiring Sodium Restriction

The Food and Nutrition Board of the National Research Council–National Academy of Sciences has estimated a safe and adequate level of sodium to be 1100 mg to 3300 mg for adults. Normally, excess sodium is excreted by the kidney in the urine or lost in perspiration, but in some illnesses, sodium is retained. When this happens, edema or hypertension or both may follow.

Edema

Normally, the body maintains a constant ratio of sodium to water. When this balance is upset, with more sodium retained, more fluid is also retained. Most of the excess sodium and fluid accumulates in the extracellular spaces (outside the cells). When fluid retention becomes visible, the condition is called *edema.* Swelling of the fingers and ankles and puffiness around the eyes are characteristic of edema. Sometimes fluid accumulates in the lungs (pulmonary edema) or in the abdominal cavity (ascites). Because of this close association between fluid and sodium, sodium restriction is effective in treating conditions in which too much fluid is retained.

Diuretics are prescribed to increase fluid and sodium excretion. Digitalis strengthens the contractions of the heart, and this promotes fluid and sodium excretion. In mild heart failure, sodium restriction alone may effectively prevent edema.

Hypertension

Hypertension is influenced by many factors, including heredity, race, body weight, activity level, cigarette smoking, psychological stress, and diet. Because the cause of essential hypertension is unknown, the methods used to prevent and treat it are controversial. There is wide agreement that achieving and maintaining ideal weight is very important in treating hypertension. However, there is controversy about the relationship of sodium to the prevention and treatment of the disorder.

For some time, sodium restriction has been prescribed in the treatment of hypertension. Its possible effectiveness has been attributed to a reduction of fluid volume and to the effects of decreased levels of sodium in sodium-sensitive persons. A moderate restriction of sodium appears to produce small decreases in blood pressure among one third to one half of hypertensives who are salt-sensitive. Yet there is increasing evidence that other nutrient substances, such as calcium, potassium, and magnesium, may have equal or more important roles in the development of hypertension.

Sources of Sodium

Food

Sodium Naturally Present in Food

Animal foods such as meat, fish, poultry, milk, and eggs have the highest natural sodium content. Milk is surprisingly high in sodium, 120 mg per 8-ounce cup, compared with fruit, which has 2 mg per ½-cup serving. Fruits contain very little sodium, and vegetables range from low to relatively high in natural sodium. Insignificant amounts are found in animal fats, vegetable oils, and cereal grains, provided no salt or sodium compound is added in processing or preparation.

Diets both high in protein (2–3 g per kg of body weight) and severely restricted in sodium (1000 mg or less) are difficult to carry out because of the high natural sodium content of animal protein foods. Special low-sodium milk may need to be used.

Sodium Added to Food

Table salt and other sodium-containing compounds used in food preservation and processing and in cooking add much sodium to the average diet (Fig. 23-1). A 3-ounce portion of fresh cooked pork contains 59 mg of sodium; an equal portion of cured cooked ham contains 1114 mg of sodium.

Table salt (sodium chloride) is 40% sodium. One level teaspoon of table salt contains approximately 2000 mg of sodium. Because moderately sodium-restricted diets limit the total amount of sodium in all food and beverages taken in a day to a total of 1000 mg to 2000 mg, it is evident that salt must be omitted from the diet or used in only very limited quantities.

The same holds true for monosodium glutamate (MSG); 1 level teaspoon contains approximately 500 mg of sodium. Salt, MSG, and other sodium compounds are used extensively in the commercial processing and preservation of food. Sodium added in this way is the greatest source of sodium in food.

The sodium content of some processed foods such as ham or potato chips is obvious. However, the sodium content of most processed foods is not quite so apparent. A few examples of these less obvious sodium additives are sodium alginate, which produces a smooth texture in ice cream and chocolate milk drinks; a salt solution, which is used in the sorting of frozen peas during processing; and sodium benzoate, which is a preservative used in some jellies.

Most canned foods, packaged mixes, frozen dinners, frozen vegetables with sauces and seasonings added, frozen waffles, pizza, and other convenience foods have sodium added in one form or another. Table 23-1 shows the sodium content of selected foods.

Water

In some communities, drinking water may have a high sodium content, as much as 200 mg or more per liter. Water softeners installed in the home add sodium. The local health department or local heart association can provide information about the sodium content of water in a particular community. In some cases, the use of distilled water may be necessary.

Medicines

The client should consult his physician before taking any unprescribed medicine or home remedy. Alkalizers for indigestion, headache remedies, cough medicines, laxatives, and others may contain sodium. A commonly used antacid contains 700 mg of sodium per dose. Home remedies such as bicarbonate of soda (sodium bicarbonate) and rhubarb and soda are high in sodium. (Chewing tobacco also contains sodium; a 2-oz plug contains approximately 960 mg.)

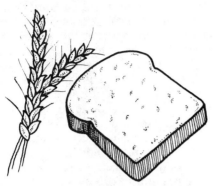

A slice of regular bread contains about 125 mg of sodium.

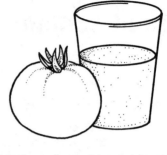

A half cup of canned tomato juice contains about 440 mg of sodium.

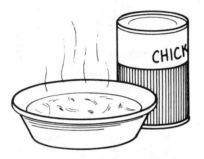

One cup of chicken noodle soup (canned, condensed, diluted with water) contains 1100 mg of sodium.

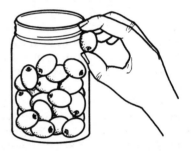

Just one large olive contains 130 mg of sodium.

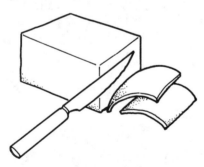

One ounce of processed American cheese contains about 400 mg sodium.

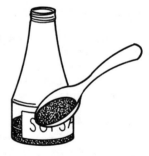

One tablespoon of soy sauce contains 1000 mg of sodium.

Fig. 23-1.   Processed foods add much sodium to the diet.

Table 23-1. Sodium Content of Selected Foods

Food	Amount	Sodium (mg)
Milk, whole, skim, or unsalted buttermilk	1 cup	122
Cultured salted buttermilk	1 cup	257
Vanilla ice cream	1 cup	105
Vanilla milkshake, thick	11 oz	317
Beef, cooked, lean	3 oz	55
Liver, calf, fried	3 oz	99
Kidney, beef, braised	3 oz	214
Corned beef	3 oz	802
Shad, baked with butter	3 oz	66
Shrimp, fried	3 oz	159
Shrimp, canned	3 oz	1955
Cheddar cheese	1 oz	176
American cheese	1 oz	406
Bleu cheese	1 oz	396
Cottage cheese	¼ cup	230
Cottage cheese, unsalted dry-curd	¼ cup	7
Green beans, frozen	½ cup	3
Chard, cooked	½ cup	71
Sauerkraut	½ cup	777
Apple	1	2
Cantaloupe	¼ melon	12
Bread, white	1 slice	114
Bread, low-sodium	1 slice	7
Cornflakes	1 cup	256
Puffed wheat	2 cups	2
Biscuit made with milk from mix	1	272
Toaster pastry, apple, frosted	1	324
Macaroni	½ cup	1
Stuffing mix, cooked	½ cup	527
Butter, salted	1 tbsp	116
Butter, unsalted	1 tbsp	2
Oil, vegetable	1 tbsp	0
Mayonnaise	1 tbsp	78
French dressing, bottled	1 tbsp	214

(The Sodium Content of your Food. USDA Home and Garden Bulletin 233. Washington, DC, U.S. Government Printing Office, 1980)

Sodium-Restricted Diets

Diet therapy aims to achieve the following: the prescribed level of sodium; adequate nutrients to meet nutritional needs; a diet that respects the client's personal food preferences and is practical and realistic; other diet modifications that may be necessary.

Diet Prescription

A sodium-restricted diet limits the amount of sodium from food and fluids to a level prescribed by the physician. The sodium level in such a diet may be as low as 200 mg or as high as 4500 mg. The physician's diet prescription will be written in grams, milligrams or milliequivalents* of sodium, stating the amount of sodium he wants the client to have each day.

The use of terms such as *low salt, salt-free,* or *salt-poor* is discouraged, since these terms do not accurately convey the level of sodium desired. The terms also falsely give the impression that table salt is the only source of sodium that needs to be considered.

The general categories of sodium restriction are as follows: 250 mg, very severe restriction; less than 1000 mg, severe restriction; 1000 mg to 2000 mg, moderate restriction; 2400 mg to 4500 mg or more, mild restriction. Because the diuretics presently used are very effective, levels of 1000 mg to 3000 mg of sodium are most commonly prescribed.

Diets severely restricted in sodium, less than 1000 mg, include only the sodium that occurs naturally in food. Even then, foods such as milk, meat, fish, poultry, and eggs have to be limited to specific amounts. In contrast, diets containing 1000 mg to 4500 mg include some salt-containing foods and/or the use of salt in

* 1 mEq sodium = 23 mg; 45 mEq sodium = 1035 mg sodium (45 × 23)

small quantities, depending on the level of restriction and the client's preferences.

Sodium-restricted diets thus differ considerably, depending on the level of restriction. It is important that the health worker find out what level of sodium is involved before attempting to assist a client with his diet. Otherwise, efforts to help may just confuse him.

Exchange Lists

A widely used method of planning sodium-restricted diets is based on the exchange system. The Exchange Lists for Meal Planning (Table A-2 in the Appendix) can be adapted for use in sodium-restricted diets (Table 23-2). Table 23-3, which summarizes the sodium content of foods in the low-sodium exchange lists, shows the approximate amount of sodium that occurs naturally in foods.

In any particular diet, the client is permitted to have a specified number of exchanges (or units) from each list. He decides which food in each list he will eat. The amount permitted from each exchange depends on nutritional needs, level of sodium restriction, food preferences, and other diet modifications such as calorie restriction. A specific diet prescription, such as a limit of 1000 mg of sodium, may be planned in a variety of ways, depending on the client's nutritional needs and food preferences. Table 23-4 shows diet plans to accommodate various needs. Any variations must be carefully planned so that the nutritive adequacy of the diet is maintained. The client should be cautioned that any changes in his diet plan must be worked out with the dietitian or diet counselor.

Milk

Because of its relatively high natural sodium content, milk is usually limited to 2 cups per day on diets containing 500 mg to 1000 mg of sodium. Skim milk, homemade unsalted buttermilk, and reconstituted evaporated milk contain the same amount of sodium as fresh whole milk. Cultured, salted buttermilk is higher in sodium and is usually omitted. Ice cream, sherbet, fountain drinks such as shakes

Table 23-2. Adapting the Exchange Lists for Meal Planning to Suit Sodium-Restricted Diets

The changes listed below eliminate foods containing salt and other sodium additives from the Exchange Lists for Meal Planning.

Foods Allowed	Foods Omitted
List 1. Milk	
Skim, whole, evaporated	Commercial foods made with milk: chocolate milk, condensed milk, ice cream, malted milk, milk mixes, milk shakes, sherbet
List 2. Vegetables	
Fresh, frozen, or canned with no salt or other sodium compounds	Canned vegetables or juices, unless canned without salt and other sodium compounds; frozen peas and lima beans if processed with salt; sauerkraut; hominy; potato chips; may be excluded because of their high natural sodium content: artichokes, beet greens, celery, Swiss chard, dandelion greens, collards, kale, mustard greens, spinach, beets, carrots, white turnips
List 3. Fruits	
Fresh, frozen, canned, or dried	Crystallized or glazed fruit, maraschino cherries, dried fruit with sodium sulfite added
List 4. Bread	
Low-sodium breads, cereals, and cereal products: bread and rolls (yeast) made without salt; quick breads made with sodium-free baking powder or potassium bicarbonate and without salt or from low-sodium dietetic mix; cooked, unsalted cereals; puffed rice, puffed wheat, shredded wheat; barley; cornmeal; cornstarch; low-sodium crackers; matzo, plain, unsalted; yeast waffles	Yeast bread, rolls, or melba toast made with salt or from commercial mixes; quick breads made with baking powder, baking soda, salt, or monosodium glutamate or from commercial mixes; quick-cooking and enriched cereals that contain a sodium compound (read labels); dry cereals except as listed; graham crackers or any other except low-sodium dietetic; salted popcorn; self-rising cornmeal; pretzels; waffles containing salt, baking powder, baking soda, or egg white.
List 5. Meat	
Meat, poultry, fish, eggs, and low-sodium cheese and peanut butter; meat or poultry: fresh, frozen, or canned low-sodium; liver (only once in 2 weeks); tongue, fresh; fish or fish fillets, fresh only—bass, bluefish, catfish, cod, eels, flounder, halibut, rockfish, salmon, sole, trout, tuna; salmon, canned low-sodium dietetic; tuna, canned low-sodium dietetic; cheese, cottage, unsalted; cheese, processed low-sodium dietetic; egg (limit 1 per day); peanut butter, low-sodium dietetic.	Brains or kidneys; canned, salted, or smoked meat: bacon, bologna, chipped or corned beef, frankfurters, ham, kosher meats, luncheon meat, salt pork, sausage, smoked tongue; frozen fish fillets; canned, salted, or smoked fish: anchovies, caviar, salted and dried cod, herring, canned salmon (except dietetic low-sodium); shellfish—clams, crabs, lobsters, oysters, scallops, shrimp; cheese except low-sodium dietetic; egg substitutes, frozen or powdered; peanut butter unless low-sodium dietetic
List 6. Fat	
Spreads, oils, cooking fats, unsalted	Salted butter or margarine, bacon and bacon fat, salt pork, olives, commercial French or other dressings except low-sodium, commercial mayonnaise except low-sodium, salted nuts

Table 23-2. *(continued)*

Foods Allowed	Foods Omitted
Miscellaneous Foods*	
Beverages: alcoholic with doctor's permission; cocoa made with milk from diet; coffee, instant, freeze-dried, or regular; coffee substitutes; lemonade; Postum; tea	Fountain beverages: instant cocoa mixes; prepared beverage mixes, including fruit-flavored powders commercial candies, cakes, cookies; commercial sweetened gelatin desserts; mixes of all types; pastries; amounts of syrup, brown sugar may have to be limited because of sodium content
Candy, homemade, salt-free, or special low-sodium; gelatin, plain unflavored; sugar, white or brown; jelly; jam; honey; syrup	
Leavening Agents	
Cream of tartar, sodium-free baking powder, potassium bicarbonate, yeast; rennet dessert powder (not tablets)	Regular baking powder, baking soda (sodium bicarbonate); rennet tablets; pudding mixes; molasses

(After American Dietetic Association: Handbook of Clinical Dietetics, p G9–G11. New Haven, Yale University Press, 1981)

* Other miscellaneous foods given in Table 22-7

and malteds, chocolate milk, and instant cocoa mixes have sodium compounds added. Ice cream or sherbet can occasionally be substituted for an appropriate quantity of milk. Other fountain beverages and drinks are usually omitted in severe and moderate sodium restriction.

A special low-sodium milk is used on diets that restrict sodium to 250 mg. It contains more potassium than regular milk and therefore cannot be used if there is reason to restrict potassium, as in some kidney conditions.

Meat, Fish, Poultry

Unless there is a protein restriction, most diets permit at least 4 to 5 ounces of meat each day. Brain, kidney, and shellfish have a higher sodium content than other meat and fish.

It is surprising to many that saltwater fish (except the shellfish listed above) as well as freshwater fish may be used in the sodium-restricted diet. However, all fresh fish should be thoroughly rinsed before being cooked, because

Table 23-3.   Sodium Content of Low-Sodium Exchange Lists *

Food	Household Measure	Sodium (approx mg)
Milk exchanges, whole, low-fat, skim	8 oz (1 cup)	120
Milk, low-sodium	8 oz (1 cup)	7
Meat exchanges	1 oz	25
Egg	1	60
Vegetable exchanges	½ cup	9
Fruit exchanges	Varies	2
Bread exchanges, low-sodium	Varies	5
Fat exchanges, unsalted	Varies	Negligible

* Foods produced, processed, or prepared without the addition of any sodium compound.

Table 23-4. 1000-mg Sodium Diet Plans (Planned to Meet Different Needs)

Food	Adult Male Recovering from Surgery Additional protein, vitamins, minerals		Business Man More meat, ¼ tsp salt		Elderly Woman Ordinary bread	
	Amount	Sodium (approx mg)	Amount	Sodium (approx mg)	Amount	Sodium (approx mg)
Milk	1 qt	480	1 cup	120	2 cups	240
Meat	9 oz cooked	225	10 oz cooked	250	5 oz	125
Egg	1	60	1	60	1	60
Vegetables	4 servings	77*	2 servings	18	3 servings	27
Fruit	4 servings	8	3 servings	6	3 servings	6
Bread	8 exchanges	40	6 exchanges	30	3 unsalted exchanges	15
					3 salted bread	450
Fat	5 exchanges	—	4 exchanges	—	3 exchanges	—
			¼ tsp salt	500		
Totals		890		984		923

* Includes average sodium value of one serving of vegetables high in natural sodium.

fish is frequently transported to market in a salt solution. If possible, fresh fish that has not been put through a brine solution should be purchased. All salted, smoked, and canned meats, fish, and poultry are avoided, including ham, bacon, luncheon meats, and sausage.

Eggs and Cheese

Eggs are usually restricted to one a day. An egg contains 60 mg of sodium, almost 2½ times the sodium content of 1 ounce of meat. Most of the sodium is in the egg white.

Cheese is high in sodium. Processed cheeses such as American cheese, cheese food, and cheese spread have twice as much sodium as cheddar cheese (see Table 23-1). Some natural cheeses, such as Roquefort, bleu, feta, camembert, and gorgonzola, are more salty than others.

On diets with only mildly restricted sodium, limited amounts of natural cheese are usually permitted: processed cheeses and highly salted natural cheeses are usually avoided in all sodium-restricted diets. Low-sodium dietetic cheeses are available. Each product must be evaluated separately to determine the amount that can be substituted for meat. Regular salted cottage cheese, including low-fat varieties, is high in sodium. A ½-cup portion contains 450 mg of sodium. Unsalted, dry-curd cottage cheese is low in sodium and may be used even on diets of 500 mg of sodium if substituted for meat.

Vegetables

The natural sodium content of vegetables ranges from approximately 9 mg per ½ cup to 70 mg per ½ cup.

High-sodium vegetables (see Table 23-2) must be omitted on diets of 500 mg of sodium or less. It is possible to allow for limited quantities on diets above 500 mg of sodium.

Vegetables should be fresh, frozen, or canned without the addition of salt or other sodium compound.

Salt is usually not added to plain frozen vegetables. However, starchy vegetables such as peas and lima beans are frequently sorted in a brine solution before being frozen. Furthermore, frozen vegetables that have sauces, mushrooms, or nuts added are much higher in sodium than the plain varieties.

All regular canned vegetables and vegetable juices have salt added. On diets of 2000 mg to 3000 mg of sodium and above, clients can reduce the sodium content of canned vegetables by rinsing them in water, straining them, and reheating them in unsalted tap water.

Fruits

Most fruits are low in sodium, approximately 2 mg per serving. Small amounts of salt are sometimes added to frozen and canned fruits to prevent darkening, and some canned and frozen fruit, as well as canned tomatoes, are dipped in sodium hydroxide so they can be easily peeled. Sodium sulfite is frequently added to dried fruit.

Breads and Cereals

Cereal grains such as wheat flour, cornmeal, barley, and rice are low in natural sodium. However, when they are made into breads, breakfast cereals, and bakery products, salt and other sodium compounds are usually added (see Table 23-1).

Unsalted bread, unsalted matzo and unsalted melba toast are generally available in food markets. Regular crackers, even though made with unsalted tops, are made with a dough that contains salt and leavening agents that contain sodium. On moderately restricted sodium diets, regular salted bread and breadstuffs are frequently permitted in limited quantities.

Cooked cereals such as farina, oatmeal, and hominy grits are low in sodium if cooked without salt; but some quick-cooking and most instant varieties of these cereals have sodium compounds added. Check labels.

Puffed rice, puffed wheat, shredded wheat, wheat germ, and some brands of granola have no sodium added. Macaroni products, rice, tapioca, white and sweet potato, corn, and dried peas and beans are also low in sodium when prepared without salt or other sodium compounds.

Fat

Oils, unsalted butter, unsalted margarine, and unsalted nuts are very low in sodium (see Table 23-1).

Miscellaneous Foods

Sugar and honey have negligible amounts of sodium. Most artificial sweeteners are composed of sodium saccharin. One popular sweetener contains 3.5 mg of sodium in a 1-g packet, a very small amount.

Sodium compounds are added to such foods as beverage mixes, fountain beverages, commercial candies, molasses, corn syrup, commercial puddings, and gelatin desserts. Soft drinks may be high in sodium owing to the sodium content of the water in the area in which they are manufactured. Low-calorie beverages artificially sweetened with sodium saccharin contain additional sodium ranging from 5 mg to 12 mg more per 8 ounces than regular soda.

Most condiments and seasonings are high in sodium.

Most convenience foods have salt and other sodium compounds added. TV dinners, frozen vegetables in seasoned sauces, mixes for baked goods, meat extenders, meat substitutes made from textured vegetable protein, seasoned bread stuffing, packaged dinners, and flavored rice mixes are high in sodium.

Mild Sodium Restriction

The sodium level of a diet of mild sodium restriction may range from 2400 mg to 4500 mg. The foods permitted depend upon the sodium level ordered by the physician. Generally speaking, light salting of food is permitted, and foods processed with moderate amounts of sodium are permitted. Highly salted foods such as

Table 23-5. Foods High in Sodium Usually Omitted on All Sodium-Restricted Diets Unless Substitutions are Made

Salty or smoked meats, such as bacon, bologna, chipped beef or corned beef, frankfurters, ham, meats koshered by salting, luncheon meats, salt pork, sausage, smoked tongue

Salty or smoked fish, anchovies, caviar, salted and dried cod, herring, sardines

Processed cheese or cheese spreads unless low-sodium dietetic

Cheese, such as Roquefort, Camembert, Gorgonzola, processed cheese

Regular peanut butter

Sauerkraut, pickles, or other vegetables prepared in brine or heavily salted

Breads and rolls with salt toppings

Regular salted popcorn, potato chips, pretzels, and other heavily salted snack foods

Olives

Salted nuts

Party spreads and dips

Canned soups, stews, and any kind of commercial bouillon; instant soup mixes

Instant cocoa mixes

Cooking wine (contains added salt)

Pickles and relishes

Celery salt, garlic salt, and onion salt

Catsup, prepared mustard

Chili sauce

Commercial seasonings made of meat and vegetable extracts

Barbecue sauces and meat sauces

Meat tenderizers

Soy sauce

Worcestershire sauce

(After Your Mild Sodium-Restricted Diet. New York, American Heart Association, 1969)

those listed in Table 23-5 are omitted unless substitutions are made.

Client Education

Food Preparation

Many clients find it difficult to accept a sodium-restricted diet. The food may taste flat, and the thought of restricting favorite foods for the rest of their lives is unpleasant. Salt is a much over-worked seasoning. Clients may not be aware of the many other ways in which food may be seasoned and flavored. Spices, herbs, and other flavoring aids are listed in Table 23-6. Examples of how the low-sodium diet may be made more palatable follow.

Meat, fish, and poultry may be made more flavorful with the use of low-sodium marinades and sauces and with the use of fruit as a flavoring aid. Low-sodium mixtures of certain wines or vinegar, vegetable oil, and permitted herbs and spices may be used as a marinade for meat

Table 23-6.   Flavor Ideas for Sodium-Restricted Diets

Dependence on salt can be reduced by use of low-sodium flavoring aids in cooking. Other spices, herbs, tasty vegetables (onion, peppers, tomato), fruit, and wine can be used to enhance the flavor of food.

May be Used

Allspice	Nutmeg
Almond extract	Onion, fresh or powder (not onion salt)
Anise seed	Orange extract
Angostura bitters	Oregano
Basil	Paprika
Bay leaf	Parsley
Bouillon cubes (low-sodium)	Pepper
Caraway seeds	Peppermint extract
Cardamon	Poppy seeds
Chili powder	Poultry seasoning
Chives	Purslane
Cinnamon	Rosemary
Cloves	Saccharin
Cumin	Saffron
Curry	Sage
Dill	Salt substitutes (only with doctor's approval)
Fennel	Savory
Garlic	Sesame seeds
Ginger	Sugar*
Horseradish (prepared without salt)	Tarragon
Juniper	Thyme
Lemon juice or extract	Turmeric
Mace	Vanilla
Maple extract	Vinegar
Marjoram	Walnut extract
Mint	Wine (not cooking wine)
Mustard, dry powder	

Avoid

Baking soda	Mustard, prepared
Barbecue sauce	Olives
Bouillon cubes, regular	Onion salt
Catsup	Pickles
Celery salt	Relishes
Chili sauce	Salad dressings (commercial)
Garlic salt	Salt
Horseradish prepared with salt	Soy sauce
Meat sauces	Worcestershire sauce
Meat tenderizers	Cooking wine
Monosodium glutamate	

* Unless limited for other reasons such as weight control.

and poultry and as a basting mixture during meat preparation. Meat, fish, or poultry may be cooked in a low-sodium tomato sauce.

A sweet–sour sauce made of diluted vinegar and sugar and seasoned with grated onion, spices, and herbs can be used to flavor vegetables. A pinch of sugar added while vegetables are cooking can also enhance flavor. Herbs may be sprinkled on vegetables after cooking.

Appetizing baked goods can be made with yeast or low-sodium baking powder, unsalted fat, and other unsalted ingredients. Low-sodium dietetic baking powder is available in food stores. It is recommended that tested recipes from low-sodium cookbooks using low-sodium baking powder be followed rather than recipes from standard cookbooks.

It is essential that the person who is responsible for food preparation in the client's household receive diet instruction along with the client. The dietitian will be alert to cultural food habits that may interfere with the diet and will provide suggestions for modifying favorite cultural foods so that they may be included. The health worker will also need to know the food habits that are part of the client's cultural background so that she can give support to the instruction being provided (see Chap. 14).

Food Labels

The importance of reading food labels depends upon the level of sodium restriction the client is on. Clients on diets of severe or moderate sodium restriction need to avoid all or most foods that have sodium compounds added. These clients should be instructed to read the labels of all foods carefully. They should avoid products that list ingredients including any of the following terms: salt, sodium, Na, soda. In some cases, a few foods containing sodium may be worked into the diet.

Some foods, such as mayonnaise and catsup, are prepared under a standard of identity (see Chap. 17). Salt may not be listed on the label. The client should be made aware that these products contain added sodium.

Persons on mild sodium restriction may not be helped by reading labels unless the sodium content of the food is listed on the label. A diet form listing permitted foods may be more useful. Clients on mildly restricted diets are usually permitted to have some foods that contain small to moderate amounts of sodium. The USDA publication *The Sodium Content of Your Food** may be a useful guide.

Low-Sodium Dietetic Foods

Under federal regulations, labels on low-sodium dietetic foods must state the milligrams of sodium per serving.

For some clients, such foods as low-sodium dietetic tuna and salmon, low-sodium dietetic canned vegetables, low-sodium cheese, and low-sodium peanut butter may prove helpful. However, dietetic foods are usually more expensive than the regular foods they replace.

The client should not assume that all low-sodium dietetic foods can be included on his diet. Some "low-sodium" foods, although lower in sodium than regular food, may still contain too much to be included in a specific diet.

Salt Substitutes

Salt substitutes should be used only with the permission of the physician. The substitutes available in drug stores and food markets contain potassium or ammonium in place of sodium. In kidney disorders, potassium salt may be prohibited, and in severe liver disease, ammonium salt must be avoided. Lite-Salt[†] contains half the sodium of regular salt and cannot be used on severely restricted diets.

Eating Out

Persons on diets restricting sodium to 500 mg to 1000 mg can eat out occasionally and keep within their diets if they choose foods carefully. However, when meals are eaten in restaurants and cafeterias on a regular basis, a sodium level

---

* USDA Home and Garden Bulletin 233. Washington, DC, U.S. Government Printing Office, 1980
† Morton Salt Co, Chicago, IL

of 3000 mg to 5000 mg is necessary to achieve variety and nutritional balance (see Table 13-5).

Potassium Replacement

The long-continued use of certain diuretics (thiazides, furosemide, and ethacrynic acid) in the treatment of hypertension and water retention may cause excessive loss of potassium. Potassium is essential to life; if loss is severe, death may follow.

Potassium can be replaced by medication and/or liberal quantities of potassium-rich foods. It is preferable to avoid potassium deficiency by means of a high-potassium diet than to use potassium supplements. Potassium medication has an unpleasant taste and is irritating to the gastrointestinal tract.

Most fruits, fresh vegetables, dried peas, beans, and lentils, and unsalted meats are good sources of potassium that are low in sodium. A medium-sized banana and 1 cup of orange juice can add more than 800 mg of potassium to the diet. (Foods high in potassium are listed in Table 24-1.)

Educational Materials

Teaching aids such as recipe pamphlets and food lists are used to instruct clients in health care facilities. Booklets prepared by the American Heart Association may be obtained by the client through his physician. Diet plans, menu suggestions, food buying and food preparation ideas, and guides for eating out are included in these booklets. The physician obtains the booklets from the local chapter of the American Heart Association. A low-sodium cookbook entitled *Cooking Without the Salt Shaker** is available from local chapters of the American Heart Association.

* American Heart Association – Northeast Ohio Affiliate. Dallas, TX, American Heart Association, 1978.

Diet Modification in Acute Cardiovascular Disorders

Symptoms such as shortness of breath, fatigue, chest pain, and abdominal distention are frequent in acute stages of cardiovascular disease. The following diet changes are made to rest the heart as much as possible:

Calories are frequently restricted, even for clients who are not obese. These smaller meals reduce the workload of the heart.

A liquid diet is given for the first 24 hours or so, since liquids are easily digested. Only small amounts of liquids are given at one time. When his condition improves, the client progresses to a soft diet.

Foods that cause gaseous discomfort are avoided. Care must be taken to determine whether the client has an intolerance for milk causing gastric distress or diarrhea.

Very hot and very cold foods are avoided. Extremes of temperature can adversely affect the cardiac muscle.

Foods containing stimulants may increase the heart rate and are usually avoided.

Some clients may need to be fed to conserve their strength.

The majority of persons admitted to coronary care units have had acute myocardial infarctions. Regardless of the consistency of a client's diet—liquid, soft, or regular—foods are usually restricted in cholesterol and modified in fat. Sodium may also be restricted.

KEYS TO PRACTICAL APPLICATION

Be sure you know the restricted sodium diet your client is following before advising him about foods he can or cannot have. Low-sodium diets differ, depending on the sodium level of the diet. Advice that conflicts with the client's diet will only confuse him.

Become aware of the sodium content of processed foods. Many clients think of sodium restriction only in terms of the salt shaker. They frequently need help recognizing processed foods that have a high sodium content.

Show the client how the restricted sodium diet has reduced his edema and body weight or decreased his blood pressure. Help him understand why these changes are beneficial to him.

Encourage the client to try new ways of flavoring food if he finds it difficult to adjust to the taste of unsalted foods. Become familiar with the many spices, herbs, and other flavoring aids that can be used.

Nonprescription medications are another unexpected and frequently overlooked source of sodium. Advise your client to discuss the use of these drugs with his physician.

Avoid use of the terms *salt-free* or *low salt* when referring to sodium-restricted diets. These terms are not accurate and give the false impression that table salt is the only food about which to be concerned.

Advise the client not to use a salt substitute without his physician's approval. Such salt substitutes may be harmful for some clients.

KEY IDEAS

Diet changes are frequently prescribed in the treatment of cardiovascular disease. Diets associated with cardiovascular disease are sodium-restricted, fat-controlled, and weight-reducing diets.

Sodium is restricted to prevent or treat edema and hypertension; restriction may also increase the effectiveness of diuretic drugs and make it possible to reduce drug dosages. The importance of sodium restriction in the prevention and treatment of hypertension is controversial.

Sources of sodium include food (natural and added sodium), water, and medications.

Animal foods — meat, fish, poultry, milk, and eggs — have a high natural sodium content; vegetables range from low in natural sodium to relatively high; fruits, animal fats, vegetable oils, and cereal grains are low in natural sodium.

The addition of salt and other sodium-containing compounds to food considerably increases the sodium content of the average diet; the addition of these sodium additives in commercial food processing is the greatest source of sodium.

The sodium content of drinking water varies considerably; distilled water may be necessary for drinking and cooking. Water softeners add much sodium to the water supply.

Antacids and other over-the-counter medications and home remedies can add much sodium to daily intake.

Sodium prescriptions should specify the level of sodium desired; terms such as *salt-free, salt-poor* and *low salt* are not

accurate and falsely give the impression that table salt is the only substance of concern.

Sodium-restricted diets differ depending upon amount of sodium permitted.

Diets that severely restrict sodium to below 1000 mg include only naturally occurring sodium; diets of 1000 mg and above include some salt-containing foods and/or the use of salt in limited quantities, depending on the level of restriction.

The Exchange Lists for Meal Planning (Table A-2 in the Appendix) can be adapted for use in sodium-restricted diets; each item within a particular exchange contains approximately the same amount of sodium as well as of protein, fat, and carbohydrate.

A diet containing a specific quantity of sodium may be planned in a number of ways, depending upon the nutritional needs, life-style, and preferences of the client.

The health worker can help the client find ways of seasoning and flavoring food without the use of salt or other sodium compounds.

Low-sodium dietetic foods are not necessary but may be useful for some clients; guidance should be given so that the client can determine whether a specific low-sodium food is suitable.

Salt substitutes should be used only with the permission of the physician.

It is unrealistic to expect a client to comply with a diet below 3000 mg of sodium if he eats out on a regular basis.

Some diuretics may cause excessive loss of potassium; prevention of potassium deficiency by means of a high-potassium diet is preferred to the use of potassium supplements, which have undesirable side-effects.

Most fruits, fresh vegetables, legumes, and meat are good sources of potassium.

In the acute stages of cardiovascular disease, changes in diet are made to rest the heart as much as possible: use of small, low-calorie meals with easily digested consistency; avoidance of gas-forming foods; and feeding of the client, if necessary.

KEYS TO LEARNING: STUDY–DISCUSSION QUESTIONS

1. Choose one of the 1000-mg sodium diet plans given in Table 23-4 and plan a day's menu. Describe the flavoring aids you might use to make the items on your menus more appealing.

2. Investigate the dietetic low-sodium foods sold in your supermarket. What kinds of low-sodium dietetic foods did you find? Check the labels for sodium content in an average serving. Are there any foods you believe might not be permitted on some sodium-restricted diets even though they are labeled low-sodium dietetic? Select one or two of these items and compare their costs with equal quantities of the regular food they are meant to replace. For example,

compare the price of low-sodium bread with that of a corresponding loaf of regular bread.

3. Prepare at home one of your favorite vegetables without adding salt or other sodium additive. Taste the unsalted food. Then divide the vegetable into two or three portions. Flavor each of these portions with a different salt substitute and taste. (Your instructor will help you obtain samples of salt substitutes.) Discuss your reaction to these flavoring aids with the class.

4. What would you tell a client if he asked for a salt substitute?

5. Select two members of your class to visit the local heart association. Obtain

information about the sodium level of the local water supply. What other nutrition services does the heart association provide for clients? Discuss your visit with the class.

6. Classify the following foods as (1) high in natural sodium, (2) low in natural sodium, or (3) high in sodium content due to sodium additives: milk, canned pears, fresh spinach, fresh pork chops, bologna, orange juice, farina, puffed wheat, chocolate malted, prepared mustard, American cheese, canned beef stew, canned tuna fish, cornflakes, broccoli, fresh mackerel.

7. Discuss with the class the experiences you have had with clients on sodium-restricted diets. What factors seem to affect their ability to adjust to sodium-restricted diets?

8. If he eats out regularly, a client on a severely or moderately restricted sodium diet cannot maintain his level of sodium restriction and at the same time eat a well-balanced and varied diet. Why?

9. Rest is one of the most important considerations in acute heart disease. How can the diet be changed to decrease the workload of the heart?

Bibliography is found at the end of Part Four.

24

Diet in Kidney Disease

KEY TERMS

albumin   A protein found in the blood as serum albumin.

anuria   Lack of urine excretion.

catheter   A tube that can be inserted into a body cavity.

degenerative   Pertaining to the deterioration of an organ.

dialysis   A process by which a liquid to be purified is passed through a semipermeable membrane and exposed to a solvent, which continuously circulates outside the membrane. Small particles pass through the membrane, but large particles do not.

filtrate   Liquid that has passed through a filter or a membrane that acts as a filter.

hematuria   The presence of blood in the urine.

oliguria   A reduced amount of urine secretion in relation to the fluid intake.

proteinuria   Protein, usually albumin, in the urine.

In early chronic kidney disease, often only moderate dietary changes are needed, whereas in acute or chronic kidney failure, diet is critical. In the past, nutritional therapy for end-stage kidney disease was aimed primarily at prolonging the client's life. Today, in addition to prolonging life, hemodialysis permits clients to maintain a near-normal degree of activity. This frequently includes a near-normal work schedule. The success of hemodialysis treatment is dependent to a large extent on the client's adherence to a prescribed diet.

Because a condition that was once 100% fatal is now treatable with dialysis, the number of clients requiring treatment has grown considerably. Some clients receive kidney transplants; others remain on dialysis indefinitely.

Physiology of the Kidney

Each kidney is composed of about 1 million functioning units called *nephrons* (Fig. 24-1). Each nephron contains a cluster of tiny blood vessels or capillaries, called a *glomerulus*, and a long, winding tubule (convoluted tubule) that extends from the glomerulus to a collecting duct. The beginning of the convoluted tubule, called *Bowman's capsule*, surrounds the glomerulus. One tiny blood vessel supplies the glomerulus with blood, and another drains it. As the blood passes through the glomerulus, a mixture of water and other small molecules (glucose, amino acids, sodium chloride, and

329

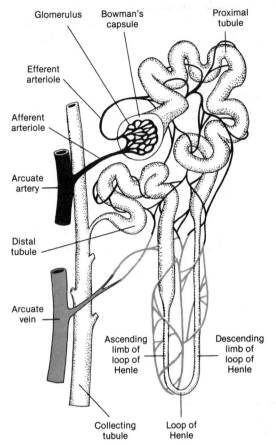

Fig. 24-1. A simplified drawing of a nephron. (Spencer RT, Nichols LW, Waterhouse HP, et al: Pharmacology and Nursing Management. Philadelphia, JB Lippincott, 1983.)

waste products) passes directly from the blood, through the capillary walls, and into Bowman's capsule. In the adult, approximately 100 ml to 120 ml of filtrate per minute are formed by the 2 million nephrons. As the filtrate passes through the convoluted tubule, approximately 99% of the water and most of the small molecules are returned to the blood. Under normal conditions, substances the body needs, such as sodium, potassium, and glucose, are returned to the bloodstream, and toxic substances are expelled in the urine. The latter include the waste products of protein metabolism: urea, uric acid, sulfate, creatinine, and organic acids. In this manner, the kidneys maintain the normal composition and volume of the blood and eliminate body wastes.

The kidney also has metabolic and hormonal functions. It is involved in the breakdown of protein, the production of ammonia (control of body acidity), glucose metabolism, and the conversion of toxic substances to harmless ones. Hormonal activities include the secretion of renin, which affects the body's blood pressure, and the secretion of the hormone erythropoietin, which stimulates the bone marrow to produce red blood cells. The kidney also plays an essential role in converting the inactive form of vitamin D to the active form necessary for normal calcium metabolism.

Kidney Diseases

When one considers the functions of the kidneys, it is not difficult to understand the serious effects of kidney failure. Excretion of poisonous wastes and regulation of water and acid–base balance are disturbed; furthermore, high blood pressure, anemia, and bone disease may follow.

Diseases of the kidney may be due to birth defects, infections, or degenerative processes such as atherosclerosis and diabetic nephropathy. Not all kidney diseases become chronic. Some may be acute, followed by healing; others may recur and eventually lead to kidney failure.

Glomerulonephritis

Glomerulonephritis is inflammation of the glomeruli. Damage to the glomeruli causes hematuria (blood in the urine) and proteinuria (protein in the urine). Other symptoms may include edema, nitrogen retention, oliguria (diminished urine output), and hypertension. Glomerulonephritis frequently follows other infections, especially those of the upper respiratory tract. Recovery is usually complete. In some cases, the disease progresses and becomes chronic, with progressive loss of kidney function.

Nephrotic Syndrome

The term *nephrotic syndrome* refers to kidney disease characterized by large quantities of protein in the urine, severe edema, low serum protein levels, elevated cholesterol and other serum lipid levels, and anemia. The disease is caused by degenerative changes in the capillaries of the kidneys that permit the passage of protein into the filtrate. Albumin (a blood serum protein) is the principal protein excreted. Sodium and water are retained. Fluid retention may be so severe that it masks the tissue wasting due to breakdown of tissue protein. The degree of malnutrition may not be apparent until the edema fluid is removed.

Kidney Failure

In kidney failure, the kidney is no longer able to excrete waste products and maintain normal blood composition. Nitrogen-containing wastes accumulate; acidosis and electrolyte abnormalities occur. The secretion of urine lessens or stops completely (anuria). Kidney failure may be acute, followed by healing, or may be chronic.

Acute Kidney Failure

Acute kidney failure involves the complete stoppage of kidney function in a person whose kidneys have been functioning adequately. The condition is most often caused by destruction of the kidney tubules due to impaired blood supply to the kidneys or to the toxic action of chemicals. Crushing accidents, severe burns, and burn shock or surgery are among the causes. Little or no urine is produced, and the client is severely ill. Dialysis is frequently employed until kidney function is restored.

Chronic Kidney Failure

Chronic kidney failure is the ultimate result of progressive kidney diseases such as chronic glomerulonephritis and of circulatory disorders and cardiac failure, which gradually lead to the permanent loss of functioning kidney tissue. Kidney function is usually expressed as the glomerular filtration rate (GFR, the quantity of filtrate formed by the kidneys per minute). As the GFR decreases, the quantity of nitrogen-containing waste products in the blood increases. When the GFR decreases to 30 ml/minute or less, symptoms appear. These may include fatigue, anemia, loss of weight, hypertension, and pain in the bones and joints. As the condition worsens, other symptoms such as nausea, vomiting, severe itching, numbness and tingling, convulsions, easy bruising, and congestive failure develop. The term *uremia* is used to describe this advanced stage of renal failure. The outcome is fatal unless dialysis or a kidney transplant is available.

Dialysis Treatment

There are two types of dialysis: hemodialysis and peritoneal dialysis.

In hemodialysis, the client's blood is circulated outside the body through a dialysis machine called a *dialyzer.* The semipermeable membranes of the dialyzer are bathed by a fluid called the *dialysate,* which removes unwanted substances, restores normal electrolyte levels, and removes excess water. A permanent opening is made surgically into the client's vascular system to provide blood flow into the dialyzer. Hemodialysis takes place 2 or 3 times a week, each treatment lasting 4 to 6 hours.

Peritoneal dialysis involves running a dialysis solution into the peritoneal (abdominal) cavity for a period of time and then draining the fluid. The peritoneal membrane acts as the semipermeable membrane, allowing for the removal of wastes and of excess electrolytes and excess fluid. The dialysate enters the abdominal cavity through a catheter inserted into the client's abdomen. Infection is a danger with this method.

Peritoneal dialysis is a slower and more gentle process than hemodialysis. Treatments last 8 to 12 hours and are carried out 3 to 5 times a week.

Dietary Treatment: General Aspects

The goals of dietary treatment are to replace nutrients being excreted excessively, to lighten the work of the kidney, and to keep the client's nutritional status as close to normal as possible. The dietary changes depend on the state of the client's kidney function; each client needs to be treated individually according to his clinical symptoms and the results of laboratory tests.

Protein Regulation

If protein is being lost in the urine, as in the nephrotic syndrome, dietary protein for the adult client is increased to levels of 100 g to 150 g.

Protein is restricted in kidney failure to about 0.6 g per kg of body weight, an average of 35 g to 40 g of protein. This is done to prevent the rapid accumulation of toxins resulting from protein metabolism.

Clients on hemodialysis require more protein, at least 1 g per kg of body weight. Those on peritoneal dialysis have even higher requirements, because their amino acid loss is greater.

Caloric Intake

Providing enough kilocalories to meet the client's energy needs is absolutely essential. If energy needs are not met, tissue protein will be broken down to supply energy. The end-products produced by the breakdown of protein tissue add to the nitrogen-containing waste products just as the breakdown of food protein does. A high caloric intake, a minimum of 35 kcal to 45 kcal per kg of body weight, is needed to promote the building of protein tissue. A liberal intake of carbohydrate and fat is also encouraged. Adequate caloric intake is difficult to achieve, because kidney disease causes nausea.

Physical activity also prevents the breakdown of muscle tissue. The client should be encouraged to be as active as his condition permits.

Water Regulation

Fluid intake is adjusted to the body's ability to eliminate fluid. (The normal intake for adults ranges from 2000 ml to 2500 ml.) As long as there is no retention of water, normal water intake is encouraged. If the kidney becomes unable to concentrate urine and excessive fluid is lost, increased intake of fluids is ordered.

In persons with acute or chronic kidney failure and in clients undergoing dialysis, fluid intake is decreased. In kidney failure, about 500 ml to 600 ml more fluid than the urine output for the previous 24 hours are permitted. In hemodialysis, fluid is restricted to prevent a weight gain of more than 1 kg between dialysis treatments. This comes to about 1 liter a day.

Sodium and Potassium Regulation

The dietary changes needed to control sodium and potassium levels depend upon the levels of these minerals in the blood and urine. Laboratory tests are made frequently and requirements determined on an individual basis. When sodium is retained in abnormal amounts, sodium intake must be restricted to prevent edema. In some stages, the kidney fails to reabsorb a sufficient amount of sodium and potassium, and extra sodium and potassium must be provided by diet and medication.

In severe kidney failure, potassium retention occurs. If potassium is allowed to accumulate without control, serious changes in heart action may occur. These changes are usually not noticeable until the patient is in extreme danger.

Calcium and Phosphorus Regulation

In advanced kidney failure, the calcium level falls and the phosphorus level rises excessively.

A major cause of this imbalance is the failure of the diseased kidney to produce the active form of vitamin D that is needed for the absorption of calcium from the intestinal tract and its decreased ability to excrete phosphorus. When serum calcium is reduced, calcium is released from the bones owing to the activity of the parathyroid hormone (PTH), which attempts to correct the imbalance between calcium and phosphorus. The elevation in phosphorus leads to the further release of calcium and phosphorus from the bones, creating a vicious cycle. *Osteodystrophy,* also called *uremic bone disease,* results.

Correcting calcium and phosphorus imbalance is difficult. Medication that binds phosphorus in the intestinal tract may be prescribed and dietary phosphorus restricted. Renal bone disease is treated with calcium supplements and substances with vitamin D hormone activity.

Vitamins and Other Minerals

Multivitamins are prescribed in chronic kidney disease. For clients on dialysis, emphasis is placed on the water-soluble vitamins: ascorbic acid, folic acid, pyridoxine, and the other B vitamins.

Iron supplements are given if serum iron levels are low. However, iron supplements may not be effective in treating the anemia of chronic kidney failure because the kidney's role in stimulating the production of red blood cells is impaired.

Dietary Treatment: Types of Diets

Diets for clients with kidney disease fall into two broad categories: the sodium-restricted, increased protein diet, and the protein-, sodium-, potassium-, phosphorus-restricted diet.

Sodium-Restricted, Increased Protein Diet

The sodium-restricted exchange system is used to plan diets when hypertension and/or edema is present (see Chap. 23). Dietary protein may be increased, normal, or moderately decreased, depending on kidney function.

Severe edema in kidney disease is sometimes partially due to the loss of protein in the urine. When this is the case, the diet is both increased in protein and restricted in sodium. Table 23-4 shows the pattern for a high-protein diet containing 900 mg of sodium used with low-sodium exchange lists. This diet supplies 125 g of protein. Because patients with kidney disease frequently experience nausea and lack of appetite, increases in protein and calories should be made gradually. A high-protein, high-calorie milk drink or a substantial bedtime snack may be more acceptable to the client than larger portions of food at meals.

If the sodium level of the diet permits, non-fat dry milk powder may be used to step up the protein without increasing the volume of food. One third of a cup of dry milk powder contains approximately 9 g of protein. It is important that the diet be adapted to the client's needs and preferences.

In severe sodium restriction (to 500 mg or less), dietary protein cannot exceed 70 g unless a low-sodium milk, Lonolac,* is used. Dialyzed low-sodium milk cannot be used if potassium is restricted. The sodium in this milk has been replaced by potassium.

Protein-, Sodium-, Potassium-, Phosphorus-Restricted Diet

Diet management in advanced kidney failure requires control of protein, sodium, potassium, phosphorus, and fluid as well as maintenance of an adequate caloric intake. Its purpose is to relieve the symptoms of uremia before dialysis is started or to prolong the client's life and alleviate symptoms if dialysis or transplantation is not possible.

* Mead Johnson laboratories, Evansville, IN 47721

Dietary control is an important aspect of dialysis treatment. Through dietary control, the quantity of waste products, electrolytes, and fluid that accumulates between treatments is limited, permitting safe removal of wastes in a reasonable period of time and reducing complications during treatment. Because dialysis removes waste products and excess electrolytes and fluid and increases the protein requirement, the diet is relatively liberal.

Protein

In uremia, the amount of protein prescribed ranges from 20 g to 60 g per day. An allowance of 35 g to 40 g is commonly used. Most of the protein is given in the form of high-quality proteins—those containing the highest percentage of essential amino acids. Milk and eggs contain the highest-quality protein. Meat also contains high-quality protein but has a higher percentage of nonessential amino acids than milk or eggs. The major protein sources in diets containing only 20 g of protein are milk and eggs. In diets permitting higher levels of protein, small amounts of meat are added.

Foods containing nonessential amino acids are reduced to as low a level as possible. This forces the body to use the nitrogen in the urea, which has accumulated in abnormal amounts, for the production of the nonessential amino acids. In this way, the urea level of the blood decreases and the distressing symptoms of uremia lessen. Foods containing protein of low biological value include breads, cereals, cereal products, vegetables, and fruit. Even the small amounts of protein in fruits must be counted.

Clients on dialysis are usually allowed 60 g to 80 g of protein daily, at least half of which should be of high biological value. The protein is best utilized when it is distributed throughout the day, divided into at least three meals.

Calories

Energy is supplied by carbohydrates and fats, which do not involve the kidneys in elimination of waste products. Maintenance of an adequate caloric intake is essential if the diet is to be effective. Because regular bread, macaroni products, cereals, and desserts made with regular flour contain protein, these foods cannot be permitted in quantities sufficient to meet energy needs on diets restricted to less than 60 g of protein.

Low-protein carbohydrate foods that are practically protein-free and low in sodium and potassium have been developed for use on low-protein diets. These products include wheat starch, low-protein baking mix, low-protein bread, low-protein pastas, and low-protein hot cereal. Recipes are available for making baked goods using the wheat starch and baking mixes.* The structure, flavor, and texture of these foods differ from those made with regular flour and are not acceptable to some clients. Moreover, these products are expensive and not easily obtained. The client will need help in learning how to obtain and use them advantageously. Such special starch products may not be necessary for clients whose protein prescription is 60 g or more.

Low-protein, low-potassium fruits and vegetables provide additional calories. Sugars and fats are used liberally to make up the remainder of the client's caloric needs.

Commercial supplements that are high in kilocalories, protein-free, and low in potassium and sodium may be used to achieve adequate kilocalorie intake. These products include Controlyte,† Polycose,‡ HyCal,§ and Cal Power.ǀ

Sodium

Sodium restriction ranges from 500 mg to 2000 mg (see Chapter 23).

Potassium

Potassium restriction ranges from 1500 mg to 3000 mg (the normal range is 2000–6000 mg).

* Cellu-Featherweight, Chicago Dietetic Supply House, LaGrange, IL; Henkel Corp, Minneapolis, MN 55435
† Doyle Pharmaceutical Co, Minneapolis, MN 55416
‡ Ross Laboratories, Columbus, OH 43216
§ Beecham-Massingill Pharmaceuticals, Melrose, MA 02176
ǀ Henkel Corp, Minneapolis, MN 55435

Potassium is distributed widely in foods (Table 24-1). Most potassium-rich foods are limited; some are omitted from the diet.

Potassium salts are highly soluble in water, so one can reduce potassium by slicing or dicing the food into small pieces, soaking it in water, and then discarding the liquid. The food is then cooked in a large quantity of fresh water, which is again discarded. This process is called *leaching*. Vegetables lend themselves well to this procedure.

Canning also reduces potassium content. Canned foods should be well drained and the liquid discarded.

Whole-grain breads and cereals have more potassium than refined varieties. Cornstarch, wheat starch, arrowroot starch, and tapioca are practically free of potassium and are used in baked goods or as thickening agents.

Tea and coffee, both regular and instant, contain significant amounts of potassium and are either omitted from the diet or severely limited. The drinking water in some areas may also be a significant source of potassium, and it may be necessary instead to use distilled water.

Salt substitutes containing potassium as well as low-sodium baking powder cannot be used when potassium is restricted. When so-

Table 24-1. Foods High in Potassium*

Calories Per Serving	Rich Sources (>400 mg [10 mEq]/Serving)	Good Sources (200–400 mg [5–10 mEq]/Serving)
<100	Banana, medium-sized, 1	Artichoke, bud or globe†
	Cantaloupe, 1 cup	Beets, cooked,† ½ cup
	Grapefruit juice, 1 cup	Beet greens,† ½ cup
	Honeydew melon, 1 cup	Blackberries, 1 cup
	Molasses, 2 tbsp	Broccoli, cooked, ½ cup
	Nectarine, large, 1	Brussels sprouts, fresh, ½ cup
	Orange juice, 1 cup	Carrots,† raw, large, 1
	Potato, baked, medium-sized, 1	Collard greens, cooked, frozen, ½ cup
	Potato, boiled, medium-sized, 1	Orange, small, 1
	Tomato juice, canned, low-sodium, 1 cup	Peach, raw, medium-sized, 1
		Pear, raw, medium-sized, 1
		Rutabaga, cooked, ½ cup
		Skim milk,† 1 cup
		Strawberries, (frozen, sliced, unsweetened, 1 cup
		Tomato, canned, low-sodium, ½ cup
		Tomato, raw, 1
		Watermelon, 2 cups
		Wheat germ, ¼ cup
		Winter squash, frozen, cooked, ½ cup

Table 24-1. *(continued)*

Calories Per Serving	Rich Sources (>400 mg [10 mEq]/Serving)	Good Sources (200–400 mg [5–10 mEq]/Serving)
100–200	Avocado, ½	Apple juice, 1 cup
	Fish,† lean types (*e.g.,* cod, halibut), 3 oz	Dried peas, beans, lentils, cooked, ½ cup
	Prunes, medium-sized, 10	Fish,† high-fat types, (*e.g.,* tuna), 3 oz
	Prune juice, ¾ cup	Lima beans, green, ½ cup
	Soybeans, cooked, ½ cup	Meat and poultry,† lean, cooked, 3 oz
		Parsnips, cooked, ½ cup
		Peaches, canned, ½ peach
		Peanut butter, unsalted, 2 tbsp
		Raisins, natural, ⅓ cup
		Sunflower seeds, hulled, unsalted, ¼ cup
		Sweet potato, canned, ½ cup
>200	Dates, medium-sized, 10	Peanuts, shelled, unsalted, ¼ cup
	Figs, dried, medium-sized, 5	

(After Suitor CW, Hunter MF: Nutrition: Principles and Application in Health Promotion, p 448. Philadelphia, JB Lippincott, 1980)
   * Other foods may contribute substantial amounts of potassium to the diet, especially if large or frequent servings are used.
   † Naturally high in sodium

dium is severely restricted, an alum baking powder that is low in potassium (Calumet*) may be used in baking bread and cakes with wheat starch.

Phosphorus

Severe phosphorus restriction is undesirable, since phosphorus is found abundantly in many nutritious foods. Instead, clients are given aluminum hydroxide medication such as Amphojel, Basaljel, and Alu-Caps. When taken with meals, the medication binds the phosphorus in the diet, causing it to be excreted in the stool. Many clients cannot tolerate the large doses

* General Foods Corp., White Plains, NY 10625

required of such medication, which is unpalatable and gives rise to side-effects such as constipation and nausea.

Control of serum phosphorus is frequently accomplished through both diet restriction and medication, with restriction ranging from 600 mg to 1200 mg per day. Milk, meat, fish, poultry, eggs, whole-grain breads and cereals, nuts, dried peas and beans, dried fruits, chocolate, and cocoa are high in phosphorus and are carefully controlled.

Fluids

Fluids include all substances that are liquid at room temperature: water, juice, milk, tea, cof-

fee, soup, soft drinks, ice, water ice, sherbet, ice cream, and gelatin dessert.

Good communication between the dietary and nursing services is essential. Attention must be given not only to the amount of fluid a client with kidney disease receives, but to the fluid itself as well. For example, orange juice and tea contain significant amounts of potassium, and canned tomato juice is high in sodium, so even small quantities of these fluids, in addition to those normally included in the diet, would give rise to problems.

Nursing care includes measures to relieve the sensation of thirst, such as frequent cleansing and lubrication of the mouth. Fluid losses, as through vomiting or diarrhea, should be accurately measured. Diversionary activities can help to take the client's mind off his thirst.

Exchange System for the Protein-, Sodium-, Potassium-Restricted Diet

The protein-, sodium-, potassium-restricted exchange lists (see Table A-3 in the Appendix) differ considerably from those described in Chapter 19. The foods are grouped according to their protein, sodium, and potassium contents. Bread, fruit, and vegetable exchange lists are divided into two or more groups to allow for the varying potassium and sodium contents of the foods in each list. Unsalted fats and low-protein bread and cereal products can be used freely.

Calories are not given for the exchanges because the caloric values of foods within the same group vary widely. For example, although they contain approximately the same protein, sodium, and potassium values, ¾ cup of heavy cream contains 624 kcal and ½ cup of whole milk contains 75 kcal.

The protein content of all fruits and vegetables is listed so that an excess of nonessential amino acids in the diet can be avoided.

Canned fruits are those canned with sugar, and vegetable exchanges are for vegetables cooked or canned without salt. Since protein foods that also are high in natural sodium—milk, eggs, and meat—are restricted, limited amounts of salted foods can frequently be used, especially if sodium is only moderately restricted. On diets restricting sodium to 1500 mg to 2000 mg, small amounts of salt may be permitted in cooking (Table 24-2).

Table 24-2. Menu for 40-g Protein, 1000-mg Sodium, and 1500-mg Potassium Diet

Breakfast
- ½ cup of cranberry juice
- 1 cup of Puffed Wheat
- ½ cup of milk
- 1 fried egg
- 2 slices of low-protein bread
- 3 tsp of salted margarine
- 2 tbsp of jam
- ½ cup of coffee

Noon Meal
- 1 oz of tuna, special diet pack
- 2 slices of low-protein bread
- 1 leaf of lettuce
- 2 tsp of salted mayonnaise
- ½ cup of unsalted canned green beans seasoned with 1 tsp of salted margarine
- ½ cup of frozen strawberries
- 3 low-protein cookies
- ½ cup of ginger ale

Evening Meal
- 1 ounce of baked chicken
- ½ cup of rice seasoned with 1 tsp of salted margarine
- ½ cup of cooked carrots seasoned with 1 tsp of salted margarine
- 2 slices of low-protein bread
- 2 tsp of salted margarine
- 1 tbsp of honey
- 1 piece of apple pie (wheatstarch crust)
- ½ cup of lemonade

(Anderson L, Dibble MV, Turkki PR et al: Nutrition in Health and Disease, 17th ed. Philadelphia, JB Lippincott, 1982)

Diet Following Kidney Transplantation

Medication used to prevent the body from rejecting the new kidney may cause complications that include the following: decreased resistance to infection; hypertension; elevated blood sugar; elevated blood lipids; obesity; and gastric ulcer. Cardiovascular disease is one of the major causes of death following kidney transplantation. Therefore, the diet currently recommended following a kidney transplant is moderately restricted in sodium (to 2000 mg), low in carbohydrate (to 120 g), high in protein (to 1.5 – 2 g per kg of body weight), and restricted in calories if weight loss is desirable. Polyunsaturated fats are used in place of saturated fats. A bland diet may also be advised to lessen irritation of the gastrointestinal tract due to steroid therapy.

Kidney Stones

Kidney stones develop when calcium salts, uric acid, and other substances crystallize out in the urinary tract and form masses. These stones, which range from the size of a pinhead to that of a walnut, obstruct the urinary system and can lead to infection. They may develop in either the kidney or the bladder. Most stones contain calcium in the form of calcium phosphate, calcium carbonate, and calcium oxalate. About 10% are composed of cystine and uric acid.

Together with medication, a diet moderately restricted in calcium and phosphorus helps control the formation of calcium phosphate stones. The diet contains 500 mg to 700 mg of calcium and 1000 mg to 1200 mg of phosphorus.

Sometimes a change in the pH of the urine is desirable. An acid urine may prevent the growth or further formation of alkaline (calcium phosphate/calcium carbonate) stones, and an alkaline urine may have the same effect on acid (cystine/uric acid) stones. Medication is usually prescribed to increase the acidity or alkalinity of the urine. In some cases, diet augments the medication. By regulation of certain foods, the urine may be made either acid or alkaline. An alkaline ash diet produces an alkaline urine; an acid ash diet produces an acid urine. Alkaline ash and acid ash foods are discussed in Chapter 10.

Client Education

The health worker plays an important role in getting the client to accept his diet. This is no easy task. The client has to make drastic changes in his eating habits; he must eat all the food served, even when he is nauseated and has no appetite; he may feel depressed; and both he and his family are under great stress. Through a positive outlook and approach, the health worker helps the client to understand why he needs the diet and to appreciate that the results of feeling better and remaining active are worth the difficulties involved.

Planning the diet is the dietitian's responsibility. The dietitian's services should be available at all times: the client may need help relieving the monotony of the diet, making the diet palatable, and planning meals for special occasions.

The problems of following restricted diets are very real. Foods must be weighed and measured; choices are limited; portion sizes of favored foods such as meats may be extremely small; and time and skill is required to prepare special foods. Many clients on dialysis do not follow their diets. After an initial period of hopefulness, they become depressed. Some express their depression by loss of appetite, whereas others overeat. Clients sometimes decide to "live it up" by eating whatever they want with the full knowledge of the serious complications that will result. The health worker must accept the client without passing judgment on him and at the same time must try to find ways to motivate him.

Self-help groups for clients with kidney disease help these persons share their frustrations and exchange ideas on how to cope with various aspects of their disease, including diet. (The National Association of Patients on Hemodialysis and Transplantation, Inc.* publishes a quarterly, "NAPHT News," written for persons with kidney disease.) The National Kidney Foundation† provides educational services for both lay and professional groups.

* 505 Northern Boulevard, Great Neck, NY 11021
† 2 Park Ave, New York, NY 10016

KEYS TO PRACTICAL APPLICATION

Encourage and persuade the client to eat all the food on his diet so he will consume adequate calories. Help him to understand that this will prevent the breakdown of body tissue, thus lightening the load on the kidney and preventing malnutrition.

See to it that the client performs the full extent of physical activity permitted by his condition. Exercise also prevents the breakdown of muscle tissue.

Correct the misconceptions about diets that require protein restriction. Most of the protein permitted should be of high biological value. Some erroneously believe that low protein means a reduction in meat, fish, and poultry in favor of cereals, vegetables, and fruit. The opposite is true.

Carefully measure fluid output as well as intake. If no allowance is made for fluid lost in vomiting and diarrhea, a client may suffer unnecessarily from thirst.

When fluids are restricted, provide good mouth care and divert the client's attention as a means of relieving his sensation of thirst.

Share what you observe about the client's eating habits with the dietitian. Let the dietitian know what foods are better accepted than others.

Show acceptance and understanding for the client who does not follow his diet. Keep trying to find ways to motivate him. Use the positive approach. Don't criticize or condemn.

KEY IDEAS

Dietary treatment in kidney disease aims to replace nutrients lost in abnormal amounts, reduce those substances in the diet that must be excreted by the kidney, and maintain as good a nutritional state as possible.

Dietary treatment varies depending on the nature and cause of the disease and the parts of the kidney affected. Diet changes depend on the level of kidney function: *Protein* is increased when albumin and other proteins are lost in the urine and is decreased when urea accumulates in the blood. *Sodium* is restricted when hypertension and edema are present. *Potassium* is increased when excessive amounts are excreted and restricted when it accumulates in the blood, as in severe kidney failure. *Phosphorus* is restricted when blood levels of phosphorus

increase and of calcium levels decrease. The imbalance between these two minerals leads to uremic bone disease. In addition to dietary phosphorus being restricted, phosphate-binding medication and supplements of calcium and vitamin D are given. *Fluid* is adjusted to the body's ability to eliminate fluid. *Iron supplements and multivitamins* are given; emphasis is placed on water-soluble vitamins for clients on dialysis.

Maintaining an adequate caloric intake is absolutely essential to prevent the breakdown of tissue protein, which adds to the accumulation of nitrogen-containing waste products and causes wasting of body tissue.

When kidney disease is characterized by loss of protein in the urine and edema, a high-protein (100–150-g), sodium-

restricted diet is ordered. A sodium-restricted exchange list is often used.

Diet management in advanced kidney failure requires the control of protein, sodium, potassium, phosphorus, and fluid. The diet for clients on dialysis is usually more liberal than for those not on dialysis.

In renal failure, protein restriction ranges from 20 g to 60 g. Most of the protein given is of high biological value. Nonessential amino acids are reduced to a minimum; this forces the body to use the nitrogen in the urea to produce nonessential amino acids. Protein is increased to 60 g to 80 g during dialysis.

To meet caloric needs in clients on protein-restricted diets, the use of special low-protein wheat starch products may be necessary. Sugars and fats are used liberally.

Potassium restriction involves limiting fruits, vegetables, meat, fish, poultry, and milk. Soaking and cooking vegetables in large quantities of water and then discarding the cooking liquid reduces the food's potassium content.

Intake of milk is limited because of a high phosphorus content. Protein foods are high in phosphorus.

Fluid orders require the careful attention and cooperation of both nursing and dietary departments.

The protein-, sodium-, potassium-restricted exchange lists differ considerably from the exchange lists used in diabetes and weight control.

Diet is sometimes used in treating kidney stones; calcium phosphate stones may be treated with a diet moderately restricted in calcium and phosphorus; acid ash and alkaline ash diets may be used together with medication to change the pH of the urine.

Compliance with such a complex diet is very difficult; encouragement, support, and understanding are needed.

KEYS TO LEARNING: STUDY – DISCUSSION QUESTIONS

1. When is protein increased in kidney disease? When is it restricted? When protein is restricted to low levels (20 – 60 g), it should be provided mostly in the form of high-quality protein, and foods containing nonessential amino acids should be reduced to a minimum. Why? What foods are used to provide needed calories?

2. Why is it essential that the client with kidney disease consume an adequate number of calories? Discuss in class the problems of nausea and lack of appetite, which frequently accompany kidney disease. Under these circumstances, what can the health professional do to promote the intake of adequate quantities of food?

3. What foods can be added to increase calories without significantly increasing protein, sodium, or potassium?

4. Both excessive loss of potassium and excessive retention of potassium can occur in kidney disease. Explain the serious effects of each condition. What foods are involved in potassium restriction? Describe the food preparation method by which the potassium content of vegetables can be reduced.

5. Fluids are restricted in kidney failure. Why? How is the permitted amount determined? Not only the amount of fluid but also the kind of fluid offered the client is important. Explain.

6. Ask the renal dietitian in your hospital to discuss ways of promoting compliance with diet among clients on dialysis.

Bibliography is found at the end of Part Four.

25

Diet in Gastrointestinal Disease

KEY TERMS

diarrhea Frequent passage of watery stools.
diverticula Abnormal sacs or pouches that form in the walls of the colon.
enteropathy Any intestinal disease.
gluten A vegetable protein found in wheat and other grains.
malabsorption Failure to absorb nutrients from the intestinal tract.
medium-chain triglycerides (MCT) A

man-made oil that is digested and absorbed differently from the usual dietary fats; MCT has been helpful in treating malabsorption disorders.
residue The material remaining in the intestinal tract after digestion has taken place.
steatorrhea Excess fat in the stools.

Stress—be it in the form of anger, worry, fear, or anxiety—is present at various times in everyone's life. However, when it is prolonged, stress may give rise to physical changes, such as reduced secretion of mucus, increased secretion of gastric acid, and contraction of the blood vessels in the stomach and duodenum. These physical changes make the gastrointestinal system susceptible to certain diseases, including peptic ulcer and ulcerative colitis (discussed more fully in Chapter 5).

There are other disorders of the gastrointestinal tract that are unrelated to emotional factors. These may be due to organic disease such as cancer, to the ingestion of toxic substances as

in food poisoning, to infection, to a lack of enzymes necessary for the digestion of certain foodstuffs, and possibly to diets lacking in fiber.

This chapter covers diet therapy in the more common diseases of the gastrointestinal tract and the accessory organs (liver, pancreas, and gallbladder). Although the accessory organs are not part of the gastrointestinal tract, they play vital roles in the digestion and absorption of food. Gastrointestinal disorders caused by cystic fibrosis and galactosemia occurring primarily in infancy and childhood are discussed in Chapter 28. Diet therapy related to surgery of the gastrointestinal tract is covered in Chapter 26.

Diseases of the Upper Gastrointestinal Tract

Peptic Ulcer

A peptic ulcer is an open sore in the gastrointestinal tract. Peptic ulcers usually occur near the pylorus, the "gate" between the stomach and small intestine. An ulcer on the stomach side of the pylorus is called a *gastric ulcer;* one on the duodenal side is called a *duodenal ulcer.* Both are known as *peptic ulcers* because of the role the enzyme pepsin plays in their development.

Under normal conditions, a healthy environment is maintained in the stomach despite the secretion of strong digestive juices by numerous glands. These juices contain hydrochloric acid (HCl) and pepsinogen (converted to the enzyme pepsin in the presence of acid), which together chemically break down food protein. Mucus, another gastric secretion, protects the lining of the stomach from being digested by HCl and pepsin. Mucus contains mucin, a substance that neutralizes acid. The mucus secretion holds acid away from the lining of the stomach and reduces the formation of pepsin.

When the acid–pepsin reaction overpowers the protective action of the mucus lining, an ulcer develops. Exactly why this occurs is not known. However, several factors appear to be involved. These include increased amounts of acid and pepsin, decreased resistance of the mucus lining due to drugs, malnutrition, or faulty production of mucus by the body, and a high degree of emotional stress. The usual symptom is a burning or gnawing pain that occurs when the stomach is empty and from 1 to 3 hours after meals. The pain is relieved by ingestion of food or nonabsorbable antacids. In some cases, hemorrhage, which may develop if the ulcer is not treated, is the first sign.

Relationship of Food to Gastric Irritation

Size of Meals. Food causes the stomach to expand. This expansion signals the release of hormones that stimulate acid secretion. Meals should be small to moderate in size to prevent excessive expansion of the stomach and excessive acid secretion. The client with an ulcer may need to have more meals than three a day to meet his caloric and nutrient needs.

Once the ulcer is healed, frequent meals may not be advised, because gastric secretion is stimulated every time food is eaten.

Protein. Protein foods both stimulate and neutralize gastric acidity. Protein foods first stimulate acid secretion, as do other foods; then the protein buffers the acid as the acid begins to break it down. However, the products that result from this breakdown of protein again stimulate gastric secretion, which is responsible for the pain experienced 1 to 3 hours after meals. To counteract this reaction, the client with an active ulcer usually takes an antacid tablet 1 hour after eating.

Although protein stimulates gastric secretion, adequate amounts of protein must be included in the diet. Protein maintains body tissue, promotes healing of the ulcer, and supports the formation of red blood cells if bleeding has occurred.

Fats and Carbohydrates. Fats depress gastric acid secretion, whereas carbohydrates do not seem to affect it one way or the other. Because fat reduces gastric acid, hourly feedings of milk and cream together with antacid medication were at one time widely used in the treatment of ulcers (Sippy diet). Modifications of this diet are prescribed in the acute stages of peptic ulcer disease, but no longer to the same extent. When milk therapy is used, whole milk or skim milk frequently replaces cream because large amounts of saturated fat are thought to increase risk of atherosclerosis.

Chemical Irritants. There is substantial evidence that certain foods cause a significant in-

crease in gastric acid or otherwise irritate the gastric mucosa. Caffeine and theobromine are stimulants that increase the secretion of gastric acid. These stimulants are found in coffee, tea, cola beverages, and chocolate. Coffee also contains an unidentified substance or substances other than caffeine that stimulate gastric secretion. Decaffeinated as well as regular coffee has this acid-promoting property.

Alcohol is only a mild stimulant but has a damaging effect on the protective mucus lining of the gastrointestinal tract, especially when taken on an empty stomach.

Meat extractives (substances that give flavor to meat) in meat-based soups and gravies also increase acid flow.

Spices and Fiber. Spices are usually avoided by persons with peptic ulcers, although controversy exists regarding their effect on gastric secretion. Opinion at the present time is that most spices can be tolerated but that individual tolerances may vary and should be respected.

Foods with a high fiber content, commonly known as *roughage,* at one time were thought to irritate ulcers. However, there is no clear-cut evidence that food that is well masticated and mixed with saliva will irritate an inflamed mucosa.

Dietary Treatment

The goal of medical treatment is to promote healing of the ulcer by reducing irritation of the gastrointestinal tract and providing adequate nutrition. Drugs decrease the secretion of acid, and nonabsorbable antacids neutralize gastric acid. Food also neutralizes acid and reduces pain for short periods of time. During acute stages, six or more small meals are provided instead of three large meals. Foods that stimulate gastric secretion are avoided.

Bland Diet. The bland diet and variations of it have been used for many years in the treatment of peptic ulcers and other gastrointestinal disorders and during treatment with steroid medication. The bland diet is low in fiber and connective tissue, restricts spices and condiments, and includes only foods that are simply pre-

pared. Foods that are fried or prepared with rich sauces and gravies are omitted. Foods that stimulate acid secretion, such as coffee (including decaffeinated), tea, chocolate and cola beverages, and meat-based soups and gravies are omitted. Alcohol is also omitted because of its damaging effect on the gastric mucosa. Table 25-1 summaries the bland diet.

The trend in recent years has been to make the bland diet as liberal as possible, tailored to the needs of the individual with few restrictions applied to all persons. This has resulted from the realization that there is a lack of scientific evidence supporting the belief that certain properties of food such as roughage and spices are irritating to the gastrointestinal tract. A number of studies indicate that the bland diet makes no significant difference in the healing of peptic ulcers.

Conservative vs. Liberal Dietary Treatment. Dietary treatments vary with the approach of the physician. The conservative or traditional view is that benefit is derived from restricting fiber or roughage, spices, and stimulants; the more liberal approach is that clients progress just as well when eating foods of their own choice. As we have seen, there is considerable disagreement as to what foods are nonirritating. Sometimes the dietary approach ordered by the physician depends upon the client's personality. Some clients expect dietary restrictions and feel more confident with them. Others may find the restrictions annoying, and an inadequate food intake as well as emotional stress may result.

Conservative treatment is still sometimes followed, for a short period, in the early treatment of bleeding ulcers. Small servings (3–6 oz) of milk, skim milk, half-and-half, or milk and cream are given every 1 to 2 hours. Simple foods such as eggs, toast, custard, cream soup, pureed fruits, and vegetables are added gradually to form three small meals.

As the client's condition improves, the hourly feedings of milk are discontinued, although milk may be given between meals. Tender meat, fish, and poultry; tender cooked or canned vegetables, such as asparagus, beets, carrots, spinach, and white potatoes; and plain desserts, such as puddings, plain cake, ice

Table 25-1.   Bland Diet

Principles

1. Low in fiber and connective tissue
2. Little or no condiments or spices, except salt in small amounts
3. No highly acidic foods
4. Foods simply prepared

Foods Used

Milk: milk, cream, buttermilk, yogurt

Cheese: cream, cottage and other soft, mild cheeses

Fats: butter or margarine

Eggs: boiled, poached, scrambled in Teflon pan or top of double boiler

Meat, fish, fowl: roast beef and lamb; broiled steak, lamb, or veal chops; stewed, broiled, or roast chicken; fresh tongue; liver; sweetbreads; baked, poached, or broiled fish

Soups: with milk or cream sauce foundation

Vegetables: potatoes, peas, squash, asparagus tips, carrots, tender string beans, beets, spinach (in severe cases these vegetables are pureed)

Fruit: orange juice, ripe bananas, avocados, baked apple (without skin), applesauce, canned peaches, pears, apricots, white cherries, stewed prunes

Bread, cereals, macaroni products: white bread and rolls, crackers, all refined cereals, macaroni, spaghetti, noodles

Desserts: custard, junket, ice cream, tapioca, rice, bread or cornstarch pudding, gelatin desserts, sponge cake, plain cookies, prune, apricot or peach whip

Beverages: milk, buttermilk, malted milk, fruit juices (if tolerated)

Foods to be Avoided

Fats: fried or fatty foods

Meat, fish: smoked and preserved meat and fish; pork

Vegetables: all raw; all cooked except those listed above

Fruits: all except those listed above

Desserts, sweets: pastries, preserves, candies

Beverages: alcoholic beverages; carbonated drinks, unless prescribed by the doctor

Condiments: pepper, other spices, vinegar, ketchup, horseradish, relishes, gravies, mustard, pickles

(Anderson L, Dibble MV, Turkki PR et al: Nutrition in Health and Disease, 17th ed, p 438. Philadelphia, JB Lippincott, 1982)

cream, and sugar cookies, are added to the foods permitted in the acute stage. This is sometimes referred to as the *convalescent bland diet.*

The full bland diet is frequently prescribed after the client's discharge from the hospital. Sometimes the convalescent stage described above is skipped and the bland diet given immediately after recovery from the acute stage. This diet may be similar to the diet plan in Table 25-1 or may be more liberal, similar to the soft

diet described in Chapter 3 except for the omission of coffee (both regular and decaffeinated), caffeine-containing beverages, and broth-based soups (pepper, chili, and other strong spices are already omitted from the soft diet). The use in the bland diet of citrus juices such as orange juice is also controversial. It may be suggested that citrus juices be diluted with water or taken at the end of a meal. Clients who experience discomfort even when these precautions are

taken should avoid the use of citrus juice. In some bland diets, ripe fresh fruits and a few raw vegetables such as tomatoes and tender salad greens may be permitted.

The client is often advised to eat three small meals and two or three between-meal feedings to avoid distending the stomach. Some physicians advise their clients to omit a bedtime feeding to avoid the excessive secretion of gastric acid during the night.

The liberal approach permits the client to make his usual food choices. However, he may need some help in selecting a nutritionally adequate diet.

Regardless of the type of dietary treatment followed, care must be taken to see that the client's nutritional needs are met. This is especially true if foods are omitted because of individual intolerances. Adequate amounts of protein and ascorbic acid are especially important, because these nutrients promote healing. If citrus fruits are not tolerated, a vitamin C supplement should be prescribed. If blood loss has occurred, supplementation of iron may also be necessary.

Client Education. Clients may need assistance in selecting meals and between-meal feedings that may be eaten in restaurants and cafeterias. Clients whose cooking facilities are limited may need help with food preparation based on their diets. The bland diet should be individualized. Food tolerances and preferences, life-styles, types of work, and work hours must be considered.

Hiatus Hernia

A hiatus hernia is a condition in which the portion of the stomach adjoining the esophagus is pushed through the diaphragm (Fig. 25-1). In some persons with this condition, the lower esophageal sphincter lacks tone and is unable to do a proper job of closing the opening between the stomach and esophagus. As a result, the stomach contents flow back, or regurgitate, into the esophagus. If this occurs repeatedly, the delicate esophageal tissue can become inflamed. Symptoms include regurgitation and

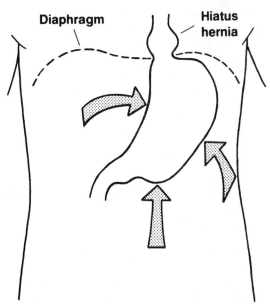

Fig. 25-1. In hiatus hernia pressure within the stomach (*arrows*) promotes regurgitation of gastric fluid into the esophagus.

"heartburn" (a sensation of burning high under the sternum). Complications such as ulceration and perforation may occur if the condition is not treated effectively.

Nutritional care is aimed at reducing pressure within the stomach, reducing gastric acidity, and increasing the tone of the lower esophageal sphincter. To achieve these goals, the client must correct obesity; eat smaller, more frequent meals; avoid constipation; take liquids between meals rather than with meals; avoid lying down for about 2 hours after eating; reduce fat intake; and avoid foods that stimulate acid secretion (coffee, tea, and alcohol). Spicy foods, carbonated beverages, and various other foods are omitted if they cause discomfort.

Indigestion

Symptoms of indigestion include "heartburn," frequent belching, and a feeling of fullness. Because these can be symptoms of organic disease, a person who experiences them frequently should seek the advice of a physician. When no organic disease is found, the condition is said to

be functional. Indigestion may be due to emotional factors, poor food habits, and hurried and irregular mealtimes (see Chap. 5).

Diseases of the Small Intestine

Malabsorption

Malabsorption refers to poor digestion and absorption of a nutrient or nutrients in the small intestine. This may be caused by increased peristalsis due to infection, a lack of digestive enzymes, a lack of bile, or defects in the lining of the small intestine. Symptoms such as loss of weight in adults, retarded growth in infants and children, abdominal bloating, abdominal cramps, diarrhea, and steatorrhea (fatty diarrhea) are frequently present.

Diarrhea

Diarrhea is a common symptom of gastrointestinal disease and not a disease in itself. It may be described as the passing of stools that are liquid or semiliquid and more frequent than normal. Because of increased peristalsis, nutrients pass too rapidly through the gastrointestinal tract to be absorbed properly. If the diarrhea continues for a prolonged period, serious losses of fluid, electrolytes, and nutrients may result.

In the acute stages of diarrhea caused by infection, a clear liquid diet (see Chap. 3) is given for a brief period and followed by a fiber-restricted diet until the client has recovered. Diarrhea resulting from lactase deficiency requires diet changes related to the cause. If the diarrhea has been long-standing, the client usually needs a high-protein, high-calorie diet supplemented by vitamins and minerals.

Lactose Intolerance

Lactose intolerance is the inability to digest lactose (milk sugar). The person with this disorder experiences bloating, flatulence (gaseousness), cramping, and sometimes diarrhea. The condition is caused by a deficiency of the enzyme lactase, which is needed to reduce lactose to glucose and galactose, the forms of sugar the body can absorb. A small percentage of infants are born with lactase deficiency. Most persons with the condition have adequate levels of lactase at birth and acquire the disease only after early childhood or as adults. It occurs most frequently among persons of African origin, Orientals, native Americans, Eskimos, and descendants of peoples who lived near the Mediterranean Sea. Lactose intolerance may also develop in persons who have undergone gastrointestinal surgery or have had gastrointestinal diseases such as celiac sprue and colitis.

For lactose intolerance of infancy, lactose-free formulas are prescribed. These may be made from soybean, meat-base, and protein mixtures. Care must be taken to avoid commercially prepared baby food products that contain milk or nonfat dry milk solids.

Most affected persons do not completely lack the enzyme lactase and can tolerate small amounts of milk (about ½ cup) with meals and in such food as butter, margarine, and baked goods. Some are able to tolerate fermented dairy products such as buttermilk, cottage cheese, and yogurt. The lactose in these products is partially changed to lactic acid by the fermentation process. Aged cheeses have very little lactose and are usually well tolerated.

For persons with severe lactose intolerance, all sources of lactose are omitted from the diet —milk and foods containing milk, such as ice cream, milk chocolate, caramel, regular margarine, creamed soups and other creamed dishes, and bakery products. The "hidden" lactose in frankfurters, luncheon meats, and salad dressings must also be avoided. Labels of commercial products must be checked carefully. Lactose may also be found in medications.

Bagels, French bread, and Italian bread are usually milk-free, as are bread, frankfurters, and

margarine sold in Jewish markets. Many diet margarines also do not contain milk.

Lact-Aid,* a commercial lactase enzyme product, can be added to milk to break down the lactose. The treated milk is sweeter than normal but is generally well accepted. Some supermarkets carry low-fat milk that has already been treated with Lact-Aid.

Milk supplies calcium and vitamins A, D, and B_2, and it is an inexpensive source of high-quality protein. As the best source of calcium in the diet, it is of central importance in maintaining a balance between calcium and phosphorus. To the degree tolerated by the client, every effort should be made to include milk and milk products or milk substitutes in the diet.

Celiac Sprue

Celiac sprue is a malabsorption disorder characterized by poor absorption of nutrients, especially fat. Because it is the gluten in protein that causes the associated problems, the disorder is also known as *gluten-induced enteropathy* (intestinal disease).

When the affected person eats food containing gluten, the mucosa of the jejunum becomes flat and thickened, losing the normal fingerlike projections of the villi and the tremendous absorptive area they provide. Absorption of fats, amino acids, vitamins, and minerals is thus greatly reduced.

Steatorrhea, the passing of stools containing undigested fat, is the most characteristic symptom. The stools are frothy, large, foul smelling, watery, and numerous. Thus, there is severe loss of all nutrients, and the resulting malnutrition is responsible for the other symptoms, such as extreme weight loss, muscle wasting, anorexia, and "pot belly."

Gluten-Free Diet

The removal of all sources of gluten in the diet brings gradual improvement in the intestinal

* SugarLo Co, P.O. Box 1017, Atlantic City, NJ 08404

mucosa. Children may respond more quickly than adults. Improvement may be quicker if fat is restricted for a month or two after the diagnosis has been made. The changes in the mucosa caused by the disease may result in poor absorption of lactose and other disaccharides as well; once the mucosa regains its normal structure, more liberal amounts of fat, lactose, and other sugars can usually be tolerated.

Gluten occurs in greatest concentration in wheat, rye, barley, and oats. Rice and corn are practically free of gluten and are well tolerated. Eliminating wheat products from the diet is not an easy task — all products made with wheat, including wheat breads and rolls, both white and whole wheat, breaded foods, stuffing, macaroni, spaghetti, noodles, hot breads, cookies, cakes, wheat cereals, and gravies and cream sauces thickened with wheat flour — must be eliminated. Because wheat flour is used widely in commercially prepared foods, labels must be read. Such products as Postum, malted milk, and Ovaltine contain cereal grains. Gluten may be present in such minor ingredients as vegetable gum, stabilizers, preparations of monosodium glutamate (MSG), hydrolyzed vegetable protein, emulsifiers, malt, and other flavorings. Clients must avoid beer and ale, which may contain cereal grain Table 25-2 summarizes a gluten-free diet.

Rice, corn, and potato and soy flour are used in place of the omitted cereal grains. The American Celiac Society does not recommend the use of wheat starch, which contains small amounts of gluten. Cornflakes, cornmeal, hominy, rice, Rice Krispies, Puffed Rice, and precooked rice cereals can be used. Gravies, cream sauces, and desserts can be thickened with cornstarch or potato flour.

Client Education

The celiac sprue client must be helped to adhere rigidly to the gluten-free diet. Even small amounts of gluten can cause damage to the mucosa. The client needs help identifying foods that contain gluten and using substitutes for

Table 25-2.   Foods Allowed on a Gluten-Free Diet

Grain Group

Breads: specially prepared using cornmeal, cornstarch, potato starch, rice flour, soy, or other bean flours
Cereals: cornmeal, cream of rice, grits, hominy; Corn or rice ready-to-eat cereals such as cornflakes. Rice
  Krispies, rice flakes, Puffed Rice

Milk Group

Milk, cream, natural cheese, plain yogurt

Fruit and Vegetable Group

Fresh, frozen, canned or dried without added thickeners

Meat Group

Legumes, nuts, seeds: plain dried peas, beans, lentils, plain nuts and nut butters, plain seeds
Meat, fish, poultry, eggs: plain fresh or frozen

Other Foods

Beverages: carbonated beverages, coffee and tea (avoid instant types), cocoa, juice drinks
Desserts: custard; fruit ice; meringue; fruit whips; gelatin; puddings made with arrowroot, cornstarch, rice,
  tapioca; rennet dessert; specially prepared baked goods
Fats; butter, margarine, mayonnaise, oils, shortening
Snacks: corn chips, olives, pickles, potato chips, popcorn
Soups: clear meat and vegetable soups, homemade soups using allowed ingredients
Sweets: corn syrup, honey, jam, jelly, molasses, sugar
Seasonings: salt, pepper, and other plain spices and herbs; vinegar; wine

  Combine allowed ingredients as desired to make many interesting foods
  Many processed not listed above are gluten-free, but you must check the label to be sure. *Avoid* any food
that contains one or more of the following ingredients: barley; flour; gluten; graham; hydrolyzed vegetable
or plant protein; malt; malted milk; millet; modified food starch; oats; rye; starch (type unspecified, or
wheat, rye, or oat starch); wheat.

(Suitor CJ, Hunter MF: Nutrition: Principles and Application in Health Promotion, p 458. Philadelphia, JB
Lippincott, 1980)

wheat flour effectively. The American Celiac Society* is a very useful resource.

Diseases of the Large Intestine

Most of the protein, carbohydrate, and fat in food is absorbed in the small intestine. It never

* American Celiac Society, 45 Gifford Ave., Jersey City, NJ 07304

reaches the colon except in situations of malabsorption, as discussed previously. Therefore, dietary treatment in diseases of the large intestine necessitates changes related to the residue of food that remains in the colon after digestion and absorption have taken place.

Residue of Food

Residue includes the tough connective tissue of meat and tissues containing plant fiber. Some foods may contribute to residue by encouraging the growth of bacteria. The bacteria and the substances they produce add to the fecal contents. Milk produces residue in this way.

Plant fiber (or roughage) is responsible for most of the residue in the colon. *Plant fiber*

refers to indigestible carbohydrate, that part of plants that is not digested by the human digestive tract. Foods containing fiber are fruits, vegetables, nuts, and whole-grain cereals and breads. All plant foods contain fiber, but the amount varies from those that are high, such as wheat bran, to those that are low, such as potato (without skins) and banana. Whole-grain cereals in the form of unprocessed bran, unrefined wheat cereals, and whole-wheat and rye flours are the most important sources of fiber in food.

A number of major diseases are associated with a lack of fiber in the diet. High-fiber diets have proved helpful in treating chronic constipation, diverticulosis, and diabetes.

Foods Low In Residue

Tender or ground meats free of tough connective tissue; fats such as butter, margarine, and oil; refined carbohydrates such as white flour, spaghetti, macaroni, noodles, rice, refined breads and cereals, and sugar add very little residue to fecal material.

Fruit and vegetable juices, though low in fiber, may be omitted from some residue-restricted diets; they contain organic acids, which may have a laxative effect.

The fiber content of fruits and vegetables can be reduced in various ways, depending on the level of restriction desired. Young, tender vegetables have less fiber than mature ones. Cooked foods have softer fiber and create less bulk than raw ones. Peels from fruits and vegetables such as apples, pears, and potatoes can be removed. Fruits and vegetables can be strained to remove much of the fiber.

Residue-Restricted Diets

Some disorders of the large intestine require a residue-restricted diet to reduce the amount of fecal material in the colon. Ulcerative colitis, acute diverticulitis, malignant and nonmalignant lesions of the colon or rectum, and hemorrhoids all call for a residue-restricted diet, as does preparation for colon surgery and the immediate postsurgical period.

Diets vary slightly from one health facility to another. The health worker should become familiar with those served in her facility.

The minimal-residue diet contains no fruits, vegetables, or whole-grain breads and cereals. Milk is often omitted. Fruit and vegetable juices may be permitted in limited amounts. This diet is followed in preparation for bowel surgery or after surgery or when the colon is so inflamed that any colon expansion or bowel movement causes pain. The diet is inadequate in some vitamins and minerals, for which supplements may be ordered.

The usual moderate-residue diet includes strained fruits and vegetables, a few cooked tender vegetables, and a few cooked or canned fruits without skins or seeds. Ripe bananas are usually permitted, as are tender whole meats. This diet is followed as the client progresses after bowel surgery or in the treatment of ulcerative colitis.

A more liberal-residue diet is ordered for clients with ulcerative colitis or other conditions that require residue restriction for an extended period of time. Strained fruits and vegetables are replaced by cooked whole tender vegetables and cooked or canned fruits without skins or seeds.

Ulcerative Colitis

Ulcerative colitis is an inflammation of the colon. The areas of ulceration may involve only part of the rectum or colon or the entire large intestine. The client may have as many as 15 to 20 stools a day. The stools are semiliquid and contain blood and mucus. The person is malnourished and underweight as a result of diarrhea and blood loss. In serious cases, surgery may be necessary. The cause of ulcerative colitis is unknown, though emotional factors appear to play an important role.

The diet is usually low in residue and as high in protein and calories as the client can tolerate. Omitting or reducing roughage prevents irritation of the colon and permits it to rest and heal. The high-protein, high-calorie diet aims to correct the malnourishment. Vitamin and mineral supplements, especially iron, are prescribed. If citrus juices and milk are not

tolerated, supplements of vitamin C and calcium are ordered.

In extremely severe attacks of ulcerative colitis, intravenous feedings may be administered to rest the colon and improve the client's nutritional status. Usually a minimal or moderate residue diet is given in the acute stage of the disease. As the client's condition improves, the diet is made more liberal. The residue-restricted diet is used during the convalescent stage of the disease.

Intolerance to milk is a frequent occurrence, believed to be due to a lactase deficiency rather than to the colitis. If milk is tolerated, it may be given in moderate quantities.

The client with ulcerative colitis is frequently a fussy eater and hard to please. He requires much patience, understanding, and encouragement from the health care team.

Diverticulosis

Diverticulosis is characterized by outpouchings, called *diverticula,* in the wall of the large intestine. Some persons may have no symptoms, whereas others may experience lower abdominal pain and distention. If the diverticula become inflamed, a condition known as *diverticulitis* develops. Bleeding of the mucosa of the colon may also occur.

It has been suggested that diverticulosis is caused by a lack of natural fiber or roughage in the diet; thus, when fecal material is small, hard, and dry, movement slows and pressure increases in the colon. This pressure forces the lining out through weak spots in the muscle covering the colon, forming pouches (Fig. 25-2).

A high-fiber diet is followed to alleviate the symptoms, though not all reports of this approach have been favorable. As little as 2 tablespoons of unprocessed wheat bran or ½ to ¾ cup of breakfast cereal high in bran (All-Bran,* Bran Buds,* or Nabisco 100% Bran†) can increase fecal bulk and promote faster movement along the digestive tract. Although raw fruits

* The Kellogg Company, Battle Creek, MI 49016
† Nabisco Brands Inc., East Hanover, NJ 07936

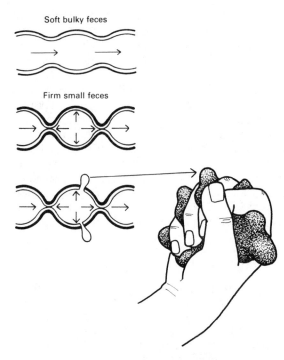

Fig. 25-2.   Diagram of the cause of diverticular disease. (Nutrition Today Magazine, Annapolis, MD. © Jan/Feb, 1976. Reprinted by permission)

and vegetables and legumes are good sources of fiber, they do not appear to be as effective as wheat bran in increasing fecal bulk. Small amounts, about 1 to 2 teaspoons, should be taken at first and increased gradually over a period of about 4 weeks until the desired amount is reached. The client should also drink plenty of fluids.

During an acute attack of diverticulitis, with fever, bleeding, and severe pain, a minimal- or moderate-residue diet is given. High-fiber foods should be discontinued if severe abdominal pain and fever develop, and the physician should be contacted.

Constipation

Constipation is the retention of feces in the colon resulting in the eventual passage of very dry, hard, or small stools. When no organic disease is found, the condition is usually attributed to poor health habits. Constipation in the elderly is often caused by a lack of muscle tone; the peristaltic waves become weak. Poor food habits and decreased activity are contributing factors.

A high-fiber diet helps prevent constipation and restore normal bowel movement if constipation exits. Whole-grain cereals and additional fruits and vegetables, both fresh and cooked, are incorporated into the diet. The addition of prunes and prune juice may be helpful.

Fluid intake should be increased to more than 1 quart a day. This is very important, since lack of fluid in a high-fiber diet can make constipation more severe.

Intestinal Gas

Symptoms of gaseousness are common. Though frequently attributed to the eating of specific foods, belching results from the swallowing of air and not from excessive gas production in the stomach.

In contrast, excessive gas in the large intestine does result from excessive gas production in the intestinal tract. The gas is produced mostly by bacterial activity on nonabsorbable carbohydrates in the colon.

Navy beans and soy beans produce appreciable quantities of gas because of the indigestible starches they contain. Persons with gastrointestinal disorders in which carbohydrates are poorly absorbed often experience excessive gas production; lactose intolerance (discussed previously) is such a disease.

The bloating feeling experienced after the ingestion of foods commonly thought to be gas-forming, such as cabbage, lettuce, and cauliflower, may be due to irritation of the gastrointestinal tract rather than to gas formation. A carefully kept diary of foods eaten and symptoms of gaseousness can help the client identify problem foods.

Diseases of the Liver

Any liver disease is devastating to the body. This is not surprising in view of the essential functions the liver performs. Nutrients, with very few exceptions, are carried by the bloodstream to the liver before they are distributed to the other tissues of the body. The liver changes the nutrients to a form that is most useful to the body; it stores some of them, such as iron, copper, vitamins A and D, and glucose in the form of glycogen; detoxifies poisonous substances; and synthesizes protein enzymes, plasma proteins, and the waste product urea from nitrogen (resulting from amino acid metabolism).

The amount of protein permitted a client —high, moderate, or low—depends upon his condition; changes are necessary as clinical status changes. Dietary treatment is complicated by the fact that, although protein is needed to rebuild damaged liver cells, protein metabolism in severe liver disease is so distorted that ammonia and other products of protein metabolism accumulate to abnormal levels in the blood. These substances are toxic to the central nervous system, and this can lead to serious complications.

Hepatitis and Early Cirrhosis

Hepatitis is an inflammation of the liver that is usually caused by a virus but may also result from the ingestion of alcohol, drugs, or other substances toxic to the liver. In hepatitis, liver cells are damaged, and replacement of the cells occurs too slowly for the organ to function normally. In milder cases, injury to liver tissue is reversible; in more severe cases, injury to liver cells is so extensive that liver failure and death result.

Cirrhosis is a term applied to all forms of liver disease in which there is extensive loss of liver cells. The cells are lost faster than they are

replaced, seriously impairing liver function. The active liver cells are replaced by scar tissue (connective tissue), which impairs blood circulation through the liver.

Cirrhosis may result from hepatitis or other causes, but it develops in 1 of every 12 chronic users of alcohol. Current research indicates that alcohol itself causes liver disease.

Dietary Treatment in Hepatitis and Early Cirrhosis

Dietary treatment in hepatitis and early cirrhosis requires a normal diet with adequate calories and a moderately high level of protein, up to 70 g to 80 g daily. Mineral and vitamin supplements are given. Achieving these goals may appear to be a simple task. However, nausea, diarrhea, fever, and fatigue interfere with food intake. Much encouragement and persuasion are needed to get the client to eat enough food. The nurse and dietitian must work closely together to provide the kinds and amounts of food most acceptable to the client and environmental conditions that promote appetite. Food intake is usually increased when six small meals are given rather than three large meals. The amount of food eaten should be carefully observed and recorded.

Meeting caloric needs is a central requirement. If calories supplied by carbohydrates and fats are not adequate, proteins from food and from body cells will be broken down to supply energy, and this will decrease the protein available for cell replacement. A calorie intake of 2500 kcal or more (approximately 35–40 kcal per kg of body weight) is offered. The level may be more than 3000 kcal if fever is high and weight loss is extensive.

Most of the energy is supplied by carbohydrate. Moderate amounts of fat are permitted unless there is obstruction of the bile duct. In such a case, fats are poorly tolerated and are restricted to 30 g to 40 g daily.

Dietary Treatment in Advanced Cirrhosis

In advanced cirrhosis, there is extensive loss of liver cells with disruption in blood flow through the liver. The liver is unable to metabolize protein normally or to detoxify the ammonia that enters the blood from the intestinal tract. As a result, ammonia and other toxins accumulate in the blood. These substances are toxic to the central nervous system, causing hepatic coma, which is characterized by symptoms of drowsiness, a fecal odor to the breath, flapping tremors of the hands and tongue when extended, and disorientation. If it is untreated, coma and finally death follow.

To reduce levels of ammonia and other protein metabolites when coma is threatened, protein in the diet is restricted. Depending on the client's condition, the prescribed protein level may range from 20 g to 60 g. The diet is similar to the protein-restricted diet used for persons with renal disease (see Chap. 24). Low-protein wheat starch products appear to be beneficial.

If hepatic coma develops, all protein is omitted. Small, frequent feedings of carbohydrate foods are given by mouth, if possible, or continuous intravenous dextrose is given to provide energy. As the client's condition improves, protein is added gradually and in small quantities. Some clients may need to restrict protein intake to 40 g to 60 g per day permanently. Here again, maintaining a sufficient calorie intake is important. If body protein is broken down to supply energy, blood ammonia levels will increase.

Ascites, an accumulation of fluid in the abdominal cavity, is a complication of cirrhosis. Sodium restriction usually stops the further accumulation of fluid and may lead to the loss of excess fluid. Severe restriction of sodium to 500 mg or even 200 mg daily may be necessary (see Chap. 23).

A very serious potential complication of cirrhosis is esophageal varices, which are enlarged blood vessels in the esophagus. Should these varices rupture, the hemorrhage (severe bleeding) that follows can threaten the client's life. Thus, coarse fibrous foods are excluded from the diet, and foods having a smooth texture are included in the diet. Meats are ground and fruits and vegetables pureed, to make them easier to swallow. If bleeding occurs, a liquid diet is substituted.

Gallbladder Disease

Gallbladder disease most frequently takes the form of cholelithiasis (gallstones) accompanied by cholecystitis (inflammation of the gallbladder). There is severe epigastric pain, indigestion, and intolerance to fatty or spicy foods, and there may be pain after the ingestion of fat and spices. Surgical removal of the gallbladder is performed if the client does not respond to medical treatment.

Before surgery, fats may be restricted if they cause pain or if steatorrhea develops owing to inadequate bile flow. Fatty meats, fish, and poultry, hard cheeses, fried foods, salad oils, salad dressings, and gravies, nuts, and rich pastries and desserts are omitted from the diet. Whole milk, butter and margarine, and eggs may be permitted in limited amounts, though eggs are omitted if they cause distress.

If the client is grossly obese, surgery is usually delayed until some weight loss has been achieved. After surgery, bile flows continuously into the small intestine. At first, the client may feel more comfortable limiting fat, but after a month or two, he may resume a normal diet. In time, a portion of the bile duct may enlarge, providing for temporary storage of bile.

Pancreatitis

Pancreatitis, or inflammation of the pancreas, may be associated with alcoholism, infection, or other disease or may be of unknown origin. Abdominal pain is the most common symptom, and nausea, vomiting, and steatorrhea may also be present.

When the pancreas is inflamed, stimulating pancreatic secretion may cause excruciating pain. Intravenous feedings usually provide nourishment during the acute stages of the disease and provide rest for the pancreas. High-carbohydrate liquids are the first oral feedings given. Later, small meals that consist of easily digested carbohydrate and protein and that are limited in fat are given. Fats are restricted because the pancreatic enzymes necessary for their digestion are missing. The diet is also bland in order to reduce the presence of dilute hydrochloric acid in the duodenum, which stimulates the flow of pancreatic juice. Pancreatic enzymes may be taken with meals and snacks. Medium chain triglycerides (MCT), a synthetic oil, may be included in the diet to provide additional calories. Pancreatic enzymes do not appear to be required for the digestion of this fat.

KEYS TO PRACTICAL APPLICATION

Learn to control stress and try to minimize it in the lives of others; prolonged stress can have a very damaging effect on health, including that of the gastrointestinal tract.

Much of what we used to believe concerning the irritating characteristics of various foods has not been supported by research. Remember this before giving advice to clients who have peptic ulcers or other gastric disorders.

Find out what type of dietary approach — conservative or liberal — has been ordered for a client with peptic ulcer. Be sure to report any aspects of the diet that may be causing anxiety. The physician will frequently permit changes that will minimize stress.

Regardless of the dietary approach used, the hospitalized client with ulcers is usually given frequent small meals. Be sure the client receives the between-

meal feedings that have been planned for him.

Respect the client's aversion to foods that cause him distress. Tolerance for foods differs greatly from person to person.

Encourage clients with a milk intolerance to seek a solution to this problem. Small amounts of milk at a time, fermented milk products, or enzyme-treated milk may be tolerated.

Be accepting of the food aversions and food-related complaints of the client with colitis. Do what you can to encourage the client to eat adequate amounts of food and to see that he

receives foods he likes to the extent possible.

When the use of bran in the diet has been ordered, caution the client to start with a small amount, increasing it gradually until the desired amount is reached, and advise him to drink plenty of water. This will help reduce the unpleasant side-effects of high-fiber diets.

Encourage the client who is experiencing nausea and vomiting to eat as much as he can, possibly small amounts at a time. Help him understand why this is important. Carefully record the amount of food consumed.

KEY IDEAS

Prolonged stress makes the gastrointestinal tract prone to disorders that may lead to diseases such as peptic ulcer and ulcerative colitis.

Factors involved in the development of peptic ulcer include increased amounts of acid and pepsin; decreased resistance of the protective mucosa; and a high degree of emotional stress.

Treatment for peptic ulcers aims to promote healing by reducing irritating conditions and providing adequate nutrition.

Use of the bland diet has declined because of a lack of scientific evidence that certain properties of food are irritating to the gastrointestinal tract.

The following foods have been found to increase gastric acidity or otherwise irritate the lining of the stomach: alcohol, coffee (regular and decaffeinated), tea, pepper, and chili powder. Meat extractives used in meat-based soups and meat drippings are thought to stimulate gastric secretion and may also be omitted from the diet.

Small, frequent feedings have been found to relieve symptoms and reduce gastric acidity; hunger is accompanied by an abundant flow of gastric juices.

Milk therapy may be used for a short period of time in the early treatment of bleeding ulcers. Prolonged use of a milk-rich bland diet is not recommended, since it may have harmful effects in clients prone to atherosclerosis or hypercalcemia.

Some physicians use the liberal approach in the treatment of peptic ulcers, believing that the client progresses just as well as or better than otherwise when eating foods of his own choice.

Dietary modifications that may relieve symptoms in hiatus hernia include correcting obesity; avoiding excessive amounts of food and excessive fat; avoiding acid-stimulating foods; drinking fluids between rather than with meals; avoiding lying down for 2 hours after eating.

Most clients with lactose intolerance can tolerate small quantities of milk at a time, fermented milk products such as yogurt and cottage cheese, or milk treated with a commercial enzyme preparation. When lactose intolerance is severe, the client must be alerted to hidden sources of lactose in the diet.

The gluten-free diet used to treat celiac

sprue requires the avoidance of all wheat, rye, oats, and barley; rice, corn, soy, and potato flours are used as substitutes for wheat flour.

Ulcerative colitis may be treated with a low-residue diet to prevent irritation and permit rest and healing; milk is frequently poorly tolerated. The client may be permitted foods of his own choice because of emotional factors.

Diverticulosis is now treated by high-fiber diets rather than by the low-residue diets used in the past. Wheat bran has been found to be the most effective form of fiber. During an acute attack of diverticulitis, a minimal- or moderate-residue diet is given.

Constipation is treated with a high-fiber diet — increased whole grains, fruits, and vegetables — and increased fluids. The laxative properties of prunes and prune juice may also be helpful.

Gas in the large intestine is produced mostly by bacterial activity on the nonabsorbable carbohydrates in the colon.

In hepatitis and early cirrhosis, the diet is moderately high in protein; in advanced cirrhosis, protein is restricted to 20 g to 60 g as a means of preventing hepatic coma. Supplying sufficient calories is extremely important at all stages of liver disease; symptoms of nausea, vomiting, and abdominal distress make the eating of adequate amounts of food difficult.

Ascites, a frequent complication of cirrhosis, requires severe sodium restriction; esophageal varices require that food be very smooth in texture — finely ground or pureed.

In gallbladder disease, fats and spices may be restricted if they cause distress. Weight loss may be required prior to gallbladder surgery. Many clients can resume a normal diet 1 to 2 months after gallbladder surgery.

Total parenteral nutrition usually provides nourishment during the acute stages of pancreatitis. When oral feedings are tolerated, the diet is very low in fat and bland to avoid stimulating the flow of pancreatic enzymes. MCT oil may be used to provide additional calories. Pancreatic enzyme medication may be taken with meals and snacks.

KEYS TO LEARNING: STUDY–DISCUSSION QUESTIONS

1. Discuss in class the relationship of emotional stress to disease of the gastrointestinal tract. What effect does it have on the functioning of the gastrointestinal tract? Do you know of other diseases that are related to stress? The control of emotional stress is beginning to receive much attention from medical authorities. Read and discuss professional articles and lay publications relating to this problem.

2. What are the basic principles in the treatment of peptic ulcer? What role does diet play in achieving these goals?

3. Ask your hospital therapeutic dietitian to discuss with the class the diet plan most frequently used in the treatment of ulcers in your hospital. What percentage of cases are being treated by the traditional approach and what percentage by the liberal approach? What changes have occurred in the diet therapy of peptic ulcer disease in recent years?

4. Plan a six-meal bland diet menu for a 37-year-old factory worker who is recovering from peptic ulcers. He works from 4:00 P.M. to 12:00 midnight.

5. Assume that you are counseling a client who has severe lactose intolerance. What foods would you advise him to avoid?

6. What effect does gluten have on the jejunal mucosa of the client with celiac sprue? What is the most characteristic symptom of this disease?

7. Plan a gluten-free menu for 1 day for a 30-year-old secretary who eats her lunch in a small luncheonette.

8. What foods contribute to residue in the intestinal tract? What foods are very low in residue?

9. Plan a five-meal menu (three meals and two between-meal feedings) for a hospitalized client on a minimum-residue diet as it is served in your hospital.

10. A 25-year-old female client with ulcerative colitis is complaining bitterly about the food served her. She chose these foods herself from the selective menu shown her the previous day. Discuss in class how this situation might be handled.

11. What foods contribute fiber or roughage to the diet? Plan a day's menu that is high in fiber. Why is fiber thought to be beneficial in the treatment of diverticular disease?

12. Discuss the dietary changes necessary in each of the following complications of cirrhosis: ascites, esophageal bleeding, and hepatic coma.

13. In your hospital, how many grams of fat are included in the low-fat diet usually served to clients with gallbladder disease? What foods supply this fat?

Bibliography is found at the end of Part Four.

Nutrition in Surgery and Following Burns

KEY TERMS

aspirate   To draw in; foreign substances may be aspirated into the nose, throat, or lungs during inhalation.

collagen   A fibrous protein found in connective tissue.

comatose   In a condition of coma, an abnormal, deep stupor.

elemental diet   A liquid formula that provides the essential nutrients in a form that is easily absorbed and leaves no residue in the intestinal tract.

parenteral   Occurring outside the gastrointestinal tract; injected into a vein or muscle or under the skin.

regurgitation   The return of solids or fluid to the mouth from the stomach.

stoma   An opening created by surgery between a body passageway and the body surface.

total parenteral nutrition   Provision of total nutritional needs intravenously via the superior vena cava.

Among the most critically ill clients are those who have undergone surgery or have experienced acute injury such as severe burns. Meeting the nutritional needs of these clients is a challenge to the health care team requiring a high degree of skill and cooperation. Without this care, recovery may be delayed or may not proceed normally. Preoperative improvement in the nutritional status of a poorly nourished client due to undergo surgery lessens the possibility of later complications. The well-nourished surgical client has many advantages: he heals more quickly, is better able to fight infection, loses less muscle tissue, and enjoys a greater sense of well-being than a client who is poorly nourished.

Nutritional Care Before Surgery

In some instances, the client's poor nutritional state may be a consequence of the disease itself, as in cancer of the stomach or the esophagus, which interferes with the intake and utilization of food. If the client is poorly nourished and if the surgery is not of an emergency nature, a high-protein, high-calorie diet may be ordered to improve his nutritional status. Methods of feeding that can improve the nutritional status of a severely malnourished client are now avail-

357

able. These methods are discussed later in this chapter.

In addition to malnourished persons, extremely obese persons are surgical risks. They may not recover from anesthesia in the normal way and may have breathing difficulties, which increase the risk of lung complications. The obese person's extra blood vessels, which nourish the adipose fatty tissue, increase the work of the heart. Furthermore, adipose tissue, which the obese person has a larger than normal amount of, heals more slowly and is more prone to infection than muscle tissue. Sometimes the physician delays surgery until the obese client loses a certain amount of weight.

A minimal-residue diet may be ordered for several days before gastrointestinal surgery to reduce the residue (material remaining after digestion) in the intestine (see Chap. 25). On the day before surgery, usually no food is permitted after the evening meal. Fluids are generally permitted until midnight.

The Body's Response to Surgery or Injury

The body's response to surgery or injury is divided into three phases. In the period immediately following surgery or injury, the *catabolic phase*, metabolism is greatly increased, with loss of body tissue resulting in a huge loss of nitrogen and potassium. Fluid and sodium are retained in the tissues owing to hormonal changes. Body fat is the primary source of energy. Peristalsis and absorption in the gastrointestinal tract are reduced.

Next comes the *anabolic phase*. Positive nitrogen balance is re-established as the lean body tissue that was lost is gradually restored. Weight is slowly regained. Excess sodium and water is excreted, and potassium is retained. Peristalsis returns to normal. This phase usually

begins within 5 to 7 days of surgery or injury but may be delayed in cases of complex surgery or severe burns.

Finally, in the *fat gain phase*, which may last for 2 to 3 months, the fat lost during the catabolic phase is restored.

Nutritional Needs Following Surgery or Acute Injury

Postoperative nutritional care includes maintenance of fluid and electrolyte balance and provision of adequate energy, protein, vitamins, and minerals.

Fluid and Electrolyte Balance

The first priority is to maintain fluid and electrolyte balance. Immediately after surgery, fluids and electrolytes are administered intravenously. No food or fluids are given by mouth until peristalsis has returned. The solutions may have 5% or 10% dextrose, amino acids, vitamins, and medications added as necessary; this provides nutritional support for persons who are in reasonably good health and who will probably be eating adequately in 3 or 4 days.

Calories

In the immediate postoperative period, intravenous solutions of 5% or 10% dextrose provide energy, although energy thus supplied falls far short of the client's needs. After surgery, an adult male weighing 70 kg (154 lb) requires 40 kcal to 70 kcal per kg of body weight, or 2800 kcal to 4900 kcal. At most, 400 kcal to 500 kcal can be administered safely in a 24-hour period by a 5% dextrose solution. During this period, body fat is the main source of energy; however, if calories are inadequate for an extended pe-

riod, wound healing and all other aspects of recovery will be hindered.

Protein

Adequate amounts of protein are essential for wound healing, to protect the liver from damage, and to promote resistance to infection. After severe injury, such as extensive burns, large amounts of muscle tissue can be lost in 1 day. After surgery, blood loss, in addition to tissue damage, results in considerable protein loss. Significant loss of protein can also result from the wasting of bone and muscle when the body is immobilized. Getting the patient up and out of bed is extremely important in promoting a positive nitrogen balance (the rebuilding of lean body tissue). In most circumstances, 1.5 g to 2 g of protein per kg of body weight is sufficient for clients who have been well-nourished. Many adult Americans ordinarily consume these amounts, which are therefore not difficult to achieve. However, in clients with poor absorption or extensive injury such as severe burns, the protein need may be well over 100 g daily, in contrast to the recommended protein allowance of 56 g for an adult male.

Vitamins and Minerals

Production of collagen, which is basic to wound healing, requires adequate amounts of ascorbic acid. Zinc is also essential for wound healing. Vitamin B_6 and other vitamins as well as various minerals are required for protein formation. Vitamin K is necessary for the normal production of prothrombin in blood clotting.

Feeding Methods Following Surgery

After surgery, most clients are able to take fluid and food by mouth in 1 to 4 days. In some cases,

however, achieving adequate nutritional intake by normal means may be impossible, and tube feedings or intravenous feedings may be necessary for extended periods of time. Although the health worker may not have direct responsibility for preparing or administering tube feedings, she may be called upon to assist with them.

The client who has been severely undernourished for many days should not be given a full diet all at one time, regardless of the method of feeding being used. Rapid refeeding may cause an overload on the heart and blood vessels and serious gastrointestinal problems. In a severely malnourished person, the amount of blood circulating in the body, the blood pressure, and the amount of blood pumped by the heart per minute are lower than normal. Also, it takes some time for digestive enzymes to be restored after surgery. Starting with one fourth the full diet and increasing the amount gradually every few days is recommended.

Progressive Hospital Diets

Following surgery, after normal peristalsis has returned, the client is given a clear liquid diet. The use of clear liquids such as broth and gelatin dessert help to determine whether fluids by mouth can be tolerated, and fluids pose fewer risks than solids should aspiration (the drawing of food into the lungs) occur as a result of vomiting. The client is then progressed to a full liquid diet, a soft or light diet, and finally a regular diet (see Chap. 3). Some clients go directly from clear liquids to a regular diet. If the client has a condition requiring a modified diet, such as diabetes or cardiovascular disease, he is given a diet appropriate to his condition.

Tube Feedings

Tube feedings are liquified foods fed through a tube inserted into the stomach or small intestine. Tube feedings are given to clients who cannot take food by mouth because, for example, they are unable to swallow, have an obstruction in the esophagus, or have undergone surgery of the mouth, neck, or esophagus. The nasogastric (nose) or orogastric (mouth) tube

requires no incision and for this reason is commonly used for short-term feeding. A gastrostomy, the creation of an opening through the abdominal wall into the stomach, is preferred for long-term use to avoid irritation of the mucous membranes. Figure 26-1 shows several routes by which tube feeding may be carried out.

There are three types of tube feeding: milk or casein-based (milk protein) formulas, blenderized formulas, and semisynthetic, fiber-free liquid diets (also called *elemental* or *chemically defined* diets). All are available in commercial form. Most hospitals use commercial formulas.

In some circumstances, calculated milk-based formulas and blenderized feedings are prepared in a health facility or at home. A *milk-based formula* is one in which some form of milk is the principal ingredient. A *blenderized formula* contains food normally included in the diet, such as meat, vegetable, fruit, pasteurized powdered egg,* and milk (the latter

* Avoid use of raw egg in making tube feedings or supplemental beverages because of the danger of salmonella food poisoning.

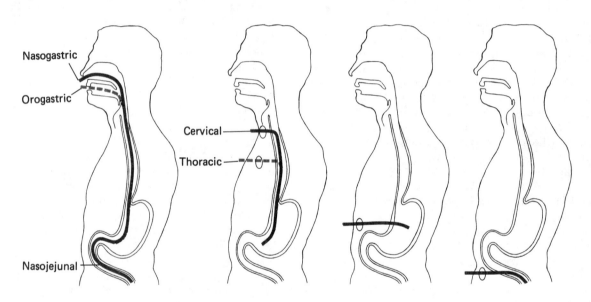

Fig. 26-1.   Various routes by which tube feedings may be administered. *(Left to right) Intragastric:* A tube is passed through nose or mouth into the stomach or jejunum and secured in place. Easily inserted by physician or trained nurse. *Esophagotomy:* A temporary or permanent opening (stoma) is constructed at one of several places to allow the tube to be introduced through the skin into the esophagus. Dependable for long-term feeding; allows apparatus to be hidden; easy to handle. *Gastrostomy:* A temporary or permanent stoma is constructed, allowing food to be introduced through the skin directly into stomach. Preferred for long-term tube feeding of children and for adults in whom use of the esophagus is not desirable. Requires partial undressing at mealtime. *Jejunostomy:* A constructed opening permitting placement of the tube directly into the jejunum. High incidence of dumping syndrome and diarrhea with use of this site. (Adapted from Suitor CW, Hunter MF: Nutrition: Principles and Application in Health Promotion. Philadelphia, JB Lippincott, 1980)

may be omitted if the client has lactose intolerance). The client who is at home may prepare his own milk-based or blenderized feeding to save money and get more variety. *Semisynthetic fiber-free liquid diets* are commercial liquid formulas that contain essential nutrients in a highly absorbable form and are free of fiber. These formulas require little digestion and leave practically no residue. They are used when there is poor absorption of nutrients or when it is desirable to rest the large intestine.

Standard tube feeding formulas contain approximately 1 kcal/ml; 1500 ml of a formula thus provide 1500 kcal. The type of tube feeding ordered and its nutritional content depend on the needs of the individual client.

Administration

Concentration and Volume. Tube feedings that have a high concentration of nutrients can cause serious problems. The intestinal tract may draw in fluid from the circulation to dilute the formula. As a result, the client may become weak, feel distended, and have diarrhea. Therefore, diluted feedings of one quarter to one half of normal strength are given during the first 24 hours in quantities of only 40 ml to 60 ml per hour. If these feedings are tolerated, the concentration and volume are gradually increased until the prescribed calorie level is reached. Volume and concentration are not increased at the same time.

Regurgitation of Stomach Contents. In elderly and comatose tube-fed clients, there is risk of aspiration pneumonia caused by the regurgitation (back-up) of the stomach contents and its aspiration (breathing in) into the lungs. The client who is lying flat is most likely to regurgitate. An elderly or unconscious client should have the head of his bed raised to a 30° angle.

Temperature. Tube feedings should not be warmed before being given. The semisynthetic liquid should be kept very cold to prevent growth of bacteria, and other commercial liquid feedings should be given at room temperature immediately after the container has been opened. Any remaining portion should be refrigerated.

Rate. Tube feedings are usually given by means of a food pump or by the gravity-drip method, both of which allow for control of the flow rate. A method in which the formula is fed as a meal through a large tube in the stomach may be followed after the client has adjusted to the tube feeding process. Jejunostomy feedings can be given only by the drip method and are given more slowly than nasogastric feedings because of an increased risk of diarrhea and other problems.

Water Intake. The client must have adequate amounts of fluid in order for the waste products of protein metabolism to be excreted in the urine. Fluid intake must be observed especially carefully in the elderly person. Close supervision and careful recording of protein intake and fluid intake and output are always necessary.

Contamination. Tube feedings provide an excellent environment for bacterial growth, which may lead to gastrointestinal infection. When a commercial tube feeding packaged in a can is opened, the top of the can should be rinsed with sterile water and the can then opened with a sterile can opener. If liquid is poured into a container, the container must be sterile for each batch of feeding. Only small batches (500 – 1000 ml) should be hung at one time. Except for unopened cans of commercial products, all tube feedings that have been in the refrigerator for 24 hours should be discarded.

Use As Oral Feedings

Except for the semisynthetic diets, commercial formula feedings are palatable when taken by mouth. The semisynthetic diets should be served well-chilled, over ice, or frozen as a slush. They should be sipped slowly and amounts increased gradually to prevent gastrointestinal problems.

Total Parenteral Nutrition

In clients with some conditions, such as severe burns and severe intestinal disease, it is not possible to provide adequate nutrition by mouth or by tube feeding for a significant period of time. In this case, a method of intravenous feeding called *total parenteral nutrition* (*parenteral* means other than through the gastrointestinal tract) is used. The total parenteral nutrition (TPN) solution contains amino acids, glucose, electrolytes, and other essential nutrients. It is given through a catheter inserted into the superior vena cava. This vein is selected because the TPN solution is highly concentrated and must enter the body in a region of high blood flow. The TPN solution is prepared under sterile conditions in the pharmacy.

TPN is sometimes associated with serious complications related to insertion of the catheter, infection, and metabolic problems. Only personnel trained and skilled in TPN should give this care; in fact, many hospitals have a specially trained TPN team that includes a physician, nurse, dietitian, and pharmacist.

Because the client on TPN is receiving nothing by mouth, the mucous lining of the oral cavity may become dry and irritated. Good oral care is a great comfort to such a client. The mouth should be moistened and cleansed and the teeth brushed regularly.

Diet Following Gastrointestinal Surgery

Gastrectomy

A gastrectomy is an operation for the removal of all or part of the stomach. Diet therapy following a gastrectomy aims at avoiding or minimizing possible postoperative problems. After surgery, the client is unable to tolerate large quantities of food at one time. After peristalsis has returned, the client is given clear liquids, in very small quantities of approximately 30 ml (1 oz) per feeding the first day increasing to 60 ml (2 oz) per feeding the second day. If these are well tolerated, he is given six to eight small feedings of easily digested foods. The feedings are limited to 3 to 4 ounces at first, the equivalent of one slice of bread and one poached egg. Volume is gradually increased until 8 to 10 ounces per feeding are taken.

Dumping Syndrome

Following a gastrectomy, the contents of the stomach tend to pass more rapidly than normal from the stomach into the intestinal tract. In order to become properly diluted, the mass of food draws water from the circulating blood, thus reducing blood volume. In addition, sugars are rapidly absorbed and overstimulate the secretion of insulin, causing very low blood sugar levels. As a result of these occurrences, the client experiences nausea, cramps, diarrhea, lightheadedness, and extreme weakness about 15 to 30 minutes after meals. This condition is known as the *dumping syndrome.*

As a means of preventing the dumping syndrome, or as therapy if it has already occurred, the diet after a gastrectomy is high in protein and fat and moderate to low in total carbohydrate. Foods permitted are low in fiber, easily digested, and free of chemical stimulants such as caffeine and spices. Concentrated sugars, such as sucrose, and foods containing them are severely restricted. For example, canned fruits and desserts such as custard must be unsweetened or artificially sweetened. Starches such as potatoes, bread, rice, and macaroni are limited to small amounts at each feeding. Moderate amounts of sugar may be tolerated after recovery.

Fluid taken with meals tends to increase the rapid movement of food. Therefore, fluid is

omitted from meals or limited to 4 ounces at each meal. Fluid may be taken 30 to 40 minutes after meals. Sometimes lactose intolerance develops after gastric surgery and requires the omission of milk from the diet.

Intestinal Surgery

Short Bowel Syndrome

Removal of a large portion of the small intestine causes loss of much of the intestinal surface through which nutrients are absorbed. This makes good nutritional status very difficult to maintain.

After surgery, the client receives TPN or elemental tube feedings. The nutrients in elemental feedings require little digestion, are readily absorbed in the upper gastrointestinal tract, and leave practically no residue. The first elemental feedings, which are very dilute, are given by nasogastric tube and gradually increased in volume and concentration. The client may then progress to low-residue tube feedings. Small oral feedings of low-fiber carbohydrate foods are gradually introduced, followed by low-fat protein foods. Fats are poorly tolerated.

It is very difficult to maintain good nutritional status in clients who have had massive intestinal resection, because changes in fluid and electrolyte balance, diarrhea, extreme weight loss, and severe malnutrition occur frequently in such clients. Very high levels of protein, energy, vitamins, and minerals are required.

Ileostomy

Serious cases of colitis may require surgery in which removal of the entire colon and rectum may be necessary. The end of the remaining ileum is attached to a small permanent opening,

the stoma, formed in the abdominal wall. Digestive wastes are eliminated through this opening into an attached pouch. Waste material in the ileum is fluid in nature and drains almost continuously. There is considerable loss of fluid, sodium, potassium, and other nutrients. Vitamin B_{12} is absorbed in only small quantities or not at all. Periodic injections of vitamin B_{12} are therefore necessary throughout the client's life.

Once he can tolerate liquids, the ileostomy client is given a very low-residue diet. Foods with higher amounts of residue are added gradually one at a time. Because weight loss is common, a high-protein, high-calorie diet is needed. Liberal fluid intake, at least 2 quarts a day, is required. Excessive fiber may need to be avoided so that the stoma does not become blocked. Foods that tend to block the stoma include dried fruit, corn, popcorn, mushrooms, membranes of citrus fruit, and coconut. Thorough chewing of food reduces the chance of blockage.

Colostomy

After the lower portion of the diseased colon has been removed, the end of the descending colon is attached to an opening created in the abdominal wall. In this part of the intestine, the intestinal contents are more formed, and some regularity in the discharge can be established.

After surgery, the client is given clear liquids followed by a very low-residue diet. Most clients are able to return to a normal diet in a short time.

Rectal Surgery

Clear liquids followed by a very low-residue diet may be ordered for a short period following rectal surgery. Sometimes a low-residue, semisynthetic diet is used. Keeping residue to a minimum delays bowel movements until healing has begun.

Nutrition in Burn Treatment

The rate of tissue breakdown and loss of body fat and other stores of nutrients are greater in serious burns than in any other disease process. Providing adequate nutritional care for the burn client is of primary importance; unless positive nitrogen balance is achieved, wound healing cannot take place. Body weight is an excellent means of evaluating the effectiveness of nutritional care.

The energy and protein needs of the burn client are much greater than normal. Energy needs range from 3000 kcal to 5000 kcal for adults and from 70 kcal to 100 kcal per kg of body weight for children; protein needs are 50% or more above normal. Greatly increased amounts of ascorbic acid are needed for wound healing, and more B vitamins than normal are needed to meet the demands of the high metabolic rate. Urinary excretion of the waste products of tissue breakdown — nitrogen and potassium — requires the ingestion of large quantities of water to hold these wastes in solution and to replace the lost body fluids.

Intravenous dextrose, electrolytes, and blood plasma are given at first. When the client can tolerate food by mouth, a high-protein, high-calorie diet is given.

For clients with extensive burns, nutritional requirements can seldom be met by oral feeding. It may be necessary to provide between 30% and 75% of the daily kilocalories intravenously or by nasogastric tube. If there is injury to the mouth, face, or respiratory or gastrointestinal tract, TPN may be required. It is important that the client receive sufficient water. The client should be made aware of his increased need for food and the ways in which this need is being met.

Recording Food Intake

Whether food and fluid are taken by mouth or by tube, the amount consumed by the client after surgery or severe injury should be carefully monitored and recorded. This is essential for the adequacy of nutritional care to be evaluated. For example, if an anorexic client is unable to eat enough food to support his recovery, the physician may decide that tube feedings are necessary.

Providing Psychological Support

Clients who are tube-fed or who receive TPN are usually critically ill and often depressed and frightened. It is not difficult to imagine the stress created by the feeding method itself; the client is denied the pleasures and the social and emotional satisfactions associated with eating.

Correct techniques, procedures, and formulas must of course be followed. However, good care goes beyond these mechanical details and considers the client's psychological needs as well. Showing kindness, understanding, concern, and encouragement is also a part of the health team's responsibility.

KEYS TO PRACTICAL APPLICATION

Check to see that diet orders are carried out accurately before surgery. Feeding a client when he should not be fed or providing the wrong diet may require a delay in surgery.

Check trays carefully. Serious complications can result if the client receives the wrong diet after surgery.

Follow instructions accurately when feeding someone who has been undernourished for many days. The severely undernourished body cannot adjust immediately to a normal amount of food. Small amounts are given at first and increased gradually.

Use sanitary techniques when preparing or handling tube feedings. Be sure that sterile equipment and sterile containers are used and that the prepared formula is properly refrigerated.

Provide good oral care for the client who is not being fed by mouth.

Record food and fluid intake accurately. This information is necessary for evaluation of the adequacy of nutritional care.

Show understanding and give encouragement to the client who is fed by tube or TPN. It is not hard to imagine the stress created by these extreme feeding methods.

KEY IDEAS

The client who is well nourished before surgery has a great advantage; when possible, the nutritional status of a poorly nourished person is built up before surgery. Weight loss may be required of the obese client.

In preparation for surgery, no food is given after the evening meal and no fluids after midnight of the day before surgery.

The body's response to surgery or injury is characterized by three phases: breakdown, recovery, and fat gain.

Maintaining fluid and electrolyte balance is the first priority after surgery.

After surgery and acute injury, the need for calories, protein, vitamins, and minerals is much higher than normal.

Body fat reserves are the primary source of

energy in the early postoperative period. However, if calories remain inadequate for long periods, protein will be used for energy rather than for repair and building of tissue, and all aspects of recovery will be hindered as a result.

In most cases, food may be taken by mouth 1 to 4 days after surgery; however, some situations require tube feeding or TPN.

Refeeding of the client who has been severely undernourished for many days should be carried out very gradually and cautiously to avoid cardiovascular overload and gastrointestinal problems.

Feeding methods after surgery include intravenous feedings of fluids, electrolytes, dextrose, amino acids, and

vitamins followed by oral feedings (progressive hospital diets or modified diets), tube feedings, or TPN.

There are three general types of tube feedings: milk or casein-based formulas, blenderized formulas, and semisynthetic fiber-free formulas (also called *elemental diets*). The type ordered and its nutritional contents depend upon the needs of the client. Commercially made feedings are usually used.

Semisynthetic, fiber-free formulas (elemental diets) require little digestion and leave practically no residue; they are used when there is poor absorption or when it is desirable to rest the large intestine. They may be given by tube or by mouth.

Serious complications, including diarrhea and aspiration pneumonia, can arise from the use of tube feedings.

Measures that can help prevent complications in the use of tube feedings include the use of very small quantities of dilute formula at first, with concentration and volume increased gradually; the avoidance of contamination of tube feeding by careful handling; and elevation of the head of the bed for elderly and comatose clients.

Clients receiving large quantities of protein need adequate fluid intake so that waste products of protein metabolism can be excreted properly.

Total parenteral nutrition (*TPN*) refers to intravenous feedings that meet the client's total nutritional needs; the solution passes through a catheter inserted into the superior vena cava, a region of high blood flow.

Good oral care for the client fed by tube or intravenously is important. Without such care, the mouth becomes dry and irritated.

The postgastrectomy diet aims at counteracting development of the "dumping syndrome": a very small volume of food is given at first and increased gradually; concentrated carbohydrate, especially sucrose, is restricted; fluids are taken 30 to 40 minutes after meals or in only very small amounts with meals.

Removal of a large portion of the small intestine entails great loss of intestinal surface through which nutrients are absorbed, making good nutritional status difficult to maintain. The client is fed by TPN or by tube for an extended period of time following surgery.

Nutritional needs of clients with severe burns are greatly above normal and are rarely met by oral feeding alone. TPN or tube feedings are necessary.

The amounts of food and fluid consumed either by mouth or by tube following surgery or severe injury should be carefully monitored and recorded.

Clients being fed by extreme measures such as tube feedings or TPN are in great need of psychological support — kindness, understanding, and encouragement.

KEYS TO LEARNING: STUDY–DISCUSSION QUESTIONS

1. Review the foods served on the clear liquid diet and on the full liquid diet (see Chap. 3). Why is the first postoperative feeding a clear liquid diet? Why is it so important that the client receive the correct diet after surgery?

2. Meeting the nutritional needs of the client is extremely important to his recovery. Why then should refeeding of the severely malnourished client be started slowly and cautiously?

3. What adverse reactions may a client experience from tube feedings? How can these be prevented? Discuss the importance of adequate water intake.

4. Why are raw eggs not used in tube feedings or supplemental beverages such as egg-nogs? What is used in their place?

5. Present to the class a case study of the nutritional care of a tube-fed client or of one on TPN. Include in your report the following information: reason client cannot take food by mouth; kind of feeding given; nutritional content (protein, fat, carbohydrate, kilocalories) of client's average daily intake; average daily fluid intake; adverse reactions, if any; and psychological outlook of client.

6. Describe the symptoms of the dumping syndrome. Why do they occur? What changes in diet help alleviate the problem?

7. What is the short bowel syndrome? When tube or oral feeding is begun, why is a semisynthetic, fiber-free (elemental) diet useful?

8. Discuss the extraordinary nutritional needs of the severely burned client. What are the methods of providing nutrients for these clients?

Bibliography is found at the end of Part Four.

27

Nutrition in Cancer and Other Special Problems

Cancer

Cancer is a general term for any malignant tumor, an abnormal growth of cells that spreads to neighboring tissue. Tumors have no useful purpose and grow at the expense of healthy tissue. Some cancer cells may break away from the original tumor and spread by the lymph or blood to distant parts of the body, a process called *metastasis*.

Cancer is the second leading cause of death in the United States. Heredity, viruses, environmental factors, and immunologic (disease resistance) factors appear to be involved in the development of cancer, but the exact cause is unknown. Surgery, radiation, and chemotherapy are the primary means of treatment. Any one or a combination of these methods may be used.

Like all cells, malignant cells require energy and nutrients to maintain themselves and to grow. This is probably responsible for the weight loss that may occur early in cancer even though the client has not changed his caloric intake or physical activity. If the disease does not respond to treatment, the continued metabolic demands of cancer cells, anorexia (loss of appetite), nausea, vomiting, and other nutrition-related problems lead to extreme weight

loss, malnutrition, and a complete collapse of bodily processes. This extreme state of malnutrition and wasting of the body is called *cancer cachexia.*

Nutritional Care

The purpose of nutritional care is to counteract the nutritional deficiencies brought on by the cancer and its treatments. Through maintenance or improvement of the client's nutritional status, the client's response to treatment as well as quality of life are improved.

Clients who are on diets high in protein and calories are better able to withstand the side-effects of the various types of cancer therapy and may be able to tolerate higher doses of drugs than clients who are not on such diets. A balanced diet can help the client maintain his strength and body weight and fight infection. Tables 27-1 and 27-2 give suggestions for increasing protein and caloric intake. These suggestions must be adapted to the needs and tolerances of the individual client.

The nutritional support selected depends on the stage of the disease, the client's nutritional status, the degree to which the gastrointestinal tract is functioning, and how well the client can chew, swallow, and feed himself. Feeding by mouth is the method of choice. Commercial food supplements are frequently added to the diet to increase caloric and protein intake. A wide variety of supplements are available: lactose-free, low-fat, high-protein, and low-sodium. Acceptance of the supplements by the client is important; it may be helpful to offer the client a tasting tray consisting of 1-ounce portions of various supplements so that he can choose the one he prefers. If sufficient calories cannot be taken by mouth, tube feedings or total parenteral nutrition (TPN) is used (see Chap. 26).

Whatever the method of feeding used, nutritional care must be individualized and adapted to the special needs of each client. The dietitian looks ahead at eating problems that are likely to result from therapy or progression of the disease and often makes changes to prevent these problems.

Table 27-1. Hints for Adding Protein to the Diet

- Protein can be added to the diet without increasing the volume of food eaten.
- Skim milk powder adds protein — try adding 2 tablespoons of dry skim milk powder to the regular amount of milk called for in recipes.
- Use fortified milk for cooking and drinking.
- Add milk powder to hot or cold cereals, scrambled eggs, soups, gravies, ground meat (for meat patties, meat balls, and meatloaf) casserole dishes, desserts, and baked goods.
- Use milk or half-and-half instead of water when making soup, cereals, instant cocoa, puddings, and canned soups. Soy formulas may also be used.
- Add diced or ground meat to soups and casseroles.
- Add grated cheese or chunks of cheese to sauces, vegetables, soups, and casseroles.
- Add cream cheese or peanut butter to butter on hot bread.
- Add cooked cubed shrimp, canned tuna, crab meat, diced ham, or sliced boiled eggs to sauces and serve over rice, cooked noodles, buttered toast, or hot biscuits.
- Choose dessert recipes that contain eggs, such as sponge and angel food cake, egg custard, bread pudding, and rice pudding.
- Add peanut butter to sauces or use it on crackers, waffles, or celery sticks.

(After Eating Hints — Recipes and Tips for Better Nutrition During Cancer Treatment, p 18. U.S. Department of Health and Human Services, National Cancer Institute, NIH Publication No. 82-2079, April, 1982)

Factors Affecting Nutritional Status

The major nutritional problem in cancer is the unwillingness or inability of the client to eat enough food. Anorexia (loss of appetite), nau-

sea and vomiting, early satiety (fullness), extreme tiredness, and pain and discomfort associated with eating all play a part. These symptoms may be caused by the disease itself or by the treatment, especially radiation and chemotherapy. Most cancer drugs cause nausea and vomiting, and many cause diarrhea.

Anorexia

Anorexia may be due in part to changes in taste sensation. The client may complain that food is tasteless or unpalatable. Some clients have a decreased ability to taste salt, sugar, and/or acid. Some find that food tastes bitter. Even the smell of food may cause nausea.

An uncomfortable sense of fullness after the first meal of the day also interferes with eating. This has been attributed to a delay in the emptying time of the stomach, possibly due to a decrease in digestive enzymes, loss of stomach muscle, and other physiological changes.

Extreme tiredness is another hindrance to eating. Loss of muscle tissue accounts for much of the weight loss that occurs in cancer, and this gives rise to fatigue, weakness, and inactivity. Chemotherapy and radiation are also very tiring, because they damage normal tissue as well as cancer cells.

Some of the following suggestions may help to increase the cancer client's food consumption:

Create a pleasant mealtime atmosphere; serve food attractively; encourage the client to eat with family and friends.

Encourage the client to suggest freely foods he thinks would appeal to him.

Have nutritious food readily available so that the client may eat when his appetite

Table 27-2. Hints for Adding Calories to the Diet

- A teaspoon of butter or margarine will add 45 kcal. Mix it into hot foods such as soups, vegetables, mashed potatoes, cooked cereal, and rice. Serve hot bread; more butter is used when it melts into it.

- Mayonnaise has 100 kcal per tablespoon, almost twice as much as salad dressing. Use it in salads, in eggs, and with lettuce on sandwiches.

- Use peanut butter (which has protein as well as calories—1 tablespoon is 90 kcal). Spread it on fruit such as apple, banana, or pear, or stuff celery with it. Add it to a sandwich with mayonnaise or cream cheese.

- Spread honey on toast, use it as a sweetner in coffee or tea, or add it to cereal in the morning.

- Sour cream and yogurt can be used on vegetables such as potatoes, beans, carrots, and squash. Try them in gravies or as a salad dressing for fruit.

- Use sour cream as a dip for fresh vegetables.

- For a good dessert, scoop it on fresh fruit, add brown sugar, and let it sit in the refrigerator for a while. One tablespoon of sour cream is 70 kcal.

- Whipping cream is about 60 kcal a tablespoon. Add it to pies, fruit, puddings, hot chocolate, jello, and other desserts.

- Add marshmallows to fruit or hot chocolate.

- Have snacks ready to eat. Nuts, dried fruits, candy, popcorn, crackers and cheese, granola, ice cream, and popsicles all make good snacks. Milk shakes add calories and are especially easy to make with a blender.

- Powdered coffee creamers add calories without volume—add them to gravy, soup, milkshakes, and hot cereals.

- Meat, chicken, and fish are higher in calories when breaded than when broiled or roasted plain.

- Add raisins, dates, or chopped nuts and brown sugar to hot or cold cereals for a snack.

(After Eating Hints—Recipes for Better Nutrition During Cancer Treatment, p 19. U.S. Department of Health and Human Services, National Cancer Institute, NIH Publication No. 82-2079, April 1982)

is good rather than according to a set meal schedule.

Alter seasonings by adding more sugar, salt, or tart flavors to food (unless these must be avoided). Encourage the client to try using herbs and other seasonings and wine and beer in cooking.

Encourage the client to try cold foods rather than hot ones. (Heat intensifies the odor of food.) Meats may be more acceptable cold than hot.

Use dairy products, legumes, and peanut butter if the client won't eat meat.

Encourage the client to eat well on days he feels well.

Encourage the client to eat small meals frequently if he feels uncomfortably full after eating small amounts of food.

Encourage the client to rest before eating when he is extremely tired. Light exercise such as a short walk may be helpful between meals.

Avoid pressuring the client to eat. This may intensify the anorexia.

Pain and Discomfort Associated with Eating

The location of the tumor is another factor that can intensify nutritional problems. Surgery of the tongue and larynx impairs swallowing, gastric surgery may cause the dumping syndrome, and tumors of the intestine and accessory organs lead to problems in digestion, absorption, and metbolism.

Pain experienced during eating due to ulceration or inflammation of the mouth and esophagus is particularly distressing. When these conditions are present, foods that are acidic, salty, spicy, dry, or very hot should be avoided. Pureed and liquid foods are most likely to be tolerated. Pain medication given at such a time as to bring relief at mealtime or a local anesthetic applied to the mouth or pharynx can improve food intake.

Radiation treatments of the head and neck may damage salivary glands so that saliva can-

not be produced. An artificial saliva, similar in composition to natural saliva, may be ordered. This is kept in a plastic squeeze bottle and used as necessary. Artificial saliva also helps reduce the severe dental decay that usually occurs after radiation of the head and neck.

When a dry mouth is a problem, moist foods or dry foods mixed with sauces, gravies, and fats should be served.

Responsibilities of the Health Team

The health worker who is aware of the eating problems that may arise in cancer will respect the likes and dislikes of the client and understand that tolerances for food may change from meal to meal. Nursing and dietary personnel must do all they can to help the client consume a reasonable amount of food. No one diet or nutrition plan can suit the needs of all clients; nutritional care must be individualized.

Problems that interfere with eating, such as pain, difficulty chewing and swallowing, and nausea, should be reported to the physician immediately so that changes can be made. The client's food intake should be checked carefully and recorded. This includes foods and beverages eaten at meals, food supplements, and food provided by family and friends. Observations should be made as inconspicuously as possible so that the client is not constantly reminded of his eating problems. He is usually well aware of them and extremely worried about them.

The Link Between Diet and Cancer

Research indicates that nutritional factors may be involved in the development of cancer. Nutritional deficiencies as well as excesses have been implicated. Some substances, such as vitamin C, vitamin A, and fiber, appear to be protective. High-fat diets have been linked to breast cancer, and high-fat, high-meat, and low-fiber diets have been linked to colon cancer.

Most of the evidence linking diet with cancer is based on comparisons of disease patterns and environmental factors (including diet) in one population group with those of

another; for example, diet and the incidence of breast cancer in Japan have been compared to these same factors in the United States. Some authorities have suggested that a diet similar to the "prudent diet" (see Chap. 13) may help reduce the incidence of cancer. This diet is reduced in fat and increased in whole grains, fruits, and vegetables.

Food Allergy

Abdominal pain, an asthmatic attack, a headache, or a rash are typical symptoms in a person with food allergy. Approximately one third of the estimated 35 million Americans suffering from allergy have a sensitivity to food. In some cases, treatment consists of the avoidance of foods that have no effect on nutritional status. However, if the offending food is a nutritionally important one or one that is widely used in food processing, treatment can be difficult, especially in the case of infants and children who are allergic to such foods as milk, wheat, or eggs.

An allergy is an adverse reaction to substances called *allergens*. This reaction causes the production of antibodies, which are proteins. In the case of an infectious disease, antibodies are protective. In allergic conditions, however, the type of antibody produced after exposure to the allergen (*e.g.,* pollen, penicillin, or pork) is not protective. When the antibodies interact with the allergen, certain chemicals are released that cause the allergic symptoms. Allergic symptoms do not usually appear at the first contact. It takes considerable exposure to an allergen before enough antibodies are formed to cause symptoms.

In the case of food allergy, antibodies trigger allergic symptoms every time a particular food is eaten. Sometimes the food does not even have to be eaten to cause symptoms—merely inhaling its aroma or having an injection of a product related to it may be enough.

Some foods that commonly cause allergic reactions are fish and seafood, berries, nuts, eggs, cereals, milk, beef, pork, chocolate, legumes such as beans and peanuts, and fresh fruits of the peach family. A person may be allergic to foods that belong to a single family of plants. For example, a person who is allergic to cantaloupe may also be allergic to pumpkin and cucumber.

The symptoms associated with food allergy are urticaria (hives), eczema, vomiting, and diarrhea. However, asthma, rhinitis (hay fever), migraine headache, angioedema (giant swellings of body tissue), and serious shock may also occur. The allergic symptoms may appear immediately or may be delayed until several hours after the food has been eaten.

Food allergies may develop in persons of any age, although infants and young children are especially susceptible. The tendency to develop an allergy appears to be inherited. Physical and emotional stress may aggravate the condition.

The food or foods causing the allergic reaction are identified by a diet history, skin tests, and elimination diets.

Food History and Skin Tests

A thorough history of foods eaten and of the occurrence of symptoms often reveals possible allergens. The patient may be asked to keep a diary of all items consumed as well as a record of symptoms. All items taken by mouth should be entered in the food diary, including beverages, gums, candies, vitamins, and over-the-counter medications.

Skin tests may be helpful in efforts to isolate suspected foods. Extracts of suspected foods are rubbed into scratches on the skin or injected under the skin. If redness or swelling occurs at the point of contact with the skin, the food is considered to be a possible allergen. However, a food giving a positive skin test is not necessarily the cause of allergic symptoms. The results of the skin tests must be evaluated in the light of information in the medical history. Skin tests may be helpful in determining what type of elimination diet (described below) should be tried.

Treatment and Counseling

Once a list of suspected foods has been established, the physician may order an *elimination diet*. This diet omits the suspected food or foods for 7 to 14 days. Relief from symptoms should occur within this time. The suspected foods are then slowly added to the elimination diet one at a time for identification of those that cause symptoms. If a food containing the allergen is consumed, symptoms appear, usually within 7 days, and subside again when the food is eliminated.

If the elimination diet fails to identify the allergen or if the allergic symptoms are very severe, an elemental diet preparation (see Chap. 26) may be given as the only source of nourishment. This diet eliminates all food allergens. Suspected foods are then added one at a time.

Once the food or foods causing the allergy have been identified, they are avoided either partially or completely. The extent to which a food is eliminated from the diet depends on its nutritional importance and the severity of the client's symptoms. Allergy to milk, wheat, or eggs, for example, is difficult to deal with because these foods are basic to the American diet and used widely in food processing.

Sometimes the changes that occur when the offending food is cooked make it more tolerable. For example, some persons who are allergic to milk or eggs may be able to tolerate small quantities of these foods in baked goods. Clients who cannot tolerate the food in any form may use a food substitute. When a substitute for a nutritionally important food is not available or is not accepted, use of vitamin and/or mineral supplements may be necessary.

Counseling for the client and his family includes their being made aware of all the sources of the food to be avoided. They need to be reminded of the hidden sources, such as dry milk powder in luncheon meats and frankfurters. The client must be instructed to read food package labels carefully to identify the allergen (Table 27-3). Foods with a standard of identity may lack an ingredient label, so the client should be informed about those that contain the offending allergen. If a substitute food can be used, such as rice flour in place of wheat

Table 27-3.   Terms on Labels Indicating the Presence of Common Allergens

Common Allergen	Terms
Milk	Casein
	Caseinate
	Casein hydrolysate
	DMS (dried milk solids)
	Lactalbumin
	Lactate solids
	Milk solid pastes
	Sweetened condensed milk
	Whey or whey solids
Egg	Albumin
	Dried egg solids
	Egg solids
	Globulin
	Ovomucin
	Vitellin
Corn	Corn solids
	Cornstarch
	Corn syrup
	Vegetable starch
Legume	Food gums from the legume family:
	Acacia gum
	Arabic gum
	Carob
	Haraya gum
	Locust bean gum
	Tragacanth
	Hydrolyzed vegetable protein
	Soy concentrate
	Soy protein
	Soya flour
	TVP (textured vegetable protein)
	Vegetable protein concentrate

(Dietary Department, University of Iowa Hospitals and Clinics: Recent Advances in Therapeutic Diets, p 107. Ames, Iowa State University Press, 1979)

flour, the client will need to know where to obtain the substitute and how to use it in food preparation.

The physician may try to desensitize the client to an allergy-causing food, especially if the food is nutritionally important. Desensiti-

zation is the development of a tolerance for an allergy-causing substance by the ingestion of controlled doses of the allergen that are minute at first and that are then increased by tiny amounts over an extended period of time. If symptoms occur, one returns to the level that does not produce symptoms.

Milk Allergy

Allergy to milk occurs most often in children under 2 years of age. Many children outgrow it. Infants who have a severe allergic reaction are given milk-free commercial infant formulas made with either soybean or meat base. These are similar in calories and nutrients to other infant formulas and provide the essentials for adequate growth.

When solid foods are added, parents must be counseled to read labels carefully to avoid foods containing nonfat dry milk. For children or adults with severe milk allergy, all foods containing milk or nonfat dry milk may have to be avoided. Clients should be alerted to hidden sources of milk, such as frankfurters, luncheon meats, and chocolate.

Supplements of calcium, vitamin D, and riboflavin are necessary for children who do not accept milk substitutes. Adults may require calcium supplements.

Wheat Allergy

Allergy to wheat requires that many foods commonly used in the American diet be avoided. Here again, the client must be made aware of hidden sources of wheat, such as malted milk; luncheon meats, frankfurters, and sausage in which wheat has been used as a filler; canned and frozen dinners; beer; and commercial soups. Some wheat flour is commonly added to rye, cornmeal, and oat breads. Rice flour, potato flour, and cornstarch may be used as a substitute for wheat flour.

Egg Allergy

Eggs are also used widely in commercial products. Baking powder and foaming beverages may contain egg white. Eggs are used in the preparation of mayonnaise, cooked salad dressing, and Hollandaise sauce; in many baked goods; in desserts such as ice cream, puddings, meringues, and candies; and in malted beverages and other preparations.

Arthritis

About 32 million persons in the United States suffer from various forms of arthritis. There is no known dietary means of preventing or curing arthritis. Nevertheless, arthritics seeking relief spend millions of dollars each year for worthless products such as filtered sea water and alfalfa tablets.

Osteoarthritis is caused by degenerative changes in the cartilage in the joints, especially of the spine and knees. The client's diet should be a normal one, adequate in all essential nutrients and moderately reduced in calories to prevent obesity if activity is restricted. If the client is already obese, a diet more restricted in calories is necessary.

Rheumatoid arthritis involves inflammation of the lining of the joints. The client is probably underweight, and if his hands are badly crippled, he may have difficulty preparing food and feeding himself. The use of special equipment for self-feeding may be recommended. (See Chap. 3.)

Aspirin and steroids, drugs often prescribed to treat arthritis, can cause gastric distress. A bland diet, antacids, and moderate sodium restriction may be advised.

Gout

Gout is an inherited disease involving abnormal metabolism of a group of compounds called

purines. The end result of this abnormality is that uric acid becomes deposited as salts in soft tissue and joints, where it causes great pain.

Drugs have replaced diet therapy in the treatment of gout. However, clients may be advised to avoid substances high in purines such as liver, kidney, sweetbread, brain, sardines, anchovies, broth, bouillon, and other meat soups and meat gravies.

The obese patient with gout should lose weight gradually. Rapid weight loss increases blood levels of uric acid and can provoke an acute attack of gout.

Hyperthyroidism

Hyperthyroidism is caused by excessive secretion of the hormone thyroxine, which regulates metabolism. In hyperthyroidism, the metabolic rate may be as much as 50% higher than normal. Symptoms include weight loss, increased appetite, nervousness, and bulging eyeballs.

Until a normal metabolic rate is established by means of medication or surgery, the diet must meet the client's increased energy needs. The client may require as many as 4000 kcal to 5000 kcal per day to prevent excessive weight loss. Stimulants such as coffee, tea, alcohol, and tobacco are omitted or limited. Substantial between-meal snacks in addition to regular meals are necessary.

Hypoglycemia

Hypoglycemia, a low blood glucose level, is a symptom rather than a disease state. It is characterized by weakness, palpitations, anxiety, sweating, and extreme hunger. In severe cases, brain function may be impaired, causing con-

fusion, amnesia, blurred vision, and finally convulsions and coma. The two general types of hypoglycemia are food-stimulated hypoglycemia, which occurs 2 to 4 hours after the person has eaten, and fasting hypoglycemia, which develops in the fasting state and is not associated with eating. (The latter type, which can be caused by drugs or various disease states, is not discussed here.)

Food-stimulated hypoglycemia may develop in early diabetes or after gastrectomy. It may also occur without evidence of organic disease (functional hypoglycemia).

Early-diabetes hypoglycemia is treated by a diabetic diet. Dietary treatment following a gastrectomy is discussed in Chapter 26.

Functional hypoglycemia resulting from an excessive production of insulin is treated with a low-carbohydrate, high-protein, moderate-fat diet. The purpose of dietary treatment is to avoid a substantial rise in blood sugar, which would stimulate the pancreas to overproduce insulin. Ingestion of proteins and fats is encouraged, because they are more slowly digested and more slowly converted to glucose than carbohydrates.

Foods containing free sugar, such as jellies, jams, desserts, and soft drinks, are omitted from the diet, and starches, such as bread, cereals, and potatoes, are limited. Milk is also limited because it contains milk sugar. Alcohol and foods containing caffeine and other stimulants are avoided because they lower blood sugar levels. Generous amounts of protein foods such as meat, fish, poultry, eggs, and cheese are taken with meals and as between-meal snacks. Food is usually divided into three meals plus three or more between-meal snacks. Each snack contains some protein food, sometimes taken together with small amounts of carbohydrates. Cheese and a few crackers or a handful of nuts is a typical between-meal snack for a hypoglycemic person.

Food and Drug Interactions

Some drugs interfere with nutritional status, and foods, in turn, may interfere with response to a drug. For example, the effectiveness of some antibiotics is reduced when they are taken with meals; in contrast, other medications, such as iron preparations, are best taken with meals to lessen gastrointestinal upset. Table 27-4 shows some drug-nutrient interactions.

Health workers should be aware of the possibility of harmful interactions between food and drugs. A drug may hinder absorption of a nutrient in the gastrointestinal tract, or it may interfere with the action of the nutrient after it is absorbed. Certain foods or dietary patterns may destroy a drug's effectiveness. Some drugs may depress appetite or induce nausea and vomiting or diarrhea. The nutritional status of clients undergoing cancer chemotherapy may be so severely upset that the therapy may have to be interrupted. Coffee, cola, and tea are examples of substances that contain stimulants (caffeine and theophylline) and thus may adversely affect persons who are sensitive to them. Aspirin and steroids can cause gastric bleeding and should therefore be taken with meals.

The client who is taking certain antidepressant drugs, monoamine oxidase inhibitors (called MAO inhibitors), should avoid foods containing tyramine, a substance formed from the amino acid tyrosine. The interaction between these drugs and tyramine causes severe hypertension and other cardiovascular changes. Some deaths have been reported. Foods rich in tyramine include yogurt, aged cheese, game, liver, dried fish, beer, ale, certain wines, chocolate, yeast, and others.

Table 27-4. Examples of Drug-Nutrient Interactions

Drugs	Indication	Possible Effects
Mineral oil	Constipation	Reduced absorption of fat-soluble vitamins
Aspirin	Rheumatoid disorders	Gastrointestinal bleeding leading to iron deficiency anemia
Thiazide diuretics	Cardiovascular disease	Increased potassium and magnesium excretion
Corticosteroids	Inflammation	Increased vitamin D metabolism leading to accelerated bone loss; decreased glucose tolerance; gastric ulceration; increased excretion of vitamin C, potassium, and zinc; increased vitamin B_6 requirement
Oral contraceptive steroids	Birth control	Reduced blood serum levels of folacin, vitamin B_6, riboflavin, and ascorbic acid; increased blood serum levels of vitamin A, iron, and copper; increased absorption of calcium

KEYS TO PRACTICAL APPLICATION

Create a pleasant mealtime atmosphere for the client with cancer, shield him from food odors that nauseate him, be alert to foods he accepts as well as to those he rejects, and provide good oral care — in short, do all you can to increase the client's food intake.

Establish a helping relationship with the cancer client; avoid nagging or pressuring him to eat.

Be sure that the client with food allergy is aware of hidden sources of the offending food.

Encourage a well-balanced diet and the maintenance of normal weight in clients with arthritis; discourage food fads promoted as cures.

Be aware of the adverse effects food and drugs may have on each other.

Be sure to check with your supervisor about the timing of medication in relation to food intake and about mixing medication with fruit juice, milk, or other foods.

KEY IDEAS

Cancer cells require energy and nutrients; they grow at the expense of healthy tissue.

The purpose of nutritional care in clients with cancer is to counteract the nutritional deficiencies caused by the cancer and the cancer treatment.

Maintaining or improving the cancer client's nutritional status will improve his response to treatment, may make possible higher doses of medication, can help maintain his strength and body weight, and can help him fight infection.

The kind of nutritional support chosen — oral, tube feeding, or TPN — depends on the client's nutritional status, the degree to which his gastrointestinal tract is functioning, and his ability to chew, swallow, and feed himself.

The major nutritional problem in cancer is the inability of the client to eat a sufficient quantity of food.

Symptoms such as anorexia, taste changes, nausea, vomiting, early satiety, extreme tiredness, and pain and discomfort associated with eating are responsible for the decline in food intake among persons with cancer.

Pureed and liquid foods are the most likely foods to be tolerated in clients with ulceration and inflammation of the mouth and esophagus; acidic, salty, spicy, and dry foods should be avoided.

When dry mouth is a problem, moist foods or dry food mixed with sauces, gravies, and fats are best tolerated.

Nutritional care in cancer must be highly individualized; no one diet or feeding program can be applied to every client.

Although dietary factors are likely to be involved in the development of cancer, the exact cause or causes have not been determined with absolute certainty; a diet low in fat and increased in whole grains, fruits, and vegetables appears to be a reasonable course to follow as a preventive measure.

Methods used to diagnose food allergy are a diary of items consumed and the occurrence of symptoms, skin tests, and elimination diets.

Treatment of food allergy involves partial or complete avoidance of the offending

food or possibly the development of a tolerance for the food through desensitization.

Counseling involves informing the client of the sources of the offending food, with special emphasis on hidden sources, and the use of substitute foods.

Diet can neither prevent nor cure arthritis; the diet for persons with arthritis should be adequate in all essential nutrients and reduced in calories for obese persons.

Drugs have replaced diet in the treatment of gout; foods high in purines are sometimes avoided.

Rapid weight loss increases blood levels of uric acid and can bring on an acute attack of gout in persons prone to the disease.

In hyperthyroidism, a high-calorie diet, 3000 kcal to 4000 kcal or more, may be necessary until a normal metabolic rate is established; foods containing stimulants are avoided or eliminated from the diet.

Functional hypoglycemia, caused by excessive production of insulin following meals, is treated with a high-protein, moderate-fat, low-carbohydrate diet; foods containing sugar, caffeine, and alcohol are omitted.

Drugs may adversely affect an individual's nutritional status, and food may interfere with a client's reaction to a drug.

KEYS TO LEARNING: STUDY – DISCUSSION QUESTIONS

1. What are the factors that interfere with eating in cancer? Discuss your own observations regarding nutritional care in cancer. What measures have you found to be helpful in improving a client's appetite?

2. What is an elimination test diet? How is it used? What test diet for food allergy is used most frequently in your hospital? What foods does it include?

3. Plan a day's menu for a 6-year-old child who is allergic to wheat.

4. Investigate and evaluate food fads associated with arthritis.

5. Rapid weight loss can be dangerous. How does this apply to gout?

Bibliography is found at the end of Part Four.

Nutrition in Diseases of Infancy and Childhood

KEY TERMS

failure to thrive   Term used to describe seriously retarded growth in infants under 18 months of age.

ketosis   A condition characterized by the accumulation of certain acids in the blood and caused by the excessive breakdown of fats.

regressive   Concerned with a turning back or return to former behavior.

seizure (*in epilepsy*)   A sudden change in consciousness; may be accompanied by convulsions.

Nutritional care of the sick infant or child involves both treatment and prevention of complications. In the case of long-term illnesses, preventive measures can improve the child's physical condition and quality of his life. For example, prevention of obesity in the child who has muscular weakness or partial paralysis of the legs may allow him to walk with crutches or braces rather than be completely dependent on a wheelchair. For the child with congenital heart disease, careful control of nutritional factors such as water balance, sodium, and calories promotes growth and development.

Most sick infants and children require a normal diet for their age. The acutely ill child may need changes to correct fluid and electrolyte balance for a short period of time. In the case of some long-term illnesses, changes in nutrient intake, such as a sodium-restricted diet for a child with congenital heart disease or the restriction of phenylalanine for a child with phenylketonuria may be necessary.

The emotional meanings of food discussed in Chapter 2 are often heightened in the sick child. His eating behavior may regress to an earlier level. The sick toddler who has been

drinking from a cup may now accept fluids only from a nursing bottle. The sick toddler who has been feeding himself may now want to be fed. Emotional tensions associated with the illness may depress the appetite of some children, whereas others may overeat. Sick children may refuse food as a way of expressing their anger or of gaining control over their lives.

Parents and health workers should try to identify the child's emotional needs and attempt to meet them in ways other than through food. Parents may be helped to be more positive and less anxious in their approach so that the child will be more relaxed. The child may be helped to handle his anger and become more involved in decisions that affect him.

The parents' desire to be involved in feeding their hospitalized child is understandable and should be respected. Choosing foods for the child and feeding him may be the only way a parent can contribute to his care. Parents should be discouraged, however, from giving "treats" of poor nutritional quality to coax the child to eat. Health workers and parents should work together in setting limits without being overly rigid.

The sick child most readily accepts foods that are familiar to him. The dietitian or nurse should obtain from the parents of a young child or from an older child himself a list of the foods he likes. Some hospitals have a special menu for the pediatric unit that usually reflects the likes of the majority of children served by the hospital.

Whether the child is in the hospital or at home, small, frequent feedings and occasional surprises may improve his food consumption. Food portions that are too large and overwhelming should be avoided. A ½-cup serving of soup, half of a peach, or half of a sandwich may be adequate for a toddler, whereas adult-sized servings may be required for a 12-year-old boy.

The company of another person may make an important difference to the sick child whose appetite is depressed. If the child is confined to bed, a friendly face or sympathetic ear can promote a better response to food. The ambulatory child will probably enjoy eating at a table with other children of the same age.

Acute Illness

Acute vomiting and diarrhea due to infection are a common cause for hospitalization of infants and young children. Moderate to severe diarrhea in this age group is extremely serious and sometimes fatal, and dehydration and fever can damage the developing nervous system.

The first need of these clients is restoration of fluid and electrolyte balance. In the infant, this may be accomplished by use of a commercial oral electrolyte–glucose solution. If sufficient fluid cannot be taken by mouth, the intravenous route is used. A careful record of fluid intake and output is important. In the young child 1 to 4 years of age, fluids such as fruit juices, and carbonated beverages are commonly given to replace lost body fluids. Solid foods with a high water content, such as sherbet, fruit ices, frozen fruit juice pop, and flavored gelatin, may also be offered.

As soon as possible after the child's needs for fluids and electrolytes have been met, calories are increased to normal to promote growth and make up for the loss of calories that has occurred during the acute stage of illness. For the infant, a diluted formula in small frequent feedings is given at first. If this is well tolerated, a standard formula and solid foods appropriate to the infant's age are added gradually. After having had severe diarrhea, some infants are not able to tolerate lactose (milk sugar) for a period of up to about 4 months. Instead, commercial lactose-free formulas are given. As the older child recovers, a soft or regular diet of easily digested foods is given. Kinds and amounts of food taken should be recorded.

In the case of mild diarrhea lasting 1 to 4 days, the infant or child is usually treated at home. Although solid food may be withheld for up to 24 hours, fluids and electrolytes must be given. The health worker should see to it that the parent understands directions for the use of commercial preparations and is advised as to the kinds of fluids that should be offered the child. The diet should be restricted no longer than necessary.

Nutritional Problems Related to Weight and Growth

Underweight

Normal rates of growth for children vary considerably. Even though a child may be thinner than other children, if he grows in height and weight at a regular rate, there is usually no cause for concern. The physician determines whether the rate of growth is so slow that it must be considered abnormal.

When an infant or child fails to grow at a normal rate, his food habits and home environment are investigated. Poor housing, inadequate parental supervision, poor sleeping arrangements, and poverty may be contributing factors. Some community nutrition programs may improve the quality and quantity of food available to the child. The WIC Program, a supplemental food program for women, infants, and preschool children; the school lunch program; and the food stamp program are services that may prove useful (see Chap. 16). Adequate sleep and rest also have an important influence on growth.

Occasionally, a child may have a poor appetite because his parents are overly concerned about the amount of food he eats. Nagging and forcing a child to eat only worsen matters. If the child has no health problems, the parents must be reassured that his appetite will improve if tensions involving his eating are reduced. The child's food choices may be very limited at first, and it may be necessary to go along with an inadequate diet for a while. When his appetite improves, small quantities of new foods can be added one at a time. Portion sizes should be small.

Failure to thrive indicates serious growth failure in infants under 18 months of age. This may be due to an underlying disease condition, the excessive loss of nutrients (due to regurgitation, diarrhea, or vomiting) or unusually high energy requirements (as in cerebral palsy).

If the infant has no disease or birth defect, it is suspected that he has not been offered enough food. He may not be fed often enough, the quantities he is given may be too small, or the formula he receives may be too dilute. Diet histories are frequently unreliable, since parents will seldom admit that their infant has not received enough food. The underlying problem is an emotionally deprived environment lacking in normal parent–child interaction. The parents may feel so overwhelmed by personal problems that they neglect the needs of the infant. In addition to growth failure, these infants show retarded motor development and little interest in their surroundings.

The infant with growth failure is usually hospitalized. His physical condition may be so poor that fluid and electrolyte balance must first be re-established. Then an adequate diet is offered. Within 3 to 5 days, the infant is usually eating more and gaining more weight than expected for his age. To the extent possible, his emotional and social needs should also be met; he should be fed and played with by experienced nursing personnel, perferably the same person, as frequently as possible.

While the infant is hospitalized, the parents receive intensive counseling to help them solve their problems. Detailed instruction about the infant's diet, the frequency of feedings, and the manner in which he should be fed are given. The infant needs to be followed on an outpatient basis, and the family should continue to receive counseling to avoid a recurrence of the problem.

Obesity

Obesity is difficult to treat in both children and adults. Because the obese child has a high likelihood of becoming an obese adult, priority should be given to the prevention of obesity in childhood (see Chaps. 16 and 20).

Very-low-calorie diets are not recommended for children and adolescents, because severe restriction of energy can retard growth. If

a child is excessively obese, a slow rate of weight loss is desirable. If a child is only moderately obese and is about to enter the adolescent growth spurt, simple prevention of further weight gain may be an appropriate goal, permitting the child to grow into his weight, as he grows taller. Parents may need to be counseled to buy less food than usual and to prepare foods that are less concentrated in calories. Fried foods, creamed dishes, rich gravies, fat-seasoned vegetables, and fat-rich or sugar-rich beverages and desserts should be eaten very sparingly.

Underactivity as well as overeating is involved in the development of obesity. In children as in adults, obesity usually develops gradually from small excesses in calories that accumulate day after day. An increase in physical activity on a regular basis should be a part of the weight control program.

The obese child requires much emotional support. He may face insults and rejection from family and friends, so acceptance and encouragement are necessary even when he does not follow his diet closely. The older child and adolescent should be involved in making decisions about their eating habits and activity patterns. They will usually readily agree to minor changes such as cutting down on between-meal snacks coupled with increased physical activity, and this may be all that is necessary to achieve desired goals.

Long-Term Illness

Cardiovascular Disease

Congenital Heart Disease

Infants with congenital heart disease tire easily, and it is difficult for them to consume normal quantities of food. Adding less water to the commercial formula concentrate will allow the infant to receive more nutrients in a smaller volume of formula. The nutritional care of these infants is complex and must be managed with great diligence. The level of nutrients supplied by a concentrated formula must be carefully planned and the formula concentrate and water carefully measured. A formula that is too concentrated can overload the kidneys or cause diarrhea and vomiting, which would be disastrous for an already seriously ill infant.

Sodium restriction is frequently necessary. When solid foods are added, unsalted strained vegetables and unsalted strained meats are appropriate. (Salt and other sodium compounds are no longer added to commercial baby foods.) The sodium-restricted diet is discussed in Chapter 23.

Nutritional care provided in the home must be adjusted to the abilities of the family. If there is doubt as to their ability to prepare formula accurately, the infant may be given a regular-strength formula with additional calories given in other ways. Feeding an infant with congenital heart disease is time-consuming, because he needs to rest frequently while eating. The parents may need help arranging the family's schedule.

Providing adequate calories and other nutrients will increase the child's strength and promote his growth, hastening the day when corrective surgery can be performed. Surgery is delayed, if possible, until the child's weight is 35 to 50 pounds.

Atherosclerosis

Children with type II hyperlipoproteinemia have a much greater risk than normal of developing early-onset cardiovascular disease. This is an inherited condition charcterized by high serum cholesterol levels. Diet therapy involves restriction of cholesterol and saturated fatty acids (see Chap. 22).

Many diet changes are needed, including restriction of animal fats (whole milk, ice cream, cheese, fatty meats, and eggs). From the preschool period on, the child will need help in coping with situations of eating outside the home.

Diabetes Mellitus

The dietary treatment of diabetes mellitus in children is discussed in Chapter 21.

Allergy

Food allergy in infants and childrn is discussed in Chapter 27.

Iron Deficiency Anemia

See Chapters 11 and 15.

Kidney Disease

Nephrosis

Childhood nephrosis is manifested by protein-uria, low serum albumin levels, high blood lipid levels, and edema.

Steroids are usually prescribed for a limited time. Because their use causes edema and sodium retention, severe sodium restriction may be ordered. The child's appetite usually is poor, and his food likes and dislikes should be respected. Very small portions should be offered at each feeding until his appetite improves. Sodium restriction may have to be eased if it seriously affects the child's intake of food. During recovery, as appetite improves, a diet high in protein (2–3 g per kg of body weight) is given to make up for protein losses in the urine and to bring the serum albumin level up to normal.

Dialysis

Dialysis is a more stressful experience for children than for adults. Height and weight are usually below normal, dialysis is required more frequently, and the required severe dietary restrictions are difficult to control. Like adults, children frequently focus their discouragement and frustrations on food.

The diet should include sufficient protein for growth and must be adequate in calories so that protein is spared for body building and not used for energy. Sodium, potassium, and fluids are restricted. The dietitian works closely with the client and his family, making every effort to have the diet be as near normal as possible. The dietitian can help parents plan for picnics and adjust the diet to allow for a slice of birthday cake or other "banned" foods on important occasions.

Children are maintained on dialysis until kidney transplantation is possible.

Epilepsy

Epilepsy is a disorder of the central nervous system. It is characterized by loss of consciousness, which may be very brief or may be more prolonged and accompanied by convulsions.

There has recently been renewed interest in the dietary treatment of epilepsy. This treatment is reported to be most effective in the control of one type of seizure that occurs in children of preschool age and makes it possible to avoid anticonvulsive drugs that have undesirable side effects. The diet is called the keto-genic diet because it produces a state of mild ketosis. Carbohydrates and proteins are restricted, and the ratio of these calories to fat calories is carefully controlled.

A ketogenic diet using medium-chain tri-glycerides (MCT*) has been developed that is much easier to manage than the original keto-genic diet. MCT is an oil that appears to produce ketosis more readily than regular fats. The diet is more palatable than previously, because less fat and more carbohydrate and protein can be included. The exchange lists described in Chapter 19 are followed for this diet. Household measures are used.

MCT oil provides 50% to 70% of the total kilocalories in the diet. The oil can be used in the preparation of such foods as milkshakes, casseroles, ice cream, and pizza. MCT should always be consumed with other foods, never by itself.

* Mead Johnson, Evansville, IN 47721

Malabsorption Disorders

Cystic Fibrosis

Cystic fibrosis is an inherited disease of the exocrine glands, those glands that excrete to the outside of the body. Characteristic of this disease is the secretion of an abnormally thick mucus, which blocks the air passages in the lungs and may plug the ducts of the liver, pancreas, and gallbladder. The sweat glands produce sweat higher in sodium chloride than normal, and this loss, expecially in hot weather, may be so extreme as to cause death. Lung problems, especially repeated infections, are the greatest threat to life. It is very likely that nutritional deficiencies contribute greatly to the occurrence of infection.

The malnutrition associated with cystic fibrosis is caused by malabsorption due to the blockage of pancreatic enzymes. The malabsorption in turn causes steatorrhea (fatty stools) and poor absorption of nutrients, especially fat-soluble vitamins and essential fatty acids. Abdominal cramps, flatulence (gas in the intestinal tract), and diarrhea are common. The affected child's growth and development are retarded. Children with acute attacks often require hospitalization.

Supplements of pancreatic enzymes are given with meals and snacks to promote digestion. Nevertheless, some degree of malabsorption continues to exist. The nutritional needs of the child with cystic fibrosis are much greater than those of the normal child because of the gastrointestinal loss of nutrients and frequent infections.

Nutritional care plays an important role in therapy. Clients who are adequately nourished are better able than poorly nourished clients to resist infection and attain improved growth and development. The diet for the client with cystic fibrosis is high in calories and protein and moderate in fat. Vitamin and mineral supplements are also given.

The tolerance for various foods, especially spicy and high-fat foods, differs greatly from one client to another. The diet must be adapted to individual needs, likes, dislikes, and tolerance for fats. When there is abnormal loss of sodium chloride in the sweat owing to activity or warm weather, extra salt is added to food, and consumption of foods such as salted crackers and pretzels is encouraged.

Special dietary products that are more readily absorbed than regular food may be given to increase caloric and protein intake. MCT is better absorbed than dietary fats. The diet may be supplemented with commercial formulas, including the semisynthetic, fiber-free diets (see Chap. 26).

Celiac Disease

Celiac disease is described in Chapter 25.

Affected infants receive rice cereal and other baby foods free of gluten. Older children are given the gluten-free diet described in Chapter 25. Care must be taken both in the hospital and at home to see that other children or well-meaning adults do not offer the affected child foods containing gluten.

Enzyme Deficiencies

Phenylketonuria and galactosemia are among a group of inherited diseases called *inborn errors of metabolism.*

Phenylketonuria

Phenylketonuria (PKU) is an inherited disease in which phenylalanine, an essential amino acid, cannot be metabolized normally owing to the lack of a liver enzyme. The result is that phenylalanine and some of its breakdown products accumulate in the blood and are excreted in the urine. These toxic substances interfere with the normal development of the central nervous system, causing mental retardation, personality changes, and other neurological disturbances.

If the disease is detected (usually by a simple test) and treated with a phenylalanine-restricted diet in the first few months of life, damage to nerve tissue can be prevented, and normal physical and intellectual development will follow. If the disorder is detected only later, mental retardation cannot be prevented, but the

child's behavior can still be somewhat improved.

There is general agreement that the diet prescribed for persons with PKU should be followed throughout infancy and early childhood. However, physicians disagree about when the diet should be discontinued.

Special consideration must be given to pregnant women with PKU, for whom adherence to the diet is essential; infants born to PKU women who are not on a phenylalanine-restricted diet are usually mentally retarded. If the diet is discontinued in childhood, it must be followed again when the client is planning to become pregnant and during pregnancy.

The purpose of diet therapy in PKU is to limit phenylalanine to the amount required to maintain an adequate blood level. Phenylalanine cannot be completely eliminated from the diet because it is an essential amino acid and is necessary for the production of body proteins. In addition, all other nutrients must be provided in amounts that will promote growth and development.

The amount of phenylalanine required varies with each infant, depending on his size and rate of growth. Changes in diet are made as the child grows. The physician's diet prescription gives the calories, grams of protein, and milligrams of phenylalanine required. A sample menu is given in Table 28-1.

All proteins contain from 4% to 6% phenylalanine. Because all foods except oils and sugars contain some protein, the diet is extremely limited. It is not possible to plan a diet that is restricted in phenylalanine and adequate in protein and calories with the use of normal foods alone. Special products have been developed that are either low in or free of phenylalanine. Lofenalac* is the product most commonly used in the United States. Lofenalac does not meet total phenylalanine requirements, so cow's milk and certain other foods are added to the diet.

An exchange system has been developed for use in the phenylalanine-restricted diet. The lists are composed mainly of fruits, vegetables, cereals, and fats; there are no lists for meat, eggs,

* Mead Johnson & Co, Evansville, IN 47721.

or milk. If the child's phenylalanine level permits, small amounts of these foods are calculated into the diet by the dietitian.

Several phenylalanine-free products are now available. They are useful in planning diets for the PKU child who is 2 years old or older.

Those responsible for the care of the infant or child are instructed by the dietitian. The cooperation of the entire family is essential, for they play a major role in controlling the disease. The dietitian maintains close contact with the parents through visits, telephone, and correspondence. The parents receive instruction about the preparation of Lofenalac and other foods. All ingredients and foods must be carefully measured or weighed, and an accurate record of the child's food intake must be kept.

The health team can help the family cope with the frustrations and fears that accompany this disease by serving as a sounding board for them and being supportive and encouraging.

In the hospital, the nursing staff must be especially careful to see that the PKU infant is offered the correct formula. Proportions of Lofenalac powder, water, and cow's milk must be carefully measured and mixed under sterile conditions. In the case of an older PKU child who is hospitalized, care must be taken to see that only the kinds and amounts of food permitted on the diet are taken. Food intake should be recorded for all PKU infants and children.

The child stays on the diet for at least 4½ years. If the decision is then made to discontinue the diet, the change to a normal diet is made gradually. Fruits, vegetables, and regular bread are permitted in unlimited amounts. Milk, meat, eggs, beans, and cheese are restricted to small or moderate amounts. Use of Lofenalac is discontinued.

Galactosemia

Galactosemia is a disorder in the metabolism of galactose, a simple sugar. In this disease, enzymes needed for the normal conversion of galactose to glucose are lacking. Galactose thus reaches abnormal blood levels and is excreted in the urine (galactosuria). If not treated, one type of galactosemia causes failure to thrive, liver disease, cataracts, and mental retardation.

Table 28-1.   Sample Menu of a Phenylalanine-Restricted Diet for a Toddler

	Phenylalanine (mg)	Protein (g)	Energy (kcal)
Approximate daily total	**384**	**25**	**1300**
16 scoops of packed dry Lofenalac	128	24	720
Add 0 oz evaporated milk	0	0	0
Add water to make 32 oz:	1 oz = 4	0.75	22.5
Breakfast			
½ grapefruit	14	0.7	59
½ cup Sugar Pops	30	0.6	43
8 oz of Lofenalac	32	6	180
Morning Snack			
4 oz of orange juice	16	0.6	60
Lunch			
½ cup of grapes (13)	14	0.5	54
4 tbsp of beef broth	16	0.5	15
4 Wheat Thins	34	0.7	32
1½ tsp of butter or fortified margarine	2	0.1	50
8 oz of Lofenalac	32	6	180
Afternoon Snack			
2 tbsp of raisins	15	0.5	58
4 oz of Lofenalac	16	3	90
Supper			
2 tbsp of raisins	15	0.5	58
2 tbsp of broccoli	14	0.4	3
2 tbsp of mushroom soup	15	0.3	17
⅓ Irish potato	29	0.6	21
1½ tsp of butter or fortified margarine	2	0.1	50
2 tbsp of cherry pie filling	6	0.2	42
8 oz of Lofenalac	32	6	180
Bedtime Snack			
5 animal crackers	33	0.7	43
4 oz of Lofenalac	16	3	90
Totals	**383**	**31**	**1325**

(After American Dietetic Association: Handbook of Clinical Dietetics, p C43. New Haven, Yale University Press, 1981)

These problems can be prevented if treatment is started within the first few days of life.

Treatment consists of the elimination of galactose from the diet. The main source of galactose is lactose, or milk sugar, which is broken down to glucose and galactose in the intestinal tract. Therefore, milk, milk products, and medications containing lactose as a filler must be avoided (foods containing lactate, lactic acid, or lactalbumin may be used), and all food labels must be read carefully. (See the section on Lactose Intolerance in Chap. 25.) Moreover, monosodium glutamate and organ meats, including liver, pancreas, and brain, also contain galactose and are omitted from the diet.

A galactose-free diet presents little difficulty during infancy, when lactose-free commercial formulas are used. As the child grows older, the diet becomes more complex. Galactose must be completely avoided, especially in the first few years of life. How strict the diet must be after early childhood is controversial. If the older child's diet is liberalized to include foods that contain small quantities of milk, his condition should be monitored.

KEYS TO PRACTICAL APPLICATION

Respect the desire of parents to become involved in feeding their hospitalized child.

Try to identify the emotional factors that frequently underlie eating problems such as poor appetite, refusal of food, or regressive behavior.

To stimulate the appetite of a poor eater, provide familiar foods, small servings, occasional surprises, and the company of other persons at mealtime.

Make sure that parents understand directions for the use of commercial preparations and special formulas in the home. Mistakes can have serious consequences.

Provide acceptance of and support for the obese child regardless of whether he follows his diet. Involve the older child or adolescent in determining how his diet and activity patterns are to be changed.

Check very carefully to see that the hospitalized PKU infant receives the correct formula and that the older PKU child receives only the kinds and amounts of food permitted on his diet.

KEY IDEAS

The emotional impact of illness may significantly affect a sick child's eating habits and attitude toward food served; health workers should try to identify the child's emotional needs and help the child and his parents meet these needs in nonfood ways.

In acute illness involving fever, vomiting, and diarrhea, restoring fluid and electrolyte balance is the first priority; a careful record of fluid intake and output is important.

When a child fails to grow at a normal rate, the cause must be determined and then corrected or treated. Possible causes include underlying disease, poverty, coaxing and nagging by parents, and an emotionally deprived environment.

Severe restriction of calories is not recommended for overweight children, because it can retard growth; instead, prevention of further weight gain or a slow rate of weight loss is desirable.

For the obese child, increasing physical activity may be more important than decreasing energy intake.

The obese child needs emotional support —
he needs to be accepted as he is, when
he fails as well as when he succeeds.

Nutritional care of chronically ill infants and
small children is time-consuming and
must be adjusted to the abilities of the
family.

Children with an inherited condition in
which cholesterol level is above normal
should consume a cholesterol-lowering
diet, restricting cholesterol and saturated
fat.

Severe sodium restriction may be ordered to
treat edema, which accompanies
nephrosis in childhood. Increased
amounts of protein are needed to make
up for protein lost in urine.

Children on dialysis must be dialyzed more
frequently than adults because they
need more protein for growth; calories
must be adequate so that body protein is
not used for energy; protein must be
limited to amounts needed for growth;
and sodium, potassium, and fluids are
usually restricted.

Creating a state of ketosis by means of diet
has been found to be helpful in
controlling certain types of epileptic
seizures in preschool children; a diet

using MCT and the exchange lists has
offered a practical means of therapy.

Malnutrition, which frequently accompanies
cystic fibrosis, is due to poor absorption
of nutrients caused by a lack of
pancreatic enzymes; commercial, easily
digested semisynthetic formulas may be
used along with regular foods to
increase caloric and protein intake, and
medication containing pancreatic
enzymes is given with meals to promote
digestion.

Phenylketonuria is an enzyme deficiency
disease in which phenylalanine, an
essential amino acid, is not metabolized
normally. Phenylalanine is restricted in
the diet to amounts needed to maintain
adequate blood levels. The formula
Lofenalac is the main source of protein
and calories; protein foods are added in
small amounts as the child grows.

Galactosemia is an inherited disease caused
by a lack of enzymes needed to convert
galactose to glucose in the body; foods
containing lactose and galactose are
avoided beginning in the first few days
of life as a means of preventing severe
mental retardation, cataracts, and other
serious consequences.

KEYS TO LEARNING: STUDY–DISCUSSION QUESTIONS

1. What changes are made in menu
planning, meal service, and feeding
techniques to promote the acceptance
of food by children in your hospital?

2. When acutely ill infants and children are
cared for in the home, parents must be
given precise instructions concerning
changes in formula, the use of
electrolyte preparations, and the types
of fluid to be given. Discuss the
importance of this.

3. Investigate community nutrition
programs in your area, and report your
findings to the class. Include such points
as who is eligible, benefits, and how

persons may become enrolled. As a
class, discuss how poorly nourished or
chronically ill infants and children can
benefit from these programs.

4. What children are at the greatest risk of
becoming obese? What measures
should be taken to prevent obesity?
Why should very-low-calorie diets be
avoided?

5. Discuss the problems involved in
obtaining adequate nourishment for an
infant or young child with congenital
heart disease.

6. What is the value of a ketogenic diet in
the treatment of epilepsy? Why is the

diet restricted in protein and
carbohydrate and high in fat?
7. Discuss the importance of nutritional
care for the patient with cystic fibrosis.
Why are pancreatic enzymes given as
medication? Increased amounts of salt
may be necessary. Why? Despite a high
caloric intake, a child with cystic fibrosis
may be undernourished. Why?
8. Plan a day's menu for a 4-year-old child
on a gluten-free diet. (See Chap. 25 for

a discussion of the gluten-free diet.)
9. What are the goals of dietary treatment
in phenylketonuria? Most protein foods
are severely restricted. How is the
body's need for protein met?
10. Why is milk excluded from the diet in
the treatment of galactosemia? What
other foods may be restricted?

Bibliography is found at the end of Part Four.

Bibliography

Part Four Diet Modifications During Illness

General References

American Dietetic Association: Handbook of Clinical Dietetics. New Haven, Yale University Press, 1981

Anderson L, Dibble MV, Turkki PR et al: Nutrition in Health and Disease, 17th ed. Philadelphia, JB Lippincott, 1982

Goodhart RS, Shils ME: Modern Nutrition in Health and Disease, 6th ed. Philadelphia, Lea & Febiger, 1980

Hodges RE: Nutrition in Medical Practice. Philadelphia, WB Saunders, 1980

Pennington JAT, Church HN: Bowes and Church's Food Values of Portions Commonly Used, 13th ed. Philadelphia, JB Lippincott, 1980

Schneider HA, Anderson CE, Coursin B (eds): Nutritional Support of Medical Practice. Hagerstown, Harper & Row, 1977

Suitor CW, Hunter MF: Nutrition: Principles and Application in Health Promotion. Philadelphia, JB Lippincott, 1980

Thiele V: Clinical Nutrition. St. Louis, CV Mosby, 1976

Chapter 19. Providing Nutritional Counseling and Care

Books and Pamphlets

Hargrave M: Nutritional Care of the Physically Disabled. Minneapolis, Sister Kenny Institute, 1979

Mason M, Wenberg BG, Welsch PK: The Dynamics of Clinical Dietetics. New York, John Wiley & Sons, 1982

Using Nutrition Labels with Food Exchange Lists. DHEW Publication No. (FDA) 77:2072. Washington, DC, U.S. Government Printing Office, 1977

Periodicals

Allaire B: Staff skills in patient/family relations. Hospitals 53:92, 1979

Butterworth T: Learning principles, practices, and peanuts. J Am Diet Assoc 62:427, 1966

Frank R: Advice from dietitions: Teaching slow learners. Diabetes Ed 8:50, 1982

Granz K: Strategies for nutritional counseling. J Am Diet Assoc 74:431, 1979

Norman RE: Ideas for teaching nutrition. J Home Ec 69:45, 1977

Patient teaching. Nursing Digest 6:1, 1978

Schneggenberger C: History-taking skills. How do you rate? Nursing '79 9:97, 1979

Zimmerman BN: Human question vs. human hurry. Am J Nurs 80:719, 1980

Chapter 20. Weight Control

Books and Pamphlets

Brownell KD: Behavior Therapy for Weight Control

—A Treatment Manual. Philadelphia, KD Brownell, 1979

Mahoney M, Mahoney K: Permanent Weight Loss: A Total Solution to the Dieter's Dilemma. New York, Norton & Co, 1976

Mayer J: Do you want to gain pounds? In: A Diet for Living. New York, David McKay, 1975

Periodicals

Barlow DH, Tillotson JL: Behavioral science and nutrition: A new perspective. J Am Diet Assoc 72:368, 1978

Bukoff M, Carlson S: Diet modifications and behavioral changes for bariatric gastric surgery. J Am Diet Assoc 78:158, 1981

Evan RJ, Hall Y: Social–psychologic perspective in motivating changes in eating behavior. J Am Diet Assoc 72:378, 1978

Experts weigh reducing potions. FDA Consumer, Oct 1979

Fergusen J: Dietitians as behavior change agents. J Am Diet Assoc 73:231, 1978

Mahoney MJ, Caggiula AW: Applying behavioral methods to nutrition counseling. J Am Diet Assoc 72:372, 1978

Nutrition and physical fitness. J Am Diet Assoc 76:437, 1980

Rogus J, Blumenthal J: Variations in dietary intake after bypass surgery for obesity. J Am Diet Assoc 79:433, 1981

Starch blockers. Nutr MD 8:3, 1982

Tullis F: Rational diet construction for mild and grand obesity. JAMA 226:70, 1973

Van Itallie TB, Yank M: Diet and weight loss. N Engl J Med 297:23, 1977

Yang SP, Martin LJ, Schneider G: Weight reduction using a protein-sparing modified fast. J Am Diet Assoc 76:343, 1980

Chapter 21. Diabetes Mellitus

Books and Pamphlets

American Diabetes Association/American Dietetic Association: Family Cookbook. Englewood, NJ, Prentice Hall, 1980

Haunz EA, Blaine M: Diabetes mellitus in adults. In Conn HF (ed): Current therapy, p 437. Philadelphia, WB Saunders, 1981

West K: Diabetes mellitus. In Schneider HA, Anderson CE (eds): Nutritional Support of Medical Practice, p 278. Hagerstown, Harper & Row, 1977

Periodicals

Anderson JW, Midgley WR, Wedman B et al: Fiber and diabetes. Diabetes Care 2:369, 1979

Bosello O, Ostuzzi R, Armellini F et al: Glucose tolerance and blood lipids in bran-fed patients with impaired glucose tolerance. Diabetes Care 3:46, 1980

Burgess BRBE: Rationale for changes in the dietary management of diabetes. J Am Diet Assoc 81:258, 1982

Crapo PA, Kolterman OG, Waldeck N et al: Postprandial hormonal responses to different types of complex carbohydrates in individuals with impaired glucose tolerance. Am J Clin Nutr 33:1723, 1980

Crapo PA, Reaven G, Olefsky J: Postprandial plasma-glucose and plasma-insulin responses to different complex carbohydrates. Diabetes 26:1178, 1977

Danowski TS, Ohlsen P, Fisher ER et al: Diabetic complications and their prevention and reversal. Diabetes Care 3:94, 1980

Etzwiler DD: Teaching allied health professionals about self-management. Diabetes Care 3:121, 1980

Friedman EA: Diabetic nephropathy is a hyperglycemic glomerulopathy. Arch Intern Med 142:1269, 1982

Jenkins DJA, Taylor RH, Wolever MS: The diabetic diet, dietary carbohydrate and differences in digestibility. Diabetologia 23:477, 1982

Koenig RJ: Correlation of glucose regulation and hemoglobin A_1C in diabetes mellitus. N Engl J Med 295:417, 1976

Lecos C: Fructose: Questionable diet aid. FDA Consumer, March 1980

Midgley W, Anderson JW: Fiber in your future. Diabetes Forecast 32:32, 1979

National Diabetes Data Group: Classification and diagnosis of diabetes mellitus and other categories of glucose tolerance. J Diabetes 28:1039, 1979

Nuttall FQ, Brunzell JD: Principles of nutrition and dietary recommendations for individuals with

diabetes mellitus: 1979. J Am Diet Assoc 75:527, 1979

Olefsky JM, Crapo P: Fructose, xylitol, and sorbitol as a sweetener in diabetes mellitus. J Am Diet Assoc 73:499, 1978

Owen OE, Boden G, Shuman CR et al: Managing insulin-dependent diabetic patients. Postgrad Med 59:127, 1976

Skyler JS, Lasky IA, Skyler DL et al: Home glucose monitoring as an aid in diabetes management. Diabetes Care 1:150, 1978

Whitehouse FW: Classification and pathogenesis of the diabetes syndrome: A historical perspective. J Am Diet Assoc 81:243, 1982

Wylie-Rosett J: Development of new educational strategies for the person with diabetes. J Am Diet Assoc 81:268, 1982

Chapter 22. Cardiovascular Disease: Atherosclerosis

Books and Pamphlets

Arteriosclerosis, 1981, Vol 1 and 2. Report of the Working Group on Arteriosclerosis of the National Heart, Lung, and Blood Institute. U.S. Dept. H.H.S. (NIH) Publication Nos. 81-2034 and 81-2035. Washington, DC, U.S. Government Printing Office, 1981

Eshleman R, Winston M: The American Heart Association Cookbook. New York, David McKay, 1979

Fact Sheet: Hyperlipoproteinemia. U.S. Dept. HHS (NIH) Publication No. 79-734. Washington, DC, U.S. Government Printing Office, 1979

Hodges RD: Diet, cholesterol, and coronary heart disease. In Nutrition in Medical Practice. Philadelphia, WB Saunders, 1980

Model Workshop on Nutrition Counseling in Hyperlipidemia. U.S. Dept. HHS (NIH) Publication No. 80-1666. Washington, DC, U.S. Government Printing Office, 1980

National Heart and Lung Institute. Dietary Management of Hyperlipoproteinemia. A Handbook for Physicians. DHEW Publication No. (NIH) 78-110. Bethesda, MD, National Institutes of Health, 1978

Nutrition Committee of the Steering Committee for Medical and Community Programs of the American Heart Association: Diet and Coronary Heart Disease. Dallas, American Heart Association, 1978

Nutrition Program Committee of the American Heart Association: Supplement to Guidelines for the Development of Nutrition Programs. Dallas, American Heart Association, 1981

Seventh Report of the National Heart, Lung and Blood Advisory Council. U.S. Dept. HHS (NIH) Publication No. 80-1673. Washington, DC, U.S. Government Printing Office, 1980

Periodicals

Castelli WP, Doyle JT, Gordon T et al: HDL cholesterol and other lipids in coronary heart disease. Circulation 55:767, 1977

Glueck CJ, Mattson F, Bierman EL et al: Diet and coronary heart disease: Another view. N Engl J Med 298:1471, 1978

Grotto AM: Is atherosclerosis reversible: J Am Diet Assoc 74:551, 1979

Grundy SM: Treatment of hypercholesterolemia. Am J Clin Nutr 30:985, 1977

Karvetti R-L: Effects of nutrition education: Changes in the diet of myocardial infarction patients. J Am Diet Assoc 79:660, 1981

Chapter 23. Cardiovascular Disease: Hypertension, Congestive Heart Failure, Acute Illness

Books and Pamphlets

American Dietetic Association: Handbook of Clinical Dietetics. New Haven, Yale University Press, 1981

American Heart Association, Northeast Ohio Affiliate: Cooking Without Your Salt Shaker. Dallas, American Heart Association, 1978

The Sodium Content of Your Food. USDA Home and Garden Bulletin 233. Washington, DC, U.S. Government Printing Office, 1980

Periodicals

Crocco SC: The role of sodium in food processing. J Am Diet Assoc 80:36, 1982

Elison RC, Newburger JW, Gross DM: Pediatric aspects of essential hypertension. J Am Diet Assoc 80:21, 1982

Frohlich ED: Physiological observations in essential hypertension. J Am Diet Assoc 80:18, 1982

Hemzacek KI: Dietary protocol for the patient who has suffered a myocardial infarction. J Am Diet Assoc 72:182, 1978

Karvetti R-L: Effects of nutrition education:

Changes in the diet of myocardial infarction patients. J Am Diet Assoc 79:660, 1981

Kris-Etherton PM, Kisloff L, Kassouf RA, Rogers C: Teaching principles and cost of sodium-restricted diets. J Am Diet Assoc 80:55, 1982

Morgan T, Gillies A, Morgan G et al: Hypertension treated by salt restriction. Lancet 1:227, 1978

Ram CVS, Garrett BN, Kaplan NM et al: Moderate sodium restriction and various diuretics in the treatment of hypertension: Effects on potassium wastage and blood pressure control. Arch Intern Med 141:1015, 1981

Shank FR et al: Perspective of food and drug administration on dietary sodium. J Am Diet Assoc 80:29, 1982

Tobian L: The relationship of salt to hypertension. Am J Clin Nutr 32:2739, 1979

Wilbur JA: The role of diet in the treatment of high blood pressure. J Am Diet Assoc 80:25, 1982

Chapter 24. Diet in Kidney Disease

Books and Pamphlets

Adelman RD, Hodges RE: Nutrition and the kidney. In Hodges RE (ed): Nutrition in Medical Practice, p 232. Philadelphia, WB Saunders, 1980

Ing TS, Kark RM: Renal disease. In Schneider HA, Anderson CE, Coursin DB (eds): Nutrition Support of Medical Practice, p 367. Hagerstown, Harper & Row, 1977

Jones W: Diet Guide for Patients on Chronic Dialysis. DHEW Publication No. (NIH) 75-685. Washington, DC, U.S. Government Printing Office, 1975

Margie JD, Anderson CF: The Mayo Clinic Renal Diet Cookbook. Bloomfield, NJ, HLF Press, Inc., 1974

Periodicals

Berger M: Dietary management of children with uremia. J Am Diet Assoc 70:498, 1977

Beto JA, Myscofski IM: Gourmet cooking workshops for dialysis patients. J Am Diet Assoc 70:626, 1977

Blackburn SL: Dietary compliance of chronic hemodialysis patients. J Am Diet Assoc 70:31, 1977

Blumenkrantz MJ, Roberts CE, Card B et al: Nutritional management of the adult patient undergoing maintenance peritoneal dialysis. J Am Diet Assoc 73:251, 1978

Bodnar DM: Rationale for nutritional requirements for patients on continuous ambulatory peritoneal dialysis. J Am Diet Assoc 80:247, 1982

Burton BT: Nutritional implications of renal disease. J Am Diet Assoc 70:479, 1977

Friedman EA, Delano BG, Butt KMH et al: Pragmatic realities in uremia therapy. N Engl J Med 298:368, 1978

Kopple JD: Nutritional management of chronic renal failure. Postgrad Med 64:135, 1978

Ritz E, Mehls O, Gilli G et al: Protein restriction in the conservative management of uremia. Am J Clin Nutr 31:1703, 1978

Shinaberger JH, Blumenkrantz MJ: Dialysis therapy and transplantation in uremia: Which to use when. Postgrad Med 64:169, 1978

Spinozzi NS, Grupe WE: Nutritional implications of renal disease. IV. Nutritional aspects of chronic renal insufficiency in childhood. J Am Diet Assoc 70:493, 1977

Chapter 25. Diet in Gastrointestinal Disease

Books and Pamphlets

Holt PR: Malabsorption. Nutrition in Disease. Columbus, OH, Ross Laboratories, 1977

Periodicals

Almy TP: Gastrointestinal illness and emotions. Carrier Foundation Letter 73, 1981

Brodribb AJM: Treatment of symptomatic diverticular disease with a high-fibre diet. Lancet 1:664, 1977

Burkett DP: Economic development not all bonus. Nutrition Today 11:11, 1976

Chapman ML: Peptic ulcer: A medical perspective. Med Clin North Am 62:39, 1978

Connell AM: Wheat bran as an etiologic factor in certain diseases: Some second thoughts. J Am Diet Assoc 71:235, 1977

Fisher RS, Cohen S: Gastroesophageal reflux. Med Clin North Am 62:3, 1978

McNutt KW: Perspective—Fiber. J Nutr Ed 8:150, 1976

Medeloff AI: Dietary fiber and human health. N Engl J Med 297:811, 1977

Chapter 26. Nutrition in Surgery and Following Burns

Periodicals

Chernoff R: Nutritional support: Formulas and delivery of enteral feeding. I. Enteral formulas. J Am Diet Assoc 79:426, 1981

Chernoff R: Nutritional support: Formulas and delivery of enteral feedings. II. Delivery systems. J Am Diet Assoc 79:430, 1981

Feldtman RW, Andrassy RJ: Meeting exceptional nutritional needs. II. Elemental enteral alimentation. Postgrad Med 64:65, 1978

McConnell E: Ten problems with nasogastric tubes and how to solve them. Nursing '79 9:78, 1979

Pennisi VM: Monitoring the nutritional care of burned patients. J Am Diet Assoc 69:531, 1976

Chapter 27. Nutrition in Cancer and Other Special Problems

Books and Pamphlets

Beaudette T: Diet, Nutrition and Cancer. Nutrition in Practice. Minneapolis, Doyle Pharmaceutical, 1981

March DC: Handbook: Interactions of Selected Drugs with Nutritional Status in Man, 2nd ed. Chicago, American Dietetic Association, 1978

National Cancer Institute: Eating Hints—Recipes and Tips for Better Nutrition During Cancer Treatment. NIH Publication No. 82-2079. Washington, DC, U.S. Government Printing Office, 1982

Talbott JA: Drug–Food Interactions. Nutrition in Disease. Columbus, OH, Ross Laboratories, 1977

Visconti JA: Drug–Food Interactions. Nutrition in Disease. Columbus, OH, Ross Laboratories, 1977

Periodicals

Carson JA, Gormican A: Disease—Medication relationship in altered taste sensitivity. J Am Diet Assoc 68:550, 1976

DeWys WD: Nutritional care of the cancer patient. JAMA 244:374, 1981

DeWys WD, Kubota TT: Enteral and parenteral nutrition in the care of the cancer patient. JAMA 246:1725, 1981

Friedman BJ: A diet free from additives in the management of allergic disease. Clin Allergy 7:417, 1977

Hartshorn EA: Food and drug interactions. J Am Diet Assoc 70:15, 1977

Hofeldt FD, Adler RA, Herman RH: Postprandial hypoglycemia. Fact or fiction? JAMA 233:1309, 1975

Meloni CR: Hypoglycemia: What kind of problem is it? Am Fam Physician 12:108, 1975

Parker C: Food allergies. Am J Nurs 80:262, 1980

Rotwein P, Giddings SJ, Permutt MA: Hypoglycemia. Diabetes Forecast 35:25, 1982

Schreier A McB, Lavenia J: The nurse's role in nutritional management of radiotherapy patients. Nurs Clin North Am 12:173, 1977

Vickers ZM, Nielsen SS, Theologides A: Food preferences of patients with cancer. J Am Diet Assoc 78:467, 1981

Welch D: Nutritional consequences of carcinogenesis and radiation therapy. J Am Diet Assoc 78:467, 1981

Chapter 28. Nutrition in Diseases of Infancy and Childhood

Books and Pamphlets

Committee on Nutrition. Pediatric Nutrition Handbook. Evanston, American Academy of Pediatrics, 1979

Fomon SJ: Nutritional Disorders of Children. Prevention, Screening, Follow-up. DHEW Publication No. (HSA) 77-5104. Washington, DC, U.S. Government Printing Office, 1977

Periodicals

Acosta PB, Blaskovics M, Cloud H et al: Nutrition in pregnancy of women with hyperphenylalaninemia. J Am Diet Assoc 80:443, 1982

American Dairy Council: Current concepts in infant nutrition. Dairy Council Digest 47:2, 1976

Beckner AS, Centerwall WR, Holt L: Effects of rapid increase of phenylalanine intake in older PKU children. J Am Diet Assoc 69:148, 1976

Berger M: Dietary management of children with uremia. J Am Diet Assoc 70:498, 1977

Heffernan JF, Trahms CM: A model preschool for patients with phenylketonuria. J Am Diet Assoc 79:306, 1981

Hubbard VS, Mangrum PJ: Energy intake and nutrition counseling in cystic fibrosis. J Am Diet Assoc 80:127, 1982

Hunt MM: Dietary care of patients with cystic fibrosis. Dietetic Currents 3:3, 1976

Palmer S, Thompson RJ: Nutrition, an integral component in health care of children. J Am Diet Assoc 69:138, 1976

Parker CE, Shaw KNF, Mitchell JB et al: Clinical experience in dietary management of phenylketonuria with a new phenylalanine-free product. J Pediatr 91:941, 1977

Pueschel SM, Hum C, Andrews M: Nutritional management of the female with phenylketonuria during pregnancy. Am J Clin Nutr 30:198, 1977

Richard K, Brady MS, Hempel J, Gresham E: Care of children with conditions characterized by high nutritional risks. J Am Diet Assoc 68:546, 1976

Spinozzi NS, Grupe WE: Implications of renal disease. IV. Nutritional aspects of chronic renal insufficiency in childhood. J Am Diet Assoc 70:493, 1977

Appendix

Table A-1. Nutritive Values of the Edible Part of Foods

(Dashes (—) denote lack of reliable data for a constituent believed to be present in measurable amount)

Item No. (A)	Foods, Approximate Measures, Units, and Weight (edible part unless footnotes indicate otherwise) (B)	Water (C) Per-cent	Food Energy (D) Cal-ories	Pro-tein (E) g	Fat (F) g	Fatty Acids Satu-rated (Total) (G) g	Unsaturated Oleic (H) g	Lino-leic (I) g	Carbo-hydrate (J) g	Calcium (K) mg	Phos-phorus (L) mg	Iron (M) mg	Potas-sium (N) mg	Vitamin A Value (O) IU	Thiamin (P) mg	Ribo-flavin (Q) mg	Niacin (R) mg	Ascorbic Acid (S) mg
	g																	
	Dairy Products (Cheese, Cream, Imitation Cream, Milk; Related Products)																	
	Butter (See Fats, Oils, and Related Products, items 103–108)																	
	Cheese																	
	Natural																	
1	Blue .... 1 oz 28	42	100	6	8	5.3	1.9	0.2	1	150	110	0.1	73	200	0.01	0.11	0.3	0
2	Camembert (3 wedges per 4-oz container) 1 wedge ... 38	52	115	8	9	5.8	2.2	0.2	tr	147	132	0.1	71	350	0.01	0.19	0.2	0
	Cheddar																	
3	Cut pieces ...... 1 oz 28	37	115	7	9	6.1	2.1	0.2	tr	204	145	0.2	28	300	0.01	0.11	tr	0
4	.... 1 cu in 17.2	37	70	4	6	3.7	1.3	0.1	tr	124	88	0.1	17	180	tr	0.06	tr	0
5	Shredded ...... 1 c 113	37	455	28	37	24.2	8.5	0.7	1	815	579	0.8	111	1200	0.03	0.42	0.1	0
	Cottage (curd not pressed down)																	
	Creamed (cottage cheese, 4% fat)																	
6	Large curd ...... 1 c 225	79	235	28	10	6.4	2.4	0.2	6	135	297	0.3	190	370	0.05	0.37	0.3	tr
7	Small curd ...... 1 c 210	79	220	26	9	6.0	2.2	0.2	6	126	277	0.3	177	340	0.04	0.34	0.3	tr
8	Low fat (2%) ..... 1 c 226	79	205	31	4	2.8	1.0	0.1	8	155	340	0.4	217	160	0.05	0.42	0.3	tr
9	Low fat (1%) ..... 1 c 226	82	165	28	2	1.5	0.5	0.1	6	138	302	0.3	193	80	0.05	0.37	0.3	tr
10	Uncreamed (cottage cheese dry curd, less than 1/2% fat) 1 c ... 145	80	125	25	1	0.4	0.1	tr	3	46	151	0.3	47	40	0.04	0.21	0.2	0
11	Cream .... 1 oz 28	54	100	2	10	6.2	2.4	0.2	1	23	30	0.3	34	400	tr	0.06	tr	0
	Mozzarella, made with—																	
12	Whole milk ...... 1 oz 28	48	90	6	7	4.4	1.7	0.2	1	163	117	0.1	21	260	tr	0.08	tr	0
13	Part skim milk .... 1 oz 28	49	80	8	5	3.1	1.2	0.1	1	207	149	0.1	27	180	0.01	0.10	tr	0
	Parmesan, grated																	
14	Cup, not pressed down 1 c ... 100	18	455	42	30	19.1	7.7	0.3	4	1376	807	1.0	107	700	0.05	0.39	0.3	0
15	Tablespoon ...... 1 tbsp 5	18	25	2	2	1.0	0.4	tr	tr	69	40	tr	5	40	tr	0.02	tr	0
16	Ounce .... 1 oz 28	18	130	12	9	5.4	2.2	0.1	1	390	229	0.3	30	200	0.01	0.11	0.1	0
17	Provolone ...... 1 oz 28	41	100	7	8	4.8	1.7	0.1	1	214	141	0.1	39	230	0.01	0.09	tr	0
	Ricotta, made with—																	
18	Whole milk ...... 1 c 246	72	430	28	32	20.4	7.1	0.7	7	509	389	0.9	257	1210	0.03	0.48	0.3	0
19	Part skim milk .... 1 c 246	74	340	28	19	12.1	4.7	0.5	13	669	449	1.1	308	1060	0.05	0.46	0.2	0
20	Romano .... 1 oz 28	31	110	9	8	—	—	—	1	302	215	—	—	160	—	0.11	tr	0

(Continued)

Table A-1. Nutritive Values of the Edible Part of Foods (Continued)

(Dashes (—) denote lack of reliable data for a constituent believed to be present in measurable amount)

						Fatty Acids												
Item No. (A)	Foods, Approximate Measures, Units, and Weight (edible part unless footnotes indicate otherwise) (B)	Water Percent (C)	Food Energy Calories (D)	Protein g (E)	Fat g (F)	Saturated (Total) g (G)	Unsaturated Oleic g (H)	Linoleic g (I)	Carbohydrate g (J)	Calcium mg (K)	Phosphorus mg (L)	Iron mg (M)	Potassium mg (N)	Vitamin A Value IU (O)	Thiamin mg (P)	Riboflavin mg (Q)	Niacin mg (R)	Ascorbic Acid mg (S)

Dairy Products (Cheese, Cream, Imitation Cream, Milk; Related Products) (Continued)

Cheese (Continued)

21	Swiss .... 1 oz	28	105	8	8	5.0	1.7	0.2	1	272	171	tr	31	240	0.01	0.10	tr	0

Pasteurized process cheese

22	American .... 1 oz	28	39	105	6	9	5.6	2.1	0.2	tr	174	211	0.1	46	340	0.01	0.10	tr	0
23	Swiss .... 1 oz	28	42	95	7	7	4.5	1.7	0.1	1	219	216	0.2	61	230	tr	0.08	tr	0
24	Pasteurized process cheese food, American ... 1 oz	28	43	95	6	7	4.4	1.7	0.1	2	163	130	0.2	79	260	0.01	0.13	tr	0
25	Pasteurized process cheese spread, American ... 1 oz	28	48	80	5	6	3.8	1.5	0.1	2	159	202	0.1	69	220	0.01	0.12	tr	0

Cream, sweet

26	Half-and-half (cream and milk) ... 1 c	242	81	315	7	28	17.3	7.0	0.6	10	254	230	0.2	314	260	0.08	0.36	0.2	2
27	... 1 tbsp	15	81	20	tr	2	1.1	0.4	tr	1	16	14	tr	19	20	0.01	0.02	tr	tr
28	Light, coffee, or table ... 1 c	240	74	470	6	46	28.8	11.7	1.0	9	231	192	0.1	292	1730	0.08	0.36	0.1	2
29	... 1 tbsp	15	74	30	tr	3	1.8	0.7	0.1	1	14	12	tr	18	110	tr	0.02	tr	tr

Whipping, unwhipped (volume about double when whipped)

30	Light .... 1 c	239	64	700	5	74	46.2	18.3	1.5	7	166	146	0.1	231	2690	0.06	0.30	0.1	1
31	... 1 tbsp	15	64	45	tr	5	2.9	1.1	0.1	tr	10	9	tr	15	170	tr	0.02	tr	tr
32	Heavy .... 1 c	238	58	820	5	88	54.8	22.2	2.0	7	154	149	0.1	179	3500	0.05	0.26	0.1	1
33	... 1 tbsp	15	58	80	tr	6	3.5	1.4	0.1	tr	10	9	tr	11	220	tr	0.02	tr	tr
34	Whipped topping, (pressurized) ... 1 c	60	61	155	2	13	8.3	3.4	0.3	7	61	54	tr	88	550	0.02	0.04	tr	0
35	... 1 tbsp	3	61	10	tr	1	0.4	0.2	tr	tr	3	3	tr	4	30	tr	tr	tr	0
36	Cream, sour .... 1 c	230	71	495	7	48	30.0	12.1	1.1	10	268	195	0.1	331	1820	0.08	0.34	0.2	2
37	... 1 tbsp	12	71	25	tr	3	1.6	0.6	0.1	1	14	10	tr	17	90	tr	0.02	tr	tr

Cream products, imitation (made with vegetable fat)

Sweet

Creamers

38	Liquid (frozen) ...... 1 c	245	77	335	2	24	22.8	0.3	tr	28	23	157	0.1	467	220[1]	0	0	tr	0
39	... 1 tbsp	15	77	20	tr	1	1.4	tr	0	2	1	10	tr	29	10[1]	0	0	tr	0
40	Powdered .... 1 c	94	2	515	5	33	30.6	0.9	tr	52	21	397	0.1	763	190[1]	0	0.16[1]	0.1	0
41	... 1 tsp	2	2	10	tr	1	0.7	tr	0	1	tr	8	tr	16	tr	0	tr	tr	0

(A)	(B)	(C)	(D)	(E)	(F)	(G)	(H)	(I)	(J)	(K)	(L)	(M)	(N)	(O)	(P)	(Q)	(R)	(S)	(T)
	Whipped topping																		
42	Frozen — 1 c	75	50	240	1	19	16.3	1.0	0.2	17	5	6	0.1	14	650[1]	0	0	0	0
	1 tbsp	4	50	15	tr	1	0.9	0.1	tr	1	tr	tr	tr	1	30[1]	0	0	0	0
44	Powdered, made with whole milk — 1 c	80	67	150	3	10	8.5	0.6	0.1	13	72	69	tr	121	290[1]	0.02	0.09	tr	1
	1 tbsp	4	67	10	tr	tr	0.4	tr	tr	1	4	3	tr	6	10[1]	tr	tr	tr	tr
46	Pressurized — 1 c	70	60	185	1	16	13.2	1.4	0.2	11	4	13	tr	13	330[1]	0	0	0	0
47	1 tbsp	4	60	10	tr	1	0.8	0.1	tr	1	tr	1	tr	1	20[1]	0	0	0	0
48	Sour dressing (imitation sour cream) made with nonfat dry milk — 1 c	235	75	415	8	39	31.2	4.4	1.1	11	266	205	0.1	380	20[1]	0.09	0.38	0.2	2
49	1 tbsp	12	75	20	tr	2	1.6	0.2	0.1	1	14	10	tr	19	tr	0.01	0.02	tr	tr
	Ice cream (see Milk desserts, frozen, items 75–80).																		
	Ice milk (see Milk desserts, frozen, items 81–83).																		
	Milk																		
	Fluid																		
50	Whole (3.3% fat) — 1 c	244	88	150	8	8	5.1	2.1	0.2	11	291	228	0.1	370	310[2]	0.09	0.40	0.2	2
51	Low fat (2%) — No milk solids added — 1 c	244	89	120	8	5	2.9	1.2	0.1	12	297	232	0.1	377	500	0.10	0.40	0.2	2
52	Milk solids added Label claims less than 10 g protein per cup — 1 c	245	89	125	9	5	2.9	1.2	0.1	12	313	245	0.1	397	500	0.10	0.42	0.2	2
53	Label claims 10 or more g protein per cup (protein fortified) — 1 c	246	88	135	10	5	3.0	1.2	0.1	14	352	276	0.1	447	500	0.11	0.48	0.2	3
54	Low fat (1%) — No milk solids added — 1 c	244	90	100	8	3	1.6	0.7	0.1	12	300	235	0.1	381	500	0.10	0.41	0.2	2
55	Milk solids added Label claims less than 10 g protein per cup — 1 c	245	90	105	9	2	1.5	0.6	0.1	12	313	245	0.1	397	500	0.10	0.42	0.2	2
56	Label claims 10 or more g protein per cup (protein fortified) — 1 c	246	89	120	10	3	1.8	0.7	0.1	14	349	273	0.1	444	500	0.11	0.47	0.2	3
57	Nonfat (skim) — No milk solids added — 1 c	245	91	85	8	tr	0.3	0.1	tr	12	302	247	0.1	406	500	0.09	0.34	0.2	2
58	Milk solids added Label claims less than 10 g protein per cup — 1 c	245	90	90	9	1	0.4	0.1	tr	12	316	255	0.1	418	500	0.10	0.43	0.2	2
59	Label claims 10 or more g protein per cup (protein fortified) — 1 c	246	89	100	10	1	0.4	0.1	tr	14	352	275	0.1	446	500	0.11	0.48	0.2	3

(Continued)

Table A-1. Nutritive Values of the Edible Part of Foods (Continued)

(Dashes (—) denote lack of reliable data for a constituent believed to be present in measurable amount)

Item No. (A)	Foods, Approximate Measures, Units, and Weight (edible part unless footnotes indicate otherwise) (B)		Water (C)	Food Energy (D)	Pro-tein (E)	Fat (F)	Fatty Acids Saturated (Total) (G)	Unsaturated Oleic (H)	Unsaturated Lino-leic (I)	Carbo-hydrate (J)	Calcium (K)	Phos-phorus (L)	Iron (M)	Potas-sium (N)	Vitamin A Value (O)	Thiamin (P)	Ribo-flavin (Q)	Niacin (R)	Ascorbic Acid (S)
		g	Percent	Calories	g	g	g	g	g	g	mg	mg	mg	mg	IU	mg	mg	mg	mg
Dairy Products (Cheese, Cream, Imitation Cream, Milk; Related Products) (Continued)																			
Milk (Continued)																			
60	Buttermilk .... 1 c	245	90	100	8	2	1.3	0.5	tr	12	285	219	0.1	371	80[3]	0.08	0.38	0.1	2
	Canned Evaporated, unsweetened																		
61	Whole milk .... 1 c	252	74	340	17	19	11.6	5.3	0.4	25	657	510	0.5	764	610[3]	0.12	0.80	0.5	5
62	Skim milk .... 1 c	255	79	200	19	1	.3	0.1	tr	29	738	497	0.7	845	1000[4]	0.11	0.79	0.4	3
63	Sweetened, condensed 1 c	306	27	980	24	27	16.8	6.7	0.7	166	868	775	0.6	1136	1000[3]	0.28	1.27	0.6	8
	Dried																		
64	Buttermilk .... 1 c	120	3	465	41	7	4.3	1.7	0.2	59	1421	1119	0.4	1910	260[3]	0.47	1.90	1.1	7
65	Nonfat instant Envelope, net wt 3.2 oz[5] 1 envelope	91	4	325	32	1	0.4	0.1	tr	47	1120	896	0.3	1552	2160[6]	0.38	1.59	0.8	5
66	Cup[7] .... 1 c	68	4	245	24	tr	0.3	0.1	tr	35	837	670	0.2	1160	1610[6]	0.28	1.19	0.6	4
	Milk beverages Chocolate milk (commercial)																		
67	Regular .... 1 c	250	82	210	8	8	5.3	2.2	0.2	26	280	251	0.6	417	300[3]	0.09	0.41	0.3	2
68	Low fat (2%) ..... 1 c	250	84	180	8	5	3.1	1.3	0.1	26	284	254	0.6	422	500	0.10	0.42	0.3	2
69	Low fat (1%) ..... 1 c	250	85	160	8	3	1.5	0.7	0.1	26	287	257	0.6	426	500	0.10	0.40	0.2	2
70	Eggnog (commercial) 1 c	254	74	340	10	19	11.3	5.0	0.6	34	330	278	0.5	420	890	0.09	0.48	0.3	4
	Malted milk, home-prepared with 1 c whole milk and 2 to 3 heaping tsp malted milk powder (about 3/4 oz)																		
71	Chocolate .... 1 c milk plus 3/4 oz powder	265	81	235	9	9	5.5	—	—	29	304	265	0.5	500	330[3]	0.14	0.43	0.7	2
72	Natural .... 1 c milk plus 3/4 oz powder	265	81	235	11	10	6.0	—	—	27	347	307	0.3	529	380	0.20	0.54	1.3	2
	Shakes, thick[8]																		
73	Chocolate, container, net wt 10.6 oz 1 container	300	72	355	9	8	5.0	2.0	0.2	63	396	378	0.9	672	260	0.14	0.67	0.4	0
74	Vanilla, container, net wt 11 oz 1 container	313	74	350	12	9	5.9	2.4	0.2	56	457	361	0.3	572	360	0.09	0.61	0.5	0
	Milk desserts, frozen Ice cream Regular (about 11% fat)																		

(A)	(B)	Measure	Grams	(C)	(D)	(E)	(F)	(G)	(H)	(I)	(J)	(K)	(L)	(M)	(N)	(O)	(P)	(Q)	(R)	(S)
75	Hardened	1/2 gal	1064	61	2155	38	115	71.3	28.8	2.6	254	1406	1075	1.0	2052	4340	0.42	2.63	1.1	6
76		1 c	133	61	270	5	14	8.9	3.6	0.3	32	176	134	0.1	257	540	0.05	0.33	0.1	1
77	Soft serve (frozen custard)	3 fl oz container	50	61	100	2	5	3.4	1.4	0.1	12	66	51	tr	96	200	0.02	0.12	0.1	tr
78		1 c	173	60	375	7	23	13.5	5.9	0.6	38	236	199	0.4	338	790	0.08	0.45	0.2	1
79	Rich (about 16% fat), hardened	1/2 gal	1188	59	2805	33	190	118.3	47.8	4.3	256	1213	927	0.8	1771	7200	0.36	2.27	0.9	5
80		1 c	148	59	350	4	24	14.7	6.0	0.5	32	151	115	0.1	221	900	0.04	0.28	0.1	1
	Ice milk																			
81	Hardened (about 4.3% fat)	1/2 gal	1048	69	1470	41	45	28.1	11.3	1.0	232	1409	1035	1.5	2117	1710	0.61	2.78	0.9	6
82		1 c	131	69	185	5	6	3.5	1.4	0.1	29	176	129	0.1	265	210	0.08	0.35	0.1	1
83	Soft serve (about 2.6% fat)	1 c	175	70	225	8	5	2.9	1.2	0.1	38	274	202	0.3	412	180	0.12	0.54	0.2	1
84	Sherbet (about 2% fat)	1/2 gal	1542	66	2160	17	31	19.0	7.7	0.7	469	827	594	2.5	1585	1480	0.26	0.71	1.0	31
85		1 c	193	66	270	2	4	2.4	1.0	0.1	59	103	74	0.3	198	190	0.03	0.09	0.1	4
	Milk desserts, other																			
86	Custard, baked	1 c	265	77	305	14	15	6.8	5.4	0.7	29	297	310	1.1	387	930	0.11	0.50	0.3	1
	Puddings																			
	From home recipe																			
	Starch base																			
87	Chocolate	1 c	260	66	385	8	12	7.6	3.3	0.3	67	250	255	1.3	445	390	0.05	0.36	0.3	1
88	Vanilla (blancmange)	1 c	255	76	285	9	10	6.2	2.5	0.2	41	298	232	tr	352	410	0.08	0.41	0.3	2
89	Tapioca cream	1 c	165	72	220	8	8	4.1	2.5	0.5	28	173	180	0.7	223	480	0.07	0.30	0.2	2
	From mix (chocolate) and milk																			
90	Regular (cooked)	1 c	260	70	320	9	8	4.3	2.6	0.2	59	265	247	0.8	354	340	0.05	0.39	0.3	2
91	Instant	1 c	260	69	325	8	7	3.6	2.2	0.3	63	374	237	1.3	335	340	0.08	0.39	0.3	2
	Yogurt																			
	With added milk solids																			
	Made with low fat milk																			
92	Fruit-flavored[9]	1 container, net wt 8 oz	227	75	230	10	3	1.8	0.6	0.1	42	343	269	0.2	439	120[10]	0.08	0.40	0.2	1
93	Plain	1 container, net wt 8 oz	227	85	145	12	4	2.3	0.8	0.1	16	415	326	0.2	531	150[10]	0.10	0.49	0.3	2
94	Made with non-fat milk	1 container, net wt 8 oz	227	85	125	13	tr	0.3	0.1	tr	17	452	355	0.2	579	20[10]	0.11	0.53	0.3	2
	Without added milk solids																			
95	Made with whole milk	1 container, net wt 8 oz	227	88	140	8	7	4.8	1.7	0.1	11	274	215	0.1	351	280	0.07	0.32	0.2	1
Eggs																				
	Eggs, large (24 oz per dozen)																			
	Raw																			
96	Whole, without shell	1 egg	50	75	80	6	6	1.7	2.0	0.6	1	28	90	1.0	65	260	0.04	0.15	tr	0

(Continued)

Table A-1. Nutritive Values of the Edible Part of Foods (Continued)

(Dashes (—) denote lack of reliable data for a constituent believed to be present in measurable amount)

Item No. (A)	Foods, Approximate Measures, Units, and Weight (edible part unless footnotes indicate otherwise) (B)	Water Per cent (C)	Food Energy Calories (D)	Protein g (E)	Fat g (F)	Saturated (Total) g (G)	Unsaturated Oleic g (H)	Unsaturated Linoleic g (I)	Carbohydrate g (J)	Calcium mg (K)	Phosphorus mg (L)	Iron mg (M)	Potassium mg (N)	Vitamin A Value IU (O)	Thiamin mg (P)	Riboflavin mg (Q)	Niacin mg (R)	Ascorbic Acid mg (S)
	Eggs (Continued)																	
97	White .... 1 white	33	15	3	tr	0	0	0	tr	4	4	tr	45	0	tr	0.09	tr	0
98	Yolk .... 1 yolk	17	65	3	6	1.7	2.1	0.6	tr	26	86	0.9	15	310	0.04	0.07	tr	0
	Cooked																	
99	Fried in butter ...... 1 egg	46	85	5	6	2.4	2.2	0.6	1	26	80	0.9	58	290	0.03	0.13	tr	0
100	Hard-cooked, shell removed 1 egg	50	80	6	6	1.7	2.0	0.6	1	28	90	1.0	65	260	0.04	0.14	tr	0
101	Poached .... 1 egg	50	80	6	6	1.7	2.0	0.6	1	28	90	1.0	65	260	0.04	0.13	tr	0
102	Scrambled (milk added) 1 egg in butter. Also omelet	64	95	6	7	2.8	2.3	0.6	1	47	97	0.9	85	310	0.04	0.16	tr	0
	Fats, Oils, and Related Products																	
	Butter																	
	Regular (1 brick or 4 sticks per lb)																	
103	Stick (1/2 cup) .... 1 stick	113	815	1	92	57.3	23.1	2.1	tr	27	26	0.2	29	3470[11]	0.01	0.04	tr	0
104	Tablespoon (about 1/8 stick) 1 tbsp	14	100	tr	12	7.2	2.9	0.3	tr	3	3	tr	4	430[11]	tr	tr	tr	0
105	Pat (1" square, 1/3" high; 1 pat 90 per lb)	5	35	tr	4	2.5	1.0	0.1	tr	1	1	tr	1	150[11]	tr	tr	tr	0
	Whipped (6 sticks or two 8-oz containers per lb)																	
106	Stick (1/2 cup) .... 1 stick	76	540	1	61	38.2	15.4	1.4	tr	18	17	0.1	20	2310[11]	tr	0.03	tr	0
107	Tablespoon (about 1/8 stick) 1 tbsp	9	65	tr	8	4.7	1.9	0.2	tr	2	2	tr	2	290[11]	tr	tr	tr	0
108	Pat (1 1/4" square, 1/3" high; 120 per lb) 1 pat	4	25	tr	3	1.9	0.8	0.1	tr	1	1	tr	1	120[11]	0	tr	tr	0
109	Fats, cooking (vegetable shortenings) 1 c	200	1770	0	200	48.8	88.2	48.4	0	0	0	0	0	—	0	0	0	0
110	1 tbsp	13	110	0	13	3.2	5.7	3.1	0	0	0	0	0	—	0	0	0	0
111	Lard 1 c	205	1850	0	205	81.0	83.8	20.5	0	0	0	0	0	0	0	0	0	0
112	1 tbsp	13	115	0	13	5.1	5.3	1.3	0	0	0	0	0	0	0	0	0	0
	Margarine																	
	Regular (1 brick or 4 sticks per lb)																	
113	Stick (1/2 cup) .... 1 stick	113	815	1	92	16.7	42.9	24.9	tr	27	26	0.2	29	3750[12]	0.01	0.04	tr	0
114	Tablespoon (about 1/8 stick) 1 tbsp	14	100	tr	12	2.1	5.3	3.1	tr	3	3	tr	4	470[12]	tr	tr	tr	0
115	Pat (1" square, 1/3" high; 1 pat 90 per lb)	5	35	tr	4	0.7	1.9	1.1	tr	1	1	tr	1	170[12]	tr	tr	tr	0
116	Soft, two 8-oz containers 1 container per lb	227	1635	1	184	32.5	71.5	65.4	tr	53	52	0.4	59	7500[12]	0.01	0.08	0.1	0

(A)	(B)	(C)	(D)	(E)	(F)	(G)	(H)	(I)	(J)	(K)	(L)	(M)	(N)	(O)	(P)	(Q)	(R)	(S)
117	Whipped (6 sticks per lb) .... 1 tbsp	14	100	tr	12	2.0	4.5	4.1	tr	3	3	tr	4	470[12]	tr	tr	tr	0
118	Stick (1/2 cup) .... 1 stick	76	545	tr	61	11.2	28.7	16.7	tr	18	17	0.1	20	2500[12]	tr	0.03	tr	0
119	Tablespoon (about 1/8 stick) ... 1 tbsp	9	70	tr	8	1.4	3.6	2.1	tr	2	2	tr	2	310[12]	tr	tr	tr	0
	Oils, salad or cooking																	
120	Corn .... 1 c	218	1925	0	218	27.7	53.6	125.1	0	0	0	0	0	—	0	0	0	0
121	1 tbsp	14	120	0	14	1.7	3.3	7.8	0	0	0	0	0	—	0	0	0	0
122	Olive .... 1 c	216	1910	0	216	30.7	154.4	17.7	0	0	0	0	0	—	0	0	0	0
123	1 tbsp	14	120	0	14	1.9	9.7	1.1	0	0	0	0	0	—	0	0	0	0
124	Peanut .... 1 c	216	1910	0	216	37.4	98.5	67.0	0	0	0	0	0	—	0	0	0	0
125	1 tbsp	14	120	0	14	2.3	6.2	4.2	0	0	0	0	0	—	0	0	0	0
126	Safflower .... 1 c	218	1925	0	218	20.5	25.9	159.8	0	0	0	0	0	—	0	0	0	0
127	1 tbsp	14	120	0	14	1.3	1.6	10.0	0	0	0	0	0	—	0	0	0	0
128	Soybean oil, hydrogenated (partially hardened) .... 1 c	218	1925	0	218	31.8	93.1	75.6	0	0	0	0	0	—	0	0	0	0
129	1 tbsp	14	120	0	14	2.0	5.8	4.7	0	0	0	0	0	—	0	0	0	0
130	Soybean-cottonseed oil blend, hydrogenated .... 1 c	218	1925	0	218	38.2	63.0	99.6	0	0	0	0	0	—	0	0	0	0
131	1 tbsp	14	120	0	14	2.4	3.9	6.2	0	0	0	0	0	—	0	0	0	0
	Salad dressings																	
	Commercial																	
	Blue cheese																	
132	Regular .... 1 tbsp	15	75	1	8	1.6	1.7	3.8	1	12	11	tr	6	30	tr	.02	tr	tr
133	Low calorie (5 cal per tsp) 1 tbsp	16	10	tr	1	0.5	0.3	tr	1	10	8	tr	5	30	tr	0.01	tr	tr
	French																	
134	Regular .... 1 tbsp	16	65	tr	6	1.1	1.3	3.2	3	2	2	0.1	13	—	—	—	—	—
135	Low calorie (5 cal per tsp) 1 tbsp	16	15	tr	1	0.1	0.1	0.4	2	2	2	0.1	13	—	—	—	—	—
	Italian																	
136	Regular .... 1 tbsp	15	85	tr	9	1.6	1.9	4.7	1	2	1	tr	2	tr	tr	tr	tr	—
137	Low calorie (2 cal per tsp) 1 tbsp	15	10	tr	1	0.1	0.1	0.4	tr	tr	1	tr	2	tr	tr	tr	tr	—
138	Mayonnaise .... 1 tbsp	14	100	tr	11	2.0	2.4	5.6	tr	3	4	0.1	5	40	tr	0.01	tr	—
	Mayonnaise type																	
139	Regular .... 1 tbsp	15	65	tr	6	1.1	1.4	3.2	2	2	4	tr	1	30	tr	tr	tr	—
140	Low calorie (8 cal per tsp) 1 tbsp	16	20	tr	2	0.4	0.4	1.0	2	3	4	tr	1	40	tr	tr	tr	—
141	Tartar sauce, regular .. 1 tbsp	14	75	tr	8	1.5	1.8	4.1	1	3	4	0.1	11	30	tr	tr	tr	tr
	Thousand Island																	
142	Regular .... 1 tbsp	16	80	tr	8	1.4	1.7	4.0	2	2	3	0.1	18	50	tr	tr	tr	tr
143	Low calorie (10 cal per tsp) 1 tbsp	15	25	tr	2	0.4	0.4	1.0	2	2	3	0.1	17	50	tr	tr	tr	tr
	From home recipe																	
144	Cooked type[13] .... 1 tbsp	16	68	1	2	0.5	0.6	0.3	2	14	15	0.1	19	80	0.01	0.03	tr	tr

(Continued)

Table A-1. Nutritive Values of the Edible Part of Foods (Continued)

(Dashes (—) denote lack of reliable data for a constituent believed to be present in measurable amount)

Item No. (A)	Foods, Approximate Measures, Units, and Weight (edible part unless footnotes indicate otherwise) (B)		Water (C) Per-cent	Food Energy (D) Cal-ories	Pro-tein (E) g	Fat (F) g	Fatty Acids Satu-rated (Total) (G) g	Unsaturated Oleic (H) g	Lino-leic (I) g	Carbo-hydrate (J) g	Calcium (K) mg	Phos-phorus (L) mg	Iron (M) mg	Potas-sium (N) mg	Vitamin A Value (O) IU	Thiamin (P) mg	Ribo-flavin (Q) mg	Niacin (R) mg	Ascorbic Acid (S) mg
		g																	
	Fish, Shellfish, Meat, Poultry, and Related Products																		
	Fish and shellfish																		
145	Bluefish, baked with butter or margarine 3 oz	85	68	135	22	4	—	—	—	0	25	244	0.6	—	40	0.09	0.08	1.6	—
	Clams																		
146	Raw, meat only 3 oz	85	82	65	11	1	—	—	—	2	59	138	5.2	154	90	0.08	0.15	1.1	8
147	Canned, solids and liquid 3 oz	85	86	45	7	1	0.2	tr	tr	2	47	116	3.5	119	—	0.01	0.09	0.9	—
148	Crabmeat (white or king), canned, not pressed down 1 c	135	77	135	24	3	0.6	0.4	0.1	1	61	246	1.1	149	—	0.11	0.11	2.6	—
149	Fish sticks, breaded, cooked, frozen (stick, 4" × 1" × ½") 1 fish stick or 1 oz	28	66	50	5	3	—	—	—	2	3	47	0.1	—	0	0.01	0.02	0.5	—
150	Haddock, breaded, fried[14] 3 oz	85	66	140	17	5	1.4	2.2	1.2	5	34	210	1.0	296	—	0.03	0.06	2.7	2
151	Ocean perch, breaded, fried[14] 1 fillet	85	59	195	16	11	2.7	4.4	2.3	6	28	192	1.1	242	—	0.10	0.10	1.6	—
152	Oysters, raw, meat only (13–19 medium Selects) 1 c	240	85	160	20	4	1.3	0.2	0.1	8	226	343	13.2	290	740	0.34	0.43	6.0	—
153	Salmon, pink, canned, solids and liquid 3 oz	85	71	120	17	5	0.9	0.8	0.1	0	167[15]	243	0.7	307	60	0.03	0.16	6.8	—
154	Sardines, Atlantic, canned in oil, drained solids 3 oz	85	62	175	20	9	3.0	2.5	0.5	0	372	424	2.5	502	190	0.02	0.17	4.6	—
155	Scallops, frozen, breaded, fried, reheated 6 scallops	90	60	175	16	8	—	—	—	9	—	—	—	—	—	—	—	—	—
156	Shad, baked with butter or margarine, bacon 3 oz	85	64	170	20	10	—	—	—	0	20	266	0.5	320	30	0.11	0.22	7.3	—
	Shrimp																		
157	Canned meat 3 oz	85	70	100	21	1	0.1	0.1	tr	1	98	224	2.6	104	50	0.01	0.03	1.5	—
158	French fried[16] 3 oz	85	57	190	17	9	2.3	3.7	2.0	9	61	162	1.7	195	—	0.03	0.07	2.3	—
159	Tuna, canned in oil, drained solids 3 oz	85	61	170	24	7	1.7	1.7	0.7	0	7	199	1.6	—	70	0.04	0.10	10.1	—
160	Tuna salad[17] 1 c	205	70	350	30	22	4.3	6.3	6.7	7	41	291	2.7	—	590	0.08	0.23	10.3	2
	Meat and meat products																		
161	Bacon (20 slices per lb, raw), broiled or fried, crisp) 2 slices	15	8	85	4	8	2.5	3.7	0.7	tr	2	34	0.5	35	0	0.08	0.05	0.8	—

(A)	(B)		(C)	(D)	(E)	(F)	(G)	(H)	(I)	(J)	(K)	(L)	(M)	(N)	(O)	(P)	(Q)	(R)	(S)
	Beef,[18] cooked																		
	Cuts braised, simmered, or pot roasted																		
162	Lean and fat (piece, 2½″ × 2½″ × ¾″)	3 oz	85	53	245	23	16	6.8	6.5	0.4	0	10	114	2.9	184	30	0.04	0.18	3.6	—
163	Lean only from item 162	2.5 oz	72	62	140	22	5	2.1	1.8	0.2	0	10	108	2.7	176	10	0.04	0.17	3.3	—
	Ground beef, broiled																		
164	Lean with 10% fat	3 oz or patty 3″ × ⅝″	85	60	185	23	10	4.0	3.9	0.3	0	10	196	3.0	261	20	0.08	0.20	5.1	—
165	Lean with 21% fat	2.9 oz or patty 3″ × ⅝″	82	54	235	20	17	7.0	6.7	0.4	0	9	159	2.6	221	30	0.07	0.17	4.4	—
	Roast, oven-cooked, no liquid added																		
	Relatively fat, such as rib																		
166	Lean and fat (2 pieces, 4⅛″ × 2¼″ × ¼″)	3 oz	85	40	375	17	33	14.0	13.6	0.8	0	8	158	2.2	189	70	0.05	0.13	3.1	—
167	Lean only from item 166	1.8 oz	51	57	125	14	7	3.0	2.5	0.3	0	6	131	1.8	161	10	0.04	0.11	2.6	—
	Relatively lean, such as heel of round																		
168	Lean and fat (2 pieces, 4⅛″ × 2¼″ × ¼″)	3 oz	85	62	165	25	7	2.8	2.7	0.2	0	11	208	3.2	279	10	0.06	0.19	4.5	—
169	Lean only from item 168	2.8 oz	78	65	125	24	3	1.2	1.0	0.1	0	10	199	3.0	268	tr	0.06	0.18	4.3	—
	Steak																		
	Relatively fat-sirloin, broiled																		
170	Lean and fat (piece, 2½″ × 2½″ × ¾″)	3 oz	85	44	330	20	27	11.3	11.1	0.6	0	9	162	2.5	220	50	0.05	0.15	4.0	—
171	Lean only from item 170	2.0 oz	56	59	115	18	4	1.8	1.6	0.2	0	7	146	2.2	202	10	0.05	0.14	3.6	—
	Relatively lean-round, braised																		
172	Lean and fat (piece, 4⅛″ × 2¼″ × ½″)	3 oz	85	55	220	24	13	5.5	5.2	0.4	0	10	213	3.0	272	20	0.07	0.19	4.8	—
173	Lean only from item 172	2.4 oz	68	61	130	21	4	1.7	1.5	0.2	0	9	182	2.5	238	10	0.05	0.16	4.1	—
	Beef, canned																		
174	Corned beef	3 oz	85	59	185	22	10	4.9	4.5	0.2	0	17	90	3.7	—	—	0.01	0.20	2.9	—
175	Corned beef hash	1 c	220	67	400	19	25	11.9	10.9	0.5	24	29	147	4.4	440	—	0.02	0.20	4.6	—
176	Beef, dried, chipped	2½ oz jar	71	48	145	24	4	2.1	2.0	0.1	0	14	287	3.6	142	—	0.05	0.23	2.7	0
177	Beef and vegetable stew	1 c	245	82	220	16	11	4.9	4.5	0.2	15	29	184	2.9	613	2400	0.15	0.17	4.7	17
178	Beef potpie (home recipe), baked[19] (piece, ⅓ of 9″ diam pie)	1 piece	210	55	515	21	30	7.9	12.8	6.7	39	29	149	3.8	334	1720	0.30	0.30	5.5	6

(Continued)

Table A-1. Nutritive Values of the Edible Part of Foods (Continued)

(Dashes (—) denote lack of reliable data for a constituent believed to be present in measurable amount)

Item No. (A)	Foods, Approximate Measures, Units, and Weight (edible part unless footnotes indicate otherwise) (B)	Water (C) Per cent	Food Energy (D) Cal ories	Pro-tein (E)	Fat (F)	Fatty Acids Satu-rated (Total) (G)	Unsaturated Oleic (H)	Lino-leic (I)	Carbo-hydrate (J)	Calcium (K)	Phos-phorus (L)	Iron (M)	Potas-sium (N)	Vitamin A Value (O)	Thiamin (P)	Ribo-flavin (Q)	Niacin (R)	Ascorbic Acid (S)
		g		g	g	g	g	g	g	mg	mg	mg	mg	IU	mg	mg	mg	mg
	Fish, Shellfish, Meat, Poultry, and Related Products (Cont.)																	
	Meat and meat products (Continued)																	
179	Chili con carne with beans, canned 1 c	255	72	340	19	16	7.5	6.8	0.3	31	82	321	4.3	594	150	0.08	0.18	3.3	—
180	Chop suey with beef and pork (home recipe) 1 c	250	75	300	26	17	8.5	6.2	0.7	13	60	248	4.8	425	600	0.28	0.38	5.0	33
181	Heart, beef, lean, braised 3 oz	85	61	160	27	5	1.5	1.1	0.6	1	5	154	5.0	197	20	0.21	1.04	6.5	1
	Lamb, cooked																	
	Chop, rib (cut 3 per lb with bone), broiled																	
182	Lean and fat 3.1 oz	89	43	360	18	32	14.8	12.1	1.2	0	8	139	1.0	200	—	0.11	0.19	4.1	—
183	Lean only from item 182 2 oz	57	60	120	16	6	2.5	2.1	0.2	0	6	121	1.1	174	—	0.09	0.15	3.4	—
	Leg, roasted																	
184	Lean and fat (2 pieces, 4⅛" × 2¼" × ¼") 3 oz	85	54	235	22	16	7.3	6.0	0.6	0	9	177	1.4	241	—	0.13	0.23	4.7	—
185	Lean only from item 184 2.5 oz	71	62	130	20	5	2.1	1.8	0.2	0	9	169	1.4	227	—	0.12	0.21	4.4	—
	Shoulder, roasted																	
186	Lean and fat (3 pieces, 2½" × 2½" × ¼") 3 oz	85	50	285	18	23	10.8	8.8	0.9	0	9	146	1.0	206	—	0.11	0.20	4.0	—
187	Lean only from item 186 2.3 oz	64	61	130	17	6	3.6	2.3	0.2	0	8	140	1.0	193	—	0.10	0.18	3.7	—
188	Liver, beef, fried[20] (slice, 6½" × 2⅜" × ⅜") 3 oz	85	56	195	22	9	2.5	3.5	0.9	5	9	405	7.5	323	45390[21]	0.22	3.56	14.0	23
	Pork, cured, cooked																	
189	Ham, light cure, lean and fat, roasted (2 pieces, 4⅛" × 2¼" × ¼")[22] 3 oz	85	54	245	18	19	6.8	7.9	1.7	0	8	146	2.2	199	0	0.40	0.15	3.1	—
	Luncheon meat																	
190	Boiled ham, slice (8 per 1 oz 8-oz pkg) 1 oz	28	59	65	5	5	1.7	2.0	0.4	0	3	47	0.8	—	0	0.12	0.04	0.7	—
	Canned, spiced or unspiced																	
191	Slice, approximately 3" × 2" × ½" 1 slice	60	55	175	9	15	5.4	6.7	1.0	1	5	65	1.3	133	0	0.19	0.13	1.8	—
	Pork, fresh,[18]																	
	Chop, loin (cut 3 per lb with bone), broiled																	

(A)	(B)	(C)	(D)	(E)	(F)	(G)	(H)	(I)	(J)	(K)	(L)	(M)	(N)	(O)	(P)	(Q)	(R)	(S)
192	Lean and fat .... 2.7 oz	78	305	19	25	8.9	10.4	2.2	0	9	209	2.7	216	0	0.75	0.22	4.5	—
193	Lean only from item 192 .... 2 oz	56	150	17	9	3.1	3.6	0.8	0	7	181	2.2	192	0	0.63	0.18	3.8	—
	Roast, oven-cooked, no liquid added																	
194	Lean and fat (piece, 2½" × 2½" × ¾") .... 3 oz	85	310	21	24	8.7	10.2	2.2	0	9	218	2.7	233	0	0.78	0.22	4.8	—
195	Lean only from item 194 .... 2.4 oz	68	175	20	10	3.5	4.1	0.8	0	9	211	2.6	224	0	0.73	0.21	4.4	—
	Shoulder cut, simmered																	
196	Lean and fat (3 pieces, 2½" × 2½" × ¼") .... 3 oz	85	320	20	26	9.3	10.9	2.3	0	9	118	2.6	158	0	0.46	0.21	4.1	—
197	Lean only from item 196 .... 2.2 oz	63	135	18	6	2.2	2.6	0.6	0	8	111	2.3	146	0	0.42	0.19	3.7	—
	Sausages (see also Luncheon meat, items 190–191)																	
198	Bologna, slice (8 per 8-oz pkg) .... 1 slice	28	85	3	8	3.0	3.4	0.5	tr	2	36	0.5	65	—	0.05	0.06	0.7	—
199	Braunschweiger, slice (6 per 6-oz pkg) .... 1 slice	28	90	4	8	2.6	3.4	0.8	1	3	69	1.7	—	1850	0.05	0.41	2.3	—
200	Brown and serve (10–11 per 8-oz pkg), browned .... 1 link	17	70	3	6	2.3	2.8	0.7	tr	—	—	—	—	—	—	—	—	—
201	Deviled ham, canned .. 1 tbsp	13	45	2	4	1.5	1.8	0.4	0	1	12	0.3	—	0	0.02	0.01	0.2	—
202	Frankfurter (8 per 1-lb pkg), cooked (reheated) .... 1 frankfurter	56	170	7	15	5.6	6.5	1.2	1	3	57	0.8	—	—	0.08	0.11	1.4	—
203	Meat, potted (beef, chicken, turkey), canned .... 1 tbsp	13	30	2	2	—	—	—	0	—	—	—	—	—	tr	—	—	—
204	Pork link (16 per 1-lb pkg), cooked .... 1 link	13	60	2	6	2.1	2.4	0.5	tr	1	21	0.3	35	0	0.10	0.04	0.5	—
	Salami																	
205	Dry type, slice (12 per 4-oz pkg) .... 1 slice	10	45	2	4	1.6	1.6	0.1	tr	1	28	0.4	—	—	0.04	0.03	0.5	—
206	Cooked type, slice (8 per 8-oz pkg) .... 1 slice	28	90	5	7	3.1	3.0	0.2	tr	3	57	0.7	—	—	0.07	0.07	1.2	—
207	Vienna sausage (7 per 4-oz can) .... 1 sausage	16	40	2	3	1.2	1.4	0.2	tr	1	24	0.3	—	—	0.01	0.02	0.4	—
	Veal, medium fat, cooked, bone removed																	
208	Cutlet (4⅛" × 2¼" × ½"), braised or broiled .... 3 oz	85	185	23	9	4.0	3.4	0.4	0	9	196	2.7	258	—	0.06	0.21	4.6	—

(Continued)

Table A-1. Nutritive Values of the Edible Part of Foods (Continued)

(Dashes (—) denote lack of reliable data for a constituent believed to be present in measurable amount)

Item No. (A)	Foods, Approximate Measures, Units, and Weight (edible part unless footnotes indicate otherwise) (B)	(g)	Water (C) Per cent	Food Energy (D) Calories	Protein (E) g	Fat (F) g	Fatty Acids Saturated (Total) (G) g	Unsaturated Oleic (H) g	Linoleic (I) g	Carbohydrate (J) g	Calcium (K) mg	Phosphorus (L) mg	Iron (M) mg	Potassium (N) mg	Vitamin A Value (O) IU	Thiamin (P) mg	Riboflavin (Q) mg	Niacin (R) mg	Ascorbic Acid (S) mg
	Fish, Shellfish, Meat, Poultry, and Related Products (Cont.)																		
	Veal (Continued)																		
209	Rib (2 pieces, 4 1/8" × 2 1/4" × 1/4"), roasted, 3 oz	85	55	230	23	14	6.1	5.1	0.6	0	10	211	2.9	259	—	0.11	0.26	6.6	—
	Poultry and poultry products																		
	Chicken, cooked																		
210	Breast, fried,[23] bones removed, 1/2 breast (3.3 oz with bones), 2.8 oz	79	58	160	26	5	1.4	1.8	1.1	1	9	218	1.3	—	70	0.04	0.17	11.6	—
211	Drumstick, fried,[23] bones removed (2 oz with bones), 1.3 oz	38	55	90	12	4	1.1	1.3	0.9	tr	6	89	0.9	—	50	0.03	0.15	2.7	—
212	Half broiler, broiled, bones removed (10.4 oz with bones), 6.2 oz	176	71	240	42	7	2.2	2.5	1.3	0	16	355	3.0	483	160	0.09	0.34	15.5	—
213	Chicken, canned, boneless, 3 oz	85	65	170	18	10	3.2	3.8	2.0	0	18	210	1.3	117	200	0.03	0.11	3.7	3
214	Chicken a la king, cooked (home recipe), 1 c	245	68	470	27	34	12.7	14.3	3.3	12	127	358	2.5	404	1130	0.10	0.42	5.4	12
215	Chicken and noodles, cooked (home recipe), 1 c	240	71	365	22	18	5.9	7.1	3.5	26	26	247	2.2	149	430	0.05	0.17	4.3	tr
	Chicken chow mein																		
216	Canned, 1 c	250	89	95	7	tr	—	—	—	18	45	85	1.3	418	150	0.05	0.10	1.0	13
217	From home recipe, 1 c	250	78	255	31	10	2.4	3.4	3.1	10	58	293	2.5	473	280	0.08	0.23	4.3	10
218	Chicken potpie (home recipe), baked,[19] piece (1/3 of 9" diam pie), 1 piece	232	57	545	23	31	11.3	10.9	5.6	42	70	232	3.0	343	3090	0.34	0.31	5.5	5
	Turkey, roasted, flesh without skin																		
219	Dark meat, piece, 2 1/2" × 1 5/8" × 1/4", 4 pieces	85	61	175	26	7	2.1	1.5	1.5	0	—	—	2.0	338	—	0.03	0.20	3.6	—
220	Light meat, piece, 4" × 2" × 1/4", 2 pieces	85	62	150	28	3	0.9	0.6	0.7	0	—	—	1.0	349	—	0.04	0.12	9.4	—
	Light and dark meat																		
221	Chopped or diced, 1 c	140	61	265	44	9	2.5	1.7	1.8	0	11	351	2.5	514	—	0.07	0.25	10.8	—
222	Pieces (1 slice white meat, 4" × 2" × 1/4" with 2 slices dark meat, 2 1/2" × 1 5/8" × 1/4"), 3 pieces	85	61	160	27	5	1.5	1.0	1.1	0	7	213	1.5	312	—	0.04	0.15	6.5	—

Fruits and Fruit Products

Columns: (A) Item No. · (B) Foods, approximate measures, units, and weight · (C) Grams · (D) Water (%) · (E) Food energy (cal) · (F) Protein (g) · (G) Fat (g) · (H) Saturated fatty acids (g) · (I) Unsaturated – Oleic (g) · (J) Unsaturated – Linoleic (g) · (K) Carbohydrate (g) · (L) Calcium (mg) · (M) Phosphorus (mg) · (N) Iron (mg) · (O) Potassium (mg) · (P) Vitamin A (IU) · (Q) Thiamin (mg) · (R) Riboflavin (mg) · (S) Niacin (mg) · (T) Ascorbic acid (mg)

(A)	(B)	(C)	(D)	(E)	(F)	(G)	(H)	(I)	(J)	(K)	(L)	(M)	(N)	(O)	(P)	(Q)	(R)	(S)	(T)
	Apples, raw, unpeeled, without cores																		
223	2¾" diam (about 3 per lb with cores) 1 apple	138	84	80	tr	1	—	—	—	20	10	14	0.4	152	120	0.04	0.03	0.1	6
224	3¼" diam (about 2 per lb with cores) 1 apple	212	84	125	tr	1	—	—	—	31	15	21	0.6	233	190	0.06	0.04	0.2	8
225	Apple juice, bottled or canned[24] 1 c	248	88	120	tr	tr	—	—	—	30	15	22	1.5	250	—	0.02	0.05	0.2	2[25]
	Applesauce, canned																		
226	Sweetened 1 c	255	76	230	tr	tr	—	—	—	61	10	13	1.3	166	100	0.05	0.03	0.1	3[25]
227	Unsweetened 1 c	244	89	100	tr	tr	—	—	—	26	10	12	1.2	190	100	0.05	0.02	0.1	2[25]
	Apricots																		
228	Raw, without pits (about 3 apricots 12 per lb with pits)	107	85	55	1	tr	—	—	—	14	18	25	0.5	301	2890	0.03	0.04	0.6	11
229	Canned in heavy syrup (halves and syrup) 1 c	258	77	220	2	tr	—	—	—	57	28	39	0.8	604	4490	0.05	0.05	1.0	10
	Dried																		
230	Uncooked (28 large or 37 1 c medium halves per cup)	130	25	340	7	1	—	—	—	86	87	140	7.2	1273	14,170	0.01	0.21	4.3	16
231	Cooked, unsweetened, fruit and liquid 1 c	250	76	215	4	1	—	—	—	54	55	88	4.5	795	7500	0.01	0.13	2.5	8
232	Apricot nectar, canned 1 c	251	85	145	1	tr	—	—	—	37	23	30	0.5	379	2380	0.03	0.03	0.5	36[26]
	Avocados, raw, whole, without skins and seeds																		
233	California, mid- and late- 1 avocado winter (with skin and seed, 3⅛" diam; wt, 10 oz)	216	74	370	5	37	5.5	22.0	3.7	13	22	91	1.3	1303	630	0.24	0.43	3.5	30
234	Florida, late summer and 1 avocado fall (with skin and seed, 3⅝" diam; wt, 1 lb)	304	78	390	4	33	6.7	15.7	5.3	27	30	128	1.8	1836	880	0.33	0.61	4.9	43
235	Banana without peel 1 banana (about 2.6 per lb with peel)	119	76	100	1	tr	—	—	—	26	10	31	0.8	440	230	0.06	0.07	0.8	12
236	Banana flakes 1 tbsp	6	3	20	tr	tr	—	—	—	5	2	6	0.2	92	50	0.01	0.01	0.2	tr
237	Blackberries, raw 1 c	144	85	85	2	1	—	—	—	19	46	27	1.3	245	290	0.04	0.06	0.6	30
238	Blueberries, raw 1 c	145	83	90	1	1	—	—	—	22	22	19	1.5	117	150	0.04	0.09	0.7	20
	Cantaloupe. See Muskmelons (item 271)																		
	Cherries																		
239	Sour (tart), red, pitted, 1 c canned, water pack	244	88	105	2	tr	—	—	—	26	37	32	0.7	317	1660	0.07	0.05	0.5	12
240	Sweet, raw, without pits 10 cherries and stems	68	80	45	1	tr	—	—	—	12	15	13	0.3	129	70	0.03	0.04	0.3	7

(Continued)

Table A-1. Nutritive Values of the Edible Part of Foods (Continued)

(Dashes (—) denote lack of reliable data for a constituent believed to be present in measurable amount)

Item No. (A)	Foods, Approximate Measures, Units, and Weight (edible part unless footnotes indicate otherwise) (B)	(g)	Water Per-cent (C)	Food Energy Cal-ories (D)	Pro-tein (E) g	Fat (F) g	Saturated (Total) (G) g	Unsaturated Oleic (H) g	Unsaturated Lino-leic (I) g	Carbo-hydrate (J) g	Calcium (K) mg	Phos-phorus (L) mg	Iron (M) mg	Potas-sium (N) mg	Vitamin A Value (O) IU	Thiamin (P) mg	Ribo-flavin (Q) mg	Niacin (R) mg	Ascorbic Acid (S) mg
Fruits and Fruit Products (Continued)																			
241	Cranberry juice cocktail, bottled, sweetened 1 c	253	83	165	tr	tr	—	—	—	42	13	8	0.8	25	tr	0.03	0.03	0.1	81[27]
242	Cranberry sauce, sweetened, canned, strained 1 c	277	62	405	tr	1	—	—	—	104	17	11	0.6	83	60	0.03	0.03	0.1	6
	Dates																		
243	Whole, without pits 10 dates	80	23	220	2	tr	—	—	—	58	47	50	2.4	518	40	0.07	0.08	1.8	0
244	Chopped 1 c	178	23	490	4	1	—	—	—	130	105	112	5.3	1153	90	0.16	0.18	3.9	0
245	Fruit cocktail, canned, in heavy syrup 1 c	255	80	195	1	tr	—	—	—	50	23	31	1.0	411	360	0.05	0.03	1.0	5
	Grapefruit																		
	Raw, medium, 3¾" diam (about 1 lb 1 oz)																		
246	Pink or red ½ grapefruit with peel[28]	241	89	50	1	tr	—	—	—	13	20	20	0.5	166	540	0.05	0.02	0.2	44
247	White ½ grapefruit with peel[28]	241	89	45	1	tr	—	—	—	12	19	19	0.5	159	10	0.05	0.02	0.2	44
248	Canned, sections with syrup 1 c	254	81	180	2	tr	—	—	—	45	33	36	0.8	343	30	0.08	0.05	0.5	76
	Grapefruit juice																		
249	Raw, pink, red or white 1 c	246	90	95	1	tr	—	—	—	23	22	37	0.5	399	(29)	0.10	0.05	0.5	93
	Canned, white																		
250	Unsweetened 1 c	247	89	100	1	tr	—	—	—	24	20	35	1.0	400	20	0.07	0.05	0.5	84
251	Sweetened 1 c	250	86	135	1	tr	—	—	—	32	20	35	1.0	405	30	0.08	0.05	0.5	78
	Frozen, concentrate, unsweetened																		
252	Undiluted, 6-fl oz can 1 c	207	62	300	4	1	—	—	—	72	70	124	0.8	1250	60	0.29	0.12	1.4	286
253	Diluted with 3 parts water by volume 1 c	247	89	100	1	tr	—	—	—	24	25	42	0.2	420	20	0.10	0.04	0.5	96
254	Dehydrated crystals, prepared with water (1 lb yields about 1 gal) 1 c	247	90	100	1	tr	—	—	—	24	22	40	0.2	412	20	0.10	0.05	0.5	91
	Grapes, European type (adherent skin), raw																		
255	Thompson Seedless 10 grapes	50	81	35	tr	tr	—	—	—	9	6	10	0.2	87	50	0.03	0.02	0.2	2
256	Tokay and Emperor, seeded types 10 grapes[30]	60	81	40	tr	tr	—	—	—	10	7	11	0.2	99	60	0.03	0.02	0.2	2

(A)	(B)	(C)	(D)	(E)	(F)	(G)	(H)	(I)	(J)	(K)	(L)	(M)	(N)	(O)	(P)	(Q)	(R)	(S)
	Grape juice																	
257	Canned or bottled .... 1 c	253	83	165	1	tr	—	—	42	28	30	0.8	293	—	0.10	0.05	0.5	tr[25]
	Frozen concentrate, sweetened																	
258	Undiluted, 6-fl oz can ... 1 can	216	53	395	1	tr	—	—	100	22	32	0.9	255	40	0.13	0.22	1.5	32[31]
259	Diluted with 3 parts water by volume ... 1 c	250	86	135	1	tr	—	—	33	8	10	0.3	85	10	0.05	0.08	0.5	10[31]
260	Grape drink, canned ..... 1 c	250	86	135	tr	tr	—	—	35	8	10	0.3	88	—	0.03[32]	0.03[32]	0.3	(32)
261	Lemon, raw, size 165, without peel and seeds (about 4 per lb with peels and seeds) ... 1 lemon	74	90	20	1	tr	—	—	6	19	12	0.4	102	10	0.03	0.01	0.1	39
	Lemon juice																	
262	Raw .... 1 c	244	91	60	1	tr	—	—	20	17	24	0.5	344	50	0.07	0.02	0.2	112
263	Canned, or bottled, unsweetened ... 1 c	244	92	55	1	tr	—	—	19	17	24	0.5	344	50	0.07	0.02	0.2	102
264	Frozen, single-strength, unsweetened, 6-fl oz can ... 1 c	183	92	40	1	tr	—	—	13	13	16	0.5	258	40	0.05	0.02	0.2	81
	Lemonade concentrate, frozen																	
265	Undiluted, 6-fl oz can ... 1 can	219	49	425	tr	tr	—	—	112	9	13	0.4	153	40	0.05	0.06	0.7	66
266	Diluted with 4⅓ parts water by volume ... 1 c	248	89	105	tr	tr	—	—	28	2	3	0.1	40	10	0.01	0.02	0.2	17
	Limeade concentrate, frozen																	
267	Undiluted, 6-fl oz can ... 1 can	218	50	410	tr	tr	—	—	108	11	13	0.2	129	tr	0.02	0.02	0.2	26
268	Diluted with 4⅓ parts water by volume ... 1 c	247	89	100	tr	tr	—	—	27	3	3	tr	32	tr	tr	tr	tr	6
	Lime juice																	
269	Raw .... 1 c	246	90	65	1	tr	—	—	22	22	27	0.5	256	20	0.05	0.02	0.2	79
270	Canned, unsweetened ... 1 c	246	90	65	1	tr	—	—	22	22	27	0.5	256	20	0.05	0.02	0.2	52
271	Muskmelons, raw, with rind, without seed cavity / Cantaloupe, orange-fleshed (with rind and seed cavity, 5" diam, 2⅓ lb) ... ½ melon with rind[33]	477	91	80	2	tr	—	—	20	38	44	1.1	682	9240	0.11	0.08	1.6	90
272	Honeydew (with rind and seed cavity, 6½" diam, 5¼ lb) ... 1/10 melon with rind[33]	226	91	50	1	tr	—	—	11	21	24	0.6	374	60	0.06	0.04	0.9	34
273	Oranges, all commercial varieties, raw / Whole, 2⅝" diam, without peel and seeds (about 2½ per lb with peel and seeds) ... 1 orange	131	86	65	1	tr	—	—	16	54	26	0.5	263	260	0.13	0.05	0.5	66

(Continued)

Table A-1. Nutritive Values of the Edible Part of Foods (Continued)

(Dashes (—) denote lack of reliable data for a constituent believed to be present in measurable amount)

Item No. (A)	Foods, Approximate Measures, Units, and Weight (edible part unless footnotes indicate otherwise) (B)	Water (C)	Food Energy (D)	Protein (E)	Fat (F)	Fatty Acids Saturated (Total) (G)	Unsaturated Oleic (H)	Linoleic (I)	Carbohydrate (J)	Calcium (K)	Phosphorus (L)	Iron (M)	Potassium (N)	Vitamin A Value (O)	Thiamin (P)	Riboflavin (Q)	Niacin (R)	Ascorbic Acid (S)
		Percent	Calories	g	g	g	g	g	g	mg	mg	mg	mg	IU	mg	mg	mg	mg
	Fruits and Fruit Products (Continued)																	
	Oranges (Continued)																	
274	Sections without membranes ... 1 c	86	90	2	tr	—	—	—	22	74	36	0.7	360	360	0.18	0.07	0.7	90
	Orange juice																	
275	Raw, all varieties ..... 1 c	88	110	2	tr	—	—	—	26	27	42	0.5	496	500	0.22	0.07	1.0	124
276	Canned, unsweetened .. 1 c	87	120	2	tr	—	—	—	28	25	45	1.0	496	500	0.17	0.05	0.7	100
	Frozen concentrate																	
277	Undiluted, 6-fl oz can	55	360	5	tr	—	—	—	87	75	126	0.9	1500	1620	0.68	0.11	2.8	360
278	Diluted with 3 parts water by volume ... 1 c	87	120	2	tr	—	—	—	29	25	42	0.2	503	540	0.23	0.03	0.9	120
279	Dehydrated crystals, prepared with water (1 lb yields about 1 gal) ... 1 c	88	115	1	tr	—	—	—	27	25	40	0.5	518	500	0.20	0.07	1.0	109
	Orange and grapefruit juice																	
	Frozen concentrate																	
280	Undiluted, 6-fl oz can	59	330	4	1	—	—	—	78	61	99	0.8	1308	800	0.48	0.06	2.3	302
281	Diluted with 3 parts water by volume ... 1 c	88	110	1	tr	—	—	—	26	20	32	0.2	439	270	0.15	0.02	0.7	102
282	Papayas, raw, 1/2" cubes ... 1 c	89	55	1	tr	—	—	—	14	28	22	0.4	328	2450	0.06	0.06	0.4	78
	Peaches																	
	Raw																	
283	Whole, 2 1/2" diam, peeled, pitted (about 4 per lb with peels and pits) ... 1 peach	89	40	1	tr	—	—	—	10	9	19	0.5	202	1330[34]	0.02	0.05	1.0	7
284	Sliced .... 1 c	89	65	1	tr	—	—	—	16	15	32	0.9	343	2260[34]	0.03	0.09	1.7	12
	Canned, yellow-fleshed, solids and liquid (halves or slices)																	
285	Syrup pack .... 1 c	79	200	1	tr	—	—	—	51	10	31	0.8	333	1100	0.03	0.05	1.5	8
286	Water pack .... 1 c	91	75	1	tr	—	—	—	20	10	32	0.7	334	1100	0.02	0.07	1.5	7
	Dried																	
287	Uncooked .... 1 c	25	420	5	1	—	—	—	109	77	187	9.6	1520	6240	0.02	0.30	8.5	29
288	Cooked, unsweetened, halves and juice ... 1 c	77	205	3	1	—	—	—	54	38	93	4.8	743	3050	0.01	0.15	3.8	5
	Frozen, sliced, sweetened																	
289	10-oz container ..... 1 container	77	250	1	tr	—	—	—	64	11	37	1.4	352	1850	0.03	0.11	2.0	116[35]
290	Cup .... 1 c	77	220	1	tr	—	—	—	57	10	33	1.3	310	1630	0.03	0.10	1.8	103[35]

416

(A)	(B)	(C)	(D)	(E)	(F)	(G)	(H)	(I)	(J)	(K)	(L)	(M)	(N)	(O)	(P)	(Q)	(R)	(S)
	Pears																	
	Raw, with skin, cored																	
291	Bartlett, 2½" diam (about 2½ per lb with cores and stems) 1 pear	164	83	100	1	1	—	—	25	13	18	0.5	213	30	0.03	0.07	0.2	7
292	Bosc, 2½" diam (about 3 1 pear per lb with cores and stems)	141	83	85	1	1	—	—	22	11	16	0.4	83	30	0.03	0.06	0.1	6
293	D'Anjou, 3" diam (about 1 pear 2 per lb with cores and stems)	200	83	120	1	1	—	—	31	16	22	0.6	260	40	0.04	0.08	0.2	8
294	Canned, solids and liquid, 1 c syrup pack, heavy (halves or slices)	255	80	195	1	1	—	—	50	13	18	0.5	214	10	0.03	0.05	0.3	3
	Pineapple																	
295	Raw, diced .... 1 c	155	85	80	1	tr	—	—	21	26	12	0.8	226	110	0.14	0.05	0.3	26
	Canned, heavy syrup pack, solids and liquid																	
296	Crushed, chunks, tidbits 1 c	255	80	190	1	tr	—	—	49	28	13	0.8	245	130	0.20	0.05	0.5	18
	Slices and liquid																	
297	Large .... 1 slice; 2¼ tbsp liquid	105	80	80	tr	tr	—	—	20	12	5	0.3	101	50	0.08	0.02	0.2	7
298	Medium .... 1 slice; 1¼ tbsp liquid	58	80	45	tr	tr	—	—	11	6	3	0.2	56	30	0.05	0.01	0.1	4
299	Pineapple juice, unsweetened, canned 1 c	250	86	140	1	tr	—	—	34	38	23	0.8	373	130	0.13	0.05	0.5	80[27]
	Plums																	
	Raw, without pits																	
300	Japanese and hybrid 1 plum .... (2⅛" diam; about 6½ per lb with pits)	66	87	30	tr	tr	—	—	8	8	12	0.3	112	160	0.02	0.02	0.3	4
301	Prune-type (1½" diam, 1 plum .... about 15 per lb with pits)	28	79	20	tr	tr	—	—	6	3	5	0.1	48	80	0.01	0.01	0.1	1
	Canned, heavy syrup pack (Italian prunes), with pits and liquid																	
302	Cup .... 1 c[36]	272	77	215	1	tr	—	—	56	23	26	2.3	367	3130	0.05	0.05	1.0	5
303	Portion .... 3 plums; 2¾ tbsp liquid[36]	140	77	110	1	tr	—	—	29	12	13	1.2	189	1610	0.03	0.03	0.5	3
	Prunes, dried,																	
	"softenized," with pits																	
304	Uncooked .... 4 extra large or 5 large prunes[36]	49	28	110	1	tr	—	—	29	22	34	1.7	298	690	0.04	0.07	0.7	1
305	Cooked, unsweetened, all 1 c[36] .... sizes, fruit and liquid	250	66	255	2	1	—	—	67	51	79	3.8	695	1590	0.07	0.15	1.5	2

(Continued)

417

Table A–1. Nutritive Values of the Edible Part of Foods (Continued)

(Dashes (—) denote lack of reliable data for a constituent believed to be present in measurable amount)

Item No. (A)	Foods, Approximate Measures, Units, and Weight (edible part unless footnotes indicate otherwise) (B)		Water Per-cent (C)	Food Energy Cal-ories (D)	Pro-tein (E)	Fat (F)	Fatty Acids Satu-rated (Total) (G)	Unsaturated Oleic (H)	Lino-leic (I)	Carbo-hydrate (J)	Calcium (K)	Phos-phorus (L)	Iron (M)	Potas-sium (N)	Vitamin A Value (O)	Thiamin (P)	Ribo-flavin (Q)	Niacin (R)	Ascorbic Acid (S)
			Per-cent	Cal-ories	g	g	g	g	g	g	mg	mg	mg	mg	IU	mg	mg	mg	mg
			g																
Fruits and Fruit Products (Continued)																			
306	Prune juice, canned or bottled	1 c 256	80	195	1	tr	—	—	—	49	36	51	1.8	602	—	0.03	0.03	1.0	5
	Raisins, seedless																		
307	Cup, not pressed down	1 c 145	18	420	4	tr	—	—	—	112	90	146	5.1	1106	30	0.16	0.12	0.7	1
308	Packet, ½ oz (1½ tbsp)	1 packet 14	18	40	tr	tr	—	—	—	11	9	14	0.5	107	tr	0.02	0.01	0.1	tr
	Raspberries, red																		
309	Raw, capped, whole	1 c 123	84	70	1	1	—	—	—	17	27	27	1.1	207	160	0.04	0.11	1.1	31
310	Frozen, sweetened, 10-oz container	1 container 284	74	280	2	1	—	—	—	70	37	48	1.7	284	200	0.06	0.17	1.7	60
	Rhubarb, cooked, added sugar																		
311	From raw	1 c 270	63	380	1	tr	—	—	—	97	211	41	1.6	548	220	0.05	0.14	0.8	16
312	From frozen, sweetened	1 c 270	63	385	1	1	—	—	—	98	211	32	1.9	475	190	0.05	0.11	0.5	16
	Strawberries																		
313	Raw, whole berries, capped	1 c 149	90	55	1	1	—	—	—	13	31	31	1.5	244	90	0.04	0.10	0.9	88
	Frozen, sweetened																		
314	Sliced, 10-oz container	1 container 284	71	310	1	1	—	—	—	79	40	48	2.0	318	90	0.06	0.17	1.4	151
315	Whole, 1-lb container (about 1¾ cups)	1 container 454	76	415	2	1	—	—	—	107	59	73	2.7	472	140	0.09	0.27	2.3	249
316	Tangerine, raw, 2⅜″ diam, size 176, without peel (about 4 per lb with peels and seeds)	1 tangerine 86	87	40	1	tr	—	—	—	10	34	15	0.3	108	360	0.05	0.02	0.1	27
317	Tangerine juice, canned, sweetened	1 c 249	87	125	1	tr	—	—	—	30	44	35	0.5	440	1040	0.15	0.05	0.2	54
318	Watermelon, raw, 4″ × 8″ wedge with rind and seeds (1/16 of 32⅔-lb melon, 10″ × 16″)	1 wedge with rind and seeds[37] 926	93	110	2	1	—	—	—	27	30	43	2.1	426	2510	0.13	0.13	0.9	30
Grain Products																			
	Bagel, 3″ diam																		
319	Egg	1 bagel 55	32	165	6	2	0.5	0.9	0.8	28	9	43	1.2	41	30	0.14	0.10	1.2	0
320	Water	1 bagel 55	29	165	6	1	0.2	0.4	0.6	30	8	41	1.2	42	0	0.15	0.11	1.4	0
321	Barley, pearled, light, uncooked	1 c 200	11	700	16	2	0.3	0.2	0.8	158	32	378	4.0	320	0	0.24	0.10	6.2	0

(A)	(B)		(C)	(D)	(E)	(F)	(G)	(H)	(I)	(J)	(K)	(L)	(M)	(N)	(O)	(P)	(Q)	(R)	(S)
	Biscuits, baking powder, 2" diam (enriched flour, vegetable shortening)																		
322	From home recipe .... 1 biscuit	28	27	105	2	5	1.2	2.0	1.2	13	34	49	0.4	33	tr	0.08	0.08	0.7	tr
323	From mix .... 1 biscuit	28	29	90	2	3	0.6	1.1	0.7	15	19	65	0.6	32	tr	0.09	0.08	0.8	tr
324	Breadcrumbs (enriched)[38] Dry, grated .... 1 c	100	7	390	13	5	1.0	1.6	1.4	73	122	141	3.6	152	tr	0.35	0.35	4.8	tr
	Soft (see White bread, items 349–350)																		
	Breads																		
325	Boston brown bread, canned, slice (3 1/4" × 1/2")[38] .... 1 slice	45	45	95	2	1	0.1	0.2	0.2	21	41	72	0.9	131	0[39]	0.06	0.04	0.7	0
	Cracked-wheat bread (3/4 enriched wheat flour, 1/4 cracked wheat)[38]																		
326	Loaf, 1 lb .... 1 loaf	454	35	1195	39	10	2.2	3.0	3.9	236	399	581	9.5	608	tr	1.52	1.13	14.4	tr
327	Slice (18 per loaf) .... 1 slice	25	35	65	2	1	0.1	0.2	0.2	13	22	32	0.5	34	tr	0.08	0.06	0.8	tr
	French or vienna bread, enriched[38]																		
328	Loaf, 1 lb .... 1 loaf	454	31	1315	41	14	3.2	4.7	4.6	251	195	386	10.0	408	tr	1.80	1.10	15.0	tr
	Slice																		
329	French (5" × 2 1/2" × 1") .... 1 slice	35	31	100	3	1	0.2	0.4	0.4	19	15	30	0.8	32	tr	0.14	0.08	1.2	tr
330	Vienna (4 3/4" × 4" × 1/2") .... 1 slice	25	31	75	2	1	0.2	0.3	0.3	14	11	21	0.6	23	tr	0.10	0.06	0.8	tr
	Italian bread, enriched																		
331	Loaf, 1 lb .... 1 loaf	454	32	1250	41	4	0.6	0.3	1.5	256	77	349	10.0	336	0	1.80	1.10	15.0	0
332	Slice (4 1/2" × 3 1/4" × 3/4") .... 1 slice	30	32	85	3	tr	tr	tr	0.1	17	5	23	0.7	22	0	0.12	0.07	1.0	0
	Raisin bread, enriched[38]																		
333	Loaf, 1 lb .... 1 loaf	454	35	1190	30	13	3.0	4.7	3.9	243	322	395	10.0	1057	tr	1.70	1.07	10.7	tr
334	Slice (18 per loaf) .... 1 slice	25	35	65	2	1	0.2	0.3	0.2	13	18	22	0.6	58	tr	0.09	0.06	0.6	tr
	Rye bread / American, light (2/3 enriched wheat flour, 1/3 rye flour)																		
335	Loaf, 1 lb .... 1 loaf	454	36	1100	41	5	0.7	0.5	2.2	236	340	667	9.1	658	0	1.35	0.98	12.9	0
336	Slice (4 3/4" × 3 3/4" × 7/16") .... 1 slice	25	36	60	2	tr	tr	tr	0.1	13	19	37	0.5	36	0	0.07	0.05	0.7	0
	Pumpernickel (2/3 rye flour, 1/3 enriched wheat flour)																		
337	Loaf, 1 lb .... 1 loaf	454	34	1115	41	5	0.7	0.5	2.4	241	381	1039	11.8	2059	0	1.30	0.93	8.5	0
338	Slice (5" × 4" × 7/8") .... 1 slice	32	34	80	3	tr	0.1	tr	0.2	17	27	73	0.8	145	0	0.09	0.07	0.6	0
	White bread, enriched[38] Soft-crumb type																		
339	Loaf, 1 lb .... 1 loaf	454	36	1225	39	15	3.4	5.3	4.6	229	381	440	11.3	476	tr	1.80	1.10	15.0	tr

(Continued)

Table A–1. Nutritive Values of the Edible Part of Foods (Continued)

(Dashes (—) denote lack of reliable data for a constituent believed to be present in measurable amount)

Item No. (A)	Foods, Approximate Measures, Units, and Weight (edible part unless footnotes indicate otherwise) (B)	Water (C)	Food Energy (D)	Pro-tein (E)	Fat (F)	Fatty Acids Satu-rated (Total) (G)	Unsaturated Oleic (H)	Lino-leic (I)	Carbo-hydrate (J)	Calcium (K)	Phos-phorus (L)	Iron (M)	Potas-sium (N)	Vitamin A Value (O)	Thiamin (P)	Ribo-flavin (Q)	Niacin (R)	Ascorbic Acid (S)
		Per-cent	Cal-ories	g	g	g	g	g	g	mg	mg	mg	mg	IU	mg	mg	mg	mg
	Grain Products (Continued)																	
	Breads (Continued)																	
340	Slice (18 per loaf) ... 1 slice	25	70	2	1	0.2	0.3	0.3	13	21	24	0.6	26	tr	0.10	0.06	0.8	tr
341	Slice, toasted ...... 1 slice	22	70	2	1	0.2	0.3	0.3	13	21	24	0.6	26	tr	0.08	0.06	0.8	tr
342	Slice (22 per loaf) ... 1 slice	20	55	2	1	0.2	0.2	0.2	10	17	19	0.5	21	tr	0.08	0.05	0.7	tr
343	Slice, toasted ...... 1 slice	17	55	2	1	0.2	0.2	0.2	10	17	19	0.5	21	tr	0.06	0.05	0.7	tr
344	Loaf, 1½ lb .... 1 loaf	680	1835	59	22	5.2	7.9	6.9	343	571	660	17.0	714	tr	2.70	1.65	22.5	tr
345	Slice (24 per loaf) ... 1 slice	28	75	2	1	0.2	0.3	0.3	14	24	27	0.7	29	tr	0.11	0.07	0.9	tr
346	Slice, toasted ...... 1 slice	24	75	2	1	0.2	0.3	0.3	14	24	27	0.7	29	tr	0.09	0.07	0.9	tr
347	Slice (28 per loaf) ... 1 slice	24	65	2	1	0.2	0.3	0.2	12	20	23	0.6	25	tr	0.10	0.06	0.8	tr
348	Slice, toasted ...... 1 slice	21	65	2	1	0.2	0.3	0.2	12	20	23	0.6	25	tr	0.08	0.06	0.8	tr
349	Cubes .... 1 c	30	80	3	1	0.2	0.3	0.3	15	25	29	0.8	32	tr	0.12	0.07	1.0	tr
350	Crumbs .... 1 c	45	120	4	1	0.3	0.5	0.5	23	38	44	1.1	47	tr	0.18	0.11	1.5	tr
	Firm-crumb type																	
351	Loaf, 1 lb .... 1 loaf	454	1245	41	17	3.9	5.9	5.2	228	435	463	11.3	549	tr	1.80	1.10	15.0	tr
352	Slice (20 per loaf) ... 1 slice	23	65	2	1	0.2	0.3	0.3	12	22	23	0.6	28	tr	0.09	0.06	0.8	tr
353	Slice, toasted ...... 1 slice	20	65	2	1	0.2	0.3	0.3	12	22	23	0.6	28	tr	0.07	0.06	0.8	tr
354	Loaf, 2 lb .... 1 loaf	907	2495	82	34	7.7	11.8	10.4	455	871	925	22.7	1097	tr	3.60	2.20	30.0	tr
355	Slice (34 per loaf) ... 1 slice	27	75	2	1	0.2	0.3	0.3	14	26	28	0.7	33	tr	0.11	0.06	0.9	tr
356	Slice, toasted ...... 1 slice	23	75	2	1	0.2	0.3	0.3	14	26	28	0.7	33	tr	0.09	0.06	0.9	tr
	Whole-wheat bread																	
	Soft-crumb type[38]																	
357	Loaf, 1 lb .... 1 loaf	454	1095	41	12	2.2	2.9	4.2	224	381	1152	13.6	1161	tr	1.37	0.45	12.7	tr
358	Slice (16 per loaf) ... 1 slice	28	65	3	1	0.1	0.2	0.2	14	24	71	0.8	72	tr	0.09	0.03	0.8	tr
359	Slice, toasted ...... 1 slice	24	65	3	1	0.1	0.2	0.2	14	24	71	0.8	72	tr	0.07	0.03	0.8	tr
	Firm-crumb type[38]																	
360	Loaf, 1 lb .... 1 loaf	454	1100	48	14	2.5	3.3	4.9	216	449	1034	13.6	1238	tr	1.17	0.54	12.7	tr
361	Slice (18 per loaf) ... 1 slice	25	60	3	1	0.1	0.2	0.3	12	25	57	0.8	68	tr	0.06	0.03	0.7	tr
362	Slice, toasted ...... 1 slice	21	60	3	1	0.1	0.2	0.3	12	25	57	0.8	68	tr	0.05	0.03	0.7	tr
	Breakfast cereals																	
	Hot type, cooked																	
	Corn (hominy) grits, degermed																	
363	Enriched .... 1 c	245	125	3	tr	tr	tr	0.1	27	2	25	0.7	27	tr[40]	0.10	0.07	1.0	0
364	Unenriched .... 1 c	245	125	3	tr	tr	tr	0.1	27	2	25	0.2	27	tr[40]	0.05	0.02	0.5	0
365	Farina, quick-cooking, enriched 1 c	245	105	3	tr	tr	tr	0.1	22	147	113[41]	(42)	25	0	0.12	0.07	1.0	0
366	Oatmeal or rolled oats 1 c	240	130	5	2	0.4	0.8	0.9	23	22	137	1.4	146	0	0.19	0.05	0.2	0
367	Wheat, rolled ...... 1 c	240	180	5	1	—	—	—	41	19	182	1.7	202	0	0.17	0.07	2.2	0
368	Wheat, whole-meal ... 1 c	245	110	4	1	—	—	—	23	17	127	1.2	118	0	0.15	0.05	1.5	0

(A)	(B)		(C)	(D)	(E)	(F)	(G)	(H)	(I)	(J)	(K)	(L)	(M)	(N)	(O)	(P)	(Q)	(R)	(S)
	Ready-to-eat																		
369	Bran flakes (40% bran), added sugar, salt, iron, vitamins	1 c	35	105	4	1	—	—	—	28	19	125	5.6	137	1540	0.46	0.52	6.2	0
370	Bran flakes with raisins, added sugar, salt, iron, vitamins	1 c	50	145	4	1	—	—	—	40	28	146	7.9	154	2200[43]	(44)	(44)	(44)	0
	Corn flakes																		
371	Plain, added sugar, salt, iron, vitamins	1 c	25	95	2	tr	—	—	—	21	(44)	9	(44)	30	(44)	(44)	(44)	(44)	13[45]
372	Sugar-coated, added salt, iron, vitamins	1 c	40	155	2	tr	—	—	—	37	1	10	(44)	27	1760	0.53	0.60	7.1	21[45]
373	Corn, oat flour, puffed, added sugar, salt, iron, vitamins	1 c	20	80	2	1	—	—	—	16	4	18	5.7	—	880	0.26	0.30	3.5	11
374	Corn, shredded, added sugar, salt, iron, thiamin, niacin	1 c	25	95	2	tr	—	—	—	22	1	10	0.6	—	0	0.33	0.05	4.4	13
375	Oats, puffed, added sugar, salt, minerals, vitamins	1 c	25	100	3	1	—	—	—	19	44	102	4.0	—	1100	0.33	0.38	4.4	13
	Rice, puffed																		
376	Plain, added iron, thiamin, niacin	1 c	15	60	1	tr	—	—	—	13	3	14	0.3	15	0	0.07	0.01	0.7	0
377	Presweetened, added salt, iron, vitamins	1 c	28	115	1	0	—	—	—	26	3	14	(44)	43	1240[45]	(44)	(44)	(44)	15[45]
378	Wheat flakes, added sugar, salt, iron, vitamins	1 c	30	105	3	tr	—	—	—	24	12	83	4.8	81	1320	0.40	0.45	5.3	16
	Wheat, puffed																		
379	Plain, added iron, thiamin, niacin	1 c	15	55	2	tr	—	—	—	12	4	48	0.6	51	0	0.08	0.03	1.2	0
380	Presweetened, added salt, iron, vitamins	1 c	38	140	3	tr	—	—	—	33	7	52	(44)	63	1680	0.50	0.57	6.7	20[45]
381	Wheat, shredded, plain	1 oblong biscuit or ½ cup spoon-size biscuits	25	90	2	1	—	—	—	20	11	97	0.9	87	0	0.06	0.03	1.1	0
382	Wheat germ, without salt and sugar, toasted	1 tbsp	6	25	2	1	—	—	—	3	3	70	0.5	57	10	0.11	0.05	0.3	1
383	Buckwheat flour, light, sifted	1 c	98	340	6	1	0.2	—	—	78	11	86	1.0	314	0	0.08	0.04	0.4	0
384	Bulgur, canned, seasoned	1 c	135	245	8	4	—	0.4	0.4	44	27	263	1.9	151	0	0.08	0.05	4.1	0
	Cake icings (see Sugars and Sweets, items 532–536)																		
	Cakes made from cake mixes with enriched flour[46]																		

(Continued)

Table A-1. Nutritive Values of the Edible Part of Foods (Continued)

(Dashes (—) denote lack of reliable data for a constituent believed to be present in measurable amount)

Item No. (A)	Foods, Approximate Measures, Units, and Weight (edible part unless footnotes indicate otherwise) (B)	(g)	Water (C) Percent	Food Energy (D) Cal-ories	Pro-tein (E) g	Fat (F) g	Fatty Acids Satu-rated (Total) (G) g	Unsaturated Oleic (H) g	Lino-leic (I) g	Carbo-hydrate (J) g	Calcium (K) mg	Phos-phorus (L) mg	Iron (M) mg	Potas-sium (N) mg	Vitamin A Value (O) IU	Thiamin (P) mg	Ribo-flavin (Q) mg	Niacin (R) mg	Ascorbic Acid (S) mg
	Grain Products (Continued)																		
	Cakes made from cake mixes with enriched flour (Continued)																		
	Angelfood																		
385	Whole cake (9¾" diam tube cake) 1 cake	635	34	1645	36	1	—	—	—	377	603	756	2.5	381	0	0.37	0.95	3.6	0
386	Piece, 1/12 of cake 1 piece	53	34	135	3	tr	—	—	—	32	50	63	0.2	32	0	0.03	0.08	0.3	0
	Coffeecake																		
387	Whole cake (7¾" × 5⅝" × 1¼"in) 1 cake	430	30	1385	27	41	11.7	16.3	8.8	225	262	748	6.9	469	690	0.82	0.91	7.7	1
388	Piece, 1/6 of cake 1 piece	72	30	230	5	7	2.0	2.7	1.5	38	44	125	1.2	78	120	0.14	0.15	1.3	tr
	Cupcakes, made with egg, milk, 2½" diam																		
389	Without icing 1 cupcake	25	26	90	1	3	0.8	1.2	0.7	14	40	59	0.3	21	40	0.05	0.05	0.4	tr
390	With chocolate icing 1 cupcake	36	22	130	2	5	2.0	1.6	0.6	21	47	71	0.4	42	60	0.05	0.06	0.4	tr
	Devil's food with chocolate icing																		
391	Whole, 2-layer cake (8" or 9" diam) 1 cake	1107	24	3755	49	136	50.0	44.9	17.0	645	653	1162	16.6	1439	1660	1.06	1.65	10.1	1
392	Piece, 1/16 of cake 1 piece	69	24	235	3	8	3.1	2.8	1.1	40	41	72	1.0	90	100	0.07	0.10	0.6	tr
393	Cupcake (2½" diam) 1 cupcake	35	24	120	2	4	1.6	1.4	0.5	20	21	37	0.5	46	50	0.03	0.05	0.3	tr
	Gingerbread																		
394	Whole cake (8" square) 1 cake	570	37	1575	18	39	9.7	16.6	10.0	291	513	570	8.6	1562	tr	0.84	1.00	7.4	tr
395	Piece, 1/9 of cake 1 piece	63	37	175	2	4	1.1	1.8	1.1	32	57	63	0.9	173	tr	0.09	0.11	0.8	tr
	White, 2-layer with chocolate icing																		
396	Whole cake (8" or 9" diam) 1 cake	1140	21	4000	44	122	48.2	46.4	20.0	716	1129	2041	11.4	1322	680	1.50	1.77	12.5	2
397	Piece, 1/16 of cake 1 piece	71	21	250	3	8	3.0	2.9	1.2	45	70	127	0.7	82	40	0.09	0.11	0.8	tr
	Yellow, 2-layer with chocolate icing																		
398	Whole cake (8" or 9" diam) 1 cake	1108	26	3735	45	125	47.8	47.8	20.3	638	1008	2017	12.2	1208	1550	1.24	1.67	10.6	2
399	Piece, 1/16 of cake 1 piece	69	26	235	3	8	3.0	3.0	1.3	40	63	126	0.8	75	100	0.08	0.10	0.7	tr
	Cakes made from home recipes using enriched flour[47]																		
	Boston cream pie with custard filling																		
400	Whole cake (8" diam) 1 cake	825	35	2490	41	78	23.0	30.1	15.2	412	553	833	8.2	734[48]	1730	1.04	1.27	9.6	2
401	Piece, 1/12 of cake 1 piece	69	35	210	3	6	1.9	2.5	1.3	34	46	70	0.7	61[48]	140	0.09	0.11	0.8	tr

(A)	(B)		(C)	(D)	(E)	(F)	(G)	(H)	(I)	(J)	(K)	(L)	(M)	(N)	(O)	(P)	(Q)	(R)	(S)
	Fruitcake, dark																		
402	Loaf, 1-lb ($7\frac{1}{2}$″ × 2″ × $1\frac{1}{2}$″)	1 loaf	454	18	1720	22	69	14.4	33.5	14.8	271	327	513	11.8	2250	540	0.72	0.73	4.9	2
403	Slice, $\frac{1}{30}$ of loaf	1 slice	15	18	55	1	2	0.5	1.1	0.5	9	11	17	0.4	74	20	0.02	0.02	0.2	tr
	Plain, sheet cake																		
	Without icing																		
404	Whole cake (9″square)	1 cake	777	25	2830	35	108	29.5	44.4	23.9	434	497	793	8.5	614[48]	1320	1.21	1.40	10.2	2
405	Piece, $\frac{1}{9}$ of cake	1 piece	86	25	315	4	12	3.3	4.9	2.6	48	55	88	0.9	68[48]	150	0.13	0.15	1.1	tr
	With uncooked white icing																		
406	Whole cake (9″square)	1 cake	1096	21	4020	37	129	42.2	49.5	24.4	694	548	822	8.2	669[48]	2190	1.22	1.47	10.2	2
407	Piece, $\frac{1}{9}$ of cake	1 piece	121	21	445	4	14	4.7	5.5	2.7	77	61	91	0.8	74[48]	240	0.14	0.16	1.1	tr
	Pound[49]																		
408	Loaf, $8\frac{1}{2}$″ × $3\frac{1}{2}$″ × $3\frac{1}{4}$″	1 loaf	565	16	2725	31	170	42.9	73.1	39.6	273	107	418	7.9	345	1410	0.90	0.99	7.3	0
409	Slice, $\frac{1}{17}$ of loaf	1 slice	33	16	160	2	10	2.5	4.3	2.3	16	6	24	0.5	20	80	0.05	0.06	0.4	0
	Spongecake																		
410	Whole cake ($9\frac{3}{4}$″diam tube cake)	1 cake	790	32	2345	60	45	13.1	15.8	5.7	427	237	885	13.4	687	3560	1.10	1.64	7.4	tr
411	Piece, $\frac{1}{12}$ of cake	1 piece	66	32	195	5	4	1.1	1.3	0.5	36	20	74	1.1	57	300	0.09	0.14	0.6	tr
	Cookies made with enriched flour[50,51]																		
	Brownies with nuts																		
	Home-prepared, $1\frac{3}{4}$″ × $1\frac{3}{4}$″ × $\frac{7}{8}$″																		
412	From home recipe	1 brownie	20	10	95	1	6	1.5	3.0	1.2	10	8	30	0.4	38	40	0.04	0.03	0.2	tr
413	From commercial recipe	1 brownie	20	11	85	1	4	0.9	1.4	1.3	13	9	27	0.4	34	20	0.03	0.02	0.2	tr
414	Frozen, with chocolate icing[52] ($1\frac{1}{2}$″ × $1\frac{3}{4}$″ × $\frac{7}{8}$″)	1 brownie	25	13	105	1	5	2.0	2.2	0.7	15	10	31	0.4	44	50	0.03	0.03	0.2	tr
	Chocolate chip																		
415	Commercial ($2\frac{1}{4}$″diam, $\frac{3}{8}$″thick)	4 cookies	42	3	200	2	9	2.8	2.9	2.2	29	16	48	1.0	56	50	0.10	0.17	0.9	tr
416	From home recipe, $2\frac{1}{3}$″ diam	4 cookies	40	3	205	2	12	3.5	4.5	2.9	24	14	40	0.8	47	40	0.06	0.06	0.5	tr
417	Fig bars, square ($1\frac{5}{8}$″ × $1\frac{5}{8}$″ × $\frac{3}{8}$″) or rectangular ($1\frac{1}{2}$″ × $1\frac{3}{4}$″ × $\frac{1}{2}$″)	4 cookies	56	14	200	2	3	0.8	1.2	0.7	42	44	34	1.0	111	60	0.04	0.14	0.9	tr
418	Gingersnaps (2″diam, $\frac{1}{4}$″ thick	4 cookies	28	3	90	2	2	0.7	1.0	0.6	22	20	13	0.7	129	20	0.08	0.06	0.7	0
419	Macaroons ($2\frac{3}{4}$″diam, $\frac{1}{4}$″thick	2 cookies	38	4	180	2	9	—	—	—	25	10	32	0.3	176	0	0.02	0.06	0.2	0
420	Oatmeal with raisins ($2\frac{5}{8}$″diam, $\frac{1}{4}$″thick)	4 cookies	52	3	235	3	8	2.0	3.3	2.0	38	11	53	1.4	192	30	0.15	0.10	1.0	tr
421	Plain, prepared from commercial chilled dough ($2\frac{1}{2}$″diam, $\frac{1}{4}$″ thick)	4 cookies	48	5	240	2	12	3.0	5.2	2.9	31	17	35	0.6	23	30	0.10	0.08	0.9	0

(Continued)

Table A-1. Nutritive Values of the Edible Part of Foods (Continued)

(Dashes (—) denote lack of reliable data for a constituent believed to be present in measurable amount)

Item No. (A)	Foods, Approximate Measures, Units, and Weight (edible part unless footnotes indicate otherwise) (B)	(g)	Water Percent (C)	Food Energy Calories (D)	Protein g (E)	Fat g (F)	Fatty Acids Saturated (Total) g (G)	Unsaturated Oleic g (H)	Linoleic g (I)	Carbohydrate g (J)	Calcium mg (K)	Phosphorus mg (L)	Iron mg (M)	Potassium mg (N)	Vitamin A Value IU (O)	Thiamin mg (P)	Riboflavin mg (Q)	Niacin mg (R)	Ascorbic Acid mg (S)
	Grain Products (Continued)																		
	Cookies made with enriched flour (Continued)																		
422	Sandwich type chocolate or vanilla (1³/₄" diam, ³/₈" thick) ... 4 cookies	40	2	200	2	9	2.2	3.9	2.2	28	10	96	0.7	15	0	0.06	0.10	0.7	0
423	Vanilla wafers, 1³/₄" diam, ¹/₄" thick ... 10 cookies	40	3	185	2	6	—	—	—	30	16	25	0.6	29	50	0.10	0.09	0.8	0
	Cornmeal																		
424	Whole-ground, unbolted, dry form ... 1 c	122	12	435	11	5	0.5	1.0	2.5	90	24	312	2.9	346	620[53]	0.46	.0.13	2.4	0
425	Bolted (nearly whole-grain), dry form ... 1 c	122	12	440	11	4	0.5	0.9	2.1	91	21	272	2.2	303	590[53]	0.37	0.10	2.3	0
	Degermed, enriched																		
426	Dry form ... 1 c	138	12	500	11	2	0.2	0.4	0.9	108	8	137	4.0	166	610[53]	0.61	0.36	4.8	0
427	Cooked ... 1 c	240	88	120	3	tr	tr	0.1	0.2	26	2	34	1.0	38	140[53]	0.14	0.10	1.2	0
	Degermed, unenriched																		
428	Dry form ... 1 c	138	12	500	11	2	0.2	0.4	0.9	108	8	137	1.5	166	610[53]	0.19	0.07	1.4	0
429	Cooked ... 1 c	240	88	120	3	tr	tr	0.1	0.2	26	2	34	0.5	38	140[53]	0.05	0.02	0.2	0
	Crackers[38]																		
430	Graham, plain (2¹/₂" square) ... 2 crackers	14	6	55	1	1	0.3	0.5	0.3	10	6	21	0.5	55	0	0.02	0.08	0.5	0
431	Rye wafers, whole-grain (1⁷/₈" × 3¹/₂") ... 2 wafers	13	6	45	2	tr	—	—	—	10	7	50	0.5	78	0	0.04	0.03	0.2	0
432	Saltines, made with enriched flour ... 4 crackers or 1 packet	11	4	50	1	1	0.3	0.5	0.4	8	2	10	0.5	13	0	0.05	0.05	0.4	0
	Danish pastry (enriched flour), plain without fruit or nuts[54]																		
433	Packaged ring, 12 oz ... 1 ring	340	22	1435	25	80	24.3	31.7	16.5	155	170	371	6.1	381	1050	0.97	1.01	8.6	tr
434	Round piece (about 4¹/₄" diam × 1") ... 1 pastry	65	22	275	5	15	4.7	6.1	3.2	30	33	71	1.2	73	200	0.18	0.19	1.7	tr
435	Ounce ... 1 oz	28	22	120	2	7	2.0	2.7	1.4	13	14	31	0.5	32	90	0.08	0.08	0.7	tr
	Doughnuts, made with enriched flour[38]																		
436	Cake type, plain (2¹/₂" diam, 1" high) ... 1 doughnut	25	24	100	1	5	1.2	2.0	1.1	13	10	48	0.4	23	20	0.05	0.05	0.4	tr
437	Yeast-leavened, glazed (3³/₄" diam, 1¹/₄" high) ... 1 doughnut	50	26	205	3	11	3.3	5.8	3.3	22	16	33	0.6	34	25	0.10	0.10	0.8	0
	Macaroni, enriched, cooked (cut lengths, elbows, shells)																		

(A)	(B)	(C)	(D)	(E)	(F)	(G)	(H)	(I)	(J)	(K)	(L)	(M)	(N)	(O)	(P)	(Q)	(R)	(S)
438	Firm stage (hot) .... 1 c 130	64	190	7	1	—	—	—	39	14	85	1.4	103	0	0.23	0.13	1.8	0
	Tender stage																	
439	Cold macaroni .... 1 c 105	73	115	4	tr	—	—	—	24	8	53	0.9	64	0	0.15	0.08	1.2	0
440	Hot macaroni .... 1 c 140	73	155	5	1	—	—	—	32	11	70	1.3	85	0	0.20	0.11	1.5	0
	Macaroni (enriched) and cheese																	
441	Canned[55] .... 1 c 240	80	230	9	10	4.2	3.1	1.4	26	199	182	1.0	139	260	0.12	0.24	1.0	tr
442	From home recipe (served hot)[56] .... 1 c 200	58	430	17	22	8.9	8.8	2.9	40	362	322	1.8	240	860	0.20	0.40	1.8	tr
	Muffins made with enriched flour[38]																	
	From home recipe																	
443	Blueberry (2 3/8″ diam, 1 1/2″ high) .... 1 muffin 40	39	110	3	4	1.1	1.4	0.7	17	34	53	0.6	46	90	0.09	0.10	0.7	tr
444	Bran .... 1 muffin 40	35	105	3	4	1.2	1.4	0.8	17	57	162	1.5	172	90	0.07	0.10	1.7	tr
445	Corn, enriched degermed cornmeal and flour (2 3/8″ diam, 1 1/2″ high)[56] .... 1 muffin 40	33	125	3	4	1.2	1.6	0.9	19	42	68	0.7	54	120[57]	0.10	0.10	0.7	tr
446	Plain (3″ diam, 1 1/2″ high) .... 1 muffin 40	38	120	3	4	1.0	1.7	1.0	17	42	60	0.6	50	40	0.09	0.12	0.9	tr
	From mix, egg, milk																	
447	Corn (2 3/8″ diam, 1 1/2″ high)[38] .... 1 muffin 40	30	130	3	4	1.2	1.7	0.9	20	96	152	0.6	44	100[57]	0.08	0.09	0.7	tr
448	Noodles (egg noodles), enriched, cooked .... 1 c 160	71	200	7	2	—	—	—	37	16	94	1.4	70	110	0.22	0.13	1.9	0
449	Noodles, chow mein, canned .... 1 c 45	1	220	6	11	—	—	—	26	—	—	—	—	—	—	—	—	—
	Pancakes (4″ diam)[38]																	
450	Buckwheat, made from mix (with buckwheat and enriched flours), egg and milk added .... 1 cake 27	58	55	2	2	0.8	0.9	0.4	6	59	91	0.4	66	60	0.04	0.05	0.2	tr
	Plain																	
451	Made from home recipe using enriched flour .... 1 cake 27	50	60	2	2	0.5	0.8	0.5	9	27	38	0.4	33	30	0.06	0.07	0.5	tr
452	Made from mix with enriched flour, egg and milk added .... 1 cake 27	51	60	2	2	0.7	0.7	0.3	9	58	70	0.3	42	70	0.04	0.06	0.2	tr
	Pies, piecrust made with enriched flour, vegetable shortening (9″ diam)																	
	Apple																	
453	Whole .... 1 pie 945	48	2420	21	105	27.0	44.5	25.2	360	76	208	6.6	756	280	1.06	0.79	9.3	9
454	Sector, 1/7 of pie .... 1 sector 135	48	345	3	15	3.9	6.4	3.6	51	11	30	0.9	108	40	0.15	0.11	1.3	2

(Continued)

Table A-1. Nutritive Values of the Edible Part of Foods (Continued)

(Dashes (—) denote lack of reliable data for a constituent believed to be present in measurable amount)

Item No. (A)	Foods, Approximate Measures, Units, and Weight (edible part unless footnotes indicate otherwise) (B)	Water (C) Per- cent	Food Energy (D) Cal- ories	Pro- tein (E) g	Fat (F) g	Fatty Acids Satu- rated (Total) (G) g	Unsaturated Oleic (H) g	Lino- leic (I) g	Carbo- hydrate (J) g	Calcium (K) mg	Phos- phorus (L) mg	Iron (M) mg	Potas- sium (N) mg	Vitamin A Value (O) IU	Thiamin (P) mg	Ribo- flavin (Q) mg	Niacin (R) mg	Ascorbic Acid (S) mg
	Grain Products (Continued)																	
	Pies (Continued)																	
	Banana cream																	
455	Whole .... 1 pie	910	2010	41	85	26.7	33.2	16.2	279	601	746	7.3	1847	2280	0.77	1.51	7.0	9
456	Sector, 1/7 of pie ..... 1 sector ...	130	54	285	6	12	3.8	4.7	2.3	40	86	107	1.0	264	330	0.11	0.22	1.0	1
	Blueberry																	
457	Whole .... 1 pie	945	51	2285	23	102	24.8	43.7	25.1	330	104	217	9.5	614	280	1.03	0.80	10.0	28
458	Sector, 1/7 of pie ..... 1 sector ...	135	51	325	3	15	3.5	6.2	3.6	47	15	31	1.4	88	40	0.15	0.11	1.4	4
	Cherry																	
459	Whole .... 1 pie	945	47	2465	25	107	28.2	45.0	25.3	363	132	236	6.6	992	4160	1.09	0.84	9.8	tr
460	Sector, 1/7 of pie ..... 1 sector ...	135	47	350	4	15	4.0	6.4	3.6	52	19	34	0.9	142	590	0.16	0.12	1.4	tr
	Custard																	
461	Whole .... 1 pie	910	58	1985	56	101	33.9	38.5	17.5	213	874	1028	8.2	1247	2090	0.79	1.92	5.6	0
462	Sector, 1/7 of pie ..... 1 sector ...	130	58	285	8	14	4.8	5.5	2.5	30	125	147	1.2	178	300	0.11	0.27	0.8	0
	Lemon meringue																	
463	Whole .... 1 pie	840	47	2140	31	86	26.1	33.8	16.4	317	118	412	6.7	420	1430	0.61	0.84	5.2	25
464	Sector, 1/7 of pie ..... 1 sector ...	120	47	305	4	12	3.7	4.8	2.3	45	17	59	1.0	60	200	0.09	0.12	0.7	4
	Mince																	
465	Whole .... 1 pie	945	43	2560	24	109	28.0	45.9	25.2	389	265	359	13.3	1682	20	0.96	0.86	9.8	9
466	Sector, 1/7 of pie ..... 1 sector ...	135	43	365	3	16	4.0	6.6	3.6	56	38	51	1.9	240	tr	0.14	0.12	1.4	1
	Peach																	
467	Whole .... 1 pie	945	48	2410	24	101	24.8	43.7	25.1	361	95	274	8.5	1408	6900	1.04	0.97	14.0	28
468	Sector, 1/7 of pie ..... 1 sector ...	135	48	345	3	14	3.5	6.2	3.6	52	14	39	1.2	201	990	0.15	0.14	2.0	4
	Pecan																	
469	Whole .... 1 pie	825	20	3450	42	189	27.8	101.0	44.2	423	388	850	25.6	1015	1320	1.80	0.95	6.9	tr
470	Sector, 1/7 of pie ..... 1 sector ...	118	20	495	6	27	4.0	14.4	6.3	61	55	122	3.7	145	190	0.26	0.14	1.0	tr
	Pumpkin																	
471	Whole .... 1 pie	910	59	1920	36	102	37.4	37.5	16.6	223	464	628	7.3	1456	22,480	0.78	1.27	7.0	tr
472	Sector, 1/7 of pie ..... 1 sector ...	130	59	275	5	15	5.4	5.4	2.4	32	66	90	1.0	208	3210	0.11	0.18	1.0	tr
473	Piecrust (home recipe) made with enriched flour and vegetable shortening, baked 1 pie shell, 9" diam	180	15	900	11	60	14.8	26.1	14.9	79	25	90	3.1	89	0	0.47	0.40	5.0	0
474	Piecrust mix with enriched flour and vegetable shortening, 10-oz pkg prepared and baked Piecrust for 2-crust pie, 9" diam	320	19	1485	20	93	22.7	39.7	23.4	141	131	272	6.1	179	0	1.07	0.79	9.9	0
475	Pizza (cheese) baked (4³/₄ " 1 sector; 1/8 of 12" diam pie)[19]	60	45	145	6	4	1.7	1.5	0.6	22	86	89	1.1	67	230	0.16	0.18	1.6	4

(A)	(B)	(C)	(D)	(E)	(F)	(G)	(H)	(I)	(J)	(K)	(L)	(M)	(N)	(O)	(P)	(Q)	(R)	(S)
	Popcorn, popped																	
476	Plain, large kernel ..... 1 c	6	25	1	tr	tr	0.1	0.2	5	1	17	0.2	—	—	—	0.01	0.1	0
477	With oil (coconut) and salt added, large kernel ... 1 c	9	40	1	2	1.5	0.2	0.2	5	1	19	0.2	—	—	—	0.01	0.2	0
478	Sugar coated .... 1 c	35	135	2	1	0.5	0.2	0.4	30	2	47	0.5	—	—	—	0.02	0.4	0
	Pretzels, made with enriched flour																	
479	Dutch, twisted (2³/₄ × 2⁵/₈") 1 pretzel	16	60	2	1	—	—	—	12	4	21	0.2	21	0	0.05	0.04	0.7	0
480	Thin, twisted (3¹/₄" × 2¹/₄" 10 pretzels × ¹/₄")	60	235	6	3	—	—	—	46	13	79	0.9	78	0	0.20	0.15	2.5	0
481	Stick (2¹/₄" long) ...... 10 pretzels	3	10	tr	tr	—	—	—	2	1	4	tr	4	0	0.01	0.01	0.1	0
	Rice, white, enriched																	
482	Instant, ready-to-serve, hot ... 1 c	165	180	4	tr	tr	tr	tr	40	5	31	1.3	—	0	0.21	(59)	1.7	0
	Long grain																	
483	Raw .... 1 c	185	670	12	1	0.2	0.2	0.2	149	44	174	5.4	170	0	0.81	0.06	6.5	0
484	Cooked, served hot .... 1 c	205	225	4	tr	0.1	0.1	0.1	50	21	57	1.8	57	0	0.23	0.02	2.1	0
	Parboiled																	
485	Raw .... 1 c	185	685	14	1	0.2	0.1	0.2	150	111	370	5.4	278	0	0.81	0.07	6.5	0
486	Cooked, served hot .... 1 c	175	185	4	tr	0.1	0.1	0.1	41	33	100	1.4	75	0	0.19	0.02	2.1	0
	Rolls, enriched[38]																	
	Commercial																	
487	Brown-and-serve (12 per 12-oz pkg), browned 1 roll	26	85	2	2	0.4	0.7	0.5	14	20	23	0.5	25	tr	0.10	0.06	0.9	tr
488	Cloverleaf or pan (2¹/₂" diam, 2" high) 1 roll	28	85	2	2	0.4	0.6	0.4	15	21	24	0.5	27	tr	0.11	0.07	0.9	tr
489	Frankfurter and hamburger (8 per 11¹/₂-oz pkg) 1 roll	40	120	3	2	0.5	0.8	0.6	21	30	34	0.8	38	tr	0.16	0.10	1.3	tr
490	Hard (3³/₄" diam, 2" high) 1 roll	50	155	5	2	0.4	0.6	0.5	30	24	46	1.2	49	tr	0.20	0.12	1.7	tr
491	Hoagie or submarine (11¹/₂" × 3" × 2¹/₂") 1 roll	135	390	12	4	0.9	1.4	1.4	75	58	115	3.0	122	tr	0.54	0.32	4.5	tr
	From home recipe																	
492	Cloverleaf (2¹/₂" diam, 2" 1 roll high)	35	120	3	3	0.8	1.1	0.7	20	16	36	0.7	41	30	0.12	0.12	1.2	tr
	Spaghetti, enriched, cooked																	
493	Firm stage, "al dente," served hot 1 c	130	190	7	1	—	—	—	39	14	85	1.4	103	0	0.23	0.13	1.8	0
494	Tender stage, served hot 1 c	140	155	5	1	—	—	—	32	11	70	1.3	85	0	0.20	0.11	1.5	0
	Spaghetti (enriched) in tomato sauce with cheese																	
495	From home recipe ..... 1 c	250	260	9	9	2.0	5.4	0.7	37	80	135	2.3	408	1080	0.25	0.18	2.3	13
496	Canned .... 1 c	250	190	6	2	0.5	0.3	0.4	39	40	88	2.8	303	930	0.35	0.28	4.5	10

(Continued)

Table A-1. Nutritive Values of the Edible Part of Foods (Continued)

(Dashes (—) denote lack of reliable data for a constituent believed to be present in measurable amount)

Item No. (A)	Foods, Approximate Measures, Units, and Weight (edible part unless footnotes indicate otherwise) (B)	Water Percent (C)	Food Energy Calories (D)	Protein g (E)	Fat g (F)	Fatty Acids Satu-rated (Total) g (G)	Unsaturated Oleic g (H)	Lino-leic g (I)	Carbo-hydrate g (J)	Calcium mg (K)	Phos-phorus mg (L)	Iron mg (M)	Potas-sium mg (N)	Vitamin A Value IU (O)	Thiamin mg (P)	Ribo-flavin mg (Q)	Niacin mg (R)	Ascorbic Acid mg (S)
	Grain Products (Continued)																	
	Spaghetti (enriched) with meat balls and tomato sauce																	
497	From home recipe ..... 1 c	70	330	19	12	3.3	6.3	0.9	39	124	236	3.7	665	1590	0.25	0.30	4.0	22
498	Canned .... 1 c	78	260	12	10	2.2	3.3	3.9	29	53	113	3.3	245	1000	0.15	0.18	2.3	5
499	Toaster pastries ...... 1 pastry	12	200	3	6	—	—	—	36	54[60]	67[60]	1.9	74[60]	500	0.16	0.17	2.1	(60)
	Waffles, made with enriched flour, 7" diam[38]																	
500	From home recipe ..... 1 waffle	41	210	7	7	2.3	2.8	1.4	28	85	130	1.3	109	250	0.17	0.23	1.4	tr
501	From mix, egg and milk added ... 1 waffle	42	205	7	8	2.8	2.9	1.2	27	179	257	1.0	146	170	0.14	0.22	0.9	tr
	Wheat flours																	
	All-purpose or family flour, enriched																	
502	Sifted, spooned ...... 1 c	12	420	12	1	0.2	0.1	0.5	88	18	100	3.3	109	0	0.74	0.46	6.1	0
503	Unsifted, spooned .... 1 c	12	455	13	1	0.2	0.1	0.5	95	20	109	3.6	119	0	0.80	0.50	6.6	0
504	Cake or pastry flour, enriched, sifted, spooned .... 1 c	12	350	7	1	0.1	0.1	0.3	76	16	70	2.8	191	0	0.61	0.38	5.1	0
505	Self-rising, enriched, unsifted, spooned ... 1 c	12	440	12	1	0.2	0.1	0.5	93	331	583	3.6	—	0	0.80	0.50	6.6	0
506	Whole-wheat, from hard wheats, stirred ... 1 c	12	400	16	2	0.4	0.2	1.0	85	49	446	4.0	444	0	0.66	0.14	5.2	0
	Legumes (Dry), Nuts, Seeds, and Related Products																	
	Almonds, shelled																	
507	Chopped (about 130 almonds) .... 1 c	5	775	24	70	5.6	47.7	12.8	25	304	655	6.1	1005	0	0.31	1.20	4.6	tr
508	Slivered, not pressed down (about 115 almonds) .... 1 c	5	690	21	62	5.0	42.2	11.3	22	269	580	5.4	889	0	0.28	1.06	4.0	tr
	Beans, dry																	
	Common varieties as Great Northern, navy, and others																	

428

(Continued)

(A)	(B)	Measure	g	(C)	(D)	(E)	(F)	(G)	(H)	(I)	(J)	(K)	(L)	(M)	(N)	(O)	(P)	(Q)	(R)	(S)
	Cooked, drained																			
509	Great Northern	1 c	180	69	210	14	1	—	—	—	38	90	266	4.9	749	0	0.25	0.13	1.3	0
510	Pea (navy)	1 c	190	69	225	15	1	—	—	—	40	95	281	5.1	790	0	0.27	0.13	1.3	0
	Canned, solids and liquid																			
	White with—																			
511	Frankfurters (sliced)	1 c	255	71	365	19	18	—	—	—	32	94	303	4.8	668	330	0.18	0.15	3.3	tr
512	Pork and tomato sauce	1 c	255	71	310	16	7	2.4	2.8	0.6	48	138	235	4.6	536	330	0.20	0.08	1.5	5
513	Pork and sweet sauce	1 c	255	66	385	16	12	4.3	5.0	1.1	54	161	291	5.9	—	—	0.15	0.10	1.3	—
514	Red kidney	1 c	255	76	230	15	1	—	—	—	42	74	278	4.6	673	10	0.13	0.10	1.5	—
515	Lima, cooked, drained	1 c	190	64	260	16	1	—	—	—	49	55	293	5.9	1163	—	0.25	0.11	1.3	—
516	Blackeye peas, dry, cooked (with residual cooking liquid)	1 c	250	80	190	13	1	—	—	—	35	43	238	3.3	573	30	0.40	0.10	1.0	—
517	Brazil nuts, shelled (6–8 large kernels)	1 oz	28	5	185	4	19	4.8	6.2	7.1	3	53	196	1.0	203	tr	0.27	0.03	0.5	—
518	Cashew nuts, roasted in oil	1 c	140	5	785	24	64	12.9	36.8	10.2	41	53	522	5.3	650	140	0.60	0.35	2.5	—
	Coconut meat, fresh																			
519	Piece (about 2″ × 2″ × ½″)	1 piece	45	51	155	2	16	14.0	0.9	0.3	4	6	43	0.8	115	0	0.02	0.01	0.2	1
520	Shredded or grated, not pressed down	1 c	80	51	275	3	28	24.8	1.6	0.5	8	10	76	1.4	205	0	0.04	0.02	0.4	2
521	Filberts (hazelnuts), chopped (about 80 kernels)	1 c	115	6	730	14	72	5.1	55.2	7.3	19	240	388	3.9	810	—	0.53	—	1.0	tr
522	Lentils, whole, cooked	1 c	200	72	210	16	tr	—	—	—	39	50	238	4.2	498	40	0.14	0.12	1.2	0
523	Peanuts, roasted in oil, salted (whole, halves, chopped)	1 c	144	2	840	37	72	13.7	33.0	20.7	27	107	577	3.0	971	—	0.46	0.19	24.8	0
524	Peanut butter	1 tbsp	16	2	95	4	8	1.5	3.7	2.3	3	9	61	0.3	100	—	0.02	0.02	2.4	0
525	Peas, split, dry, cooked	1 c	200	70	230	16	1	—	—	—	42	22	178	3.4	592	80	0.30	0.18	1.8	—
526	Pecans, chopped or pieces (about 120 large halves)	1 c	118	3	810	11	84	7.2	50.5	20.0	17	86	341	2.8	712	150	1.01	0.15	1.1	2
527	Pumpkin and squash kernels, dry, hulled	1 c	140	4	775	41	65	11.8	23.5	27.5	21	71	1602	15.7	1386	100	0.34	0.27	3.4	—
528	Sunflower seeds, dry, hulled	1 c	145	5	810	35	69	8.2	13.7	43.2	29	174	1214	10.3	1334	70	2.84	0.33	7.8	—
	Walnuts																			
	Black																			
529	Chopped or broken kernels	1 c	125	3	785	26	74	6.3	13.3	45.7	19	tr	713	7.5	575	380	0.28	0.14	0.9	—
530	Ground (finely)	1 c	80	3	500	16	47	4.0	8.5	29.2	12	tr	456	4.8	368	240	0.18	0.09	0.6	—
531	Persian or English, chopped (about 60 halves)	1 c	120	4	780	18	77	8.4	11.8	42.2	19	119	456	3.7	540	40	0.40	0.16	1.1	2

Table A-1. Nutritive Values of the Edible Part of Foods (Continued)

(Dashes (—) denote lack of reliable data for a constituent believed to be present in measurable amount)

Item No. (A)	Foods, Approximate Measures, Units, and Weight (edible part unless footnotes indicate otherwise) (B)		Water Per-cent (C)	Food Energy Cal-ories (D)	Pro-tein (E)	Fat (F)	Fatty Acids			Carbo-hydrate (J)	Calcium (K)	Phos-phorus (L)	Iron (M)	Potas-sium (N)	Vitamin A Value (O)	Thiamin (P)	Ribo-flavin (Q)	Niacin (R)	Ascorbic Acid (S)
							Satu-rated (Total) (G)	Unsaturated Oleic (H)	Lino-leic (I)										
		g	Per-cent	Cal-ories	g	g	g	g	g	g	mg	mg	mg	mg	IU	mg	mg	mg	mg
Sugars and Sweets																			
	Cake icings																		
	Boiled, white																		
532	Plain .... 1 c	94	18	295	1	0	0	0	0	75	2	2	tr	17	0	tr	0.03	tr	0
533	With coconut .... 1 c	166	15	605	3	13	11.0	0.9	tr	124	10	50	0.8	277	0	0.02	0.07	0.3	0
	Uncooked																		
534	Chocolate made with milk and butter 1 c	275	14	1035	9	38	23.4	11.7	1.0	185	165	305	3.3	536	580	0.06	0.28	0.6	1
535	Creamy fudge from mix 1 c and water	245	15	830	7	16	5.1	6.7	3.1	183	96	218	2.7	238	tr	0.05	0.20	0.7	tr
536	White .... 1 c	319	11	1200	2	21	12.7	5.1	0.5	260	48	38	tr	57	860	tr	0.06	tr	tr
	Candy																		
537	Caramels, plain or chocolate 1 oz	28	8	115	1	3	1.6	1.1	0.1	22	42	35	0.4	54	tr	0.01	0.05	0.1	tr
	Chocolate																		
538	Milk, plain .... 1 oz	28	1	145	2	9	5.5	3.0	0.3	16	65	65	0.3	109	80	0.02	0.10	0.1	tr
539	Semisweet, small pieces 1 c or 6-oz pkg (60 per oz)	170	1	860	7	61	36.2	19.8	1.7	97	51	255	4.4	553	30	0.02	0.14	0.9	0
540	Chocolate-coated peanuts 1 oz	28	1	160	5	12	4.0	4.7	2.1	11	33	84	0.4	143	tr	0.10	0.05	2.1	tr
541	Fondant, uncoated 1 oz (mints, candy corn, other)	28	8	105	tr	1	0.1	0.3	0.1	25	4	2	0.3	1	0	tr	tr	tr	0
542	Fudge, chocolate, plain 1 oz	28	8	115	1	3	1.3	1.4	0.6	21	22	24	0.3	42	tr	0.01	0.03	0.1	tr
543	Gum drops .... 1 oz	28	12	100	tr	tr	—	—	—	25	2	tr	0.1	1	0	0	tr	tr	0
544	Hard .... 1 oz	28	1	110	0	tr	—	—	—	28	6	2	0.5	1	0	0	0	0	0
545	Marshmallows .... 1 oz	28	17	90	1	tr	—	—	—	23	5	2	0.5	2	0	0	tr	tr	0
	Chocolate-flavored beverage powders (about 4 heaping tsp per oz)																		
546	With non-fat dry milk .. 1 oz	28	2	100	5	1	0.5	0.3	tr	20	167	155	0.5	227	10	0.04	0.21	0.2	1
547	Without milk .... 1 oz	28	1	100	1	1	0.4	0.2	tr	25	9	48	0.6	142	—	0.01	0.03	0.1	0
548	Honey, strained or 1 tbsp extracted	21	17	65	tr	0	0	0	0	17	1	1	0.1	11	0	tr	0.01	0.1	tr
549	Jams and preserves ..... 1 tbsp	20	29	55	tr	tr	—	—	—	14	4	2	0.2	18	tr	tr	0.01	tr	tr
550	1 packet	14	29	40	tr	tr	—	—	—	10	3	1	0.1	12	tr	tr	tr	tr	tr
551	Jellies .... 1 tbsp	18	29	50	tr	tr	—	—	—	13	4	1	0.3	14	tr	tr	0.01	tr	1
552	1 packet	14	29	40	tr	tr	—	—	—	10	3	1	0.2	11	tr	tr	tr	tr	1

(A)	(B)		(C)	(D)	(E)	(F)	(G)	(H)	(I)	(J)	(K)	(L)	(M)	(N)	(O)	(P)	(Q)	(R)	(S)
	Syrups																		
	Chocolate-flavored syrup or topping																		
553	Thin type .... 1 fl oz or 2 tbsp	38	32	90	1	1	0.5	0.3	tr	24	6	35	0.6	106	tr	0.01	0.03	0.2	0
554	Fudge type .... 1 fl oz or 2 tbsp	38	25	125	2	5	3.1	1.6	0.1	20	48	60	0.5	107	60	0.02	0.08	0.2	tr
	Molasses, cane																		
555	Light (first extraction) .... 1 tbsp	20	24	50	—	—	—	—	—	13	33	9	0.9	183	—	0.01	0.01	tr	—
556	Blackstrap (third extraction) .... 1 tbsp	20	24	45	—	—	—	—	—	11	137	17	3.2	585	—	0.02	0.04	0.4	—
557	Sorghum .... 1 tbsp	21	23	55	—	—	—	—	—	14	35	5	2.6	—	—	—	0.02	tr	—
558	Table blends, chiefly corn, light and dark .... 1 tbsp	21	24	60	0	0	0	0	0	15	9	3	0.8	1	0	0	0	0	0
	Sugars																		
559	Brown, pressed down .. 1 c	220	2	820	0	0	0	0	0	212	187	42	7.5	757	0	0.02	0.07	0.4	0
	White																		
560	Granulated .... 1 c	200	1	770	0	0	0	0	0	199	0	0	0.2	6	0	0	0	0	0
561	.... 1 tbsp	12	1	45	0	0	0	0	0	12	0	0	tr	tr	0	0	0	0	0
562	.... 1 packet	6	1	23	0	0	0	0	0	6	0	0	tr	tr	0	0	0	0	0
563	Powdered, sifted, spooned into cup .... 1 c	100	1	385	0	0	0	0	0	100	0	0	0.1	3	0	0	0	0	0
	Vegetable and Vegetable Products																		
	Asparagus, green																		
	Cooked, drained																		
	Cuts and tips (1½"–2" lengths)																		
564	From raw .... 1 c	145	94	30	3	tr	—	—	—	5	30	73	0.9	265	1310	0.23	0.26	2.0	38
565	From frozen .... 1 c	180	93	40	6	tr	—	—	—	6	40	115	2.2	396	1530	0.25	0.23	1.8	41
	Spears (½" diam at base)																		
566	From raw .... 4 spears	60	94	10	1	tr	—	—	—	2	13	30	0.4	110	540	0.10	0.11	0.8	16
567	From frozen .... 4 spears	60	92	15	2	tr	—	—	—	2	13	40	0.7	143	470	0.10	0.08	0.7	16
568	Canned, spears (½" diam at base) .... 4 spears	80	93	15	2	tr	—	—	—	3	15	42	1.5	133	640	0.05	0.08	0.6	12
	Beans																		
	Lima, immature seeds, frozen, cooked, drained																		
569	Thick-seeded types (Fordhooks) .... 1 c	170	74	170	10	tr	—	—	—	32	34	153	2.9	724	390	0.12	0.09	1.7	29
570	Thin-seeded types (baby limas) .... 1 c	180	69	210	13	tr	—	—	—	40	63	227	4.7	709	400	0.16	0.09	2.2	22
	Snap																		
	Green																		
	Cooked, drained																		
571	From raw (cuts and French style) .... 1 c	125	92	30	2	tr	—	—	—	7	63	46	0.8	189	680	0.09	0.11	0.6	15

(Continued)

Table A-1. Nutritive Values of the Edible Part of Foods (Continued)

(Dashes (—) denote lack of reliable data for a constituent believed to be present in measurable amount)

Item No. (A)	Foods, Approximate Measures, Units, and Weight (edible part unless footnotes indicate otherwise) (B)		Water Per-cent (C)	Food Energy Cal-ories (D)	Pro-tein (E)	Fat (F)	Fatty Acids Satu-rated (Total) (G)	Unsaturated Oleic (H)	Lino-leic (I)	Carbo-hydrate (J)	Calcium (K)	Phos-phorus (L)	Iron (M)	Potas-sium (N)	Vitamin A Value (O)	Thiamin (P)	Ribo-flavin (Q)	Niacin (R)	Ascorbic Acid (S)
		g	Percent	Calories	g	g	g	g	g	g	mg	mg	mg	mg	IU	mg	mg	mg	mg
	Vegetable and Vegetable Products (Continued)																		
	Beans, snap, green, cooked, drained (Continued)																		
	From frozen																		
572	Cuts .... 1 c	135	92	35	2	tr	—	—	—	8	54	43	0.9	205	780	0.09	0.12	0.5	7
573	French style .... 1 c	130	92	35	2	tr	—	—	—	8	49	39	1.2	177	690	0.08	0.10	0.4	9
574	Canned, drained solids 1 c (cuts)	135	92	30	2	tr	—	—	—	7	61	34	2.0	128	630	0.04	0.07	0.4	5
	Yellow or wax																		
575	Cooked, drained From raw (cuts and French style) 1 c	125	93	30	2	tr	—	—	—	6	63	46	0.8	189	290	0.09	0.11	0.6	16
576	From frozen (cuts) .. 1 c	135	92	35	2	tr	—	—	—	8	47	42	0.9	221	140	0.09	0.11	0.5	8
577	Canned, drained solids 1 c (cuts)	135	92	30	2	tr	—	—	—	7	61	34	2.0	128	140	0.04	0.07	0.4	7
	Beans, mature (see Beans, dry, items 509-515, and Blackeye peas, dry, item 516)																		
	Bean sprouts (mung)																		
578	Raw .... 1 c	105	89	35	4	tr	—	—	—	7	20	67	1.4	234	20	0.14	0.14	0.8	20
579	Cooked, drained ..... 1 c	125	91	35	4	tr	—	—	—	7	21	60	1.1	195	30	0.11	0.13	0.9	8
	Beets																		
	Cooked, drained, peeled																		
580	Whole beets (2" diam) 2 beets	100	91	30	1	tr	—	—	—	7	14	23	0.5	208	20	0.03	0.04	0.3	6
581	Diced or sliced ...... 1 c	170	91	55	2	tr	—	—	—	12	24	39	0.9	354	30	0.05	0.07	0.5	10
	Canned, drained solids																		
582	Whole beets, small .... 1 c	160	89	60	2	tr	—	—	—	14	30	29	1.1	267	30	0.02	0.05	0.2	5
583	Diced or sliced ...... 1 c	170	89	65	2	tr	—	—	—	15	32	31	1.2	284	30	0.02	0.05	0.2	5
584	Beet greens, leaves and stems, cooked, drained 1 c	145	94	25	2	tr	—	—	—	5	144	36	2.8	481	7400	0.10	0.22	0.4	22
	Blackeye peas, immature seeds, cooked and drained																		
585	From raw .... 1 c	165	72	180	13	1	1	—	—	30	40	241	3.5	625	580	0.50	0.18	2.3	28
586	From frozen .... 1 c	170	66	220	15	1	1	—	—	40	43	286	4.8	573	290	0.68	0.19	2.4	15
	Broccoli, cooked, drained																		
	From raw																		
587	Stalk, medium size ... 1 stalk	180	91	45	6	1	1	—	—	8	158	112	1.4	481	4500	0.16	0.36	1.4	162
588	Stalks cut into 1/2"pieces 1 c	155	91	40	5	tr	tr	—	—	7	136	96	1.2	414	3880	0.14	0.31	1.2	140
	From frozen																		
589	Stalk (4 1/2"–5"long) ... 1 stalk	30	91	10	1	tr	tr	—	—	1	12	17	0.2	66	570	0.02	0.03	0.2	22

(A)	(B)		(C)	(D)	(E)	(F)	(G)	(H)	(I)	(J)	(K)	(L)	(M)	(N)	(O)	(P)	(Q)	(R)	(S)
590	Chopped	1 c	185	92	50	5	1	—	—	9	100	104	1.3	392	4810	0.11	0.22	0.9	105
	Brussels sprouts, cooked, drained																		
591	From raw, 7–8 sprouts (1 1/4"–1 1/2" diam)	1 c	155	88	55	7	1	—	—	10	50	112	1.7	423	810	0.12	0.22	1.2	135
592	From frozen	1 c	155	89	50	5	tr	—	—	10	33	95	1.2	457	880	0.12	0.16	0.9	126
	Cabbage																		
	Common varieties																		
	Raw																		
593	Coarsely shredded or sliced	1 c	70	92	15	1	tr	—	—	4	34	20	0.3	163	90	0.04	0.04	0.2	33
594	Finely shredded or chopped	1 c	90	92	20	1	tr	—	—	5	44	26	0.4	210	120	0.05	0.05	0.3	42
595	Cooked, drained	1 c	145	94	30	2	tr	—	—	6	64	29	0.4	236	190	0.06	0.06	0.4	48
596	Red, raw, coarsely shredded or sliced	1 c	70	90	20	1	tr	—	—	5	29	25	0.6	188	30	0.06	0.04	0.3	43
597	Savoy, raw, coarsely shredded or sliced	1 c	70	92	15	2	tr	—	—	3	47	38	0.6	188	140	0.04	0.06	0.2	39
598	Cabbage, celery (also called pe-tsai or wongbok), raw, 1" pieces	1 c	75	95	10	1	tr	—	—	2	32	30	0.5	190	110	0.04	0.03	0.5	19
599	Cabbage, white mustard (also called bokchoy or pakchoy), cooked, drained	1 c	170	95	25	2	tr	—	—	4	252	56	1.0	364	5270	0.07	0.14	1.2	26
	Carrots																		
	Raw, without crowns and tips, scraped																		
600	Whole (7 1/2" × 1 1/8", or 18 strips, 2 1/2"–3" long)	1 carrot or 18 strips	72	88	30	1	tr	—	—	7	27	26	0.5	246	7930	0.04	0.04	0.4	6
601	Grated	1 c	110	88	45	1	tr	—	—	11	41	40	0.8	375	12,100	0.07	0.06	0.7	9
602	Cooked (crosswise cuts), drained	1 c	155	91	50	1	tr	—	—	11	51	48	0.9	344	16,280	0.08	0.08	0.8	9
	Canned																		
603	Sliced, drained solids	1 c	155	91	45	1	tr	—	—	10	47	34	1.1	186	23,250	0.03	0.05	0.6	3
604	Strained or junior (baby food)	1 oz (1 3/4–2 tbsp)	28	92	10	tr	tr	—	—	2	7	6	0.1	51	3690	0.01	0.01	0.1	1
	Cauliflower																		
605	Raw, chopped	1 c	115	91	31	3	tr	—	—	6	29	64	1.3	339	70	0.13	0.12	0.8	90
	Cooked, drained																		
606	From raw (flower buds)	1 c	125	93	30	3	tr	—	—	5	26	53	0.9	258	80	0.11	0.10	0.8	69
607	From frozen (flowerets)	1 c	180	94	30	3	tr	—	—	6	31	68	0.9	373	50	0.07	0.09	0.7	74
608	Celery, Pascal type, raw / Stalk, large outer (8" × 1 1/2" at root end)	1 stalk	40	94	5	tr	tr	—	—	2	16	11	0.1	136	110	0.01	0.01	0.1	4

(Continued)

433

Table A-1. Nutritive Values of the Edible Part of Foods (Continued)

(Dashes (—) denote lack of reliable data for a constituent believed to be present in measurable amount)

Item No. (A)	Foods, Approximate Measures, Units, and footnotes (B)	Weight (edible part unless indicated otherwise) g	Water (C) Per cent	Food Energy (D) Calories	Pro-tein (E) g	Fat (F) g	Fatty Acids Saturated (Total) (G) g	Unsaturated Oleic (H) g	Linoleic (I) g	Carbo-hydrate (J) g	Calcium (K) mg	Phos-phorus (L) mg	Iron (M) mg	Potas-sium (N) mg	Vitamin A Value (O) IU	Thiamin (P) mg	Ribo-flavin (Q) mg	Niacin (R) mg	Ascorbic Acid (S) mg
	Vegetable and Vegetable Products (Continued)																		
	Celery, Pascal type, raw (Continued)																		
609	Pieces, diced ... 1 c	120	94	20	1	tr	—	—	—	5	47	34	0.4	409	320	0.04	0.04	0.4	11
	Collards, cooked, drained																		
610	From raw (leaves without stems) 1 c	190	90	65	7	1	—	—	—	10	357	99	1.5	498	14,820	0.21	0.38	2.3	144
611	From frozen (chopped) 1 c	170	90	50	5	1	—	—	—	10	299	87	1.7	401	11,560	0.10	0.24	1.0	56
	Corn, sweet																		
	Cooked, drained																		
612	From raw, ear (5" × 1¾") 1 ear[61]	140	74	70	2	1	—	—	—	16	2	69	0.5	151	310[62]	0.09	0.08	1.1	7
	From frozen																		
613	Ear (5" long) 1 ear[61]	229	73	120	4	1	—	—	—	27	4	121	1.0	291	440[62]	0.18	0.10	2.1	9
614	Kernels 1 c	165	77	130	5	1	—	—	—	31	5	120	1.3	304	580[62]	0.15	0.10	2.5	8
	Canned																		
615	Cream style 1 c	256	76	210	5	2	—	—	—	51	8	143	1.5	248	840[62]	0.08	0.13	2.6	13
	Whole kernel																		
616	Vacuum pack 1 c	210	76	175	5	1	—	—	—	43	6	153	1.1	204	740[62]	0.06	0.13	2.3	11
617	Wet pack, drained solids 1 c	165	76	140	4	1	—	—	—	33	8	81	0.8	160	580[62]	0.05	0.08	1.5	7
	Cowpeas (see Blackeye peas, Items 585–586)																		
	Cucumber slices, ⅛" thick (large, 2⅛" diam; small, 1¾" diam)																		
618	With peel 6 large or 8 small slices	28	95	5	tr	tr	—	—	—	1	7	8	0.3	45	70	0.01	0.01	0.1	3
619	Without peel 6½ large or 9 small pieces	28	96	5	tr	tr	—	—	—	1	5	5	0.1	45	tr	0.01	0.01	0.1	3
620	Dandelion greens, cooked, drained 1 c	105	90	35	2	1	—	—	—	7	147	44	1.9	244	12,290	0.14	0.17	—	19
621	Endive, curly (including escarole), raw, small pieces 1 c	50	93	10	1	tr	—	—	—	2	41	27	0.9	147	1650	0.04	0.07	0.3	5
	Kale, cooked, drained																		
622	From raw (leaves without stems and midribs) 1 c	110	88	45	5	1	—	—	—	7	206	64	1.8	243	9130	0.11	0.20	1.8	102
623	From frozen (leaf style) 1 c	130	91	40	4	1	—	—	—	7	157	62	1.3	251	10,660	0.08	0.20	0.9	49

(A)	(B)	(C)	(D)	(E)	(F)	(G)	(H)	(I)	(J)	(K)	(L)	(M)	(N)	(O)	(P)	(Q)	(R)	(S)
	Lettuce, raw																	
	Butterhead, as Boston types																	
624	Head, 5″ diam ... 1 head[63]	220	95	25	2	tr	—	—	—	4	57	42	3.3	430	1580 0.10	0.10	0.5	13
625	Leaves ... 1 outer, 2 inner, or 3 heart leaves	15	95	tr	tr	tr	—	—	—	tr	5	4	0.3	40	150 0.01	0.01	tr	1
	Crisphead, as Iceberg																	
626	Head, 6″ diam ... 1 head[64]	567	96	70	5	1	—	—	—	16	108	118	2.7	943	1780 0.32	0.32	1.6	32
627	Wedge, 1/4 of head ... 1 wedge	135	96	20	1	tr	—	—	—	4	27	30	0.7	236	450 0.08	0.08	0.4	8
628	Pieces, chopped or shredded ... 1 c	55	96	5	tr	tr	—	—	—	2	11	12	0.3	96	180 0.03	0.03	0.2	3
629	Looseleaf (bunching varieties including romaine or cos), chopped or shredded pieces ... 1 c	55	94	10	1	tr	—	—	—	2	37	14	0.8	145	1050 0.03	0.04	0.2	10
630	Mushrooms, raw, sliced or chopped ... 1 c	70	90	20	2	tr	—	—	—	3	4	81	0.6	290	tr 0.07	0.32	2.9	2
631	Mustard greens, without stems and midribs, cooked, drained ... 1 c	140	93	30	3	1	—	—	—	6	193	45	2.5	308	8120 0.11	0.20	0.8	67
632	Okra pods (3″ × 5/8″), cooked ... 10 pods	106	91	30	2	tr	—	—	—	6	98	43	0.5	184	520 0.14	0.19	1.0	21
	Onions																	
	Mature																	
	Raw																	
633	Chopped ... 1 c	170	89	65	3	tr	—	—	—	15	46	61	0.9	267	tr[65] 0.05	0.07	0.3	17
634	Sliced ... 1 c	115	89	45	2	tr	—	—	—	10	31	41	0.6	181	tr[65] 0.03	0.05	0.2	12
635	Cooked (whole or sliced), drained ... 1 c	210	92	60	3	tr	—	—	—	14	50	61	0.8	231	tr[65] 0.06	0.06	0.4	15
636	Young green, bulb (3/8″ diam) and white portion of top ... 6 onions	30	88	15	tr	tr	—	—	—	3	12	12	0.2	69	tr 0.02	0.01	0.1	8
637	Parsley, raw, chopped ... 1 tbsp	4	85	tr	tr	tr	—	—	—	tr	7	2	0.2	25	300 tr	0.01	tr	6
638	Parsnips, cooked (diced or 2″ lengths) ... 1 c	155	82	100	2	1	—	—	—	23	70	96	0.9	587	50 0.11	0.12	0.2	16
	Peas, green																	
	Canned																	
639	Whole, drained solids ... 1 c	170	77	150	8	1	—	—	—	29	44	129	3.2	163	1170 0.15	0.10	1.4	14
640	Strained (baby food) ... 1 oz (1 3/4 to 2 tbsp)	28	86	15	1	tr	—	—	—	3	3	18	0.3	28	140 0.02	0.03	0.3	3
641	Frozen, cooked, drained ... 1 c	160	82	110	8	tr	—	—	—	19	30	138	3.0	216	960 0.43	0.14	2.7	21
642	Peppers, hot, red, without seeds, dried (ground chili powder, added seasonings) ... 1 tsp	2	9	5	tr	tr	—	—	—	1	5	4	0.3	20	1300 tr	0.02	0.2	tr
	Peppers, sweet (about 5 per lb, whole), stem and seeds removed																	

(Continued)

435

Table A-1. Nutritive Values of the Edible Part of Foods (Continued)

(Dashes (—) denote lack of reliable data for a constituent believed to be present in measurable amount)

Item No. (A)	Foods, Approximate Measures, Units, and Weight (edible part unless footnotes indicate otherwise) (B)	(g)	Water Per-cent (C)	Food Energy Cal-ories (D)	Pro-tein (E)	Fat (F)	Fatty Acids Satu-rated (Total) (G)	Unsaturated Oleic (H)	Lino-leic (I)	Carbo-hydrate (J)	Calcium (K)	Phos-phorus (L)	Iron (M)	Potas-sium (N)	Vitamin A Value (O)	Thiamin (P)	Ribo-flavin (Q)	Niacin (R)	Ascorbic Acid (S)
		g	Per-cent	Cal-ories	g	g	g	g	g	g	mg	mg	mg	mg	IU	mg	mg	mg	mg
Vegetable and Vegetable Products (Continued)																			
	Peppers, sweet (Continued)																		
643	Raw .... 1 pod	74	93	15	1	tr	—	—	—	4	7	16	0.5	157	310	0.06	0.06	0.4	94
644	Cooked, boiled, drained 1 pod	73	95	15	1	tr	—	—	—	3	7	12	0.4	109	310	0.05	0.05	0.4	70
	Potatoes, cooked																		
645	Baked, peeled after baking (about 2 per lb, raw) 1 potato	156	75	145	4	tr	—	—	—	33	14	101	1.1	782	tr	0.15	0.07	2.7	31
	Boiled (about 3 per lb, raw)																		
646	Peeled after boiling ... 1 potato	137	80	105	3	tr	—	—	—	23	10	72	0.8	556	tr	0.12	0.05	2.0	22
647	Peeled before boiling ... 1 potato	135	83	90	3	tr	—	—	—	20	8	57	0.7	385	tr	0.12	0.05	1.6	22
	French-fried, strip (2 to 3½" long)																		
648	Prepared from raw ... 10 strips	50	45	135	2	7	1.7	1.2	3.3	18	8	56	0.7	427	tr	0.07	0.04	1.6	11
649	Frozen, oven-heated ... 10 strips	50	53	110	2	4	1.1	0.8	2.1	17	5	43	0.9	326	tr	0.07	0.01	1.3	11
650	Hashed brown, prepared from frozen 1 c	155	56	345	3	18	4.6	3.2	9.0	45	28	78	1.9	439	tr	0.11	0.03	1.6	12
	Mashed, prepared from— Raw																		
651	Milk added .... 1 c	210	83	135	4	2	0.7	0.4	tr	27	50	103	0.8	548	40	0.17	0.11	2.1	21
652	Milk and butter added 1 c	210	80	195	4	9	5.6	2.3	0.2	26	50	101	0.8	525	360	0.17	0.11	2.1	19
653	Dehydrated flakes (without milk), water, milk, butter, and salt added 1 c	210	79	195	4	7	3.6	2.1	0.2	30	65	99	0.6	601	270	0.08	0.08	1.9	11
654	Potato chips (1¾" × 2½" oval cross section) 10 chips	20	2	115	1	8	2.1	1.4	4.0	10	8	28	0.4	226	tr	0.04	0.01	1.0	3
655	Potato salad, made with cooked salad dressing 1 c	250	76	250	7	7	2.0	2.7	1.3	41	80	160	1.5	798	350	0.20	0.18	2.8	28
656	Pumpkin, canned .... 1 c	245	90	80	2	1	—	—	—	19	61	64	1.0	588	15,680	0.07	0.12	1.5	12
657	Radishes, raw 4 radishes	18	95	5	tr	tr	—	—	—	1	5	6	0.2	58	tr	0.01	0.01	0.1	5
658	Sauerkraut, canned, solids 1 c and liquid	235	93	40	2	tr	—	—	—	9	85	42	1.2	329	120	0.07	0.09	0.5	33
	Southern peas (see Blackeye peas, items 585–586)																		

(A)	(B)	(C)	(D)	(E)	(F)	(G)	(H)	(I)	(J)	(K)	(L)	(M)	(N)	(O)	(P)	(Q)	(R)	(S)
	Spinach																	
659	Raw, chopped .... 1 c	55	91	15	2	tr	—	—	2	51	28	1.7	259	4460	0.06	0.11	0.3	28
	Cooked, drained																	
660	From raw .... 1 c	180	92	40	5	1	—	—	6	167	68	4.0	583	14,580	0.13	0.25	0.9	50
	From frozen																	
661	Chopped .... 1 c	205	92	45	6	1	—	—	8	232	90	4.3	683	16,200	0.14	0.31	0.8	39
662	Leaf .... 1 c	190	92	45	6	1	—	—	7	200	84	4.8	688	15,390	0.15	0.27	1.0	53
663	Canned, drained solids .. 1 c	205	91	50	6	1	—	0.1	7	242	53	5.3	513	16,400	0.04	0.25	0.6	29
	Squash, cooked																	
664	Summer (all varieties), diced, drained .... 1 c	210	96	30	2	tr	—	—	7	53	53	0.8	296	820	0.11	0.17	1.7	21
665	Winter (all varieties), baked, mashed .... 1 c	205	81	130	4	1	—	—	32	57	98	1.6	945	8610	0.10	0.27	1.4	27
	Sweet potatoes																	
	Cooked (raw, 5" × 2", about 2½ per lb)																	
666	Baked in skin, peeled .. 1 potato	114	64	160	2	1	—	—	37	46	66	1.0	342	9230	0.10	0.08	0.8	25
667	Boiled in skin, peeled .. 1 potato	151	71	170	3	1	—	—	40	48	71	1.1	367	11,940	0.14	0.09	0.9	26
668	Candied, 2½" × 2" piece 1 piece	105	60	175	1	3	2.0	0.8	36	39	45	0.9	200	6620	0.06	0.04	0.4	11
	Canned																	
669	Solid pack (mashed) .. 1 c	255	72	275	5	1	—	—	63	64	105	2.0	510	19,890	0.13	0.10	1.5	36
670	Vacuum pack, piece (2¾" × 1") .... 1 piece	40	72	45	1	tr	—	—	10	10	16	0.3	80	3120	0.02	0.02	0.2	6
	Tomatoes																	
671	Raw (2⅗" diam, 3 per 12 oz pkg) .... 1 tomato[66]	135	94	25	1	tr	—	—	6	16	33	0.6	300	1110	0.07	0.05	0.9	28[67]
672	Canned, solids and liquid 1 c	241	94	50	2	tr	—	—	10	14[68]	46	1.2	523	2170	0.12	0.07	1.7	41
673	Tomato catsup .... 1 c	273	69	290	5	1	—	—	69	60	137	2.2	991	3820	0.25	0.19	4.4	41
674	.... 1 tbsp	15	69	15	tr	tr	—	—	4	3	8	0.1	54	210	0.01	0.01	0.2	2
	Tomato juice, canned																	
675	Cup .... 1 c	243	94	45	2	tr	—	—	10	17	44	2.2	552	1940	0.12	0.07	1.9	39
676	Glass (6 fl oz) ...... 1 glass	182	94	35	2	tr	—	—	8	13	33	1.6	413	1460	0.09	0.05	1.5	29
677	Turnips, cooked, diced .. 1 c	155	94	35	1	tr	—	—	8	54	37	0.6	291	tr	0.06	0.08	0.5	34
	Turnip greens, cooked, drained																	
678	From raw (leaves and stems) .... 1 c	145	94	30	3	tr	—	—	5	252	49	1.5	—	8270	0.15	0.33	0.7	68
679	From frozen (chopped) .. 1 c	165	93	40	4	tr	—	—	6	195	64	2.6	246	11,390	0.08	0.15	0.7	31
680	Vegetables, mixed, frozen, cooked .... 1 c	182	83	115	6	1	—	—	24	46	115	2.4	348	9010	0.22	0.13	2.0	15

Miscellaneous Items

Baking powders for home use

Sodium aluminum sulfate

(Continued)

Table A-1. Nutritive Values of the Edible Part of Foods (Continued)

(Dashes (—) denote lack of reliable data for a constituent believed to be present in measurable amount)

Item No. (A)	Foods, Approximate Measures, Units, and Weight (edible part unless footnotes indicate otherwise) (B)	Weight g	Water Per-cent (C)	Food Energy Calories (D)	Pro-tein g (E)	Fat g (F)	Fatty Acids Satu-rated (Total) g (G)	Fatty Acids Unsaturated Oleic g (H)	Fatty Acids Lino-leic g (I)	Carbo-hydrate g (J)	Calcium mg (K)	Phos-phorus mg (L)	Iron mg (M)	Potas-sium mg (N)	Vitamin A Value IU (O)	Thiamin mg (P)	Ribo-flavin mg (Q)	Niacin mg (R)	Ascorbic Acid mg (S)
	Miscellaneous Items (Continued)																		
	Baking powders for home use (Continued)																		
681	With monocalcium phosphate monohydrate 1 tsp	3.0	2	5	tr	tr	0	0	0	1	58	87	—	5	0	0	0	0	0
682	With monocalcium phosphate monohydrate, calcium sulfate 1 tsp	2.9	1	5	tr	tr	0	0	0	1	183	45	—	—	0	0	0	0	0
683	Straight phosphate 1 tsp	3.8	2	5	tr	tr	0	0	0	1	239	359	—	6	0	0	0	0	0
684	Low-sodium 1 tsp	4.3	2	5	tr	tr	0	0	0	2	207	314	—	471	0	0	0	0	0
685	Barbecue sauce 1 c	250	81	230	4	17	2.2	4.3	10.0	20	53	50	2.0	435	900	0.03	0.03	0.8	13
	Beverages, alcoholic																		
686	Beer 12 fl oz	360	92	150	1	0	0	0	0	14	18	108	tr	90	—	0.01	0.11	2.2	—
	Gin, rum, vodka, whisky																		
687	80-proof 1½-fl oz jigger	42	67	95	—	—	0	0	0	tr	—	—	—	1	—	—	—	—	—
688	86-proof 1½-fl oz jigger	42	64	105	—	—	0	0	0	tr	—	—	—	1	—	—	—	—	—
689	90-proof 1½-fl oz jigger	42	62	110	—	—	0	0	0	tr	—	—	—	1	—	—	—	—	—
	Wines																		
690	Dessert 3½-fl oz glass	103	77	140	tr	0	0	0	0	8	8	—	—	77	—	0.01	0.02	0.2	—
691	Table 3½-fl oz glass	102	86	85	tr	0	0	0	0	4	9	10	0.4	94	—	tr	0.01	0.1	—
	Beverages, carbonated, sweetened, nonalcoholic																		
692	Carbonated water 12 fl oz	366	92	115	0	0	0	0	0	29	—	—	—	—	0	0	0	0	0
693	Cola-type 12 fl oz	369	90	145	0	0	0	0	0	37	—	—	—	—	0	0	0	0	0
694	Fruit-flavored sodas and Tom Collins mixer 12 fl oz	372	88	170	0	0	0	0	0	45	—	—	—	—	0	0	0	0	0
695	Ginger ale 12 fl oz	366	92	115	0	0	0	0	0	29	—	—	—	0	0	0	0	0	0
696	Root beer 12 fl oz	370	90	150	0	0	0	0	0	39	—	—	—	0	0	0	0	0	0
	Chili powder (see Peppers, hot, red, item 642)																		
	Chocolate																		
697	Bitter or baking 1 oz	28	2	145	3	15	8.9	4.9	0.4	8	22	109	1.9	235	20	0.01	0.07	0.4	0
	Semisweet (see Candy, chocolate, item 539)																		
698	Gelatin, dry 1 7-g envelope	7	13	25	6	tr	0	0	0	0	—	—	—	—	—	—	—	—	—
699	Gelatin dessert prepared with gelatin dessert powder and water 1 c	240	84	140	4	0	0	0	0	34	—	—	—	—	—	—	—	—	—
700	Mustard, prepared, yellow 1 tsp or individual serving pouch or cup	5	80	5	tr	tr	—	—	—	tr	4	4	0.1	7	—	—	—	—	—

(A)	(B)	(C)	(D)	(E)	(F)	(G)	(H)	(I)	(J)	(K)	(L)	(M)	(N)	(O)	(P)	(Q)	(R)	(S)
	Olives, pickled, canned																	
701	Green .... 4 medium, 3 extra large, or 2 giant[69]	16	78	15	tr	2	0.2	1.2	0.1	tr	8	2	0.2	7	40	—	—	—
702	Ripe, Mission .... 3 small or 2 large[69]	10	73	15	tr	2	0.2	1.2	0.1	tr	9	1	0.1	2	10	tr	—	4
	Pickles, cucumber																	
703	Dill, medium, whole (3³/₄"long, 1¹/₄"diam) .... 1 pickle	65	93	5	tr	tr	—	—	—	1	17	14	0.7	130	70	0.01	tr	1
704	Fresh-pack, slices (1¹/₂" diam, ¹/₄" thick) ..... 2 slices	15	79	10	tr	tr	—	—	—	3	5	4	0.3	—	20	tr	tr	1
705	Sweet, gherkin, small, whole (about 2¹/₂"long, ³/₄" diam) .... 1 pickle	15	61	20	tr	tr	—	—	—	5	2	2	0.2	—	10	tr	tr	1
706	Relish, finely chopped, sweet ..... 1 tbsp	15	63	20	tr	tr	—	—	—	5	3	2	0.1	—	—	—	—	—
	Popcorn (see items 476–478)																	
707	Popsicle, 3-fl oz size .... 1 popsicle	95	80	70	0	0	0	0	0	18	0	—	tr	—	0	0	0	0
	Soups																	
	Canned, condensed																	
	Prepared with equal volume of milk																	
708	Cream of chicken ...... 1 c	245	85	180	7	10	4.2	3.6	1.3	15	172	152	0.5	260	610	0.27	0.7	2
709	Cream of mushroom ..... 1 c	245	83	215	7	14	5.4	2.9	4.6	16	191	169	0.5	279	250	0.34	0.7	1
710	Tomato .... 1 c	250	84	175	7	7	3.4	1.7	1.0	23	168	155	0.8	418	1200	0.25	1.3	15
	Prepared with equal volume of water																	
711	Bean with pork ...... 1 c	250	84	170	8	6	1.2	1.8	2.4	22	63	128	2.3	395	650	0.08	1.0	3
712	Beef broth, bouillon, consummé ..... 1 c	240	96	30	5	0	0	0	0	3	tr	31	0.5	130	tr	0.02	1.2	—
713	Beef noodle .... 1 c	240	93	65	4	3	0.6	0.7	0.8	7	7	48	1.0	77	50	0.07	1.0	tr
714	Clam chowder, Manhattan-type (with tomatoes, without milk) ..... 1 c	245	92	80	2	3	0.5	0.4	1.3	12	34	47	1.0	184	860	0.02	1.0	—
715	Cream of chicken ..... 1 c	240	92	95	3	6	1.6	2.3	1.1	8	24	34	0.5	79	410	0.05	0.5	tr
716	Cream of mushroom ..... 1 c	240	90	135	2	10	2.6	1.7	4.5	10	41	50	0.5	98	70	0.12	0.7	tr
717	Minestrone .... 1 c	245	90	105	5	3	0.7	0.9	1.3	14	37	59	1.0	314	2350	0.05	1.0	—
718	Split pea .... 1 c	245	85	145	9	3	1.1	1.2	0.4	21	29	149	1.5	270	440	0.15	1.5	1
719	Tomato .... 1 c	245	91	90	2	3	0.5	0.5	1.0	16	15	34	0.7	230	1000	0.05	1.2	12
720	Vegetable beef .... 1 c	245	92	80	5	2	—	—	—	10	12	49	0.7	162	2700	0.05	1.0	—
721	Vegetarian .... 1 c	245	92	80	2	2	—	—	—	13	20	39	1.0	172	2940	0.05	1.0	—
	Dehydrated																	
722	Bouillon cube (¹/₂") .... 1 cube	4	4	5	1	tr	—	—	—	tr	—	—	—	4	—	—	—	—
	Mixes																	
	Unprepared																	
723	Onion .... 1¹/₂-oz pkg	43	3	150	6	5	1.1	2.3	1.0	23	42	49	0.6	238	30	0.03	0.3	6

(Continued)

Table A-1. Nutritive Values of the Edible Part of Foods (Continued)

(Dashes (—) denote lack of reliable data for a constituent believed to be present in measurable amount)

Item No. (A)	Foods, Approximate Measures, Units, and Weight (edible part unless footnotes indicate otherwise) (B)	Weight g	Water Percent (C)	Food Energy Calories (D)	Protein g (E)	Fat g (F)	Fatty Acids Saturated (Total) g (G)	Oleic g (H)	Linoleic g (I)	Carbohydrate g (J)	Calcium mg (K)	Phosphorus mg (L)	Iron mg (M)	Potassium mg (N)	Vitamin A Value IU (O)	Thiamin mg (P)	Riboflavin mg (Q)	Niacin mg (R)	Ascorbic Acid mg (S)
	Miscellaneous Items (Continued)																		
	Soups, dehydrated, mixes (Continued)																		
	Prepared with water																		
724	Chicken noodle ..... 1 c	240	95	55	2	1	—	—	—	8	7	19	0.2	19	50	0.07	0.05	0.5	tr
725	Onion ..... 1 c	240	96	35	1	1	—	—	—	6	10	12	0.2	58	tr	tr	tr	tr	2
726	Tomato vegetable with noodles ..... 1 c	240	93	65	1	1	—	—	—	12	7	19	0.2	29	480	0.05	0.02	0.5	5
727	Vinegar, cider ..... 1 tbsp	15	94	tr	tr	0	0	0	0	1	1	1	0.1	15	—	—	—	—	—
728	White sauce, medium, with enriched flour ..... 1 c	250	73	405	10	31	19.3	7.8	0.8	22	288	233	0.5	348	1150	0.12	0.43	0.7	2
	Yeast																		
729	Baker's, dry, active ..... 1 pkg	7	5	20	3	tr	—	—	—	3	3	90	1.1	140	tr	0.16	0.38	2.6	tr
730	Brewer's, dry ..... 1 tbsp	8	5	25	3	tr	—	—	—	3	17[20]	140	1.4	152	tr	1.25	0.34	3.0	tr

Footnotes to table 1

[1] Vitamin A value is largely from beta-carotene used for coloring. Riboflavin value for items 40–41 applies to products with added riboflavin.

[2] Applies to product without added vitamin A. With added vitamin A, value is 500 International Units (IU).

[3] Applies to product without added vitamin A.

[4] Applies to product with added vitamin A. Without added vitamin A, value is 20 IU.

[5] Yields 1 qt fluid milk when reconstituted according to package directions.

[6] Applies to product with added vitamin A.

[7] Weight applies to product with label claim of 1⅓ cups equal 3.2 oz.

[8] Applies to products made from thick shake mixes and those that do not contain added ice cream. Products made from milk shake mixes are higher in fat and usually contain added ice cream.

[9] Content of fat, vitamin A, and carbohydrate varies. Consult the label when precise values are needed for special diets.

[10] Applies to product made with milk containing no added vitamin A.

[11] Based on year-round average.

[12] Based on average vitamin A content of fortified margarine. Federal specifications for fortified margarine require a minimum of 15,000 IU vitamin A per pound.

[13] Fatty acid values apply to product made with regular-type margarine.

[14] Dipped in egg, milk or water, and breadcrumbs; fried in vegetable shortening.

[15] If bones are discarded, value for calcium will be greatly reduced.

[16] Dipped in egg, breadcrumbs, and flour or batter.

[17] Prepared with tuna, celery, salad dressing (mayonnaise type), pickle, onion, and egg.

[18] Outer layer of fat on the cut was removed to within approximately ½" of the lean. Deposits of fat within the cut were not removed.

[19] Crust made with vegetable shortening and enriched flour.

[20] Regular-type margarine used.

[21] Value varies widely.

[22] About one-fourth of the outer layer of fat on the cut was removed. Deposits of fat within the cut were not removed.

[23] Vegetable shortening used.

[24] Also applies to pasteurized apple cider.

[25] Applies to product without added ascorbic acid. For value of product with added ascorbic acid, refer to label.

[26] Based on product with label claim of 45% of U.S. RDA in 6 fl oz.

[27] Based on product with label claim of 100% of U.S. RDA in 6 fl oz.

[28] Weight includes peel and membranes between sections. Without these parts the weight of the edible portion is 123 g for item 246 and 118 g for item 247.

[29] For white-fleshed varieties, value is about 20 IU per cup; for red-fleshed varieties, 1080 IU.

[30] Weight includes seeds. Without seeds, weight of the edible portion is 57 g.

[31] Applies to product without added ascorbic acid. With added ascorbic acid, based on claim that 6 fl oz of reconstituted juice contains 45% or 50% of the U.S. RDA, value is 108 mg or 120 mg for a 6-fl oz can (item 258), 36 or 40 for 1 cup of diluted juice (item 259).

[32] For products with added thiamin and riboflavin but without added ascorbic acid, values would be 0.60 mg for thiamin, 0.80 mg for riboflavin, and trace for ascorbic acid. For products with only ascorbic acid added, value varies with the brand. Consult the label.

[33] Weight includes rind. Without rind, the weight of the edible portion is 272 g for item 271 and 149 g for item 272.

[34] Represents yellow-fleshed varieties. For white-fleshed varieties, value is 50 IU for 1 peach, 90 IU for 1 cup of slices.

[35] Value represents products with added ascorbic acid. For products without added ascorbic acid, value is 116 mg for a 10-oz container, 103 mg for 1 cup.

[36] Weight includes pits. After removal of the pits, the weight of the edible portion is 258 g for item 302, 133 g for item 303, 43 g for item 304, and 213 g for item 305.

[37] Weight includes rind and seeds. Without rind and seeds, weight of the edible portion is 426 g.

[38] Made with vegetable shortening.

[39]Applies to product made with white cornmeal. With yellow cornmeal, value is 30 IU.

[40]Applies to white varieties. For yellow varieties, value is 150 IU.

[41]Applies to products that do not contain disodium phosphate. If disodium phosphate is an ingredient, value is 162 mg.

[42]Value may range from less than 1 mg to about 8 mg depending on the brand. Consult the label.

[43]Applies to product with added nutrient. Without added nutrient, value is trace.

[44]Value varies with the brand. Consult the label.

[45]Applies to product with added nutrient. Without added nutrient, value is trace.

[46]Excepting angelfood cake, cakes were made from mixes containing vegetable shortening; icings, with butter.

[47]Excepting spongecake, vegetable shortening was used for cake portion; butter, for icing. If butter or margarine was used for cake portion, vitamin A values would be higher.

[48]Applies to product made with a sodium aluminum-sulfate type baking powder. With a low-sodium-type baking powder containing potassium, value would be about twice the amount shown.

[49]Equal weights of flour, sugar, eggs, and vegetable shortening.

[50]Products are commercial unless otherwise specified.

[51]Made with enriched flour and vegetable shortening except for macaroons, which do not contain flour or shortening.

[52]Icing made with butter.

[53]Applies to yellow varieties; white varieties contain only a trace.

[54]Contains vegetable shortening and butter.

[55]Made with corn oil.

[56]Made with regular margarine.

[57]Applies to product made with yellow cornmeal.

[58]Made with enriched degermed cornmeal and enriched flour.

[59]Product may or may not be enriched with riboflavin. Consult the label.

[60]Value varies with the brand. Consult the label.

[61]Weight includes cob. Without cob, weight is 77 g for item 612, 126 g for item 613.

[62]Based on yellow varieties. For white varieties, value is trace.

[63]Weight includes refuse of outer leaves and core. Without these parts, weight is 163 g.

[64]Weight includes core. Without core, weight is 539 g.

[65]Value based on white-fleshed varieties. For yellow-fleshed varieties, value is 70 IU for item 633, 50 IU for item 634, and 80 IU for item 635.

[66]Weight includes cores and stem ends. Without these parts, weight is 123 g.

[67]Based on year-round average. For tomatoes marketed from November through May, value is about 12 mg, from June through October, 32 mg.

[68]Applies to product without calcium salts added. Value for products with calcium salts added may be as much as 63 mg for whole tomatoes, 241 mg for cut forms.

[69]Weight includes pits. Without pits, weight is 13 g for item 701, 9 g for item 702.

[70]Value may vary from 6 to 60 mg.

(From USDA Home and Garden Bulletin No. 72. Washington, DC, 1981)

(Anderson L, Dibble MV, Turkki PR et al: Nutrition in Health and Disease, 17th ed. Philadelphia, JB Lippincott, 1982)

Table A-2.   Exchange Lists for Meal Planning

List 1—Milk Exchanges

Includes **nonfat,** low-fat, and whole milk. One exchange of milk contains 12 g of carbohydrate, 8 g of protein, a trace of fat, and 80 kcal.

This list shows the kinds and amounts of milk or milk products to use for 1 milk exchange. Those that appear in **bold type** are **nonfat.** Low-fat and whole milk contain saturated fat.

Nonfat fortified milk	1 cup
Skim or nonfat milk	1 cup
Powdered (nonfat dry, before adding liquid)	⅓ cup
Canned, evaporated-skim milk	½ cup
Buttermilk made from skim milk	1 cup
Yogurt made from skim milk (plain, unflavored)	1 cup
Low-fat fortified milk	
1%-fat fortified milk (omit ½ fat exchange)	1 cup
2%-fat fortified milk (omit 1 fat exchange)	1 cup
Yogurt made from 2% fortified milk (plain, unflavored) (omit 1 fat exchange)	1 cup
Whole milk (omit 2 fat exchanges)	
Whole milk	1 cup
Canned, evaporated whole milk	½ cup
Buttermilk made from whole milk	1 cup
Yogurt made from whole milk (plain, unflavored)	1 cup

List 2—Vegetable Exchanges

One exchange of vegetables contains about 5 g of carbohydrate, 2 g of protein, and 25 kcal.

This list shows the kinds of **vegetables** to use for 1 vegetable exchange. One exchange is ½ cup.

Asparagus	**Greens**
Bean sprouts	**Beets**
Beets	**Chard**
Broccoli	**Collards**
Brussels sprouts	**Dandelion**

Cabbage	**Kale**
Carrots	**Mustard**
Cauliflower	**Spinach**
Celery	**Turnip**
Cucumbers	**Mushrooms**
Eggplant	**Okra**
Green pepper	**Onions**
Rhubarb	**Tomatoes**
Rutabaga	**Tomato juice**
Sauerkraut	**Turnips**
String beans, green or yellow	**Vegetable juice cocktail**
Summer squash	**Zucchini**

The following **raw vegetables** may be used as desired:

Chicory	**Lettuce**
Chinese cabbage	**Parsley**
Endive	**Radishes**
Escarole	**Watercress**

Starchy vegetables are found in the bread exchange list.

List 3—Fruit Exchanges

One exchange of fruit contains 10 g of carbohydrate and 40 kcal.

This list shows the kinds and amounts of **fruits** to use for 1 fruit exchange.

Apple	1 small
Apple juice	⅓ cup
Applesauce (unsweetened)	½ cup
Apricots, fresh	2 medium
Apricots, dried	4 halves
Banana	½ small
Berries	
Blackberries	½ cup
Blueberries	½ cup
Raspberries	½ cup
Strawberries	¾ cup
Cherries	10 large
Cider	⅓ cup

Table A-2.   Exchange Lists for Meal Planning (Continued)

Dates	2		Rye or pumpernickel	1 slice
Figs, fresh	1		Raisin	1 slice
Figs, dried	1		Bagel, small	½
Grapefruit	½		English muffin, small	½
Grapefruit juice	½ cup		Plain roll, bread	1
Grapes	12		Frankfurter roll	½
Grape juice	¼ cup		Hamburger bun	½
Mango	½ small		Dried bread crumbs	3 tbsp
Melon			Tortilla, 6″	1
Cantaloupe	¼ small		**Cereal**	
Honeydew	⅛ medium		**Bran flakes**	½ cup
Watermelon	1 cup		**Other ready-to-eat unsweetened cereal**	¾ cup
Nectarine	1 small		**Puffed cereal (unfrosted)**	1 cup
Orange	1 small		**Cereal (cooked)**	½ cup
Orange juice	½ cup		**Grits (cooked)**	½ cup
Papaya	¾ cup		**Rice or barley (cooked)**	½ cup
Peach	1 medium		**Pasta (cooked): spaghetti, noodles, macaroni**	½ cup
Pear	1 small		**Popcorn (popped, no fat added)**	3 cups
Persimmon, native	1 medium		**Cornmeal (dry)**	2 tbsp
Pineapple	½ cup		**Flour**	2½ tbsp
Pineapple juice	⅓ cup		**Wheat germ**	¼ cup
Plums	2 medium		**Crackers**	
Prunes	2 medium		**Arrowroot**	3
Prune juice	¼ cup		**Graham, 2½″ square**	2
Raisins	2 tbsp		**Matzoh, 4″ × 6″**	½
Tangerine	1 medium		**Oyster**	20

Cranberries may be used as desired if no sugar is added.

List 4—Bread Exchanges

Includes **bread, cereal, and starchy vegetables.**

One exchange of bread contains 15 g of carbohydrate, 2 g of protein, and 70 kcal.

This list shows the kinds and amounts of breads, cereals, starchy vegetables, and prepared foods to use for 1 bread exchange. Those that appear in **bold type** are **low-fat.**

Pretzels, 3⅛″ × ⅛″ diameter	25
Rye wafers, 2″ × 3½″	3
Saltines	6
Soda, 2½″ square	4
Dried beans, peas, and lentils	
Beans, peas, lentils (dried and cooked)	½ cup
Baked beans, no pork (canned)	¼ cup
Starchy vegetables	
Corn	⅓ cup
Corn on the cob	1 small
Lima beans	½ cup
Parsnips	⅔ cup

Bread

White (including French and Italian)	1 slice
Whole wheat	1 slice

Table A-2.   Exchange Lists for Meal Planning (Continued)

Peas, green (canned or frozen)	½ cup
Potato, white	1 small
Potato (mashed)	½ cup
Pumpkin	¾ cup
Winter squash, acorn or butternut	½ cup
Yam or sweet potato	¼ cup

Prepared foods

Biscuit 2″ diameter (omit 1 fat exchange)	1
Corn bread, 2″ × 2″ × 1″ (omit 1 fat exchange)	1
Corn muffin, 2″ diameter (omit 1 fat exchange)	1
Crackers, round butter type (omit 1 fat exchange)	5
Muffin, plain, small (omit 1 fat exchange)	1
Potatoes, french-fried, length 2″ to 3½″ (omit 1 fat exchange)	8
Potato or corn chips (omit 2 fat exchanges)	15
Pancake, 5″ × ½″ (omit 1 fat exchange)	1
Waffle, 5″ × ½″ (omit 1 fat exchange)	1

List 5—Meat Exchanges
Lean Meat

One exchange of lean meat (1 oz) contains 7 g of protein, 3 g of fat, and 55 kcal.

This list shows the kinds and amounts of **lean meat** and other protein-rich foods to use for 1 low-fat meat exchange.

Beef: baby beef (very lean), chipped beef, chuck, flank steak, tenderloin, plate ribs, plate skirt steak, round (bottom, top), all cuts of rump, spare ribs, tripe	1 oz
Lamb: leg, rib, sirloin, loin (roast and chops), shank, shoulder	1 oz
Pork: leg (whole rump, center shank), ham, smoked (center slices)	1 oz
Veal: leg, loin, rib, shank, shoulder, cutlets	1 oz

Poultry: meat without skin of chicken, turkey, cornish hen, guinea hen, pheasant	1 oz
Fish: Any fresh or frozen	
Canned salmon, tuna, mackerel, crab, and lobster	¼ cup
Clams, oysters, scallops, shrimp	5 or 1 oz
Sardines, drained	3
Cheeses containing less than 5% butterfat	1 oz
Cottage cheese, dry and 2% butterfat	¼ cup
Dried beans and peas (omit 1 bread exchange)	½ cup

Medium-Fat Meat

For each exchange of medium-fat meat, omit ½ fat exchange.

This list shows the kinds and amounts of medium-fat meat and other protein-rich foods to use for 1 medium-fat meat exchange.

Beef: ground (15% fat), corned beef (canned), rib eye, round (ground commercial)	1 oz
Pork: loin (all cuts tenderloin), shoulder arm (picnic), shoulder blade, Boston butt, Canadian bacon, boiled ham	1 oz
Liver, heart, kidney, and sweetbreads (these are high in cholesterol)	1 oz
Cottage cheese, creamed	¼ cup
Cheese: mozzarella, ricotta, farmer's cheese, Neufchatel	1 oz
Parmesan	3 tbsp
Egg (high in cholesterol)	1
Peanut butter (omit 2 additional fat exchanges)	2 tbsp

High-Fat Meat

For each exchange of high-fat meat, omit 1 fat exchange.

This list shows the kinds and amounts of high-fat meat and other protein-rich foods to use for 1 high-fat meat exchange.

Table A-2.   Exchange Lists for Meal Planning (Continued)

Beef: brisket, corned beef (brisket), ground beef (more than 20% fat), hamburger (commercial), chuck (ground commercial), roasts (rib), steaks (club and rib)	1 oz	Pecans†	2 large whole
Lamb: breast	1 oz	**Peanuts†**	
Pork: spare ribs, loin (back ribs), pork (ground), country-style ham, deviled ham	1 oz	**Spanish**	20 whole
		Virginia	10 whole
Veal: breast	1 oz	**Walnuts**	6 small
Poultry: capon, duck (domestic), goose	1 oz	**Nuts, other†**	6 small
Cheese: cheddar types	1 oz	Margarine, regular stick	1 tsp
Cold cuts	4½″ × ⅛″ slice	Butter	1 tsp
Frankfurter	1 small	Bacon fat	1 tsp

Bacon, crisp — 1 strip
Cream, light — 2 tbsp
Cream, sour — 2 tbsp
Cream, heavy — 1 tbsp
Cream cheese — 1 tbsp
French dressing‡ — 1 tbsp
Italian dressing‡ — 1 tbsp
Lard — 1 tsp
Mayonnaise‡ — 1 tsp
Salad dressing, mayonnaise type‡ — 2 tsp
Salt pork — ¾″ cube

List 6 — Fat Exchanges

One exchange of fat contains 5 g of fat and 45 kcal.

This list shows the kinds and amounts of fat-containing foods to use for 1 fat exchange. To plan a diet low in saturated fat, select only those exchanges that appear in **bold type; they are polyunsaturated.**

Margarine, soft, tub or stick*	1 tsp
Avocado (4″ in diameter)†	⅛
Oil, corn, cottonseed, safflower, soy, sunflower	1 tsp
Oil, olive†	1 tsp
Oil, peanut†	1 tsp
Olives†	5 small
Almonds†	10 whole

* Made with corn, cottonseed, safflower, soy, or sunflower oil only.
† Fat content is primarily monounsaturated.
‡ If made with corn, cottonseed, safflower, soy, or sunflower oil, can be used on fat-modified diet.

(Based on material in the *Exchange Lists for Meal Planning* prepared by Committees of the American Diabetes Association, Inc. and The American Dietetic Association in cooperation with the National Institute of Arthritis, Metabolism and Digestive Diseases and the National Heart and Lung Institute, National Institutes of Health, Public Health Service, U.S. Department of Health, Education and Welfare.)

Table A-3.   Abbreviated Exchange Lists for Protein-, Sodium-, and Potassium-Controlled Diets

Unless otherwise noted, foods grouped together are similar in their content of protein, sodium, and potassium.

Low-Sodium Meat List

Average values: protein, 8 g; Na, 30 mg; K, 100 mg

Egg	1 medium
Meat: beef, lamb, fresh pork, veal, organ meats	1 oz
Poultry, without skin: chicken, duck, goose, turkey	1 oz

Table A-3. Abbreviated Exchange Lists for Protein-, Sodium-, and Potassium-Controlled Diets (Continued)

Fish, fresh or unsalted waterpack	1 oz
Shellfish	
Clams	¼ cup, or 4–5
Oysters	⅓ cup, or 3–4 small
Shrimp	1 oz

Dairy List

Average values: protein, 4 g; Na, 70 mg; K, 185 mg	
Cream, half & half	½ cup
Cream, heavy whipping	¾ cup
Ice cream (chocolate, vanilla, strawberry)	¾ cup
Milk (whole, low-fat, skim, chocolate)	½ cup
Evaporated whole or skim milk	¼ cup

Note: One serving of milk is *4* fluid ounces, not *8* ounces.

Bread, Cereal, and Starch Lists

Regular

Average values: protein, 2 g; Na, 200 mg; K, 30 mg	
Bread (white enriched, cracked wheat, French, Italian, American rye)	1 slice
Doughnut	1 small
Graham cracker	2 squares
Hamburger or hotdog bun	½ large
Muffin, plain	1 small
Sugar wafers	5 wafers

Vanilla wafers	10 wafers
Dry cereals: portion sizes vary widely	

Low-Sodium

Average values: protein, 2 g; Na, 5 mg; K, 30 mg	
Low-sodium crackers	4 small
Low-sodium white bread	1 slice
Salt-free matzoh cracker	1 (6″) square
Salt-free Venus wheat wafers	4
Cereals and rice cooked without salt (avoid seasoned mixes)	½ cup
Dry cereals	
Frosted Mini Wheats	3 biscuits
Spoon Size Shredded Wheat	⅓ cup
Puffed wheat or rice	1 cup
Low-sodium corn-flakes	1 cup
Pasta cooked without salt	⅓ cup

Fruit List #1

Average values: protein, 0.5 g; Na, 5 mg; K, 100 mg	
Apple, fresh	1 small
Apple juice	½ cup
Applesauce	½ cup
Blueberries, fresh or frozen	¾ cup
Cherries	8 large
Grape juice, frozen, diluted 1:3	1 cup
Orange, fresh	½ small (2½″ diameter)
Pear, fresh	½ large (3″ diameter)
Pear halves, canned	2 small halves

Table A-3. Abbreviated Exchange Lists for Protein-, Sodium-, and Potassium-Controlled Diets (Continued)

Pineapple chunks	½ cup
Prunes, dried	2 medium
Strawberries, fresh	6 large
Tangerine, fresh	1 medium (2½″ diameter)
Watermelon, diced	½ cup

Fruit List #2

Average values: protein, 0.6 g; Na, 5 mg; K, 175 mg

Apricots, fresh	2 medium
Banana, fresh	3″ piece
Dates	4 medium
Fruit cocktail, canned	½ cup
Grapefruit juice (canned, fresh, or frozen)	½ cup
Peach halves, canned	2 medium halves
Prune juice	⅓ cup
Raisins, dried	2 tbsp

Fruit List #3

Average values: protein, 0.7 g; Na, 5 mg; K, 250 mg

Apple, fresh	1 large (3½″ diameter)
Apple juice	1 cup
Banana	5″ piece
Cantaloupe, fresh	⅙ (5″ diameter)
Orange juice (canned, fresh, or frozen	½ cup
Papaya, fresh	⅓ medium (3½″ diameter)

Vegetable List #1

Average values: protein, 1 g; Na, 10 mg; K, 100 mg

Asparagus, fresh cooked	4 medium spears
Asparagus, frozen, cooked	3 medium spears
Aspargus, low-sodium, canned	⅓ cup
Beans (snap or wax), fresh cooked, canned, frozen	½ cup
Cucumber, raw, pared	10 slices
Cabbage (all varieties), raw or cooked, shredded	½ cup
Carrots, low-sodium, canned	½ cup
Cauliflower, fresh cooked	½ cup
Lettuce (all varieties), chopped	½ cup
Mustard greens, frozen, cooked	½ cup
Onion, raw or cooked, sliced	½ cup
Pepper, sweet green, cooked	1

Vegetable List #2

Average values: protein, 1 g; Na, 20 mg; K, 170 mg

Beets, fresh slices, cooked or low-sodium, canned	½ cup
Carrots, fresh, diced, cooked	½ cup
Celery, raw or cooked, diced	1 stalk or ½ cup
Eggplant, diced, cooked	½ cup
Mushrooms, raw	½ cup or 3–4 small
Okra, fresh slices, cooked	½ cup
Parsnips, diced, cooked	⅓ cup
Pepper, sweet green, raw	1
Radishes, raw	10 medium
Rutabagas, sliced, cooked	½ cup

Table A-3.   Abbreviated Exchange Lists for Protein-, Sodium-, and Potassium-Controlled Diets (Continued)

Squash, summer, sliced	½ cup
Squash, winter, boiled and mashed	⅓ cup
Turnips, cubed, cooked	½ cup

Vegetable List #3

Average values: protein, 1 g; Na, 15 mg; K, 250 mg

Avocado, raw	¼ small
Beet greens, cooked	½ cup
Carrot, raw	1 (7″) long
Chard, fresh, cooked	½ cup
Potato, pared, sliced, cooked	½ cup
Squash, winter, baked	¼ cup
Tomato, cooked	⅓ cup
Tomato, raw, unpeeled	1 small
Tomato, low-sodium, canned	½ cup

Vegetable List #4

Average values: protein, 2.5 g; Na, 20 mg; K, 200 mg, but varies widely

Artichoke, cooked	1 medium
Broccoli, fresh or frozen, cooked	½ cup
Collard greens, fresh or frozen, cooked	½ cup
Corn, fresh, cut off cob, or low-sodium canned	½ cup
Peas, frozen or low-sodium canned	½ cup
Potato, baked	1 (2¼″)
Spinach, fresh or frozen, cooked	½ cup
Sweet potato, baked	1 (5″ × 2″)

Free List

Fats Unsalted
Butter, unsalted
Low-sodium French dressing
Lard
Margarine, unsalted
Vegetable oil
Shortening
Whipping cream, 1 tbsp, unwhipped
Low-Protein Products
Arrowroot
Cornstarch
Low-protein bread
Low-protein cereal, pasta, rusks, Aproten
Wheatstarch cookies
Nondairy Products
Coffee-Mate, 1 tbsp
Dessert topping, frozen powder or pressurized
D'Zerta whipped topping
Spices, Seasonings, and Flavorings
All dry spices and herbs
Diazest
Garlic, fresh
Liquid Smoke, Wright's
Tabasco sauce
Vinegar, distilled
Sweets
Cranberry sauce, ¼ cup
Danish dessert, ½ cup
Gum drops
Hard candy
Honey
Jam, preserves
Jelly
Jelly beans
Sugar, white, granulated, or powdered

Table A-3.   Abbreviated Exchange Lists for Protein-, Sodium-, and Potassium-Controlled Diets (Continued)

Note: The foods in the free list can be added to diets that are controlled in protein, sodium, and/or potassium as desired unless the amount allowed is specified.

Commercial low-electrolyte, high-calorie supplements that may be useful when protein, sodium, and/or potassium intake must be restricted:

Amin-Aid—flavored essential amino acids (including histidine), carbohydrate, and soybean oil

Cal-Power—flavored colored liquid glucose

Controlyte—hydrolysed cornstarch with vegetable oil

Hy-Cal—flavored, colored liquid glucose

Lipomul oral—corn oil emulsion

Polycose—hydrolyzed cornstarch

Sumacal—flavored, colored liquid glucose

(Condensed from *A Guide to Protein Controlled Diets for Dietitians, ed. 2.* Diet Therapy Committee. Los Angeles: Los Angeles District of the California Dietetic Association, 1977. Used with permission)

Index

Numbers followed by an *f* indicate a figure; *t* indicates tabular material.